Revision Notes in Psychiatry

Revision Notes in Psychiatry

2nd edition

BASANT K. PURI
MA, PhD, MB, BChir, BSc (Hons) MathSci, MRCPsych, DipStat, MMath
Senior Lecturer/Consultant in Psychiatry and Imaging, MRC CSC, Imperial College London;
Honorary Consultant in Imaging, Department of Imaging, Hammersmith Hospital, London

ANNE D. HALL
BA, MB, BCh, MRCPsych
Consultant Psychiatrist, South Kensington and Chelsea Mental Health Centre, Chelsea and
Westminster Hospital, London

A member of the Hodder Headline Group
LONDON

First published in Great Britain in 1998
Second edition published in 2004 by
Arnold, a member of the Hodder Headline Group,
338 Euston Road, London NW1 3BH

http://www.arnoldpublishers.com

Distributed in the United States of America by
Oxford University Press Inc.,
198 Madison Avenue, New York, NY10016
Oxford is a registered trademark of Oxford University Press

Whilst the advice and information in this book are believed to be true and
accurate at the date of going to press, neither the author[s] nor the publisher
can accept any legal responsibility or liability for any errors or omissions
that may be made. In particular, (but without limiting the generality of the
preceding disclaimer) every effort has been made to check drug dosages;
however it is still possible that errors have been missed. Furthermore,
dosage schedules are constantly being revised and new side-effects
recognized. For these reasons the reader is strongly urged to consult the
drug companies' printed instructions before administering any of the drugs
recommended in this book.

British Library Cataloguing in Publication Data
A catalogue record for this book is available from the British Library

Library of Congress Cataloging-in-Publication Data
A catalog record for this book is available from the Library of Congress

ISBN   0 340 76131 8

1 2 3 4 5 6 7 8 9 10

Commissioning Editor:	Serena Bureau
Development Editor:	Layla Vandenbergh
Production Controller:	Deborah Smith
Cover Design:	Stewart Larking

Typeset in 10/12pt Minion by Phoenix Photosetting, Chatham, Kent
Printed and bound in Malta

What do you think about this book? Or any other Arnold title?
Please send your comments to feedback.arnold@hodder.co.uk

Contents

Preface to the Second Edition

In preparing the second edition of this book, we have taken the opportunity to update much of the information contained therein. As is evident from the increased size of this edition, we have also greatly expanded many chapters; this has happened partly to furnish the reader with more background material that puts the key facts in their proper context, and partly in line with the latest syllabi for the examinations for Parts I and II of the Membership of the Royal College of Psychiatrists. These *Revision Notes* should also prove useful in preparing for similar postgraduate examinations in psychiatry in other parts of the English-speaking world.

BKP
ADH

Preface to the First Edition

This book aims to provide detailed revision notes covering all the important basic sciences and clinical topics required for postgraduate psychiatry examinations. To this end, the current syllabus for both parts of the examinations for the Membership of the Royal College of Psychiatrists has been followed closely. It should be emphasized, however, that this book is not meant to be a replacement for either wider reading, or, more importantly, clerking and following-up patients.

BKP
ADH

Basic psychology

PRINCIPLES OF LEARNING THEORY

Definition of learning

Learning is a change in behaviour as a result of prior experience. It does not include behaviour change caused by maturation or temporary conditions (e.g. drug effects or fatigue).

Learning may occur through associations being made between two or more phenomena. Two forms of such associative learning are recognized: *classical conditioning* and *operant conditioning*. *Cognitive learning* is a more complex process in which current perceptions are interpreted in the context of previous information in order to solve unfamiliar problems. Evidence that learning can also take place through the observation and imitation of others has led to the development of the observational learning theory.

Classical conditioning

DEFINITION AND INTRODUCTION

Classical conditioning (respondent learning) was first described by the Russian physiologist Ivan Petrovich Pavlov (1849–1936) in 1927. (Although Pavlov was awarded a Nobel prize, that was in 1904 for his work on digestion.) Following several repetitions of pairing of light (or a bell sounding) followed by the presentation of food to a dog, it was found that just switching on the light led to salivation. The dog had been conditioned to associate the light with food. Food was acting as the *unconditioned stimulus* (US), eliciting the reflex response of salivation without new learning being involved. The response to the unconditioned stimulus is known as the *unconditioned response* (UR). The light would not normally have elicited the response of salivation, but was now a *conditioned stimulus* (CS) that had elicited the response through its association with an unconditioned stimulus. The *conditioned response* (CR) is the learned or acquired response to a conditioned stimulus. This is shown diagrammatically in Figure 1.1. Thus, in Pavlov's experiments, salivation was both an unconditioned response before conditioning, and a conditioned response after conditioning.

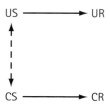

Figure 1.1 *Diagram showing the processes associated with classical conditioning. US = unconditioned stimulus; UR = unconditioned response; CS = conditioned stimulus; CR = conditioned response.*

CONCEPTS

Acquisition stage

The acquisition stage of conditioning is the period during which the association is being acquired between the conditioned stimulus and the unconditioned stimulus with which it is being paired.

Timing

- *Delayed conditioning.* In delayed conditioning the onset of the conditioned stimulus precedes that of the unconditioned stimulus and the conditioned stimulus continues until the response occurs. Delayed conditioning is optimal when the delay between the onsets of the two stimuli is around half a second.
- *Simultaneous conditioning.* In simultaneous conditioning the onset of both stimuli is simultaneous and the conditioned stimulus continues until the response occurs. It is less successful than delayed conditioning.
- *Trace conditioning.* In trace conditioning the conditioned stimulus ends before the onset of the unconditioned stimulus and the conditioning becomes less effective as the delay between the two increases.
- *Backward conditioning.* In backward conditioning the presentation of the conditioned stimulus occurs after that of the unconditioned stimulus.

Higher-order conditioning

In higher-order conditioning the conditioned stimulus is paired with a second (or third, etc.) conditioned stimulus, which on presentation by itself elicits the original conditioned response. In other words, the original conditioned stimulus now acts as the unconditioned stimulus in the new pairing. If there is just a second conditioned stimulus, then this gives rise to second-order conditioning. A third conditioned stimulus gives rise to third-order conditioning, and so on. Higher-order (that is, second-order or above) conditioning is weaker than first-order conditioning; in general, the higher the order, the weaker the conditioning.

Extinction

Extinction is the gradual disappearance of a conditioned response and occurs when the conditioned stimulus is repeatedly presented without the unconditioned stimulus. It does not entail the complete loss of the conditioned stimulus. Following extinction, if an experimental animal is allowed to rest, a weaker conditioned response re-emerges; this is known as *partial recovery*.

Generalization

Generalization is the process whereby, once a conditioned response has been established to a given stimulus, that response can also be evoked by other stimuli that are similar to the original conditioned stimulus.

Discrimination

Discrimination is the differential recognition of, and response to, two or more similar stimuli.

Incubation

Incubation is the increase in strength of conditioned responses resulting from repeated brief exposure to the conditioned stimulus.

Stimulus preparedness

Stimulus preparedness refers to the fact that some stimuli are more likely to become conditioned stimuli than are others.

The case of Little Albert

In 1920 the American psychologist John Broadus Watson (1878–1958) and his research assistant Rosalie Rayner described the experimental induction of a phobia, using classical conditioning, in an 11-month-old boy known as Little Albert. Following several episodes of pairing in which the presentation of a white rat was accompanied by a loud noise caused by striking a steel bar, the boy developed a fear of the rat in the absence of the frightening noise. This was then repeated with a rabbit, and then generalized to any furry mammal.

Operant conditioning (instrumental learning)

DEFINITION AND INTRODUCTION

Operant conditioning (or instrumental learning) is particularly associated with Skinner (1953, 1969) although much of the groundwork for the underlying theory was carried out by Thorndike (1911). Burrhus Frederic Skinner (1904–90) and Edward Lee Thorndike (1874–1949) were American psychologists. A voluntary behaviour is engaged in because its occurrence is reinforced by being rewarded. Such behaviour is independent of stimuli and was termed *operant behaviour* by Skinner. An alternative type of behaviour, termed *respondent behaviour* by Skinner, refers to behaviour that is dependent on known stimuli.

CONCEPTS

Trial-and-error learning/behaviour

Thorndike described experiments in which hungry cats were placed in puzzle boxes. By chance, in time a cat would effect an escape, for example by pressing on a lever, and reach some visible food outside the box. Less time would be needed to carry out the same behaviour in later trials. This is trial-and-error learning or behaviour.

Law of effect

Thorndike's law of effect holds that voluntary behaviour that is paired with subsequent reward is strengthened.

Skinner box

Skinner developed the experimental procedures of Thorndike, creating the Skinner box. Operant conditioning can be demonstrated using a Skinner box in which, for example, every time the animal presses a lever a pellet of food is released. If hungry rats are placed in it, random trial-and-error learning leads to the lever being pressed, the conditioned response, to obtain the reinforcing stimulus of the reward of food pellets. If, after many repetitions of this pairing, the conditioned response is no longer reinforced, then the conditioned response abates; that is, extinction occurs. Following extinction, if the animal is allowed to rest, a weaker conditioned response can re-emerge; this is partial recovery. Discrimination (see above) can also occur.

Observational learning (vicarious learning/modelling)

DEFINITION AND INTRODUCTION

Observational learning (or modelling), also known as vicarious learning (or modelling), is the learning of behaviours and skills that can occur by observation without direct reinforcement. The occurrence of the observational learning of aggressive behaviour in humans has been demonstrated by Bandura.

CONCEPTS

The bobo doll experiments

Albert Bandura (1925–present), a Canadian psychologist working at Stanford, USA, carried out the bobo doll experiments. (Bobo dolls are inflatable, balloon-like objects, shaped like eggs, which bob back up after being knocked down, owing to the presence of extra weighting in the dolls' 'bottoms'.) Bandura made a film of one of his female students verbally and physically attacking a bobo doll, including hitting it with a hammer. This film was then shown to groups of kindergartners. The children liked the film and when let out to play in an area containing a new bobo doll and some toy hammers, they proceeded verbally and physically to imitate the actions of the young woman in Bandura's film.

Bandura pointed out that a change in behaviour in the children had occurred without rewards being received for approximations to the new behaviour. He termed this phenomenon, which clearly differed from classical and operant learning, *observational learning* or modelling; his theory is referred to as social learning theory.

To deal with the criticism that a bobo doll is made to be hit, Bandura repeated the bobo doll experiments, this time substituting a live clown for the doll. Again, the children imitated the actions of the young woman, to the extent of kicking and punching a live clown, and hitting him with (toy) hammers.

Optimal conditions for observational learning

1 The subject sees that the behaviour observed is being reinforced.
2 Owing to perceived similarity, the subject must believe that he/she can emit the response necessary to obtain reinforcement (self-efficacy).

Steps involved in the modelling process

According to Bandura, the following steps are involved in the modelling process.

1 *Attention.* Successful observational learning is more likely to occur in association with the following factors:
   - optimal arousal
   - an attractive model
   - a prestigious model
   - a colourful and dramatic model
   - a model who appears to be like the observer.

In contrast, unsuccessful observational learning is more likely to occur in association with the following factors:

- low arousal (e.g. sleepiness)
- over-arousal
- the presence of distracting stimuli.

2 *Retention.*
3 *Reproduction.* The translation of what has been remembered into behaviour.
4 *Motivation.* See the section below on concepts of extinction and reinforcement in explaining behaviour.

Cognitive learning

DEFINITION

The notion of a mental model of reality is central to the cognitive approach to psychology. Cognition involves the reception, organization and utilization of information. Cognitive learning is an active form of learning in which mental cognitive structures (cognitive maps) are formed. These allow mental images to be formed which allow meaning and structure to be given to the internal and external environment.

MECHANISMS

Cognitive learning can occur in the following ways:

- *Insight learning.* The learning occurs apparently out of the blue, because of an understanding of the relationship between various elements relevant to a problem.
- *Latent learning.* Cognitive learning takes place but is not manifested except in certain circumstances such as the need to satisfy a basic drive.

ASSIMILATION THEORY

The assimilation theory of cognitive learning is based on the following concepts:

- Learning in humans is influenced by prior knowledge.
- Human learning is manifested by a change in the meaning of experience rather than a purely behavioural change.
- Those involved in teaching should help their students reflect on their experiences.
- Those involved in teaching should construct new meanings.

Concepts of extinction and reinforcement in explaining behaviour

EXTINCTION

Extinction has been defined above.

REINFORCEMENT

A *positive reinforcer* is a reinforcing reward stimulus (e.g. food and water, money in humans) which increases the probability of occurrence of the operant behaviour. A *negative reinforcer* is an aversive stimulus (e.g. an electric shock, fear) whose removal increases the probability of occurrence of the operant behaviour. For example, a Skinner box may be arranged so that, in order to avoid an aversive stimulus, the animal must press a lever. Learning this response is called *avoidance conditioning*. *Escape conditioning* is a variety of negative reinforcement in which the response learnt provides complete escape from the aversive stimulus (very resistant to extinction).

Primary reinforcement occurs through reduction of needs deriving from basic drives (e.g. food and drink). *Secondary reinforcement* derives from association with primary reinforcers (e.g. money, tokens).

SCHEDULES OF REINFORCEMENT

In *continuous reinforcement*, reinforcement takes place following every conditioned response. This leads to the maximum response rate.

In *partial reinforcement*, only some of the conditioned responses are reinforced.

- In a *fixed interval schedule*, reinforcement occurs after a fixed interval of time. It is poor at maintaining the conditioned response; the maximum response rate typically occurs only when the reinforcement is expected.
- In a *variable interval schedule*, reinforcement occurs after variable intervals. It is very good at maintaining the conditioned response.
- In a *fixed ratio schedule*, reinforcement occurs after a fixed number of responses. It is good at maintaining a high response rate.
- In a *variable ratio schedule*, reinforcement occurs after a variable number of responses. It is very good at maintaining a high response rate.

PUNISHMENT

Punishment is the situation that occurs if an aversive stimulus is presented whenever a given behaviour occurs, thereby reducing the probability of occurrence of this response. The removal of the aversive stimulus then allows it to act as a negative reinforcer rather than a punisher.

MOTIVATION

In observational learning theory, Bandura has put forward the following motives that encourage observational learning:

- *Past reinforcement.* This is similar to the types of reinforcement that are recognized in classical and operant learning theory.
- *Promised reinforcements.* These are incentives which can be imagined.
- *Vicarious reinforcement.* This refers to the sight and recollection of the model that is being reinforced.

Negative motivations that inhibit observational learning include:

- past punishment
- promised punishment – that is, threats
- vicarious punishment.

Bandura contends that punishment is less effective than reinforcement.

Clinical applications of behavioural treatments

RECIPROCAL INHIBITION

This holds that relaxation inhibits anxiety so that the two are mutually exclusive (Wolpe, 1958) and in fact does not hold true. It can be used in treating conditions associated with anticipatory anxiety (e.g. phobias). Patients identify increasingly greater anxiety-evoking stimuli, to form an anxiety hierarchy. During systematic desensitization the person is successfully exposed (in reality or in imagination) to these stimuli in the hierarchy, beginning with the least anxiety-evoking one, each exposure being paired with relaxation.

HABITUATION

Habituation is an important component of the behavioural treatment of obsessive–compulsive disorder using exposure and response prevention. The ultimate aim of exposure techniques is to reduce the discomfort associated with the eliciting stimuli through habituation.

For example, Vaughan and Tarrier (1992) have described the use of *image habituation training* in the therapy of patients suffering from post-traumatic stress disorder. Image habituation training involved the generation by the patient of verbal descriptions of the traumatic event, which were recorded onto audiotape. After the initial training session with the therapist, homework sessions of self-directed exposure in which the person visualized the described event in response to listening to the audiotape recordings were carried out. There were significant decreases in anxiety between and within homework sessions, suggesting that habituation did occur and was responsible for improvement. Treatment gains were maintained at six-month follow-up.

CHAINING

In (response) chaining, the components of a more complex desired behaviour are first taught and then connected in order to teach the latter. Chaining may be conceptualized in the following two different ways.

1   Responses function as discriminative stimuli for subsequent responses.
2   Responses produce stimuli that function as discriminative stimuli for subsequent responses.

Chaining can be used in, for example, people with learning difficulties. Thvedt et al. (1984) studied stimulus functions in chaining. Twenty-four adults with learning difficulties learned a chain of circuit board assembly responses consisting of placing resistors in the board and pressing switches. Lights came on after switch responses. After learning the chain, each subject was exposed to three experimental conditions (counterbalanced):

- altered stimulus location
- altered stimulus sequence
- missing stimulus.

This study lent some support for the second conceptual position given above (i.e. that responses produce stimuli that function as discriminative stimuli for subsequent responses).

SHAPING

In shaping, successively closer approximations to the desired behaviour are reinforced in order to achieve the latter. It finds application clinically in the management of behavioural disturbances in people with learning difficulties and in the therapy of patients suffering from psychoactive substance use disorder.

For example, Preston *et al.* (2001) have used shaping to attempt to bring about cocaine abstinence by successive approximation. Cocaine-using methadone-maintenance patients were randomized to standard contingency management (abstinence group of size 49) or to a contingency designed to increase contact with reinforcers (shaping group of size 46). For eight weeks, both groups earned escalating-value vouchers based on thrice-weekly urinalyses: the abstinence group earned vouchers for cocaine-negative urines only; the shaping group earned vouchers for each urine specimen with a 25% or greater decrease in cocaine metabolite (during the first three weeks) and then for negative urines only (during the final five weeks). Cocaine use was found to be lower in the shaping group, but only in the last five weeks, when the response requirement was identical. Thus, the shaping contingency appeared to prepare patients better for abstinence. (A second phase of the study showed that abstinence induced by escalating-value vouchers can be maintained by a non-escalating schedule, suggesting that contingency management can be practical as a maintenance treatment.)

CUEING

Cueing is the process of helping the learner to focus attention on the important or relevant stimuli to render the essential learning characteristics distinct from the other stimuli; it consists of any action which separates figure from ground (see below). The use of cueing can decrease learning times. For example, in reading matter and pictorial presentations, visual cues can be given using any of the following strategies:

highlighting	implosions
underlining	bordering
arrows	texture
contrasting colours	novelty
animation	size
explosions	labelling.

A famous example is that of *Clever Hans*. Hans was a horse, belonging to Mr Von Osten, which appeared capable of carrying out a range of intellectual tasks normally associated with humans, such as the arithmetical operations of addition, subtraction, multiplication and division of natural numbers and fractions, reading and spelling. Answers were communicated by means of tapping out the answer with one of his feet. For example, if asked to calculate '2 + 3', Clever Hans would tap his foot five times and then stop. Pfungst (1907/1911), in conjunction with the Berlin psychologist Carl Stumpf, designed a set of experiments which showed that Clever Hans was, in fact, being cued to give the correct answer by the questioner. The questioner, consciously or unconsciously, would provide Clever Hans with visual cues, such as subtle changes in facial expression and posture. For example, in the above example, as Clever Hans reached five foot taps, he could pick up visual cues showing how the tension in the questioner was rising. As soon as the fifth tap was executed, the sense of relief in the questioner was also apparent in visual cues, and the horse knew this was when to stop tapping.

A clinical example of the therapeutic use of cueing is in unilateral neglect, following a cerebral lesion. Robertson *et al.* (1992) based their therapeutic intervention on the experimental finding that limb activation contralateral to a cerebral lesion appears to reduce visual neglect. (There is controversy as to whether this is the result of perceptual cueing or of hemispheric activation.) In the treatment of unilateral left neglect, Robertson *et al.* found that treatment focused on cueing for left arm activation, without explicit instructions for perceptual anchoring, gave positive results.

ESCAPE CONDITIONING

As mentioned above, in escape conditioning the animal learns to escape from an unpleasant or punishing stimulus by making a new response. For example, rodents can be trained to escape from electric shocks by pressing a button.

This is a form of negative reinforcement, in which the reinforcement is getting away from an aversive stimulus. It is a special form of operant conditioning, consisting of a conditioning procedure in which successive occurrences of a response repeatedly terminate a negative reinforcing stimulus.

Escape conditioning may be used in the treatment of alcoholism. For example, Glover and McCue (1977) found that a group of patients with alcoholism, when treated with partially reinforced electrical escape conditioning, had a significantly better outcome on follow-up than a control group which showed a parallel level of motivation and were treated by conventional methods. No sex differences in outcome were found for either group. In the experimental group treated with escape conditioning, better prognosis was associated with higher social class and older age, and poorer prognosis with single marital status. There were no variations in outcome for age in the control group. In the age range 20 to 40 years, escape conditioning did not show better results than conventional therapies, but with subjects above this age range it was significantly superior.

AVOIDANCE CONDITIONING

As mentioned above, in avoidance conditioning the animal learns to avoid an unpleasant or punishing stimulus by making a new response. For example, rodents can be trained to avoid electric shocks by pressing a button.

Like escape conditioning, avoidance conditioning is a form of negative reinforcement, in which the reinforcement is getting away from an aversive stimulus. Avoidance conditioning may be considered to be a special case of operant conditioning under intermittent reinforcement.

Avoidance conditioning, and indeed also escape conditioning, may be used in the treatment of enuresis. For example, Hansen (1979) described a twin-signal device that provided both escape and avoidance conditioning in enuresis control.

SELF-CONTROL THERAPY

Bandura helped to develop the therapeutic technique of self-control therapy, based on concepts of self-regulation. It may be used as part of a treatment package for the cessation of smoking, in countering over-eating, and in helping students to improve their ability to study. The components are as follows.

- *Behavioural charts.* This involves keeping a record of one's behaviour based on self-observation. For example, in attempting to improve study habits prior to an examination, a student may make a record of how much time is spent studying each day, how many books are (re-)read, and how many past or sample examination papers are fully attempted. Such a record could be graphical or in the form of a behavioural diary. In the case of the latter, further relevant details should be noted, which may offer insight into cues associated with the desired (or undesired) behaviour. For example, the student may find that he or she accomplishes more when in a library compared with being at home, and accomplishes least when in a room with a television switched on.
- *Environmental planning.* Based on the behavioural chart and diary, changes to one's environment can be planned. For example, to continue with the example of the student, he or

she may plan to spend more time in a library and in study groups with others also sitting the same examination, and less time at home with the television switched on.

- *Self-contracts.* A contract can be written down (perhaps witnessed by the therapist), stipulating the reward to oneself for accomplishing certain tasks, and the punishment for not doing so. For example, in the case of the student, the contract might state 'If I fully revise chapters 1 to 4 from my revision book next week, then I shall reward myself by buying my favourite recording of Beethoven's Fifth Piano Concerto; if I fail to achieve this goal, then I shall … [state some unpleasant but necessary task or chore].'

MODELLING THERAPY

Bandura also developed modelling therapy. Here, a person suffering from a difficulty coping with a certain situation watches somebody else cope perfectly easily with the same situation, and then in turn is able to cope by means of observational learning. An example of the use of modelling therapy is in the treatment of phobias.

PHENOMENA OF VISUAL AND AUDITORY PERCEPTION

Perception

Definition
Perception is an active process involving the awareness and interpretation of sensations received through sensory organs.

Thresholds

- *Absolute threshold* is the minimum energy required to activate the sensory organ.
- *Difference threshold* of two sources of a sensory modality is the minimum difference that has to exist between the intensities of the two sources to allow them to be perceived separately.

Weber's law
The increase in stimulus intensity needed to allow two sources of intensity to be perceived as being different is directly proportional to the value of the baseline intensity.

Fechner's law
Weber's law is an approximation which fails to hold over a large range of stimulus intensities. A better, though again not perfect, approximation is provided by Fechner's law which holds that sensory perception is a logarithmic function of stimulus intensity.

Signal detection theory
This holds that perception does not depend solely on stimulus intensity but is also a function of biophysical factors and psychological factors such as motivation, previous experiences, and expectations.

Perceptual organization

Perception is an active process in which there is a search for meaning. A number of perceptual phenomena are described in Gestalt psychology:

- The whole perception is different from the sum of its parts.
- According to the 'law of simplicity', the percept corresponds to the simplest stimulation interpretation.
- According to the 'law of closure', partial outlines are perceived as whole.
- According to the 'law of continuity', interrupted lines (for example) are seen as continuous.
- According to the 'law of similarity', like items are grouped together.
- According to the 'law of proximity', adjacent items are grouped together.
- There is figure–ground differentiation.

Note that *Gestalt* is a German word meaning shape or form.

FIGURE–GROUND DIFFERENTIATION

Patterns are perceived as figures differentiated from their background with contours and boundaries, thus simulating objects. Thus the relevant perceptual system needs to make a 'decision' as to how to differentiate correctly between the figure that is being perceived and its background. In doing so, the following features characterize figure and ground, particularly in respect of visual stimuli:

- The figure is more conspicuous than the ground.
- The figure appears more like an object in its own right.
- The ground does not appear to be an object, but rather generally formless.
- The ground extends past the figure.
- The perception is of the figure being 'in front of' the ground.
- The contour or outline that differentiates figure from ground is perceived as belonging to the figure rather than the ground.

An example of a visual figure–ground relationship is shown in Figure 1.2. It may not be obvious, the first time this is looked at, what information it conveys. In fact, the figure consists of the spaces between the objects (the ground). Armed with this knowledge, it is immediately clear that a word of importance to examination candidates is depicted.

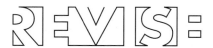

Figure 1.2   *Visual example of a figure/ground relationship (see text).*

An example of an ambiguous, reversible, visual figure–ground relationship is that of the Rubin vase, shown in Figure 1.3. (This was devised by the Danish psychologist Edgar Rubin.) Here, the figure may be the vase and the ground the faces. Alternatively, the two faces may be considered to be the figure and the vase shape in between them the ground.

Figure–ground differentiation is not confined to visual stimuli. An example involving auditory stimuli is that of hearing a particular conversation over background noise.

OBJECT CONSTANCY

This is the tendency to perceive objects as unchanged under different conditions:

- *Shape constancy.* The perception of an object's shape is constant regardless of the viewing angle.
- *Size constancy.* The perception of an object's size is constant regardless of the viewing distance.

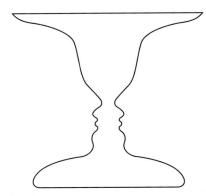

Figure 1.3 *Visual example of a reversible figure/ground relationship – the Rubin vase.*

- *Lightness/colour constancy.* The perception of an object's shade/colour is constant regardless of the lighting conditions.
- *Location constancy.* The perception of an object's spatial position is constant regardless of the viewer's movement.

For example, when walking or running through a room, all the walls and the ceiling and floor are perceived as each having a rectangular shape, in spite of the fact that the shapes projected on the retina are those of non-static non-rectangles.

DEPTH PERCEPTION

A three-dimensional visual perception is formed from two-dimensional retinal images as a result of multiple cues such as binocular vision and convergence, relative size and brightness, motion parallax, object interposition, and linear perspective.

PERCEPTUAL SET

Perceptual set is a motivational state of mind in which certain aspects of stimuli are perceived according to expectation. This can be associated with a change in the perception threshold. The way in which stimuli are perceived is influenced by personality and individual values, and past experiences. Perceptual set was described in his book *Becoming* in 1955 by the American psychologist Gordon Willard Allport (1897–1967).

Relevance of visual perceptual theory to psychopathology

ILLUSIONS

Illusions are misperceptions of real stimuli that are influenced by the perceptual set and suggest an active search for meaning. With respect to visual perceptual theory, illusions can arise from the following phenomena:

- *Difficulties in figure/ground differentiation.* An example is an ambiguous figure such as the Rubin vase.
- *Changes in object constancy.* For example, perceptual constancy may change as a result of different lighting conditions, giving rise to visual illusions.

- *Difficulties in depth perception.* This can occur, for example, owing to ocular problems. Abnormal ocular lens accommodation can give rise to abnormalities in monocular cueing, while defects in the ability of the eyes properly to converge can cause abnormalities in binocular cueing.

HALLUCINATIONS

Hallucinations are false sensory perceptions occurring in the absence of real external stimuli. They are perceived as being located in objective space and as having the same realistic qualities as normal perceptions.

According to visual perceptual theory, the majority of the processing that comprises perception takes place within the brain rather than in the sense organs themselves. Therefore, any factors that adversely affect neuronal processing within the brain may cause the subject to experience hallucinations. Such factors (described in later chapters) include cerebral lesions, psychoactive substances, and toxic states.

Furthermore, on the basis of visual perceptual theory it would also be predicted that abnormalities in the sense organs themselves or in primary perceptual functioning could also give rise to hallucinations. Evidence exists to support this contention. For instance, visual hallucinations, in the absence of other psychopathology, have been reported in association with ocular disease with visual loss in Charles Bonnet syndrome ('visual hallucinations of the blind'). An auditory analogue to visual perceptual theory also exists; an example of auditory impairment being associated with auditory hallucinations is the report of the association of musical hallucinations with hearing impairment.

OTHER PSYCHOPATHOLOGY

An *agnosia* is an inability to interpret and recognize the significance of sensory information, which does not result from impairment of the sensory pathways, mental deterioration, disorders of consciousness and attention or, in the case of an object, a lack of familiarity with the object. Abnormalities in the way in which visual perceptual systems (functioning according to visual perceptual theory) interact with systems of the brain associated with functions such as learning and memory can give rise to agnosias.

In schizophrenia, depersonalization, derealization, temporal lobe epilepsy and acute brain syndromes, there is disturbance of perception, particularly depth perception and perceptual constancy.

Development of visual perception

The development of human visual perception is an illustration of a constitutional–environmental interaction. In general, complex visual stimuli, such as human faces, are preferred. The early developmental stages are as follows.

- Birth – the ability to discriminate brightness and to carry out eye tracking; visual acuity impaired, with focusing fixed at 0.2 m
- 2 months – depth perception (as evidenced by visual cliff experiments)
- 4 months – accommodation and colour vision
- 6 months – 6:6 acuity.

The following visual processes appear to be innate:

visual scanning	fixating
tracking	figure–ground discrimination.

In contrast, the following visual processes appear to be learnt:

size constancy	depth perception
shape constancy	shape discrimination.

Culturally sanctioned distress states

Reports of cultural and ethnic variation in the experience of hallucinations (Al-Issa, 1977; Schwab, 1977) suggest that hallucinations are not necessarily pathological phenomena, while reports of hallucinatory experiences in the general population provide additional evidence that psychosis is on a continuum with normality (Johns et al., 2002); cognitive psychological models have attempted to explain how anomalous experiences are transformed into psychotic symptoms (Garety et al., 2001). Visual and auditory phenomena can occur in culturally sanctioned distress states without necessarily being pathognomonic of mental disorder. A few examples follow.

NOCTURNAL HALLUCINATIONS IN ULTRA-ORTHODOX JEWISH ISRAELI MEN

Greenberg and Brom (2001) reported that hallucinations that occur predominantly at night were found in 122 out of a sample of 302 ultra-orthodox Jewish Israeli men referred for psychiatric evaluation. Most of those with nocturnal hallucinations were in their late teens, were seen only once or twice, were brought in order to receive an evaluation letter for the Israeli army, and had a reported history of serious learning difficulties. The nocturnal hallucinatory experiences were predominantly visual, and the images were frightening figures from daily life or from folklore. Many of the subjects were withdrawn, monosyllabic, reluctant interviewees. Greenberg and Brom suggested that this cultural group's value on study at Yeshivas away from home places significant pressure on teenage boys with mild or definite subnormality, possibly precipitating the phenomenon at this age in this sex. Although malingering had to be considered as a possible explanation in many cases owing to the circumstances of the evaluation, short-term and long-term follow-up on a limited sample allowed this explanation to be dismissed in a significant number of cases. They therefore suggested that these nocturnal hallucinations are a culture-specific phenomenon.

ISOLATED SLEEP PARALYSIS WITH VISUAL HALLUCINATIONS AMONG NIGERIAN STUDENTS

Ohaeri et al. (1992) reported the results of a cross-sectional study of the pattern of isolated sleep paralysis among the entire population of nursing students at the Neuropsychiatric Hospital in Abeokuta, Nigeria, consisting of 58 males and 37 females. Forty-four per cent of the students (both male and female) admitted having experienced this phenomenon. The findings largely supported the results of a similar study of Nigerian medical students, except that there was a slight male preponderance among those who had the experience. Visual hallucination was the most common perceptual problem associated with the episodes, and all the affected subjects were most distressed by the experience. The popular, culturally sanctioned, view in Africa is that this distress state associated with visual phenomena is caused by witchcraft.

MU-GHAYEB

Mu-Ghayeb is a traditional bereavement reaction that occurs in Oman following a sudden unexpected death. The deceased relative or friend may be seen as an unearthly figure at night. During the daytime, the deceased may be seen, normally clothed, in circumstances that are difficult to authenticate; for instance, sitting in a motor vehicle that passes by at speed. These visual phenomena are consistent with the belief in traditional Omani society that after such a sudden untimely 'death' the 'deceased' continue to be alive; they are expected to be resurrected to a strange, ghostly existence, with nocturnal wanderings interleaving episodes of sleeping naked in caves during the day. This belief in the return of the dead persists even after an elaborate ritual of burial and a prescribed period of mourning. The deceased are expected to leave the grave after burial and join their families when the spell placed on them by a sorcerer is broken or counteracted. Although the Mu-Ghayeb belief is inconsistent with their Islamic religion, this culture-specific response to bereavement may be explained in terms of sudden and untimely death which used to be rife in the seafaring Omani society (Al-Adawi *et al.*, 1997).

AUDITORY AND VISUAL HALLUCINATIONS RELATED TO BEREAVEMENT IN THE CARIBBEAN

Long-lasting auditory and visual hallucinations may occur in individuals living in, or originally from, the Caribbean, following the death of a relative, such that these auditory and visual phenomena may not be pathognomonic of mental disorder. An example is given in a case report by Boran and Viswanathan (2000) relating to an American patient originally from Jamaica:

Mrs G, a 28-year-old woman who was eight weeks pregnant, was hospitalized on an obstetrics–gynaecology unit of a university hospital with a diagnosis of mild hyperemesis gravidarum. The patient had no prior psychiatric history, including no history of alcohol or substance abuse, and no significant medical history. She lived with her mother and sister. A psychiatric consultation was requested because the person had auditory and visual hallucinations.

The patient was hearing someone knocking at the door and was seeing a man sitting in the chair next to her bed when there was nobody else in the room. When asked about the hallucinations, she said that she and her family believed that after death the spirit of the dead person was still among them. If the dead one was somebody who had always helped them in difficult moments of their life, then he or she continued to do so by 'showing up' and being of comfort. Such was 'Uncle Pete', the man the patient saw when she was admitted, and who appeared to the family on several other difficult occasions.

Mrs G's mental status examination was unremarkable except for the hallucinations. The medical workup did not reveal any organic causes for her symptoms. She showed no distress or impairment of functioning as a result of the belief. With the patient's permission, we spoke to her mother and sister by telephone. They reported that Uncle Pete had also appeared to them and confirmed that neither Mrs G nor others in the family had any prior psychiatric history.

The nurse assigned by the medical staff to watch the patient in the hospital also told the psychiatric consultant about her own family spirit, who was similar to Uncle Pete in many ways. The patient and the nurse were both from Jamaica and came to the United States with their families as children. The patient's symptoms were determined to be culturally based beliefs, and there was no evidence of psychosis. No psychiatric sequelae appeared in the patient's subsequent hospital course.

INFORMATION PROCESSING AND ATTENTION

Information processing

Information processing is concerned with the way in which external signals arriving at the sense organs are converted into meaningful perceptual experiences.

Data-driven processing
The processing is initiated by the arrival of data. The simplest scheme for classifying and recognizing patterns is template matching, in which recognition is achieved by matching the external signal against the internal template.

Conceptually driven processing
This applies when data input is incomplete. The processing starts with the conceptualization of what might be present and then looks for confirmatory evidence, thereby biasing the processing mechanisms to give the expected results. Conceptually driven data (schema) are essential to perception. However, they can lead to misperceptions.

Attention

Attention is an intensive process in which information selection takes place. Types include:

- *Selective/focused attention.* One type of information is attended to while additional distracting information is ignored; e.g. the cocktail party effect. In dichotic listening studies in which subjects attend to one channel evidence indicates that the unattended channel is still being processed and the listener can switch rapidly if appropriate.
- *Divided attention.* At least two sources of information are attended to simultaneously. Performance is inefficient. Loss of performance is called 'dual-task interference'.
- *Sustained attention.* The environment is monitored over a long period of time. Performance deteriorates with time.
- *Controlled attention.* Effort is required. It has been suggested that a defect of controlled attention might underlie symptoms of schizophrenia.
- *Automatic attention.* The subject becomes skilled at a task and therefore little conscious effort is required.
- *Stroop effect.* An automatic process is so ingrained that it interferes with controlled processing.

FACTORS AFFECTING MEMORY

Memory

Memory comprises encoding/registration, storage and retrieval of information.

- *Encoding/registration.* This is the transformation of physical information into a code that memory can accept.
- *Storage.* This is the retention of encoded information. According to the multi-store model of Atkinson and Shriffrin (1968), which has now been superseded, memory storage can be

considered to be made up of sensory memory, short-term memory and long-term memory. This modal model is shown in Figure 1.4.

- *Retrieval.* This is the recovery of information from memory when needed.

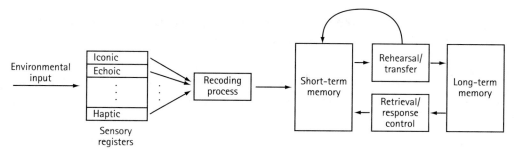

Figure 1.4 *The multi-store modal model of memory.* (After Atkinson & Shriffrin, 1968).

Influences upon memory

According to the multi-store modal model, sensory memory has a large capacity; sensory information is retained here in an unprocessed form in peripheral receptors. Sensory memory is a very short-lived (fade time 0.5 s) trace of the sensory input. Visual input is briefly retained as a mental image called an 'icon'; this is known as an *iconic memory*. The sensory memory for auditory information is called an *echoic memory*, while that for information from touch is called a *haptic memory*. Sensory memory is considered to give an accurate account of the environment as experienced by the sensory system. It holds a representation of the stimulus so that parts of it can be attended to, processed, and transferred into more permanent memory stores.

Those aspects of sensory information that are the object of active attention are transferred into a temporary working memory called the *short-term memory*. Encoding is mainly acoustic; visual encoding rapidly fades. This is the memory used temporarily to hold a telephone number, for example, until dialled; it is lost in 20 s unless rehearsed. Short-term (primary or working) memory consists of a small finite number (seven ± two) of registers which can be filled only by data entering one at a time. According to the *displacement principle*, when the registers are full the addition of a new datum leads to the displacement and loss of an existing one. The probability of correctly recalling an item of information is greater if it is one of the first items to be encountered, even if more than seven items have been presented; this is known as the *primacy effect*. Similarly, the *recency effect* refers to the finding that the probability of correctly recalling an item of information is increased if it is one of the most recent items to be encountered. Those items having an intermediate serial position are least likely to be recalled accurately, and this overall phenomenon is referred to as the *serial position effect*. Whereas the recency effect can be accounted for in terms of the comparatively short interval of time elapsing before recall, the primary effect is more difficult to explain, and may be caused by greater rehearsal of these first items. Retrieval from short-term memory is considered to be effortless and error-free.

Rehearsal is not as necessary in approximately 5% of children possessing a photographic memory, known in psychology as *eidetic imagery*, in whom a detailed visual image can be retained for over half a minute.

Long-term memory stores information more or less permanently and theoretically may have unlimited capacity, although there may be limitations on retrieval. Input and retrieval take longer and are more effortful than for short-term memory. Some motivation is required to encode information into long-term memory. Schizophrenia and depression affect memory at this level.

Optimal conditions for encoding, storage and retrieval of information

ENCODING/REGISTRATION

Conrad (1964) showed that confusion occurs between acoustically similar letters presented against background noise. For example, the letter P is more likely to be incorrectly recalled as V (which is acoustically similar) than as the letter R (which is visually similar). Baddeley (1966a) then went on to demonstrate that acoustically similar words are also more difficult to recall immediately (a test of short-term memory) than are semantically similar words. For example, the sequence rat–mat–cat–cap (which are acoustically similar words) is more difficult to recall immediately than the sequence large–big–huge–grand (which is semantically similar). However, in a test of long-term memory, Baddeley (1966b) found a semantic similarity effect rather than a phonological similarity effect. So, in terms of the parameters studied, it appeared that encoding or registration for short-term memory is better for semantically similar word sequences than for phonologically (acoustically) similar words, while encoding or registration for long-term memory is better for phonologically (acoustically) similar word sequences than for semantically similar words.

Semantic encoding has been shown to aid short-term memory in respect of trigrams (three-letter sequences). Increased memory span has been demonstrated for meaningful trigrams, such as CNN–CIA–NBC, than for meaningless trigrams, such as AUM–GLB–CDX (Bower & Springston, 1970).

With respect to iconic memory encoding, a preceding or subsequent visual sensory presentation of data at a similar energy level (that is, brightness) to that of the index presentation leads to a masking of the index presentation so that it is not registered. The term for this phenomenon is *energy masking* and it occurs at the level of the retina. Another form of masking that has been described is *pattern masking*, in which the preceding or subsequent visual presentation is of data visually similar to that of the index presentation. Pattern masking occurs at a deeper level of visual information processing than the retinal level. The deduction of the relative depth of level of visual processing at which energy masking and pattern masking occur followed from the finding that, whereas the former can take place only when the index presentation and the masking presentation are both to the same eye, the latter can take place even when the index presentation is to one eye and the corresponding masking presentation is to the other eye (Turvey, 1973). With respect to rapidly changing picture presentations, it appears to take about 100 ms for a scene to be understood and no longer be susceptible to ordinary visual masking, and a further 300 ms or so to be no longer susceptible to conceptual masking (from a succeeding picture representation, for example) (Potter, 1976).

So far as the registration of two auditory stimuli is concerned, experiments in which two sounds are presented to subjects and in which the just noticeable interval between noise pulses is compared with the level of the second noise pulse demonstrate that confusion occurs between the echoic image of the first auditory presentation and the onset of the second auditory presentation, unless either a sufficient time interval is allowed for the echoic image of the first presentation to fade before presenting the second stimulus, or the volume of the second stimulus is increased (Plomp, 1964).

As with visual masking (see above), so *binaural masking* has also been demonstrated. A masking sound presented soon after an index sound interferes with detection; this interference is greater when both stimuli are presented to the same ear than when the masking sound is presented to the contralateral ear following the presentation of the index auditory stimulus (Deatherage & Evans, 1969).

In studies of auditory encoding of stimuli and their serial position, a *suffix effect* occurs. This refers to the auditory encoding error that occurs when there is a categorical similarity between the penultimate and ultimate speech-like sounds heard (Crowder, 1971; Ayres *et al.*, 1979).

Elaborating meaning appears to improve encoding of the written word. For instance, your encoding of the text of each of the remaining chapters of this book is likely to be better if you look at some questions specifically related to these chapters before reading each of them. (Suitable questions may be found in the companion books of multiple choice questions (MCQs) and extended matching items (EMIs).) When you read the actual chapters after being primed with the need to search for the answers, you are more likely to elaborate parts of each of these chapters, and encode the information better (Frase, 1975; Anderson, 1980).

STORAGE

One of many examples of findings that are not consistent with the multi-store modal model of memory is that of the finding of positive recency effects in delayed free recall. According to the model, a *continuous distraction procedure*, such as counting backwards between the presentation of items such as unrelated words, should prevent the subject from rehearsing the items and should replace these items in short-term memory. However, in practice the serial position curve shows both a primacy effect and a recency effect under such circumstances (Tzeng, 1973). There also does not appear to be a positive (or negative) relationship between the amount of rehearsal of presented items and how well they are recalled from short-term memory (Craik & Watkins, 1973; Glenberg *et al.*, 1977).

Gillund and Shiffrin (1981) found that the free recall of complex pictures was better than that of words. Many further studies have confirmed a *picture superiority effect*. In general, pictures are remembered and recalled better than words, and non-verbal information storage of pictures and designs is found to be more stable over a period of hours and days than is the storage of words (e.g Hart & O'Shanick, 1993). Simple pictures appear to be better remembered than complex pictures; the *asymmetric confusability effect* is manifested in the finding that there is a greater accuracy in recognition testing of same versus changed stimulus in simple rather than complex pictures (Pezdek & Chen, 1982).

RETRIEVAL

Retrieval of information from the long-term memory is error prone but is improved if the information being stored is organized. *Hierarchical organization* is particularly useful in this regard, perhaps because it improves the search process within long-term memory (Bower *et al.*, 1969).

Another optimal condition for retrieval of information is to arrange that the context within which the information is to be retrieved is similar to that within which it was encoded (Estes, 1972).

Memory information processing

PRIMARY WORKING MEMORY STORAGE CAPACITY

Working memory refers to the temporary storage of information in connection with performing other, more complex, tasks (Baddeley, 1986). In the multi-store modal model of memory, it is the short-term memory (or short-term store) that acts as a key working memory system to allow information to transfer into the long-term memory (or long-term store) and thereby allow learning to take place.

As mentioned above, a number of findings, such as the lack of a positive (or negative) relationship between the amount of rehearsal of presented items and how well they are recalled from short-term memory (Craik & Watkins, 1973), cast doubt on the validity of the multi-store modal model of memory, and in particular on the assumption implicit in this model that holding information in short-term memory (or the short-term store) necessarily leads to information transfer into long-term memory (or the long-term store). Furthermore, since in this modal model the short-term memory (store) acts as the working memory that is essential for learning, it would be expected that patients with short-term memory (store) impairment should manifest impaired long-term learning. However, Shallice and Warrington (1970) described the case of a patient with a severely affected short-term memory (store) who nonetheless had a normal long-term learning capacity; this person had a memory span of just two digits and almost no recency effect in the free-recall task (in which the subject is asked to recall as many of a previously presented list of unrelated words as he/she can, in any order). Moreover, when a short-term memory (store) deficit is experimentally induced in normal subjects by giving them digits to rehearse concurrently with a grammatical reasoning task, even with eight digits the reasoning time increases by only around 50% and the error rate remains around 5% (the same as with fewer digits to rehearse) (Baddeley & Hitch, 1974), and this in spite of the fact that a digit load of eight should have totally filled the short-term memory (store) according to the multi-store modal model. Tasks using a similar digit load concurrent with comprehension and free-recall learning also show that the long-term memory (store) can be impaired but that the recency effect still occurs, again contrary to the modal model prediction.

In response to these difficulties, Baddeley and Hitch formulated the working memory model shown diagrammatically in Figure 1.5. The *central executive* is an attentional controller which is supported by two active slave systems, the *articulatory* or *phonological loop*, responsible for the maintenance of speech-based information, and the *visuospatial scratch-pad* or *sketch-pad*, which can hold and manipulate information in the visuospatial domain. This model was compatible with the findings mentioned in the previous paragraph. For example, concurrent verbal (articulatory) activity and visual or spatial activity appear to interfere with two different systems. Subjects using a mnemonic based on spatial location to remember word lists have better recall of the lists than those who use a simple rote rehearsal procedure, but this advantage disappears if the former subjects are required to carry out a visuospatial task concurrently (Baddeley & Lieberman, 1980). Again, a patient with gross impairment of digit span would be hypothesized to have a defect of their phonological loop functioning; if there were no co-existent impairment of the functioning of the central executive or visuospatial sketch-pad, then normal learning should still be possible.

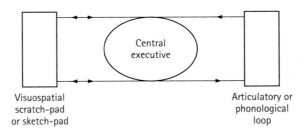

Figure 1.5 *The working memory model of Baddeley and Hitch.* (After Baddeley & Hitch, 1974).

Working memory capacity can be measured using a task in which, after reading a series of sentences, the subject is required to recall the last word of each of these sentences (Daneman & Carpenter, 1980). This task therefore requires both comprehension and recall (as opposed to just recall in the simple word-span task).

There is a strong positive correlation between working memory tests and intelligence quotient (IQ) tests. Furthermore, standard intelligence quotient tests appear to be more susceptible to the subject's previous knowledge, whereas working memory tests appear to have a greater relationship to the speed of processing (Kyllonen & Christal, 1990).

In terms of the model of working memory of Baddeley and Hitch (1974), the central executive is a limited-capacity system which provides the link between the two slave systems (see Figure 1.5) and long-term memory; it is responsible for planning and selecting strategies (Baddeley, 1986). The visuospatial scratch-pad or sketch-pad appears to have a visual component, which is concerned with such factors as shape and colour, and a spatial component, which is concerned with location (Baddeley & Lieberman, 1980; Baddeley, 1986). The articulatory or phonological loop also appears to be made up of two components: a memory store which can hold phonological information for one to two seconds; and an articulatory control process (or processor) (Baddeley, 1986; Paulesu *et al.*, 1993). Memory traces in the phonological loop can be refreshed by means of subvocal articulation. (Subvocal or vocal articulation may also be used to provide an input into this slave system upon the visual presentation of objects by the subject articulating the names of those objects.) The phonological loop is held to provide the basis for digit span. In particular, the number of items retained in the digit span is believed to be a function of both the rate of fading of the memory trace in the phonological loop and the rate of refreshing of memory traces by means of subvocal articulation. The size of the storage capacity can be reduced in the following ways:

- *The phonological similarity effect.* This involves trying to remember items with similar sounding names.
- *Presenting irrelevant spoken material.* This gains access to the store and corrupts the memory trace.
- *The word length effect.* As the length of the words increases, the memory span decreases, presumably because of the longer time required for longer words to be rehearsed, leading to a greater probability of memory trace decay.
- *Articulatory suppression.* This requires a subject repeatedly to articulate an irrelevant speech sound which interferes with subvocal rehearsal.

THE PRINCIPLE OF CHUNKING

Chunking increases the amount of information stored in 'short-term memory registers' (in the multi-modal model) by allowing one entry to cover several items. While the number of chunks is restricted, their content is not. With the help of long-term memory, new material can be recoded thereby increasing the content of chunks.

For example, British trainee and qualified psychiatrists are unlikely to require eight 'registers' in order to remember the letters MRCPSYCH. Similarly, the string DSMIVTRICDEEG can readily be split into the chunks DSM-IV-TR, ICD, and EEG.

It has been suggested that the acquisition of skills through practice may involve the grouping of sets of mental entities (be they motor or perceptual) as chunks (Newell & Rosenbloom, 1981).

SEMANTIC MEMORY

Semantic memory refers to the subject's knowledge of facts, language, concepts, and the like, and is an aspect of long-term/secondary memory that is consistent with the finding that verbal information is stored in terms of meaning rather than exact words (Tulving, 1972). It is easier to remember words paired with meanings (Bower, 1972), and to recall words synonymous to those in a given list (Sachs, 1967). Therefore semantic encoding is a more efficient way than simple rehearsal of transferring information from the 'short-term memory' to the long-term/secondary one.

EPISODIC MEMORY

Episodic memory is an aspect of long-term/secondary memory that refers to the memory for events. It provides a continually changing and updated record of autobiographical material (Tulving, 1972).

SKILLS MEMORY

Skills memory, or procedural memory, is an aspect of long-term/secondary memory that supports skilled performance.

OTHER ASPECTS OF LONG-TERM/SECONDARY MEMORY

Ryle (1949) distinguished between procedural knowledge and *declarative knowledge*; whereas the former referred to knowledge that supported the performance of tasks, the latter referred to factual knowledge. Tulving (1985) distinguished between *autonoetic awareness* (or remembering) and *noetic awareness* (or knowing).

The process of forgetting and the influence of emotional factors on retrieval

Forgetting from long-term/secondary memory is usually the result of retrieval failure rather than storage failure. This explains why forgotten memories can be recovered under hypnosis, and also the 'tip of the tongue' experience.

THEORIES OF FORGETTING

Under the multi-modal model of memory, forgetting from long-term memory could be caused by interference or trace decay.

According to the *interference theory*, forgetting by interference is item-dependent. There are two main types. In *proactive* interference/inhibition, previous learning is likely to impair subsequent learning. In *retroactive* interference/inhibition, new learning is likely to impair previous learning.

According to the *decay theory*, memories fade with time. The longer the item remains in the memory system, the weaker its strength. New material has a high trace strength while older has a low trace strength. Forgetting by decay is time-dependent.

EMOTIONAL FACTORS AND RETRIEVAL

Emotional factors can influence retrieval from long-term memory in the following ways:

- Emotionally charged situations are rehearsed and organized more than non-emotionally charged ones. Retrieval is facilitated.
- Negative emotions and anxiety hinder retrieval.
- Retrieval of events and emotions is more likely to be successful if it occurs in the same context as that in which the original events and emotions occurred; this is known as *state-dependent learning*.
- Repression of emotionally charged material hinders retrieval.

The processes of interference, schemata and elaboration

INTERFERENCE

Retroactive interference refers to the negative effect of new learning on retrieval of prior knowledge. It has been demonstrated in many experimental trials, for example by Slamecka (1960). In contrast, proactive interference refers to the negative effect of prior knowledge on new learning.

SCHEMATA

A schema (plural schemata) may be defined as a mental model or representation, built up through experience, about a person, an object, a situation, or an event (Searleman & Herrmann, 1994). The roles of schemata include (Morton & Bekerian, 1986):

- interpretation of sensory data
- retrieval of information from memory
- organization of actions
- determination of goals
- determination of behaviour
- allocation of processing resources
- directing overall processing in attentional, perceptual and memory systems.

They help to integrate information that is currently being experienced with the subject's long-term past in a single representation (Groeger, 1997).

It has been suggested that lack of the schemata needed to help organize episodic memory may help explain the origin of *infantile amnesia*, which is the inability of humans to access their early childhood memories (Schachtel, 1947). In contrast, the organization of retrieval cues into stable *retrieval schemata* has been put forward as being part of the explanation of the occurrence of exceptional memory performance, in the *skilled memory theory* (Ericsson & Kintsch, 1995).

ELABORATION

As mentioned earlier in this chapter, elaboration appears to improve encoding of new information. Methods of elaboration include:

- semantic processing
- forming complex images
- attempting to answer questions based on the material to be learned.

FACTORS AFFECTING THOUGHT

The relationship of thought to language

Early work in psychology suggested that thought could not occur independently of language. It was held that children, on learning to speak, simply articulated their thoughts until they learned to suppress the vocalization, whence thought simply became concealed speech. Watson (1913) argued that (unarticulated) thought consisted of laryngeal motor habits. This gained support from the electrophysiological finding of Jacobsen (1932) that mental activities ('thought') were accompanied by electrical activity in the musculature of the throat.

There is much evidence that stands in opposition to this early theory. To give just two examples:

- Many infrahuman animals appear to be able to think but do not appear to possess language.
- Temporary paralysis of all voluntary muscles with D-tubocurarine is not associated with an inability to think (Smith *et al.*, 1947).

CONCEPTS

Concepts are the properties or relationships that given object classes or ideas have in common. They constitute a means of grouping what otherwise would form too wide a variety of disparate items or ideas for efficient thought and communication.

- Concrete concepts refer to objects. For example, the concept 'book' refers to objects having properties shared by most books, such as having pages, containing information, having a title, having authors, and so on.
- Abstract concepts refer to abstract ideas, such as honesty, integrity and justice. Concepts of activities include drinking, walking, cycling, and so on.

PROTOTYPES

Prototypes are idealized forms. For instance, the prototypical book might be considered to have the shape of this book with: a front cover having a title; a back cover; multiple pages in between the covers mostly containing printed words arranged into sentences, paragraphs, subsections, sections and chapters; some diagrams interspersed amongst the words; a title page and list of contents at the beginning; an index at the end. According to the prototype theory, the acquisition of prototypes occurs through repeated exposure.

Reasoning

DEDUCTIVE REASONING

This is reasoning based on deduction, the domains of which include:

- relational inferences
- propositional inferences
- syllogisms
- multiply quantified inferences.

Relational inferences are based on relations such as:

Is equal to, denoted by $=$
Is greater than, denoted by $>$
Is less than, denoted by $<$
Is greater than or equal to, denoted by $\geq$
Is less than or equal to, denoted by $\leq$
After
Before
To the right of
To the left of.

Propositional inferences are based on relations such as:

Negation, denoted by $-$
Conjunction, denoted by $\&$
Disjunction, denoted by $\vee$
Implication, denoted by $\rightarrow$
Bi-implication, denoted by $\leftrightarrow$.

(Note that these are the symbols used in logic. In ordinary mathematics other symbols are often used, for instance $\Rightarrow$ for implication.)

Syllogisms are based on pairs of statements or premises, each of which contains one quantifier, such as:

The universal quantifier ('for all'), denoted by $\forall$
Some
The existential quantifier ('there exist(s)'), denoted by $\exists$.

Multiply quantified inferences are based on statements or premises that contain more than one quantifier. (Such statements in turn can be converted into sets of statements that each contain only one quantifier.)

The arithmetic symbols used in formal reasoning statements can be reduced to just three:

The zero symbol, denoted by 0
The successor symbol, denoted by $'$
The addition symbol, denoted by $+$.

In addition, it is convenient to include:

The multiplication symbol, denoted by $\cdot$.

For example, the statement that every (real) number possesses a square root may be formally stated as:

$$\forall x_0 \exists x_1 (x_1 \cdot x_1) = x_0$$

Some have argued that human cerebral deductive reasoning is dependent on the formal rules of inference, as used in formal logic (e.g. Braine *et al.*, 1984); these are known as *formal rule theories*. In contrast, other cognitive scientists such as Johnson-Laird (1993) have argued that deductive reasoning (and indeed also inductive reasoning) is a semantic process rather similar to that carried out when searching for counterexamples; this is known as the *mental model theory*.

As an example, suppose that we consider the following deductive reasoning problem relating to the relative positions of various chapters of this book:

- The chapter on schizophrenia comes after the chapter on social sciences.
- The chapter on social psychology comes before the chapter on social sciences.
- What is the positional relationship between the chapter on schizophrenia and the chapter on social psychology?

The only model containing all three chapters that is consistent with these statements is:

social psychology   social sciences   schizophrenia

So the answer to the question is that the chapter on schizophrenia comes after the chapter on social psychology. There is just one model corresponding to the statements, and the problem has a valid answer, and so this is known as a *one-model problem with a valid answer*. Now consider the following problem:

- The chapter on schizophrenia comes after the chapter on social psychology.
- The chapter on social sciences comes after the chapter on social psychology.
- What is the positional relationship between the chapter on schizophrenia and the chapter on social sciences?

There are now two models containing all three chapters that are consistent with these statements:

social psychology   social sciences   schizophrenia

and

social psychology   schizophrenia   social sciences

In this particular case, there are two models, and there is no positional relationship between the chapter on schizophrenia and the chapter on social sciences that is common to both models. We say that there is no valid answer. This case is a *multiple-model problem with no valid answers*.

Formal rule theories predict that one-model problems are more difficult than multiple-model problems with valid answers. In contrast, the mental model theory predicts that multiple-model problems with no valid answers are more difficult than multiple-model problems with valid answers, which in turn are themselves more difficult than one-model problems. Experimental evidence supports the mental model theory (e.g. Byrne & Johnson-Laird, 1989).

INDUCTIVE REASONING

In inductive reasoning, a general statement is derived by inductive arguments from many instances. An elementary example is given from number theory in mathematics. Consider the following (correct) equations:

$$1 = 1$$
$$1 + 2 = 3$$
$$1 + 2 + 2^2 = 7$$
$$1 + 2 + 2^2 + 2^3 = 15$$
$$1 + 2 + 2^2 + 2^3 + 2^4 = 31$$
$$1 + 2 + 2^2 + 2^3 + 2^4 + 2^5 = 63.$$

Consider the values of the positive integers (whole numbers) on the right-hand side of each equation. We have:

$$1 = 2 - 1 = 2^1 - 1$$
$$3 = 2^2 - 1$$
$$7 = 2^3 - 1$$
$$15 = 2^4 - 1$$
$$31 = 2^5 - 1$$
$$63 = 2^6 - 1.$$

So here we have the following pattern that appears to be emerging:

$$1 + 2 + 2^2 + 2^3 + \ldots + 2^{n-1} = 2^n - 1 \qquad (1.1)$$

(This may also be written as $2^0 + 2^1 + 2^2 + 2^3 + \ldots + 2^{n-1} = 2^n - 1$.)

We have six instances in which equation (1.1) is true. What we shall now do is use inductive reasoning to prove that the general statement, equation (1.1), is itself true.

Let S represent the set of positive integers (positive whole numbers, such as 1, 2, 3, etc.) for which the formula given in equation (1.1) is correct. Now, when $n = 1$, the left-hand side of this formula is

1, while the right-hand side is $2^1 - 1 = 2 - 1 = 1$. Since $1 = 1$, the formula is correct for $n = 1$. Therefore, the integer 1 belongs to the set S. Assume now that equation (1.1) is true for a fixed positive integer k. Then we have:

$$1 + 2 + 2^2 + \ldots + 2^{k-1} = 2^k - 1 \quad (1.2)$$

Now we need to show that our formula holds for the positive integer $k + 1$. If we add 2^k to each side of equation (1.2), we obtain:

$$\begin{aligned}
1 + 2 + 2^2 + \ldots + 2^{k-1} + 2^k &= 2^k - 1 + 2^k \\
&= 2^k + 2^k - 1 \\
&= 2 \cdot 2^k - 1 \\
&= 2^1 \cdot 2^k - 1 \\
&= 2^{k+1} - 1
\end{aligned}$$

So this means that equation (1.1) is true when $n = k + 1$. Therefore $k + 1$ belongs to S. Hence whenever the positive integer k belongs to S, then $k + 1$ belongs to S. But we know that 1 belongs to S. Hence, by inductive reasoning, it follows that S must contain all positive integers. So the formula shown in equation (1.1), initially hypothesized on just six instances, has been shown to hold for all positive integers (infinite in number) by inductive reasoning.

Problem–solving strategies

ALTERNATIVE REPRESENTATIONS

One method of problem-solving is to represent the given data in a different way. For example, we have seen two different representations in the last two examples. In the first of these, in which a problem relating to the relative order of chapters of this book was set, a diagrammatic representation was used, in which the data were, as it were, visualized. In the most recent example, on the other hand, in which inductive reasoning was being used, it was more convenient to use symbolic representation. In a similar fashion, in elementary mathematics, problem-solving can also sometimes be carried out using a more geometric approach or a more algebraic approach.

EXPERTISE

The way in which problems are represented by experts tends to differ from the representations used by inexperienced people. For instance, the way in which the reader (assumed to be clinically competent and qualified) might diagnose a central nervous system lesion in a patient would likely be different and more efficient (and more likely to be correct) than the methods employed by relatively inexperienced third-year medical students; the recall of the person's symptoms and signs would also tend to be better for the reader. In particular, compared with a beginner, an expert's memory would tend to have more potential representations of the problem that he or she can draw upon to solve it. Experts are also more likely to be able to invoke heuristics (see below) that are not available to novices.

COMPUTER SIMULATIONS

Computer simulations may be used to study the way in which representations and heuristics are employed in problem-solving.

Algorithms

In a general sort of way, an algorithm consists of a specific sequence of steps that need to be carried out according to precise instructions in order to solve a given problem. For example, suppose you were to stop reading right now and take a pencil and paper and calculate the value of 22 divided by 7 to three decimal places, using long division. The correct answer is 3.143. The method you used to carry out this calculation involved a mechanical use of the rules of long division; no deep thought is required but, rather, a simple adherence to the simple rules of this method of problem-solving. This is a characteristic feature of algorithms.

More precisely, an algorithm is any process that can be carried out by a Turing machine. A Turing machine is a simple, mechanical calculating device invented by the British mathematician Alan Turing (1912–54). At its most basic, a Turing machine can be imagined to be an infinitely long tape segmented into squares. Starting at any one square, the Turing machine can do the following:

1 Stop the computation.
2 Move one square to the right.
3 Move one square to the left.
4 Write S_0 to replace whatever is in the square being scanned.
5 Write S_1 to replace whatever is in the square being scanned.

.
.
.

$n + 4$ Write S_n to replace whatever is in the square being scanned.

This may seem, at first sight, to be a rather primitive machine that can only handle addition and subtraction, say. In fact, however, it can carry out multiplication, division, and the calculation of square roots and other power functions. Indeed, it may be the case that, in principle, a Turing machine can carry out any calculation that a powerful modern supercomputer can.

Heuristics

As mentioned above, heuristics are strategies that can be applied to problems and that often give the correct answer (or 'goal state') more quickly than simple algorithms; they are not guaranteed to work, however. Such heuristic techniques are not usually available to novices, whereas experts can access these during problem-solving. As an example, at one stage of his career the author of this chapter had cause to devise a method of accurately quantifying cerebral ventricular volumes in serial magnetic resonance scans that had been accurately matched using subvoxel registration, a feat that had not hitherto been accomplished. A heuristic of the type 'consider an analogous problem that you know you can solve' was used first, and then this solution was generalized to allow the required equations to be arrived at.

FACTORS AFFECTING PERSONALITY

Derivation of nomothetic and idiographic theories

The terms *nomothetic* and *idiographic* in respect of the study of people were introduced by Wilhelm Windelband, the German philosopher who taught at Heidelberg and initiated axiological neo-

Kantianism. He distinguished between the study of whole populations (the nomothetic approach) and the study of individuals (the idiographic approach).

The nomothetic approach to personality considers that personality theory should be at least partly based on the study of the common features and differences between people. For instance, personality has been defined by Wiggins (1979) as being:

> ... that branch of psychology which is concerned with providing a systematic account of the ways in which individuals differ from one another.

In contrast, the idiographic approach attempts to gain an understanding of personality in the context of each individual's unique existence. According to Tyrer and Ferguson (2000):

> The idiographic approach focuses on the uniqueness of the individual and as such can provide a rich, multifaceted description of subtle areas of personal attributes and behaviour. Numerous strands are brought together to build up a portrait which cannot be confused with any other. The case history is the most obvious example and has been used with effect to describe processes, which can then be generalized to explain similar psychological mechanisms in others.

An influential early proponent of the idiographic approach was Gordon Allport (1937), but the nomothetic approach has prevailed.

Trait and state approaches

Traits are 'broad, enduring, relatively stable characteristics used to assess and explain behavior' (Hirschberg, 1978).

The study of traits has a long history. Aristotle (in his *Nicomachean Ethics* of the fourth century BCE) regarded determinants of moral and immoral behaviour to include the following phenomena, which we might regard as being traits:

Cowardice
Modesty
Vanity.

The Greek physician Galen of Pergamum (129 to *circa* 199/200; Greek: Claudios Galenos; Latin: Claudius Galenus) regarded the four Hippocratic humours as forming the basis for his four temperaments:

Choleric
Melancholic
Phlegmatic
Sanguine.

The German philosopher Immanuel Kant (1724–1804) placed these four temperaments along the following two dimensions:

Activity
Feelings.

Thus, a choleric temperament corresponded to strong activity and a phlegmatic temperament corresponded to weak activity. Similarly, a sanguine temperament corresponded to strong feelings and a melancholic temperament corresponded to weak feelings.

The German physiologist and psychologist Wilhelm Wundt (1832–1920), whom most regard as the father of experimental psychology, superimposed the following two dimensions on the four temperaments:

Srong *versus* weak emotions
Changeable (or rapid changes) *versus* unchangeable activity (or slow changes).

Thus, a choleric temperament was unstable (strong emotion) and changeable (rapid changes); a melancholic temperament was unstable and unchangeable; a phlegmatic temperament was stable (weak emotions) and unchangeable; and a sanguine temperament was stable and changeable.

A major impetus was given to the scientific study of the trait approach to personality research by developments in statistical techniques, particularly the use of systematic collection of data and the discovery of correlational and factor analytic techniques. Raymond Cattell and colleagues (1970) have developed the Sixteen Personality Factor Questionnaire (or 16PF) which measures 16 primary factors along 16 dimensions. These are as follows:

Trait A: Outgoing/warmhearted *versus* reserved/detached
Trait B: Intelligence
Trait C: Unemotional/calm *versus* emotional/changeable
Trait E: Assertive/dominant *versus* humble/cooperative
Trait F: Cheerful/lively *versus* sober/taciturn
Trait G: Conscientious/persistent *versus* expedient/undisciplined
Trait H: Venturesome/socially bold *versus* shy/retiring
Trait I: Tough-minded/self-reliant *versus* tender-minded/sensitive
Trait L: Suspicious/sceptical *versus* trusting/accepting
Trait M: Imaginative/Bohemian *versus* practical/conventional
Trait N: Shrewd/discreet *versus* forthright/straightforward
Trait O: Guilt-prone/worrying *versus* resilient/self-assured
Trait Q1: Radical/experimental *versus* conservative/traditional
Trait Q2: Self-sufficient/resourceful *versus* group-dependent/affiliative
Trait Q3: Controlled/compulsive *versus* undisciplined/lax
Trait Q4: Tense/driven *versus* relaxed/tranquil.

In contrast, Hans Eysenck's rating studies initially only yielded two dimensions, and more recently the following three dimensions (following a factor analysis of items) (see Eysenck & Eysenck, 1991):

Extraversion (that is, extraversion *versus* introversion)
Neuroticism
Psychoticism.

The first two of these dimensions were derived by Eysenck (1944) following the study of 700 soldiers in a military hospital suffering from various 'neurotic' disorders and complaints (such as 'headaches', 'sex anomalies' and 'narrow interests'). *Extraversion* is associated with traits such as:

Sociable
Lively
Dominant
Care-free
Active
Assertive
Sensation-seeking
Venturesome
Surgent.

Introversion is associated with the opposite traits. *Neuroticism* is associated with traits such as:

Anxious
Depressed
Emotional
Guilt feelings
Irrational
Low self-esteem
Moody
Shy
Tense.

Psychoticism, which is orthogonal to (and therefore independent of) extraversion and neuroticism in the revised Eysenck factor analysis-based model of personality, is associated with traits such as:

Aggressive
Antisocial
Cold
Creative
Egocentric
Impersonal
Impulsive
Tough-minded
Unempathetic.

In contrast to traits, which refer to stable phenomena related to behaviour and ideas relating to enduring dispositions, states are unstable short-term features of the individual. An example of a state variable is a temporary short-term feeling of anxiety in someone who normally scores highly on the extraversion dimension.

Trait and state approaches can be combined. For example, Figure 1.6 shows a model (based on Michael Eysenck, 1982) of the adverse effects of anxiety on information processing and performance; this model in turn is based on the more complex model of Spielberger (1966).

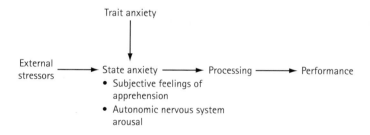

Figure 1.6 *Eysenck's state-trait model showing the effects of anxiety on performance.* (After Eysenck, 1982).

Construct theory

The personal construct theory of George Kelly (an American engineer who went on to become a clinical psychologist) is based on the proposition that behaviour in humans is anticipatory rather than reactive (Kelly, 1955). Kelly considered every man to be a scientist, interpreting the world on the basis of past experience. Constructs are created and predictions made accordingly. A system of constructs results, unique in each individual, existing at various levels of consciousness, those formed at earlier developmental stages being unconscious. Each construct has a range of convenience, some are specific (e.g. chewy versus tender), whereas others have a wider range of convenience. Constructs are arranged into hierarchies. Superordinate constructs are central to the individual's sense of identity, subordinate constructs less so.

According to this theory, anxiety results when the individual is presented with events outside his or her range of personal constructs. Hostility comprises imposition of constructs upon another.

The main points relating to construct systems are as follows:

- Individuals' construct systems make the world more predictable and thereby make it easier to negotiate one's way around.
- Individuals' construct systems are not static but may grow and be modified in response to circumstances. For example, suppose you were under the impression that professors of psychiatry are honest, intelligent people of integrity who care deeply about the need to help discover the aetiology of various types of mental illness and who wish to help find the best treatments for such illnesses. If you were then to discover that a couple of such professors were in fact utterly dishonest, cruel, selfish and psychopathic, with little or no real commitment to academic excellence but ready to steal the fruits of the work of others, then your construct system in this regard would be challenged. In these circumstances, you could alter your construct system in one of these ways:
    - *Adaptation.* Your construct system could be changed to reflect your new experience.
    - *Immunization.* You could try to maintain your belief system by having thoughts such as 'There must be some important reason that I am not privy to which explains why they seemed to act in such an evil way.'
- The construct system of an individual represents the truth as uniquely understood and experienced by that person.
- A construct system is not necessarily internally consistent.
- Since construct systems are partly a function of prior experience, they affect expectations and behaviour.
- Constructs representing core values and the most important relationships of a person are more firmly held and of greater importance that those related to less important matters.
- The degree to which one individual can relate to and understand the construct system of another person is a function to his/her empathy with the latter.

Humanist approaches

Humanistic approaches pay particular attention to those qualities that differentiate humans from non-human animal species. The Association for Humanistic Psychology lists the following five basic postulates:

Man, as man, supersedes the sum of his parts.
Man has his being in a human context.
Man is aware.
Man has choice.
Man is intentional.

Self-actualization is held to be a core individual motivational force.

ROGERS' SELF THEORY

Each individual has a drive to fulfil himself or herself and develop an ideal self within a phenomenal field of subjective experience. The most important aspect of personality is the congruence between the individual's view of himself or herself and reality, and the person's view of himself or herself compared with the ideal self. If an individual acts at variance with the personal self image, anxiety, incongruence and denial result. The congruent individual is able to grow (self-actualization) and achieve a personal potential both internally and socially.

MASLOW

Abraham Maslow is considered to be another leading founder of the humanist approach. Maslow's hierarchy of needs is considered in the next section of this chapter. Transient episodes of self-actualization have been termed 'peak experiences' by Maslow (1970); they are described in terms such as:

Aliveness
Beauty
Effortlessness
Goodness
Perfection
Self-sufficiency
Truth
Uniquenss
Wholeness.

Characteristics of self-actualizers according to Maslow (1967) include:

- They accept themselves and other people for what they are.
- They are highly creative.
- They have a good sense of humour.
- They tend to be problem-centred rather than self-centred.
- They are able to tolerate uncertainty.
- They exhibit spontaneous thought.
- They exhibit spontaneous behaviour.
- Even though they do not make an effort to be unconventional, nevertheless they are resistant to enculturation.
- They have the capacity to consider life objectively.
- They form deep and satisfying relationships with relatively few others.

Behaviours that Maslow (1967) considered may lead to self-actualization include:

Being honest
Assuming responsibility
Working hard at the tasks decided upon
Becoming fully absorbed and concentrating fully, experiencing life as a child does
Identifying one's defences and giving them up
Being prepared to try new things
Evaluating experiences personally without being swayed by the opinions of others
Being willing to be unpopular.

Psychoanalytic approaches

Behaviour and feelings are explained by unconscious drives and conflicts. The *id* is held to be derived from the *libido*. Irrational, impulsive instincts are unable to postpone gratification, and are present at birth. The *ego* develops as the child grows. A conscious mind balances the demands of the *id* with the realities of the outside world. Anxiety results if the *ego* is unable to control the energies of the *id*. The *superego* comprises the internalization of the views of parents and society, like a conscience. The *id*, *ego* and *superego* are in balance with each other.

FREUD'S STAGES OF PSYCHOSEXUAL DEVELOPMENT

- *Oral stage:* age 0 to 1 year
  - Gratification through sucking, biting
  - Failure to negotiate leads to oral personality traits: moodiness, generosity, depression and elation, talkativeness, greed, optimism, pessimism, wishful thinking, narcissism
- *Anal stage:* age 1 to 3 years
  - The anus and defaecation are sources of sensual pleasure
  - Failure to negotiate leads to anal personality traits: obsessive–compulsive personality, tidiness, parsimony, rigidity and thoroughness
- *Phallic stage:* age 3 to 5 years
  - Genital interest, relates to own sexuality; Oedipus/Electra complex
  - Failure to negotiate leads to hysterical personality traits: competitiveness and ambitiousness
- *Latency stage:* age 5 to 12 years
- *Genital stage:* age 12 to 20 years
  - Gratification from normal relations with people
  - Able to relate to a partner.

ERIKSON'S STAGES OF DEVELOPMENT

Age (years)	*Sense of:*
0–1	Trust/security
1–4	Autonomy
4–5	Initiative
5–11	Duty/accomplishment
11–15	Identity
15–adult	Intimacy
Adulthood	Generativity
Maturity	Integrity

Epigenesis is the process of development of the *ego* through these stages.

Situationist approach

The external situation is considered the most powerful determinant of behaviour. Situationists maintain that traits *result* from differences in learning experiences. Behaviour changes according to the situation an individual finds himself (or herself) in. Proponents dismiss the trait theory. Mischel (1983) argues against the existence of any stable personality dimension because of poor correlation between behaviour or attitudes in one situation compared with another.

Interactionist approach

Interactionism holds that behaviour depends upon both the situation and the person (or personality traits) as well as their mutual interaction. Endler (1983) was a prominent advocate of the interactionist approach, arguing that behaviour is:

> ... a function of a continuous multidirectional process of person-by-situation interactions; cognitive, motivational and emotional factors have important determining roles on behaviour, regarding the person side; and the perception or psychological meaning that the situation has for the person is an essential determining factor of behaviour.

Inventories

Personality inventories are questionnaires in which the same questions are put to each person.

16PF

As mentioned above, Cattell and colleagues (1970) developed the 16PF (16 Personality Factor questionnaire) which measures 16 primary factors along 16 dimensions. It was based on the use of factor analysis to identify these 16 basic personality traits, which are listed above, from an initial list of over 3000 personality trait names of Allport and Odbert (1936). Over 100 questions (with yes/no answers) were then selected to allow these traits to be measured. For example, the following question helps to assess trait E (assertive/dominant *versus* humble/cooperative):

> Do you tend to keep in the background on social occasions?

An affirmative reply would give the subject a point on the humble/cooperative end of the trait E scale, while a negative reply would give a point on the assertive/domain end.

The 16PF gives scores on various personality characteristics such as:

Dominance
Emotional stability
Self-control.

MMPI

The opinions of experts (usually working in psychiatry) were garnered in generating the categories for subjects on whom the Minnesota Multiphasic Personality Inventory or MMPI was developed. The final version of the MMPI contains over 550 (567 in one recent version) statements (or questions), relating to:

Attitudes
Emotional reactions
Physical symptoms
Psychological symptoms.

The person being tested is asked to answer true, false, or cannot say to each statement. An example of such a statement is:

> At times my thoughts have raced ahead faster that I could speak them.

An affirmative response to this statement would yield a higher score on the hypomania (Ma) scale. Scores are obtained for several scales from the MMPI as follows (with their abbreviations):

Lie/social desirability (L)
Frequency/distress (F)
Correction/defensiveness (K)
Hypochondriasis (Hs)
Depression (D)
Hysteria (Hy)
Psychopathic deviancy (Pd)
Paranoia (Pa)
Psychasthenia (Pt)
Schizophrenia (Sc)
Hypomania (Ma)
Social introversion–extraversion (Si)
Masculinity–femininity (Mf).

The first three of these scales are used for validity purposes. They include the following statements:

- L scale:
  - Once in a while I think of things too bad to talk about.
  - At times I feel like swearing.
  - I do not always tell the truth.
  - Once in a while I put off until tomorrow what I ought to do today.
  - I would rather win than lose in a game.
  - I do not like everyone I know.
- F scale:
  - Evil spirits possess me at times.
  - When I am with people I am bothered by hearing very queer things.
  - My soul sometimes leaves my body.
  - Someone has been trying to poison me.
  - Someone has been trying to rob me.
  - Everything tastes the same.
  - My neck spots with red often.
  - Someone has been trying to influence my mind.
- K scale:
  - Often I can't understand why I have been so cross and grouchy.
  - At times my thoughts have raced ahead faster than I could speak them.
  - Criticism or scolding hurts me terribly.
  - I certainly feel useless at times.
  - I have never felt better in my life than I do now.
  - What others think of me does not bother me.
  - I find it hard to make talk when I meet new people.
  - I frequently find myself worrying about something.

Tyrer and Ferguson (2000) have made the following comment:

> ... the individual scales ... show a considerable degree of intercorrelation. The scales themselves have unfortunately been labelled using standard psychiatric nosology (e.g. paranoia, schizophrenia and hypomania) which can lead to confusion with Axis I diagnosis. They should more properly be regarded as indicative of the presence of specific personality attributes. Although the MMPI is currently used in

candidate-selection procedures, its principal value would appear to be in the study of clinically abnormal personalities where interpretation by an experienced psychologist is required.

In addition to the problem of the intercorrelation of many scales, another problem with the MMPI is that responses may change over time. (This is a problem relating to reliability.) The same person taking the MMPI at baseline and then a few days later may score differently overall and on different scales.

CPI

The California Psychological Inventory or CPI employs some of the same statements as the MMPI. In the development of the CPI, the opinions of non-experts, such as the peers of the test subjects, were used. The CPI is constructed to measure less 'abnormal' personality traits than the MMPI (in 'normal' people), such as:

Dominance
Independence
Responsibility
Self-acceptance
Socialization
Flexibility
Masculinity–femininity.

In total, the CPI has over 450 (480 in one recent version) true/false items, of which many (178 in the same recent version) are from the MMPI, and yields 15 scales that measure personality and three scales that are used to eliminate response bias. Overall, the CPI yields the following three broad *vector scales*:

Internality/externality
Norm-favoring/norm-questioning
Self-fulfilled/dispirited.

The CPI was given to 13 000 individuals and separate scores were obtained for males and females. The mean scores for each scale were obtained. The scores of subjects now taking the CPI can be compared with the mean scores for these original 13 000 individuals.

OTHER INVENTORIES

Other personality inventories include:

* Children's Personality Questionnaire
* Differential Personality Inventory
* Edwards Personality Inventory
* Eysenck Personality Inventory
* Eysenck Personality Questionnaire
* Maudsley Personality Inventory
* Neo Personality Inventory
* Omnibus Personality Inventory.

The Maudsley Personality Inventory (MPI) was superseded by the Eysenck Personality Inventory (EPI), which in turn was superseded by the Eysenck Personality Questionnaire (EPQ) which measures psychoticism and contains a lie scale.

LIMITATIONS OF INVENTORIES

There are several limitations on the use of personality inventories.

- There are limitations imposed by the cultural origins of the questionnaires. For example, in assessing the answers to the MMPI and the CPI, it needs to be borne in mind that these questionnaires were created for American subjects. One of the statements on the F scale of the MMPI is that 'Evil spirits possess me at times'; in some cultures it is accepted as perfectly normal that 'evil spirits' should 'possess' a person, while in other cultures such terminology might be normal but not to be taken literally.
- Deliberate faking. Subjects may deliberately try to come across as possessing (or not possessing) a particular personality trait. Lie scales are often included to try to detect for this.
- Questionnaires are susceptible to response sets – subjects may exhibit a systematic tendency to respond to test questions.
- The inventories tend to have a low validity, particularly in respect of predictive validity.
- A social desirability bias may occur, in which subjects may have an unconscious tendency to give socially desirable responses that make them look good.
- The inventories only rarely allow an assessment of the underlying reasons for the responses to questions.
- The responses depend on an accurate knowledge, on the part of the subjects, of their beliefs, behaviour, abilities and feelings.
- The responses depend on a willingness, on the part of the subjects, to make known their beliefs, behaviour, abilities and feelings.
- Questionnaires are susceptible to contamination by relatively minor changes in the mental state of the subject.
- The dimensions chosen by psychologists in creating questionnaires may be difficult to relate to personality disorder categories used by psychiatrists.

Rating scales

There are several rating scales that may be used for the assessment of personality disorder. The following are all structured interview schedules.

SAP

The Standardized Assessment of Personality or SAP is carried out by a trained clinical interviewer. A personality profile is obtained from an informant. An ICD-10 diagnosis is obtained.

SCID II

The Structured Clinical Interview for DSM-III-R Personality Disorders or SCID II is carried out by a clinician and yields DSM diagnoses.

SIDP

The Structured Interview for DSM-III Personality Disorders or SIDP is carried out by a psychologist or psychiatrist and yields DSM-III-R diagnoses.

PAS

The Personality Assessment Schedule or PAS yields five diagnostic categories:

Sociopathic
Schizoid
Passive dependent
Anankastic
Normal.

It assesses 24 dimensions of personality and should be carried out by a trained clinical interviewer.

PDE

The Personality Disorder Examination or PDE yields DSM diagnoses.

IPDE

The International Personality Disorder Examination for DSM-IV and ICD-10 personality disorders or IPDE is carried out by trained interviewers and covers DSM-IV(-TR) and ICD-10 operational criteria.

Repertory grid

George Kelly devised the repertory grid or role construct repertory (REP) test. This grid assesses personality based on an individual's personal constructs. A typical grid might consist of ten rows (excluding rows containing headings), which need to be filled in by the subject. The subject begins by naming specific people who fit into given categories, such as a happy person, and a successful person. These form columns that cross the rows. Other columns correspond to other people, such as the subject's father, mother, the subject himself or herself, children, spouse or partner, etc. There is now a grid of, say, ten rows and around ten columns. On each row, three cells are circled; no two rows contain the same three circles. These correspond to three different individuals. Row by row, the subject must now decide for the three individuals concerned what description shows how two of these three individuals are similar and how they differ from the third individual. The former description is placed in a column (column 1) on the left-hand side of the grid, while the latter description is similarly placed in a column (column 2) on the right-hand side of the grid. A code is used to fill in the circles (e.g. 1 for similarity, as in the column 1 description, 2 for difference, as in column 2, and 0 if neither column 1 nor column 2 applies). Then the rest of the grid is filled in. There are many scoring systems available, although the grid itself overall gives an indication of how the subject views others.

Q-sort schedule

This is an *ipsative method*, that is, one which compares alternatives within an individual, in which the rater (or coder) sorts statements into a standard distribution. Jack Block (1961, 1971) used it in his research on childhood development. A deck of cards was produced in which each card contained a word or phrase. An individual was described by sorting this deck into piles corresponding to how closely the card descriptions were deemed to apply to the subject. The Q-sort schedule is designed to apply across different individuals and over time, over different ages.

FACTORS AFFECTING MOTIVATION

Extrinsic theories and homeostasis

Theories based on instincts were replaced by a drive reduction theory in which the motivation of behaviour is to reduce the level of arousal associated with a basic drive (biological drive, such as hunger and thirst) in order to maintain homeostatic control of the internal somatic environment.

- Hull developed a theory in which *primary biological drives* are activated by needs which arise from homeostatic imbalance acting via brain receptors.
- Mowrer developed the notion of *secondary drives* (e.g. anxiety) which result from generalization and conditioning.

Hypothalamic systems and satiety

An example of a primary biological drive is provided by hypothalamic systems and satiety. In rat experiments, the hypothalamic ventromedial nucleus acts as a satiety centre, with hyperphagia occurring if it is ablated, while the lateral hypothalamus contains a hunger centre, with aphagia occurring if it is ablated. (See Chapter 13.)

Intrinsic theories

Whereas extrinsic theories require reduction of drive externally, intrinsic theories propose that the activity engaged in has its own intrinsic reward.

Optimal arousal
An example is offered by optimal arousal, in which the subject attains an optimal level of arousal to achieve optimal performance. In general a moderate level of arousal leads to an optimum degree of alertness and interest, and therefore to a comparatively high efficiency of performance. High and low arousal lead to reduced performance and are described in the inverted-U shape of the Yerkes–Dodson curve.

Cognitive dissonance
According to this theory, first formulated by Festinger, discomfort occurs when two or more cognitions are held but are inconsistent with each other. The individual is motivated to achieve cognitive consistency and may change one or more of the cognitions.

Attitude–discrepant behaviour
When attitude and behaviour are inconsistent (attitude-discrepant behaviour), alteration of attitude helps bring about cognitive consistency.

Need for achievement (nAch)
McClelland formulated a need for achievement (nAch) to explain pleasure resulting from mastery.

Curiosity drive

Whereas the homeostatic model predicts that once physiological needs such as thirst and hunger have been satisfied, or aversive stimuli such as pain have successfully been avoided, and the body returned to its normal state, the organism should no longer be motivated and should be quiescent, in practice this is not the case. Humans and other mammals, for example, have been noted to seek stimulation actively. A curiosity drive has been proposed to help explain this phenomenon, in which the organism has drives to:

- explore new environments
- investigate objects
- manipulate objects (if appropriate)
- seek changing sensory stimulation (and avoid sensory deprivation)
- seek sensation.

Maslow's hierarchy of needs

This unified theory, relating to self-actualization, integrates both extrinsic and intrinsic theories of motivation. A hierarchy of needs is described in which those with survival importance take precedence over others:

- self-actualization needs (highest)
- aesthetic needs
- cognitive needs
- self-esteem needs
- love and belonging needs
- safety needs
- physical/physiological needs (lowest).

FACTORS AFFECTING EMOTION

Types of emotion

An emotion is a mental feeling or affection having cognitive, physiological and social concomitants. Plutchik has classified them into eight primary emotions:

Disgust
Anger
Anticipation
Joy
Acceptance
Fear
Surprise
Sadness.

Any two adjacent emotions can give rise to a secondary emotion. For example, the secondary emotion of love is derived from the primary emotions of joy and acceptance. Similarly, submission results from acceptance and fear, disappointment from surprise and sadness, contempt from disgust and anger, and so on.

Components of emotional response

The main components of emotional response are:

- subjective awareness
- physiological changes
- behaviour.

James–Lange theory

According to this theory, the experience of emotion is secondary to the somatic responses (e.g. sweating, increased cardiac rate, increased arousal) to the perception of given emotionally important events. For example, if an arachnophobe becomes aroused, experiences increased activity of the sympathetic nervous system and runs away after seeing a spider, the feelings of anxiety and fear are the result of the increased sympathetic activity and running away, and not primarily because of the emotion-evoking stimulus.

Cannon criticized this theory. It was argued that similar physiological changes can accompany different emotions. Also, pharmacologically induced simulation of such physiological changes is usually not accompanied by these emotions. The experience of emotions can be shown to be independent of somatic responses, sometimes occurring before the somatic responses.

Cannon–Bard theory

This holds that, following the perception of an emotionally important event, both the somatic responses and the experience of emotion occur together. In neurophysiological terms, the perceived stimulus undergoes thalamic processing, and signals are then relayed both to the cerebral cortex, leading to the experience of emotion, and to other parts of the body, such as the autonomic nervous system, leading to somatic responses.

This theory can be criticized on the basis of the observation that there are stimuli (e.g. sudden danger) which can lead to increased sympathetic activity before the emotion is experienced. Conversely, the experience of emotions sometimes occurs before the somatic response.

Schachter's cognitive labelling theory and cognitive appraisal

According to this theory, the conscious experience of an emotion is a function of the stimulus, of somatic or physiological responses, and of cognitive factors such as the cognitive appraisal of the situation and input from long-term memory. The influence of cognitive factors on the conscious experience of emotion was demonstrated in an experiment by Schachter and Singer (1962) in which subjects were injected with adrenaline. Their cognitive appraisal of the current situation, based on observation of others, influenced the conscious experience of emotion. Thus cognitive cues were important in their interpretation of arousal.

STRESS

Stress results when demand exceeds resources. An individual's response to a stressful situation is affected by biological susceptibility and personality characteristics.

Physiological and psychological aspects

Physiological effects of stress include: physical disorders (ulcers, cardiac disease and hypertension); and immune response changes. Other physical disorders have also been attributed to emotional stress; examples are migraine, eczema, asthma and allergies.

Situational factors

These include life events, daily hassles/uplifts, conflict and trauma (see Chapter 29).

Life events
These are changes in a person's life that require readjustment. They are ranked in order from most to least stressful. The most stressful include: death of spouse; divorce; marital separation; gaol term; death of close family member; personal illness; and marriage. The scale has been found to be universally applicable to people in both underdeveloped and Western countries. Many conditions, both physical and mental, show an excess of life events in the months preceding onset.

Vulnerability and invulnerability

Type A behaviour is related to increased proneness to heart disease. Such behaviour includes: competitiveness; striving for achievement; time urgency; difficulty relaxing; impatience; and anger. It is possible to modify such behaviour.

Type B individuals do not exhibit the above characteristics. They can relax more easily and are slow to anger.

Stress-resistant people are those who view change as a challenge, and feel they have more control over events.

Coping mechanisms

Although the following mechanisms, used to cope with stress, are conscious, they relate to unconscious defence mechanisms too (given in parentheses):

- concentration only on the current task (denial)
- empathy (projection)
- logical analysis (rationalisation)
- objectivity (isolation)
- playfulness (regression)
- substitution of other thoughts for disturbing ones (reaction formation)
- suppression of inappropriate feelings (repression).

Learned helplessness

Seligman found that dogs given unavoidable electric shocks suffered a number of phenomena which he considered were similar to depression, such as reduced appetite, disturbed sleep and reduced sex drive. He called this learned helplessness.

The cognitive theory of depression is based largely on this concept. Further work has found that individuals who believe that they have no personal control over events are much more likely to develop learned helplessness, whereas those believing that nobody could have controlled the outcome are unlikely to do so. Thus a person's attribution of what is occurring influences the likelihood of developing major depression in cognitive terms.

Locus of control

Rotter differentiated those who see their lives as being under their own control (internal locus of control) from those who see their lives as being controlled externally (external locus of control).

BIBLIOGRAPHY

Al-Adawi, S., Burjorjee, R. & Al-Issa, I. 1997: Mu-Ghayeb: a culture-specific response to bereavement in Oman. *International Journal of Social Psychiatry* 43:144–151.

Al-Issa, I. 1977: Social and cultural aspects of hallucinations. *Psychological Bulletin* 84:570–587.

Allport, G.W. 1937: *Personality: A psychological interpretation*. New York: Holt, Rinehart & Winston.

Allport, G.W. 1955: *Becoming: Basic Considerations for a Psychology of Personality*. New Haven, CT: Yale University Press.

Allport, G.W. & Odbert H.S. 1936: Trait names: a psycholexical study. *Psychological Monographs* 47, no. 211.

Anderson, J.R. 1980: *Cognitive Psychology and its Implications*. San Francisco: Freeman.

Atkinson, R.C. & Shriffrin, R.M. 1968: Human memory: a proposed system and its control processes. In Spence, K.W. & Spence, J.T. (eds) *The Psychology of Learning and Memory*, vol. 2. New York: Academic Press.

Atkinson, R.L., Atkinson, R.C. & Smith, E.E 1990: *Introduction to Psychology*, 10th edn. San Diego: Harcourt Brace Jovanovich.

Ayres, T.J., Jonides, J., Reitman, J.S., Egan, J.C. & Howard, D.A. 1979: Differing suffix effects for the same physical suffix. *Journal of Experimental Psychology: Human Learning and Memory* 5:315–321.

Baddeley, A.D. 1966a: Short-term memory for word sequences as a function of acoustic, semantic and formal similarity. *Quarterly Journal of Experimental Psychology* 18:362–365.

Baddeley, A.D. 1966b: The influence of acoustic and semantic similarity on long-term memory for word sequences. *Quarterly Journal of Experimental Psychology* 18:302–309.

Baddeley, A.D. 1986: *Working Memory*. Oxford: Oxford University Press.

Baddeley, A.D. & Hitch, G. 1974: Working memory. In: Bower, G.A. (ed.) *The Psychology of Learning and Motivation*, vol. 8. New York: Academic Press.

Baddeley, A.D. & Lieberman, K. 1980: Spatial working memory. In: Nickerson, R.S. (ed.) *Attention and Performance*, vol. 8. Hillsdale, NJ: Erlbaum.

Bandura, A. & Walters, R.H. 1963: *Social Learning and Personality Development*. New York: Holt, Rinehart & Winston.

Block, J. 1961: *The Q-sort Method in Personality Assessment and Psychiatric Research*. Springfield, IL: Charles C. Thomas.

Block, J. 1971: *Lives Through Time*. Berkeley, CA: Bancroft Books.

Boran, M. & Viswanathan, R. 2000: Separating subculture from psychopathology. *Psychiatric Services* 51:678.

Bower, G.H. 1972: Mental imagery and associative learning. In: Gregg, L.W. (ed.) *Cognition in Learning and Memory*. New York: John Wiley.

Bower, G.H. & Springston, F. 1970: Pauses as recoding points in letter series. *Journal of Experimental Psychology* 83:421–430.

Bower, G.H., Clark, M., Winzenz, D. & Lesgold, A. 1969: Hierarchical retrieval schemes in recall of categorical word lists. *Journal of Verbal Learning and Verbal Behavior* 8:323–343.

Braine, M.D.S, Reiser, B.J. & Rumain, B. 1984: Some empirical justification for a theory of natural propositional logic. In *The Psychology of Learning and Motivation*, vol. 18. New York: Academic Press.

Byrne, R.M.J. & Johnson-Laird, P.N. 1989: Spatial reasoning. *Journal of Memory and Language* 28:564–575.

Cattell, R.B., Eber, H.W. & Tatsuoka, M.M. 1970: *Handbook for the Sixteen Personality Factor Questionnaire.* Champaign, IL: Institute for Personality and Ability Testing.

Conrad, R. 1964: Acoustic confusion in immediate memory. *British Journal of Psychology* 55:75–84.

Craik, F.I.M. & Watkins, M.J. 1973: The role of rehearsal in short-term memory. *Journal of Verbal Learning and Verbal Behavior* 12:599–607.

Crowder, R.G. 1971: The sound of vowels and consonants in immediate memory. *Journal of Verbal Learning and Verbal Behavior* 10:587–596.

Daneman, M. & Carpenter, P.A. 1980: Individual differences in working memory and reading. *Journal of Verbal Learning and Verbal Behavior* 19:450–466.

Deatherage, B.H. & Evans, T.R. 1969: Binaural masking: backward, forward and simultaneous effects. *Journal of the Acoustical Society of America* 46:362–371.

Endler, N.S. 1983: Interactionism: a personality model but not yet a theory. In Page, M.M. (ed.) *Nebraska Symposium on Motivation 1982: Personality – current theory and research.* Lincoln, NE: University of Nebraska Press.

Ericsson, K.A. & Kintsch, W. 1995: Long-term working memory. *Psychological Review* 102:211–245.

Estes, W.K. 1972: An associative basis for coding and organization in memory. In: Melton, A.W. & Martin, E. (eds) *Coding Processes in Human Memory.* Washington, DC: Winston.

Eysenck, H.J. 1944: Types of personality: a factorial study of 700 neurotic soldiers. *Journal of Mental Science* 90:851–961.

Eysenck, H.J. & Eysenck, S.B.G. 1991: *The Eysenck Personality Questionnaire-Revised.* Sevenoaks: Hodder & Stoughton.

Eysenck, M.W. 1982: *Attention and Arousal: Cognition and Performance.* New York: Springer.

Frase, L.T. 1975: Prose processing. In: Bower, G.H. (ed.) *The Psychology of Learning and Motivation*, vol. 9. New York: Academic Press.

Garety, P., Kuipers, E., Fowler, D. *et al.* 2001: A cognitive model of the positive symptoms of psychosis. *Psychological Medicine* 31:189–195.

Gillund, G. & Shiffrin, R.M. 1981: Free recall of complex pictures and abstract words. *Journal of Verbal Learning and Verbal Behavior* 20:575–592.

Glenberg, A.M., Smith, S.M. & Green, C. 1977: Type I rehearsal: maintenance and more. *Journal of Verbal Learning and Verbal Behavior* 16:339–352.

Glover, J.H. & McCue, P.A. 1977: Electrical aversion therapy with alcoholics: a comparative follow-up study. *British Journal of Psychiatry* 130:279–286.

Greenberg, D. & Brom, D. 2001: Nocturnal hallucinations in ultra-orthodox Jewish Israeli men. *Psychiatry* 64:81–90.

Groeger, J.A. 1997: *Memory and Remembering: Everyday Memory in Context.* Edinburgh: Longman.

Hansen, G.D. 1979: Enuresis control through fading, escape, and avoidance training. *Journal of Applied Behavioural Analysis* 12:303–307.

Hart, R.P. & O'Shanick, G.J. 1993: Forgetting rates for verbal, pictorial, and figural stimuli. *Journal of Clinical and Experimental Neuropsychology* 15:245–265.

Hirschberg, N. 1978: A correct treatment of traits. In London, H. (ed.) *Personality: A New Look at Metatheories.* New York: Macmillan.

Jacobsen, E. 1932: The electrophysiology of mental activities. *American Journal of Psychology* 44:677–694.

Johns, L.C., Nazroo, J.Y., Bebbington, P. & Kuipers, E. 2002: Occurrence of hallucinatory experiences in a community sample and ethnic variations. *British Journal of Psychiatry* 180:174–178.

Johnson-Laird, P.N. 1993: *Human and Machine Thinking*. Hillsdale, NJ: Erlbaum.

Kelly, G.A. 1955: *The Psychology of Personal Constructs*. New York: Norton.

Kyllonen, P.C. & Christal, R.E. 1990: Reasoning ability is (little more than) working-memory capacity. *Intelligence* 14:389–433.

Maslow, A.H. 1967: Self-actualization and beyond. In Bugental J.F.T (ed.) *Challenges of Humanistic Psychology*. New York: McGraw-Hill.

Maslow, A.H. 1970: *Motivation and Personality*, 2nd edn. Philadelphia: W.B. Saunders.

Mischel, W. 1983: Alterations in the pursuit of predictability and consistency of persons: stable data that yield unstable interpretations. *Journal of Personality* 51:578–604.

Morton, J. & Bekerian, D.A. 1986: Three ways of looking at memory. In Sharkey N.E. (ed.) *Advances in Cognitive Science* vol. 1. Chichester: Ellis Horwood.

Mu-Ghayeb 1997: A culture-specific response to bereavement in Oman. *International Journal of Social Psychiatry* 43:144–151.

Newell, A. & Rosenbloom, P.S. 1981: Mechanisms of skill acquisition and the law of practice. In Anderson, J.R. (ed.) *Cognitive Skills and their Acquisition*. Hillsdale, NJ: Erlbaum.

Ohaeri, J.U., Adelekan, M.F., Odejide, A.O. & Ikuesan, B.A. 1992: The pattern of isolated sleep paralysis among Nigerian nursing students. *Journal of the National Medical Association* 84:67–70.

Paulesu, E., Frith, C.D. & Frackowiak, R.S.J. 1993: The neural correlates of the verbal component of working memory. *Nature* 362:342–345.

Pezdek, K. & Chen, H.C. 1982: Developmental differences in the role of detail in picture recognition memory. *Journal of Experimental Child Psychology* 33:207–215.

Pfungst, O. 1907. *Das Pferd des Herrn von Osten (Der Kluge Hans). Ein Beitrag zur experimentellen Tier- und Menschen-Psychologie*. Leipzig: Johann Ambrosius Barth. [Translated into English by C.L. Rahn, with a prefatory note by J.R. Angell, as Pfungst, O. 1911: *Clever Hans (The Horse of Mr Von Osten): A Contribution to Experimental Animal and Human Psychology*. New York: Henry Holt.]

Plomp, R. 1964: Rate of decay of auditory sensation. *Journal of the Acoustical Society of America* 36:277–282.

Potter, M.C. 1976: Short-term conceptual memory for pictures. *Journal of Experimental Psychology: Human Learning and Memory* 2:509–522.

Preston, K.L., Umbricht, A., Wong, C.J. & Epstein, D.H. 2001: Shaping cocaine abstinence by successive approximation. *Journal of Consulting Clinical Psychology* 69:643–654.

Robertson, I.H., North, N.T. & Geggie, C. 1992: Spatiomotor cueing in unilateral left neglect: three case studies of its therapeutic effects. *Journal of Neurological and Neurosurgical Psychiatry* 55:799–805.

Ryle, G. 1949: *The Concept of Mind*. London: Hutchinson.

Sachs, J.D.S. 1967: Recognition memory for syntactic and semantic aspects of connected discourse. *Perception and Psychophysics* 2:437.

Schachtel, E.G. 1947: On memory and childhood amnesia. *Psychiatry* 10:1–26.

Schachter, S. & Singer, J.E. 1962: Cognitive, social and physiological determinants of emotional state. *Psychological Review* 69:379–399.

Schwab, M.E. 1977: A study of reported hallucinations in a southeastern county. *Mental Health and Society* 4:344–354.

Searleman, A. & Herrmann, D. 1994: *Memory from a Broader Perspective*. New York: McGraw-Hill.

Shallice, T. & Warrington, E.K. 1970: Independent functioning of verbal memory stores: a neuropsychological study. *Quarterly Journal of Experimental Psychology* 22:261–273.

Skinner, B.F. 1953: *Science and Human Behavior*. New York: Macmillan.

Skinner, B.F. 1969: *Contingencies of Reinforcement*. New York: Appleton–Century–Crofts.

Slamecka, N.J. 1960: Retroactive inhibition of connected discourse as a function of practice level. *Journal of Experimental Psychology* 59:104–108.

Smith, S.M., Brown, H.O., Thomas, J.E.P & Goodman, L.S. 1947: The lack of cerebral effects of D-tubocurarine. *Anesthesiology* 8:1–14.

Spear, P.D., Penrod, S.D. & Baker, T.B. 1988: *Psychology: Perspectives on Behaviour*. New York: John Wiley.

Spielberger, C.D. 1966: The effects of anxiety on complex learning and academic achievement. In Spielberger, C.D. (ed.) *Anxiety: Current Trends in Theory and Research*, vol. 1. London: Academic Press.

Thvedt, J.E., Zane, T. & Walls, R.T. 1984: Stimulus functions in response chaining. *American Journal of Mental Deficiency* 88:661–667.

Thorndike, E.L. 1911: *Animal Intelligence*. New York: Macmillan.

Tulving, E. 1972: Episodic and semantic memory. In: Tulving, E. & Donaldson, W. (eds) *The Organization of Memory*. New York: Academic Press.

Tulving, E. 1985: Memory and consciousness. *Canadian Psychology* 26:1–12.

Turvey, M.T. 1973: On peripheral and central processes in vision: inferences from an information-processing analysis of masking with patterned stimuli. *Psychological Review* 80:1–52.

Tyrer, P. & Ferguson, B. 2000: Classification of personality disorder. In: Tyrer, P. (ed.) *Personality Disorders: Diagnosis, Management and Course*. Oxford: Butterworth–Heinemann.

Tzeng, O.J.L. 1973: Positive recency effects in delayed free recall. *Journal of Verbal Learning and Verbal Behavior* 12:436–439.

Vaughan, K. & Tarrier, N. 1992: The use of image habituation training with post-traumatic stress disorders. *British Journal of Psychiatry* 161:658–664.

Watson, J.B. 1913: Psychology as the behaviorist views it. *Psychological Review* 20:158–177.

Wiggins, J.S. 1979: A psychological taxonomy of trait-descriptive terms: the interpersonal domain. *Journal of Personality and Social Psychology* 37:395–412.

Wolpe, J. 1958: *Psychotherapy by Reciprocal Inhibition*. Palo Alto: Stanford University Press.

2

Social psychology

ATTITUDES AND HOW THEY ARE AFFECTED

DEFINITION

The definition of an attitude has been given variously as: 'a mental and neural state of readiness, organized through experience, exerting a directive or dynamic influence upon the individual's response to all objects and situations with which it is related' (Allport); and 'an enduring organization of motivational, emotional, perceptual, and cognitive processes with respect to some aspect of the individual's world' (Krech & Crutchfield). They are mutually consistent and internally consistent.

COMPONENTS

Attitudes are based on beliefs, a tendency to behave in an observable way, and also have affective components which are the most resistant to change. A change in one of these three components leads to changes in the other two.

When predicting behaviour, situational variables must be taken into account. Otherwise measured attitudes are poor predictors of behaviour.

Measurement of attitude

Thurstone scale

This is a dichotomous scale indicating agreement/disagreement with presented and previously ranked statements. Disadvantages of this scale include:

- Different response patterns may result in the same mean score.
- The set-up is unwieldy.
- The ranking may be biased.

Likert scale

This is a five-point scale indicating level of agreement with presented statements. Its advantages include the fact that it has increased sensitivity compared with the dichotomous Thurstone scale; and that it is more easily administered. A disadvantage is that different response patterns may result in the same mean score.

Semantic differential scale

This is a bipolar visual analogue scale. Its advantages include:

- ease of use
- good test–retest reliability.

Its disadvantages include:

- possible occurrence of positional response bias
- no consistent meaning attributed to a midpoint mark.

Attitude change

A change in one of the three components of attitude leads to changes in the other two.

The origin of attitudes can be by means of the processes of learning: classical conditioning, operant conditioning, and observational learning. Superimposed on these are cognitive processes such as appraisal and modification in the light of new information.

Attitudes can be modified by either central pathways, entailing the consideration of new information, or by peripheral pathways involving the presentation of cues. Advertising uses both pathways.

The *balance theory* of Heider holds that each individual attempts to organize his or her attitudes, perceptions and beliefs so that they are in harmony or balance with each other.

Persuasive communication

The factors to consider are those concerned with the communicator, the recipient and the message being communicated.

Communicator

Characteristics of persuasive communicators include:

- attractiveness
- audience identification with the communicator
- credibility
- expertise
- genuine motivation
- being an opinion leader
- non-verbal communication
- views of reference groups.

Recipient

High self-esteem and intelligence of the recipient increase the likelihood that complex communications will be persuasive.

Message

Key aspects relating to the message and attitude change include:

- Message repetition can be a persuasive influence leading to attitude change.
- Explicit messages are more persuasive for the less intelligent and implicit messages for the more intelligent recipient.
- Interactive personal discussions are more persuasive than mass media communication.
- One-sided communications are more persuasive for those who are less intelligent and/or already favourably disposed to the message.
- Two-sided presentations are more effective with intelligent and neutral recipients.
- A low-anxiety recipient is more influenced by a high-fear message, and vice versa.

Cognitive consistency and dissonance

When cognitive dissonance occurs, the individual feels uncomfortable, may experience increased arousal, and is motivated to achieve cognitive consistency. This may occur by changing one or more of the cognitions involved in the dissonant relationship, changing the behaviour which is inconsistent with the cognition(s), or adding new cognitions which are consonant with pre-existing ones. Cognitive consistency can also be achieved, when attitude and behaviour are inconsistent (attitude discrepant behaviour), by altering attitude.

SELF-PSYCHOLOGY

Self-concept

This is a set of attitudes that the individual holds about himself/herself. It does not necessarily correspond to reality. Self-theory was developed by Rogers.

Self-esteem

This is one's own evaluation of self-worth and feeling accepted by others. Those lacking in self-esteem have feelings of worthlessness, alienation and lack of acceptance by others, whereas those with high self-esteem are more socially active, less prejudiced, more risk-taking and warmer in social relationships. It is learned and so may change with experience.

Self-esteem may be raised by identification with a group. For example, deaf individuals who identify with other deaf people have a higher self-esteem, on average, than those who do not. In turn, the raised self-esteem can help to compensate for problems relating to *personal identity*.

Self-image

Self-image is a set of beliefs held about oneself, based on achievements and social interactions, which influences personal meaning and behaviour.

Self-perception theory

An individual infers what his or her attitude must be by observation of his or her own behaviour, in a similar way to how other people infer the individual's behaviour.

Self-perception theory provides a better explanation than cognitive dissonance theory for behaviour that lies within the general range of behaviours acceptable to the individual.

INTERPERSONAL ISSUES

Interpersonal attraction

In general, humans seek the company of others to whom they are attracted. In difficult situations this may allow assessment by social comparisons, taking note of the opinions of others (*social comparison theory* – Festinger). An alternative theory is that seeking the company of others leads to *arousal reduction* (Epley).

Theories of interpersonal attraction include:

- *Reinforcement theory*. Reciprocal reinforcement of the attractions occurs with rewards in both directions (Newcomb). Conversely, punishments diminish the probability of interpersonal attraction.
- *Social exchange theory*. People prefer relationships that appear to offer an optimum cost–benefit ratio (Homans).
- *Equity theory*. The preferred relationships are those in which each feels that the cost–benefit ratio of the relationship for each person is approximately equal (Hatfield & Traupmann).
- *Proxemics*. This relates to interpersonal space/body buffer zone.

Factors predisposing to interpersonal attraction include proximity, familiarity, similarity of interests and values, exposure, perceived competence, reciprocal liking and self-disclosure, and physical attractiveness. Similarity is more important than complementarity, although the latter increases in importance with time.

According to the *matching hypothesis*, pairing occurs such that individuals seek others who have a similar level of physical attractiveness.

Attribution theory

Attribution theory (Heider) deals with the rules people use to infer the causes of observed behaviour.

- *Internal or dispositional attribution*. This is the inference that the person is primarily responsible for his or her behaviour.
- *External or situational attribution*. This is the inference that the cause of a behaviour is external to the person.
- *Primary (fundamental) attribution error*. When inferring the cause of other people's behaviour there is a bias towards dispositional rather than situational attribution.

Theory of mind

In primate research, theory of mind refers to the ability of primates to *mentalize* their fellows. In humans, the ('cold') theory of mind refers to the ability of most normal people to comprehend the thought processes of others (such as their attention, feelings, beliefs, false beliefs and knowledge).

Research into children tends to suggest that, at the age of 3 years, normal human children do not acknowledge false belief as they have difficulty in differentiating belief from world. Formulating a theory of mind appears not to be inevitable, but relies on cognitive changes that occur at around the age of 4 years. It has been suggested that a failure to acquire a theory of mind is associated with disorders such as autism.

A 'hot' theory of mind entails constructing the meaningful intentions and evaluative attitudes (such as fear, surprise and pleasure) of others. The latter can be inferred from facial expressions.

LEADERSHIP, SOCIAL INFLUENCE, POWER AND OBEDIENCE

Leadership

Lewin *et al.* distinguished between the following leadership styles:

- *autocratic*: abandon task in leader's absence; good for situations of urgency
- *democratic*: yields greater productivity unless a highly original product is required
- *laissez-faire*: appropriate for creative, open-ended, person-oriented tasks.

Social facilitation

This refers to the way in which tasks and responses are facilitated when carried out in the presence of others (Allport; Harlow). For it to occur, the others do not necessarily have to be engaging in the same task. Facilitation also occurs if the others are simply observing; this has been called the *audience effect* (Dashiell).

Social power

French and Raven described the following five types of social power:

- *authority*: power derived from role
- *reward*: power derived from ability to allocate resources
- *coercive*: power to punish
- *referent*: charismatic and liked by others
- *expert*: power derives from skill, knowledge and experience.

Conformity

Two types of conformity to the actions and opinions of others have been identified (Duetsch & Gerard):

- *Informational social influence.* An individual conforms to the consensual opinion and behaviour of the group both publicly and in his/her own thoughts (evident with ambiguous stimuli).
- *Normative social influence.* An individual publicly conforms to the consensual opinion and behaviour of the group but has a different view in his/her own mind. The individual conforms to the group under social pressure to avoid *social rejection*.

Self-reliant, intelligent, expressive, socially effective individuals are least vulnerable to group pressure.

Obedience to authority

Milgram found that most subjects would obey an experimenter's orders to administer what they believed to be increasingly powerful electrical shocks to others, right up to the maximum voltage available. Factors that increased the rate of obedience included:

- the presence of the experimenter
- the belief that the prior agreement was binding on the subject
- increasing distance from the apparently suffering person.

INTER-GROUP BEHAVIOUR

Stereotypes

A stereotype is an over-generalized inference about a person or group of people in which they are all assumed to possess particular traits or characteristics.

The use of *schemata* (working stereotypes) is inevitable until further experience either refines or discredits them. Many stereotypes are benign but may be resistant to change. However, stereotypes can become self-perpetuating and self-fulfilling.

Stigma

Definition and example
Stigma is an attribute of an individual which marks him or her as being unacceptable, inferior or dangerous and 'spoils' identity. For example, psychiatric disorders are highly stigmatized in societies which value rationality.

- *Enacted stigma* is the experience of discrimination of an individual who bears a stigma.
- *Felt stigma* is the fear of discrimination of an individual who bears a stigma.

Development
Stigma first appears during the psychoanalytic stage of latency, approximately corresponding with Erikson's stage of industry versus inferiority, during which children develop a strong awareness of the ways in which they are similar to and differ from others.

Prejudice

Definition and example
Prejudice is a preconceived set of beliefs held about others who are 'pre-judged' on this basis; the negative meaning of the term is the one usually used. It is not amenable to discussion and is resistant to change. Prejudiced individuals may behave in ways that create stereotyped behaviour which sustains their prejudice.

For example, racism or racial prejudice is the dogmatic belief that one 'race' is superior to another one, and that there exist identifiable 'racial characteristics' that influence cognition, achievement, behaviour, etc.

Discrimination is the enactment of prejudice. (In the case of racism, the enactment is also termed 'racialism'.)

Some causes of prejudice

- The person holding the prejudice is rigid in his or her beliefs and does not tolerate weaknesses in others. This is sometimes referred to by sociologists as an authoritarian personality.
- There is scapegoating of the victims of the prejudice.
- There is stereotyping of the victims of the prejudice.

Reducing prejudice

Cook showed that the following conditions need to be satisfied in order to reduce prejudice:

- equal status
- the potential for personal acquaintance
- exposure to non-stereotypical individuals
- a social environment favouring equality
- co-operative effort.

THE PHENOMENON OF AGGRESSION

Aggression is behaviour intended to harm others. We may distinguish between:

- *hostile aggression*: the sole intent is to inflict injury
- *instrumental aggression*: the intention is to obtain reward or inflict suffering.

Explanations of aggression

Psychoanalytic
Aggression is viewed as a basic instinct.

Social learning theory
Aggression is viewed as a learned response. It is learned through observation, imitation and operant conditioning.

Operant conditioning
Positive reinforcers can include victim suffering and material gains. The consequences of aggression play an important role in shaping future behaviour.

Ethology
Some ethologists believe that humans and animals are innately aggressive. Animal studies show that certain behaviours inhibit aggression:

- maintaining a distance
- evoking a social response incompatible with aggression
- familiarity.

Frustration–aggression hypothesis

This proposes that preventing a person reaching his or her goal induces an aggressive drive resulting in behaviour intended to harm the one causing the frustration. Expressing this aggression reduces the aggressive drive.

Arousal

Emotional arousal can increase aggression.

Influence of television

It is known that children imitate observed aggression. Some studies suggest a relationship between exposure to violence on television and aggressive behaviour in boys, but not in girls. It may be that this is because aggressive behaviour in boys, but not in girls, is socially reinforced.

Ways in which filmed violence may increase aggressive behaviour include:

- teaching aggressive styles of conduct
- increasing arousal
- desensitizing people to violence
- reducing restraint on aggressive behaviour
- distorting views about conflict resolution.

THE CONCEPT OF ALTRUISM

The concept of the type of interpersonal co-operation known as altruism refers to an act (or acts) which are motivated by the desire to benefit another person (or persons) rather than oneself.

Altruism may be considered to be a higher defence mechanism is which the individual deals with emotional conflict or internal or external stressors by dedication to meeting the needs of others. Unlike the self-sacrifice sometimes characteristic of reaction formation, the individual receives gratification either vicariously or from the response of others (DSM-IV-TR).

Altruism can also be explained on the basis of social exchange theory (see above).

It has been suggested that failure to exclude an ulterior motive means that, strictly speaking, altruism cannot be said to have occurred under these circumstances. Indeed, there may be personal rewards of a private nature that occur as a result of acting in this way; for instance, a person may feel virtuous.

BIBLIOGRAPHY

Atkinson, R.L., Atkinson, R.C. & Smith, E.E. 1990: *Introduction to Psychology*, 10th edn. San Diego: Harcourt Brace Jovanovich.

Bandura, A. & Walters, R.H. 1963: *Social Learning and Personality Development*. New York: Holt, Rinehart & Winston.

Spear, P.D., Penrod, S.D. & Baker, T.B. 1988: *Psychology: Perspectives on Behaviour*. New York: John Wiley.

3

Neuropsychological processes

MEMORY

SENSORY MEMORY

The anatomical correlate of iconic memory is probably visual association cortex, while that of echoic memory is probably auditory association cortex.

SHORT–TERM MEMORY

The anatomical correlate of auditory verbal short-term memory is the left (dominant) parietal lobe, while that of visual verbal short-term memory is possibly the left temporo-occipital area. That of non-verbal short-term memory is possibly the right (non-dominant) temporal lobe.

EXPLICIT MEMORY

This requires a deliberate act of recollection and can be reported verbally. It includes declarative memory and episodic memory, which are probably stored separately, since it is possible to lose one type of memory while retaining the other. *Declarative* memory involves knowledge of facts whereas *episodic* memory involves memory of autobiographical events. Explicit memory involves the medial temporal lobes, particularly the hippocampus, entorhinal cortex, subiculum and parahippocampal cortex. Damage to these structures results in an inability to store new memory; they have been termed *bottleneck structures*. Memory probably passes from medial temporal lobe structures after a few weeks/months to longer-term storage in the cortex.

The amygdala may be involved in the emotional charging of information. It may also be a bottleneck structure.

IMPLICIT MEMORY

This is recalled automatically without effort and is learned slowly through repetition. It is not readily amenable to verbal reporting. It comprises *procedural* knowledge, that is, knowing *how*. Its storage requires functioning of the cerebellum, amygdala and specific sensory and motor systems used in the learned task. For example, the basal ganglia are involved in learning motor skills. Classical and operant learning involve implicit memory.

LANGUAGE

Cerebal dominance

Cerebral dominance for language is as follows:

- In 99% of right-handers the left cerebral hemisphere is dominant.
- In 60% of left-handers the left cerebral hemisphere is dominant.

In early life there is plasticity for cerebral dominance for language before the functions are established.

Speech and language areas

Broca's area

This is the motor speech area, occupying the opercular and triangular zones of the inferior frontal gyrus (BA 44 and 45). It is involved in coordinating the organs of speech to produce coherent sounds. In lesions confined to this area in the dominant hemisphere, speech comprehension is intact and muscles involved in speech production work normally, but production of speech is affected.

Wernicke's area

This is the sensory speech and language area, occupying the posterior part of the auditory association cortex (BA 42 and 22) of the superior temporal gyrus. It is usually larger in the left hemisphere. It is involved in making sense of speech and language.

Angular gyrus

This part of the brain (BA 39) has abundant connections with the somatosensory, visual, and auditory association cortices. Lesions here produce inability to read or write.

Pathways

- *Understanding spoken language (hearing)*: spoken word →auditory cortex → auditory association cortex → Wernicke's area → hear and comprehend speech.
- *Understanding written language (reading)*: written word → visual cortex → visual association cortex → angular gyrus → Wernicke's area → read and comprehend.
- *Speaking*: thought/cognition → Wernicke's area → Broca's area → motor speech areas → speech.
- *Writing*: thought/cognition → Wernicke's area → angular gyrus → motor areas → write.

Dysphasias

Damage to brain areas involved with speech and language results in dysphasia; the type of dysphasia is determined by the areas of the brain involved.

Receptive dysphasia

Damage to Wernicke's area disrupts the ability to comprehend language, either written or spoken. In addition to loss of comprehension, the person also is unaware that his or her dysphasic speech is difficult for others to follow. Speech is normal in rhythm and intonation (because Broca's area is intact), but the content is abnormal. Words used have lost their meaning; empty words (e.g. 'thing', 'it') and paraphrasias are used liberally. Thus damage to Wernicke's area results in a *fluent receptive dysphasia*.

Expressive dysphasia

Damage to Broca's area results in loss of rhythm, intonation and grammatical aspects of speech. Comprehension is normal (because Wernicke's area is intact) and the person is aware that his or her speech is difficult for others to follow, resulting in distress and frustration. Speech is slow and hesitant, often lacking connecting words. Speech sounds agrammatical and articulation may be crude, probably because of the close proximity of Broca's area to motor areas. Thus damage to Broca's area results in *dysfluent expressive dysphasia*.

Conduction dysphasia

Damage to the arcuate fasciculus results in a conduction dysphasia in which the person cannot repeat what is said by another. Comprehension and verbal fluency remain intact.

Global dysphasia

This results from global left hemispheric dysfunction, and shows a combination of all the above.

PERCEPTION

Perception relates to the means by which the brain makes representations of the external environment.

Agnosia is the inability to interpret and recognize the significance of sensory information, which does not result from impairment of the sensory pathways, mental deterioration, disorders of consciousness and attention, or, in the case of an object, a lack of familiarity with the object.

Visual perception

- Shape, colour and spatial orientation are recognized in the occipital lobes. A lesion at this level results in *pseudoagnosia*.
- Visuospatial elements are drawn together into complete percepts (objects seen as a whole) in the right parietal lobe. Meaning is not yet attributed to the objects. A lesion at this level results in *apperceptive agnosia*.
- The meaning of objects is then accessed from the left parietal lobe (which itself accesses meaning from semantic memory) and processed in parieto-occipital areas. A lesion at this level results in *associative agnosia*.

OTHER AGNOSIAS

- *Prosopagnosia* is an inability to recognize faces. In advanced Alzheimer's disease a person may misidentify his or her own mirrored reflection – the mirror sign.

- In *agnosia for colours*, the person is unable correctly to name colours, although colour sense is still present.
- In *simultanagnosia*, the person is unable to recognize the overall meaning of a picture whereas its individual details are understood.
- *Agraphognosia* or *agraphaesthesia* is tested by asking the person to identify, with closed eyes, numbers or letters traced on his or her palm; this disorder is present if the person is unable to identify such writing.
- In *anosognosia*, there is a lack of awareness of disease, particularly of hemiplegia (most often following a right parietal lesion).
- *Autotopagnosia* is the inability to name, recognize or point on command to parts of the body.
- In *astereognosia*, objects cannot be recognized by palpation.
- In *finger agnosia*, the person is unable to recognize individual fingers.
- *Topographical disorientation* can be tested using a locomotor map-reading task in which the person is asked to trace out a given route by foot.
- In *hemisomatognosis* or *hemidepersonalization*, the person feels that a limb (which in fact is present) is missing.

Apraxias

Apraxia is an inability to perform purposive volitional acts, which does not result from paresis, incoordination, sensory loss or involuntary movements.

- *Constructional apraxia* is closely associated with *visuospatial agnosia*. There is an inability to construct a figure.
- In *dressing apraxia*, there is an inability to dress.
- In *ideomotor apraxia*, there is an inability to carry out progressively more difficult tasks.
- In *ideational apraxia*, there is an inability to carry out a coordinated sequence of actions.

FRONTAL LOBE FUNCTIONS

PREFRONTAL CORTEX

This is probably involved in the following functions:

- problem-solving
- perceptual judgement
- memory
- programming and planning of sequences of behaviour
- verbal regulation
- level of response emission
- adaptability of response pattern
- tertiary level of motor control.

FRONTAL EYE FIELDS

These are involved in voluntary eye movements.

MOTOR AND PREMOTOR CORTEX

These are probably involved in the following functions:

- primary and secondary levels of motor control
- design fluency.

BROCA'S AREA

This is involved in expressive speech.

ORBITAL CORTEX

This is probably involved in the following functions:

- personality
- social behaviour.

FRONTAL LOBE LESIONS

These may cause:

- personality change – disinhibition, reduced social and ethical control, sexual indiscretions, poor judgement, elevated mood, lack of concern for the feelings of other people, and irritability
- perseveration
- utilization behaviour
- pallilalia
- impairment of attention, concentration and initiative
- aspontaneity, slowed psychomotor activity
- motor Jacksonian fits
- urinary incontinence
- contralateral spastic paresis
- aphasia
- primary motor aphasia
- motor agraphia
- anosmia
- ipsilateral optic atrophy.

GERSTMANN'S SYNDROME

This is caused by dominant parietal lobe lesions and consists of:

- dyscalculia
- agraphia
- finger agnosia
- right–disorientation.

BIBLIOGRAPHY

Smith, E.E., Nolen-Hoeksema, S., Frederickson, B.L. *et al.* (eds) 2003: *Atkinson and Hilgard's Introduction to Psychology (with Lecture Notes and InfoTrac)*, 14th edn. Florence, KT: Wadsworth.

4

Human growth and development

CONCEPTUALIZING DEVELOPMENT

BASIC CONCEPTS

Human development involves an interaction between nature and nurture.

Stage theories propose that development occurs in a progressive sequence reflecting maturation. Examples include: Piaget's cognitive stages; Freud's psychosexual stages; and Kohlberg's stage theory. Maturation refers to the orderly changes in behaviour that result from biological development and whose timing and form are relatively independent of external experience. Maturational tasks are influenced by: biological growth; the drive for independence; and other people's general expectations.

GENE–ENVIRONMENT INTERACTIONS

These interactions determine all psychological characteristics, such as intelligence. Genetic factors determine the inherited potential, while environmental factors determine the degree to which this potential is fulfilled.

With respect to intelligence, while it is generally agreed that there is a genetic component to intelligence, there is disagreement about the degree of environmental influence on it. The correlation coefficient for intelligence quotient (IQ) between monozygotic twins is 0.86 compared with 0.60 for dizygotic twins. Using factor analysis, Spearman identified a general factor, g, and a specific factor, s, of intelligence; it was proposed that the level of g was associated with how intelligent the individual was.

HISTORICAL MODELS

The historical developmental models of Freud and Erikson are described in Chapter 33. Social-learning models lay emphasis on the way in which environmental influences affect subsequent behaviour. The most influential theory of cognitive development is that of Piaget (see below).

ATTACHMENT AND BONDING

Attachment theory

This comes from the work of Bowlby. *Attachment* refers to the tendency of infants to remain close to certain people (attachment figures) with whom they share strong positive emotional ties. Monotropic attachment is when the attachment is to one individual, usually the mother. Polytropic attachment is less common. Attachment usually takes place from infant to mother. In contrast, neonatal–maternal *bonding* takes place in the opposite direction. Both processes can start immediately after birth.

Some behaviourists consider attachment to result from the mother acting as a conditioned reinforcer. This theory was challenged by Harlow who, using cuddly and wire artificial surrogate mothers and infant rhesus monkeys, found that attachment is a function of the requirement to be in contact with a soft object (contact comfort), which provides security. Other studies have found that warm or rocking artificial surrogate mothers are preferred to colder or still surrogates, respectively.

Lorenz considered attachment to result from imprinting whereby geese, during a critical period soon after hatching, persistently follow the first nearby moving object encountered. There is no evidence that imprinting occurs in primates.

Bowlby considered infant attachment to take place in the context of a warm, intimate and continuous relationship with the care-giver in which there is reciprocal satisfaction. The attachment process takes an average of 6 months to become fully established. Bonding is stronger if there is tactile contact as soon as possible after birth. The mother's attachment behaviour is reinforced by infant smiling, movement and crying. *Attachment behaviours* are the signs of distress shown by the child when separated from his or her attachment figure, and include:

- crying when the care-giver (usually mother) leaves the room
- attempting to follow her
- clinging hard when distressed
- hugging her
- being more playful and talkative in her company
- using her as a secure base from which exploration can take place.

These start to occur at about the age of 6 months and decrease visibly by 3 years. Prior to this age separation is tolerated without distress.

Attachment abnormalities

INSECURE ATTACHMENT

There is chronic clinginess and ambivalence towards the mother. Clinically this may be relevant, as it may be a precursor to:

- childhood emotional disorders (including school refusal)
- disorders (such as agoraphobia) starting in adolescence and adulthood.

AVOIDANT ATTACHMENT

A distance is kept from the mother, who may sometimes be ignored. Clinically, avoidant attachment caused by rejection by the mother may be relevant as it may be a precursor to:

- poor social functioning in later life (including aggression).

SEPARATION ANXIETY

This is the fear an infant shows of being separated from his or her care-giver. Holding a comfort object or transitional object (Winnicott) may help with separation.

The rate of disappearance of separation anxiety varies with the child's:

- experiences of previous separations (real or threatened)
- handling by mother
- perception of whether mother will die or depart
- temperament.

ACUTE SEPARATION REACTION

After starting to form attachments, at around 6 months to 2 years of age, separation from mother leads to the following reaction (in the order given):

1 protest – including crying and searching behaviour
2 despair – apathy and misery with an apparent belief that mother may not return
3 detachment – emotionally distant from (and indifferent to) mother.

Stranger anxiety

This refers to a fear of strangers shown by infants usually between the ages of 8 months and 1 year. It is not necessarily part of attachment behaviour and may occur independently of separation anxiety.

Maternal deprivation

Following a failure to form adequate attachments, for example because of prolonged maternal separation or rejecting parents, the effects of maternal deprivation may include:

- developmental language delay
- indiscriminate affection-seeking
- shallow relationships
- enuresis
- aggression
- lack of empathy
- social disinhibition
- attention-seeking and overactivity in school
- poor growth – deprivation dwarfism.

FAMILY RELATIONSHIPS AND PARENTING PRACTICE

Child-rearing practice

Table 4.1 (after Baumrind, 1967) shows how the parents of three groups of children have been found to score on the four dimensions of:

- control – by the parents of the child's activities and behaviour
- maturity demands – of the child to act at his/her ability level
- communication – clarity of parent–child communication
- nurturance – parental nurturance towards the child.

Table 4.1 *The way in which parents of three groups of children score on the dimensions of control, maturity demands, communication and nurturance*

	Control	Maturity demands	Communication	Nurturance
Group I	↑↑	↑↑	↑↑	↑↑
Group II	↑	→	↓	↓↓
Group III	↓↓	↓↓	↓↓	↑

The three groups of children were:

- Group I: the most mature and competent
- Group II: moderately self-controlled and self-reliant but somewhat withdrawn and distrustful
- Group III: the most immature and dependent.

Family structure

In the UK and US, around 25% of children are not living with both biological parents by the age of 16 years. If orthodox families are defined as those nuclear families in which there are two parents with a small number of children, then non-orthodox family structures may or may not be relevant so far as healthy psychosocial development of the child is concerned (see Table 4.2).

Table 4.2 *Consequences of family structure*

Single parent
↑ Behavioural and emotional problems (particularly if no other support)

Extended family
Not harmful

Two lesbian parents
Not harmful

Large family size
↑ Behavioural and educational problems
↓ Intelligence

ORDINAL POSITION IN FAMILY

The oldest child has a slight advantage in intellectual development. This also applies to an only child. Twins show delayed language development.

Distorted family function

Dysfunctional families may manifest:

- discord
- overprotection of children by parents
- rejection of the child(ren)
- enmeshment, whereby parents may be over-involved in their children's feelings and lives
- disengagement, whereby parents may be under-involved in their children's feelings and lives
- triangulation, in which exclusive alliances are formed within the family; e.g. father/daughter (although this may for example be helpful in preventing father from leaving home)
- communication difficulties owing to ambiguous or incongruous communications
- myths created within the family.

Marital conflicts may cause the parents to need to have a child with a problem who can act as a scapegoat (until he or she leaves home).

Impact of bereavement

The death of a parent leads to initial bereavement reactions, which may include prolonged sadness, crying and irritability during childhood. In addition:

- Young children may exhibit functional enuresis and/or temper tantrums.
- Older children (especially girls) my have sleep disturbance and/or clear-cut depressive reactions.
- School performance may be impaired (possibly temporarily).

Impact of parental divorce

Parental divorce is associated with an increased rate of disturbance in children (greater than following parental bereavement). Protective factors include:

- amicable arrangements for access following the divorce
- good parental relationship with the child
- good relationships of the child with other siblings
- the child's temperament.

Impact of intrafamilial abuse

Sexual abuse

Child sexual abuse is 'the involvement of dependent, developmentally immature children and adolescents in sexual activities that they do not fully comprehend, are unable to give informed consent to, and that violate the social taboos of family roles' (Schechter & Roberge, 1976).

The findings of a study by Cosentino *et al.* (1995) suggest that sexual abuse in preadolescent girls is associated with sexual behaviour problems. This study compared a group of sexually abused girls, aged 6–12 years, with two demographically comparable control groups, girls from a child psychiatry outpatient department, and girls from a general paediatric clinic. Compared to both control groups, sexually abused girls manifested more sexual behaviour problems: masturbating openly and excessively, exposing their genitals, indiscriminately hugging and kissing strange adults and children, and attempting to insert objects into their genitals. Abuse by fathers or stepfathers involving intercourse was associated with particularly marked sexual behaviour disturbances. There was a subgroup of sexually abused girls who tended to force sexual activities on siblings and peers.

All of these girls had experienced prolonged sexual abuse (>2 years) involving physical force which was perpetrated by a parent.

Recognized sequelae of sexual abuse include:

- anxiety states and anxiety-related symptoms (e.g. sleep disturbance, nightmares, psychosomatic complaints, and hypervigilance), re-enactments of the victimization, and post-traumatic stress disorder (Goodwin, 1985; Green, 1985)
- depression (Gaensbauer & Sands, 1979; Sgroi, 1982)
- dissociation (Kluft, 1985; Putnam, 1985)
- paranoid reactions and mistrust (Green, 1978; Herman, 1981)
- excessive reliance on primitive defence mechanisms (e.g. denial, projection, dissociation, and splitting) (Green, 1978)
- borderline personality disorder (especially in females) (Herman *et al.*, 1989)
- inability to control sexual impulses (precocious sexual play with high sexual arousal) (Cosentino *et al.*, 1995; Friedrich & Reams, 1987; Yates, 1982)
- weakened gender identity (a tendency to reject their maleness or femaleness) (Aiosa-Karpas *et al.*, 1991)
- increased incidence of homosexuality (Finkelhor, 1984)
- increased incidence of molesting children (the cycle of abuse may continue – there is a high incidence of sexual abuse in the backgrounds of male and female child molesters) (McCarty, 1986; Seghorn *et al.*, 1987)
- drug and alcohol abuse (Herman, 1981)
- eating disorders (Oppenheimer *et al.*, 1985).

Physical abuse/non-accidental injury

Non-accidental injury can be defined as occurring 'when an adult inflicts a physical injury on a child more severe than that which is culturally acceptable' (Graham, 1991). Recognized sequelae of physical abuse (which overlap with those of sexual abuse) include:

- anxiety states and anxiety-related symptoms (e.g. sleep disturbance, nightmares, psychosomatic complaints, and hypervigilance), re-enactments of the victimization, and post-traumatic stress disorder (Goodwin, 1985; Green, 1985)
- depression (Gaensbauer & Sands, 1979; Sgroi, 1982)
- dissociation (Kluft, 1985; Putnam, 1985)
- paranoid reactions and mistrust (Green, 1978; Herman, 1981)
- excessive reliance on primitive defence mechanisms (e.g. denial, projection, dissociation, and splitting) (Green, 1978)
- borderline personality disorder (especially in females) (Herman *et al.*, 1989)
- aggressive and destructive behaviour at home and school (George & Main, 1979; Green, 1978)
- cognitive and developmental impairment (Elmer & Gregg, 1967; Oates, 1986)
- delayed language development (Martin, 1972)
- neurological impairment (Green *et al.*, 1981)
- abusive behaviour with their own children (the cycle of abuse may continue) (Steele, 1983).

TEMPERAMENT

Temperament can be defined as early-appearing, biologically rooted, basic personality dimensions (Zuckerman, 1991).

Individual temperamental differences

In the New York Longitudinal Study, Thomas and Chess (Chess & Thomas, 1984; Thomas & Chess, 1977) identified the following nine categories of temperament describing how children behave in daily life situations:

Activity level
Rhythmicity (regularity of biological functions)
Approach or withdrawal to new situations
Adaptability in new or altered situations
Sensory threshold of responsiveness to stimuli
Intensity of reaction
Quality of mood
Distractibility
Attention span/persistence.

In terms of the impact of individual temperamental differences on parent–child relationships, the above nine categories have been found to cluster as follows:

- *Easy child* pattern – characterized by regularity, positive approach responses to new stimuli, high adaptability to change, and expressions of mood that are mild/moderate in intensity and predominantly positive.
- *Difficult child* pattern – characterized by irregularity in biological functions, negative withdrawal responses to new situations, non-adaptability or slow adaptability to change, and intense, frequently negative expressions of mood.
- *Slow-to-warm-up child* – characterized by a combination of negative responses of mild intensity to new situations with slow adaptability after repeated contact.

Origins, typologies and stability of temperament

Medieval personality theorists relied on a temperament typology based on the balance of the humours, but twentieth and twenty-first century theorists have put the strongest emphasis on environmental causation models. Acceptance of the concept of biologically rooted personality dimensions is a fairly recent stage in the history of scientific psychology and psychiatry (Bates *et al.*, 1995). The following are important points to note:

- Temperament is a theoretical construct – it is more useful to think of specific dimensions of temperament, e.g. activity level, sociability, negative emotionality, or distractibility.
  Temperament concepts can be defined at the following three levels (Bates, 1989):
  - as patterns of surface behaviour
  - as a pattern of nervous system responses
  - as having inborn genetic roots.
- There is an increased understanding of the biological processes involved in temperament. Since concepts of temperament typically focus on individual differences in emotion, attention and activity (Bates, 1989), the neural basis of temperament can be thought of as emerging from the brain systems supporting emotion, attention and activity:
  - limbic structures
  - association cortex
  - motor cortical areas.

- Environmental influences affect how the biological bases of temperament are expressed. For example, Gunnar (1994) showed how sensitive, responsive care-givers could enhance otherwise highly inhibited preschoolers' likelihood of approaching novel stimuli.
- Concepts of temperament can be useful in helping people solve problems. When the processes of linkage between temperament and the evolution of character and personality are understood better, this should assist prevention and treatment.

The stability of temperament and its relationship to the evolution of character and personality have been demonstrated in a number of studies. Characteristics of temperament in infants and preschool-age children predict adjustment in middle childhood and adolescence. For example, Caspi and Silva (1995) showed how temperamental qualities at the of age 3 years predict personality traits in young adulthood. In an unselected sample of over 800 subjects, the following five temperament groups were identified when the children were aged 3 years:

Under-controlled
Inhibited
Confident
Reserved
Well-adjusted.

These groups were reassessed at the age of 18 years. The findings in the young adults were as follows:

- Under-controlled children scored high on measures of impulsivity, danger seeking, aggression, and interpersonal alienation (as young adults).
- Inhibited children scored low on measures of impulsivity, danger seeking, aggression, and social potency.
- Confident children scored high on impulsivity.
- Reserved children scored low on social potency.
- Well-adjusted children continued to exhibit normative behaviours.

PIAGET'S MODEL OF COGNITIVE DEVELOPMENT

Piaget believed that infantile and childhood intellectual development involve interactions with the outside world (for example through play). These lead to certain outcomes:

- New cognitive structures (*schemes*) are constructed incorporating new information.
- In the presence of suitable existing schemes:

  - *assimilation:* new information is incorporated into appropriate existing schemes
  - *accommodation:* there is modification of existing scheme(s).

Piaget identified the following four stages of cognitive development:

Sensorimotor
Preoperational
Concrete operational
Formal operational.

SENSORIMOTOR STAGE

This is the first stage and occurs from birth to 2 years of age. *Circular reactions* are repeated voluntary motor activities, for example shaking a toy, occurring from around 2 months. They are classified as follows:

- *primary circular reactions* – from 2 to 5 months (approximately), when they have no apparent purpose
- *secondary circular reactions* – from 5 to 9 months (approximately), when experimentation and purposeful behaviour are gradually manifested
- *tertiary circular reactions* – from 1 year to 18 months (approximately), which include the creation of original behaviour patterns and the purposeful quest for novel experiences.

During this stage the infant comes to distinguish himself/herself from the environment. Thought processes exhibit *egocentrism*, in which the infant believes that everything happens in relation to him/her. Until around 6 months the infant believes that an object hidden from view no longer exists. *Object permanence* is fully developed after around the age of 18 months.

PREOPERATIONAL STAGE

This is the second stage and occurs from age 2 to 7 years. During this stage the child learns to use the symbols of language. Certain thought processes are exhibited during this stage.

- *Animism*. Life, thoughts and feelings are attributed to all objects, including inanimate ones.
- *Artificialism*. Natural events are attributed to the actions of people.
- *Authoritarian morality*. It is believed that wrongdoing, including breaking the rules of a game, should be punished according to the degree of the damage caused, whether accidental or not, rather than according to motive; negative events are perceived as punishments.
- *Creationism*. A teleological approach is taken in which, for example, stars and the moon exist in order to provide light at night.
- *Egocentrism*. This is as in the sensorimotor stage.
- *Finalism*. All things have a purpose.
- *Precausal reasoning*. This is based on internal schemes rather than the results of observation; so that, for example, the same volume of liquid poured from one container to another with a different height and diameter may be considered to have changed volume.
- *Syncretism*. Everything is believed to be connected with everything else.

CONCRETE OPERATIONAL STAGE

This is the third stage and occurs from age 7 to around 12–14 years of age. During this stage the child demonstrates logical thought processes and more subjective moral judgements.

An understanding of the *laws of conservation* of, initially, number and volume, and then weight, is normally achieved. Reversibility and some aspects of classification are mastered.

FORMAL OPERATIONAL STAGE

This is the final stage and occurs from the age of around 12–14 years of age onwards. It is characterized by the achievement of being able to think in the abstract, including the ability systematically to test hypotheses.

LANGUAGE DEVELOPMENT

Language can be defined as the sum of the skills required to communicate verbally (Graham, 1991).

Normal childhood development

- In the first hours postnatally, the baby learns to distinguish his/her mother's voice.
- By 3 to 4 months babbling occurs.
- By 8 months repetitive babbling occurs.
- By 12 months the baby has usually acquired the equivalent designations 'mama', 'dada' (no matter what language the parent speaks) and one additional word.
- By 18 months a 20- to 50-word vocabulary is expressed in single-word utterances.
- By 2 years, two- or three-word utterances can be strung together with some understanding of grammar. These are telegraphic utterances omitting grammatical morphemes (small units of meaning signifying the plural, for example).
- At an average age of 3 years, the child can usually understand a request containing three parts.

Environmental influences and communicative competence

- *Bilingual home.* Being brought up in a home in which two languages are spoken is not a disadvantage unless there is another cause of slowed language development.
- *Family size.* Larger family size is associated with slower speech development.
- *Pregnancy.* Intrauterine growth retardation is associated with slower language development. Prolonged second-stage labour is associated with slower language development.
- *Sex.* Early language development in girls is slightly greater than in boys.
- *Social class.* Being middle-class is associated with relatively faster language development.
- *Stimulation.* Although the capacity for language and grammar may be built-in, speech and language are not achieved in the usual manner if children are deaf or are not spoken to.
- *Twins.* Being a twin is associated with slower speech development.

MORAL DEVELOPMENT

Kohlberg's stage theory

Kohlberg presented a set of stories, each containing a moral dilemma, to various individuals of various ages and backgrounds. Questions were posed concerning the moral dilemmas. On the basis of the reasons given for the answers, Kohlberg formulated a theory of moral development consisting of six developmental stages of moral judgement categorized into three levels (I to III).

Preconventional morality (Level I)
This is the level at which the moral judgements of children up to the age of 7 years mainly lie.

- *Stage 1: Punishment orientation.* Rules are obeyed in order to avoid punishment.
- *Stage 2: Reward orientation.* Rules are conformed to in order to be rewarded.

Conventional morality (Level II)
This is the level at which most moral judgements of children lie by the age of 13 years.

- *Stage 3: Good-boy/good-girl orientation.* Rules are conformed to in order to avoid the disapproval of others.

- *Stage 4: Authority orientation*. Laws and social rules are upheld in order to avoid the censure of authorities and because of guilt about not doing one's duty.

Postconventional morality (Level III)
This level, which may never be reached even in adulthood, requires individuals to have achieved the later stages of Piaget's formal operational stage.

- *Stage 5: Social contract orientation*. Actions are guided by principles generally agreed to be essential for public welfare. These principles are upheld in order to maintain the respect of peers and self-respect.
- *Stage 6: Ethical principle orientation*. Actions are guided by principles chosen oneself, usually emphasizing dignity, equality and justice. These principles are upheld in order to avoid self-condemnation.

Relationship to the development of social perspective taking

Social perspective taking is the ability to take the perspective of others. It is a skill that may be seen at the following levels:

- *perceptual role-taking*: the ability to take into account how a perceptual array appears to another person when that person's perspective differs from one's own
- *cognitive role-taking*: the ability to take into account the thoughts of another person when they differ from one's own
- *affective role-taking*: the ability to take into account the feelings of another person when they differ from one's own.

   In addition to being necessary to being able to emphathize with others, social perspective taking was considered by Kohlberg as being necessary to develop higher stages of moral reasoning.

DEVELOPMENT OF FEARS IN CHILDHOOD AND ADOLESCENCE

Fear is an unpleasant emotional state (a feeling of apprehension, tension or uneasiness) caused by a realistic current or impending danger that is recognized at a conscious level. It differs from anxiety in that in the latter the cause is vague or not as understandable. However, fear and anxiety are terms that are often used interchangeably.

Development of fear with age

The types of fear that develop in childhood and adolescence differ with age (Marks, 1987):

- At 6 months, fear of novel stimuli begins (such as fear of strangers), reaching a peak at 18 months to 2 years.
- At 6–8 months, fear of heights begins, and becomes worse when walking starts.
- At 3–5 years, common fears are those of animals, the dark, and 'monsters'.
- At 6–11 years, fear of shameful social situations (such as ridicule) begins.
- In adolescence, fear of death, failure, social gatherings (such as parties) and thermonuclear war may be particularly evident.

Possible aetiological and maintenance mechanisms

Unconscious conflict
Sigmund Freud (1926/1959) suggested that psychological anxiety is a signal phenomenon and that neurotic anxiety starts as the remembrance of realistic anxiety/fear related to a real danger. Each stage of life was considered to have age-appropriate determinants of anxiety/fear, including, with increasing age:

Fear of birth
Fear of separation from the mother
Fear of castration
Fear of the superego – fear of its anger or punishment
Fear of the superego – fear of its loss of love
Fear of the superego – fear of death.

Learned response
Fear/anxiety may become associated with particular situations by means of learning.

Lack of control
Fear/anxiety may occur when an individual feels helpless in a situation beyond his or her control.

SEXUAL DEVELOPMENT

Sex determination

Sex determination is primarily as a result of the sex chromosomes (XX female and XY male). Gonad formation is first indicated in the embryo by the appearance of an area of thickened epithelium on the medial aspect of the mesonephric ridge during week five. Various factors affect subsequent differentiation of the genital organs into male ones (epididymis, ductus (vas) deferens, ejaculatory ducts, penis, and scrotum) or female ones (fallopian tubes, uterus, clitoris, and vagina) during ontogeny.

Y chromosome
In mammals, testis determination is under the control of the testis-determining factor borne by the Y chromosome. SRY, a gene cloned from the sex-determining region of the human Y chromosome, has been equated with the testis-determining factor in humans.

Degree of ripeness of the ovum at fertilization
Over-ripeness of the ovum at fertilization is associated with a reduced number of primordial germ cells. This in turns leads to a masculinizing effect on genetic females.

Endocrine actions
Androgens and oestrogens can modify the process of sexual differentiation, while in twin pregnancy with fetuses of opposite sex and anastomosed placental circulations, the genetically male fetus may have a masculinizing effect on the genetically female fetus. A genetically female fetus may also be masculinized (and be born with either ambiguous or male genitalia) by fetal androgen from another source (e.g. in congenital adrenal (suprarenal) hyperplasia). Similarly, a genetically male fetus with a Y chromosome and testes may develop female genitalia in the absence of fetal androgen (e.g. in enzyme deficiency) or if androgen receptors are defective (e.g. in testicular feminization).

Changes at puberty

Puberty consists of a series of physical and physiological changes which convert a child into an adult who is capable of sexual reproduction.

Physical changes
These include:

- growth spurt
- change in body proportions
- development of sexual organs
- development of secondary sexual characteristics.

Tanner described a standardized system for recording breast, pubic hair and genital maturation:

- *Onset in girls.* In 95%, onset occurs at between 9 and 13 years. The first sign is:
  - breast formation – in 80%
  - pubic hair growth – in 20%
  - In Western countries menarche occurs at a mean age of 13.5 years.
- *Onset in boys.* In 95%, onset occurs at between 9.5 and 13.5 years. The first sign is usually testicular and scrotal enlargement, followed by growth of the penis and pubic hair. On average, the first ejaculation occurs at around 13 years.

Physiological changes
A raising of the threshold for gonadohypothalamic negative feedback precedes the onset of puberty. An increase in suprarenal androgen release (adrenarche) usually begins between the ages of 6 and 8 years; these hormones lead to the growth of sexual hair and skeletal maturation.

GENDER IDENTITY

This is an individual's perception and self-awareness with respect to gender. It is usually established by the age of 3 or 4 years and usually remains firmly established thereafter.

GENDER/SEX TYPING

This is the process by which individuals acquire a sense of gender and gender-related cultural traits appropriate to the society and age into which they are born. It usually begins at an early age with male and female infants being treated differently, for example with respect to the choice of their clothing.

GENDER ROLE

This is the type of behaviour that an individual engages in that identifies him or her as being male or female, for example with respect to the type of clothes worn and the use of cosmetics.

SEXUAL BEHAVIOUR

Sexual drive
This is the need to achieve sexual pleasure through genital stimulation. It exists from birth to middle childhood and increases again during adolescence as a result of increased androgen secretion.

Childhood sexuality
This may manifest itself in normal children as:

- sex play in infancy
- erections in boys
- vaginal lubrication in girls
- masturbation – which may involve orgasm
- exploratory encounters with other children.

Masturbation
This is the predominant mode of sexual expression for most adolescent males and probably fewer adolescent females.

Sexual orientation

This is the erotic attraction that an individual feels. Its shaping is a developmental process associated with certain patterns of childhood experience and activity. Superimposed on this, there are arguments for and against the theory that human sexual orientation is biologically determined.

The term 'homosexuality' is associated with the following behavioural dimensions:

- sexual fantasy
- sexual activity
- sense of identity
- social role.

The first of these is the most important dimension in assessing homosexual orientation. If present, it does not necessarily imply sexual activity with others, as in individuals who are homosexual in orientation and celibate.

It should be noted that there is no non-human mammalian species in which predominant or exclusive homosexuality occurs in the way it does in humans.

MODERN ARGUMENTS IN FAVOUR OF BIOLOGICAL DETERMINISM OF SEXUAL ORIENTATION

Endocrine
On the basis of rat and human experiments, Dorner (1986, 1989) has hypothesized that 21-hydroxylase deficiency represents a genetic predisposition to female homosexuality in heterozygous forms (homozygous forms lead to congenital adrenal hyperplasia) while in males 21-hydroxylase deficiency and/or prenatal stress leads to an overall inhibition in the effects of androgen on brain differentiation and to male homosexuality. Among their experiments on humans, Dorner and colleagues studied the effects of oestrogen infusion on LH secretion and reported that, in contrast to heterosexual men, homosexual men manifest a positive oestrogen feedback effect on LH secretion, which was said to provide evidence that homosexual men have a predominantly female-differentiated brain. Furthermore, as a result of ACTH provocation tests on the suprarenal (adrenal) glands, Dorner reported that female homosexuals display significantly increased ratios of 17a-hydroxyprogesterone/cortisol and androstenedione/cortisol after ACTH stimulation compared with female heterosexual control subjects.

Neuroanatomical
LeVay (1991) reported histological differences in the interstitial nuclei of the anterior hypothalamus between homosexual and heterosexual men, suggesting that sexual orientation may be mediated by

the central nervous system. The anterior hypothalamus of the brain is known to participate in the regulation of male-typical sexual behaviour. The volumes of four cell groups in this region (interstitial nuclei of the anterior hypothalamus (INAH) 1, 2, 3, and 4) were measured in postmortem tissue from three subject groups: women, men who were presumed to be heterosexual, and homosexual men. No differences were found between the groups in the volumes of INAH 1, 2, or 4. As had been previously reported, INAH 3 was found to be more than twice as large in the heterosexual men as in the women. It was also, however, more than twice as large in the heterosexual men as in the homosexual men. This finding indicates that INAH is dimorphic with sexual orientation, at least in men.

A second neuroanatomical difference was reported by Allen and Gorski (1992). On the basis of the examination of 90 postmortem brains, it was found that the midsagittal plane of the anterior commissure in homosexual men was 18% larger than in heterosexual women and 34% larger than in heterosexual men. This finding of a difference in a structure not known to be related to reproductive functions supports the hypothesis that factors operating early in development differentiate sexually dimorphic structures and functions of the brain in a global fashion.

Genetic

Bailey and Pillard (1991) found evidence of heritability of homosexuality in a study of monozygotic (MZ) and dizygotic (DZ) twins. Homosexual male probands with MZ cotwins, DZ cotwins, or adoptive brothers were recruited. Of the relatives whose sexual orientation could be rated, 52% (29/56) of MZ cotwins, 22% (12/54) of DZ cotwins, and 11% (6/57) of adoptive brothers were homosexual. Childhood gender non-conformity did not appear to be an indicator of genetic loading for homosexuality.

In a second genetic study, Hamer *et al.* (1993) reported a linkage between DNA markers on the X chromosome and male sexual orientation. Pedigree and linkage analyses on 114 families of homosexual men were carried out. Increased rates of homosexual orientation were found in the maternal uncles and male cousins of these subjects, but not in their fathers or paternal relatives, suggesting the possibility of sex-linked transmission in a portion of the population. DNA linkage analysis of a selected group of 40 families in which there were two gay brothers and no indication of non-maternal transmission revealed a correlation between homosexual orientation and the inheritance of polymorphic markers on the X chromosome in approximately 64 percent of the sib-pairs tested. The linkage to markers on Xq28 had a multipoint lod score of 4.0.

ARGUMENTS AGAINST BIOLOGICAL DETERMINISM OF SEXUAL ORIENTATION

Endocrine

Gooren *et al.* (1990) have argued that oestrogen feedback cannot be used to assess the status of brain differentiation in primates in the same way as it can in the rat. For example, sexual differentiation of the control of LH secretion occurs in the mouse, hamster, and guinea pig but not in primates. Among their experiments on humans, Gooren and colleagues studied directly the control of LH secretion in homosexuals and transsexuals compared with heterosexuals. Following oestrogen exposure, the response of LH to LHRH was not positive in male homosexuals, transsexuals and heterosexuals; it was positive in female homosexuals, transsexuals (prior to treatment) and heterosexuals; moreover, a positive LH response to oestrogen infusion in homosexual men was not found.

Neuroanatomical

LeVay (1991) pointed out that his sample contained no homosexual women and that AIDS patients may constitute an unrepresentative sample of homosexual men. Moreover, some presumed heterosexual men had relatively small INAH 3 nuclei (within the homosexual range) and some presumed homosexual men had relatively large INAH 3 nuclei (within the heterosexual range). The effect might have resulted from AIDS (although there was no effect of AIDS on the volume of the three other INAH nuclei examined and the size difference in INAH 3 was present when the homosexual men were compared with heterosexual AIDS patients).

Genetic

King (1993) has pointed out that the result of Hamer *et al.* (1993) is preliminary. Their evidence is based on a small, highly selected group of homosexual men. The result is purely statistical. The gene is hypothetical and has not been cloned, and the linkage has been observed in only one series of families.

ADOLESCENCE

Adolescence is a time of transitions, representing a developmental phase between middle childhood/latency and adulthood, but its boundaries are difficult to demarcate clearly. In his model of cognitive development, Piaget viewed adolescence as the final, formal operational stage of development; the adolescent has a greater capacity to focus on himself/herself. The pubertal changes of adolescence have been considered above.

Conflict with parents and authority

Theories of why conflict between adolescents and parents and other authority figures often occurs include:

- cognitive developmental models
- Erikson's stages of psychosocial development
- ethological and sociobiological models
- social learning theory
- equity theory
- separation–individuation.

Cognitive developmental models
The adolescent has newly acquired powers of hypothetical reasoning which enable him or her to consider and articulate alternatives to the status quo.

Erikson's stages of psychosocial development
In his fifth psychosocial developmental stage (identity versus role confusion), Erikson considered adolescence to be a time of identity formation during which the individual pursues personal autonomy. This pursuit is associated with the potential for conflict with parents and other authority figures.

Ethological and sociobiological models
Conflict at the time of pubertal changes is considered to be adaptive, prompting the individual to spend more time with his or her peers. It forms part of the status realignments of entry into adulthood.

Social learning theory
Adolescents may be considered to have experienced vicarious exposure to problem-solving occurring via conflict. Witnessing their parents giving in to their children's conflicting demands may be considered to provide intermittent reinforcement to the children.

Equity theory
According to equity theory the preferred relationships, particularly those of an intimate nature, between any two given people are those in which each feels that the cost–benefit ratio of the relationship for each person is approximately equal. It has been argued that the amount of emotional investment of both the adolescent and the parent(s) in their relationship means they both wish to preserve it. As the adolescent pursues autonomy, this can lead to occasional conflicts, but these are usually not fervent enough to destroy the relationship.

Separation–individuation
It has been argued that adolescence can be considered to represent a second separation–individuation phase, in which continued biological, motor and social development now allow the adolescent to move away from a dependent relationship with the parent(s) to take his or her own place in society. However, social and psychological pulls towards dependency mean that the separation–individuation may entail ambivalence and conflict.

Affective stability and 'turmoil'

Successive developments in the psychological understanding of affective stability and 'turmoil'in adolescence have been provided by Anna Freud, Erikson, and Offer and Offer.

Anna Freud
A rapid oscillation between excess and asceticism during adolescence was described by Anna Freud (1936/1946). Affective instability and behaviour swings were considered to be caused by:

- the drives stimulated by sexual maturity
- pubertal endocrine changes
- instability of the newly stressed defences of the ego against these drives.

Erikson
Erikson (1959) characterized adolescence as manifesting 'adolescent turmoil' and a maladaptive, temporary state of 'identity diffusion', which he implied all adolescents passed through.

Offer and Offer
Offer and Offer (1975) showed that, in general, adolescence is a time of less turmoil and upheaval than previously thought. They studied a cohort of American males who had been aged 14 years in 1962. Sixty-one of these adolescents were studied intensively and followed-up into adulthood. They came mainly from intact families, and there were no serious drug problems or major delinquent activity. Seventy-four per cent went to college during the first year after high-school graduation. They showed no significant difference in basic values from that of their parents.

Normal and abnormal adolescent development

Offer and Offer

Offer and Offer (1975) identified the following three adolescent developmental routes (the percentages given are those of the sample of adolescents they studied; the remaining 21% could not be classified easily, but were closer to the first two categories than to the third one):

- *Continuous growth* (23%). Eriksonian intimacy was achieved and shame and guilt could be displayed. Major separation, death and severe illness were less frequent. Their parents encouraged independence.
- *Surgent growth* (35%). The adolescents in this group were 'late-bloomers'. They were more likely than the first group to have frequent depressive and anxious moments. Although often successful, they were less introspective and not as action-oriented as the first group. There were more areas of disagreement with their parents.
- *Tumultous growth* (21%). Recurrent self-doubt and conflict with their families occurred in this group. Their backgrounds were less stable than in the first two groups. The arts, humanities and social sciences were preferred to professional and business careers.

Block and Haan

Block and Haan (1971) used factor analysis to isolate the following groups among a cohort of 84 male adolescents studied longitudinally to adulthood:

- ego-resilient adolescents
- belated adjustors – similar to the surgent group of Offer and Offer
- vulnerable over-controllers
- anomic extroverts – less inner life and relatively uncertain values
- unsettled under-controllers – given to impulsivity.

A similar cohort of 86 females was divided into:

- female prototype
- cognitive type – individuals tend to be intellectualized in the way problems are negotiated
- hyperfeminine repressors – similar to hysterical personality disorder
- dominating narcissists
- vulnerable under-controllers
- lonely independents.

ADAPTATIONS IN ADULT LIFE

Pairing

Even in Western countries, it appears that there are a number of constraints which govern the choice of mate in much the same way as elders or parents do in arranged marriages.

Homogamous mate selection

Pairing tends to occur within the same socioeconomic, religious and cultural group (Eshelman, 1985).

Reinforcement theory
People are attracted to those who reinforce the attraction with rewards. This process is a reciprocal one with rewards also passing in the opposite direction and further reinforcing the interpersonal attraction (Newcomb, 1956).

Social exchange theory
People have a preference for relationships that appear to offer an optimum cost–benefit ratio: maximum benefits such as love with minimum costs such as time spent with each other (Homans, 1961).

Equity theory
As mentioned above, this is a modification of the social exchange theory in which the preferred relationships, particularly of an intimate nature, between two people are those in which each feels that the cost–benefit ratio of the relationship for each person is approximately equal (Hatfield & Traupmann, 1981).

Matching hypothesis
According to this hypothesis, heterosexual pairing tends to occur in such a way that, although ideally a person would prefer to pair with the most attractive people (Huston, 1973), in practice individuals seek to pair with others who have a similar level of physical attractiveness rather than the most attractive (Berscheid & Walster, 1974). This is felt by the individual to lead to a greater probability of acceptance by the other person, a lower probability of rejection, and a lower probability of losing the partner to another person in the future.

Cultural differences
People in Asian and African countries tend to value home-keeping potential and a desire for home and children in mate selection, while people in Western countries tend to value love, character and emotional maturity. Chastity is rated very highly in some countries (such as India and China) and cultures (such as orthodox/traditional Jewish, Christian and Islamic communities) and very low in others (such as Australia, New Zealand, North America, South America, and Scandinavia – excluding their traditional observant religious groups) (Buss et al., 1990).

Cross-cultural constancies
Across cultures, men prefer mates who are physically attractive, while women prefer mates who show ambition, industriousness and other signs of earning power potential (Buss et al., 1990).

Parenting

Parenting is a complex, dyadic process that is influenced by a range of factors, including:

- cultural beliefs of the parent about child-rearing (Maccoby & Martin, 1983)
- genetic – temperamental characteristics of the parent (i.e. genetic factors influencing the provision of parenting) (Perusse et al., 1994)
- genetic – temperamental characteristics of the child (i.e. genetic factors influencing the elicitation of parenting) (Bell, 1968).

Furthermore, reporting bias is likely, with parents stressing the similarity with which they treat their children, and children emphasizing the differences in parental treatment that they perceive (Plomin et al., 1994).

Abusive parenting is a strong predictor of later psychopathology. On the other hand, parental warmth and support buffers children against externalizing and antisocial behaviour (Hetherington & Clingempeel, 1992) and is positively associated with a child's self-esteem (Bell & Bell, 1983).

Grief, mourning and bereavement

Definitions

- *Grief* describes those psychological and emotional processes, expressed both internally and externally, that accompany bereavement.
- *Mourning* describes those culture-bound social and cognitive processes through which one must pass in order that grief be resolved, allowing one to return to more normal functioning. The word is often used, less strictly, as being synonymous with grief.
- *Bereavement* is a term that can apply to any loss event, from the loss of a relative by death, to unemployment, divorce or loss of a pet. It refers to being in the state of mourning.

SYMPTOMATOLOGY OF NORMAL GRIEF

- There is initial shock and disbelief – 'a feeling of numbness'.
- Increasing awareness of the loss is associated with painful emotions of sadness and anger. The anger may be denied.
- There may be irritability
- Somatic distress may include sleep disturbance, early morning waking, tearfulness, loss of appetite, weight loss, loss of libido, and anhedonia.
- Identification phenomena may arise: the mannerisms and characteristics of the deceased are taken on.

In 1944, Lindemann read to the centenary meeting of the American Psychiatric Association the results of his study of 101 bereaved individuals, many of whom had lost loved ones in the tragic Coconut Grove nightclub fire in Boston, MA. He identified the following five points as being pathognomonic of acute grief:

- somatic distress
- preoccupation with the image of the deceased
- guilt
- hostile reactions
- loss of patterns of conduct.

Note that grief is not seen in babies if a parent/care-giver dies prior to the development of attachment behaviour.

BEREAVEMENT

Parkes described the following five stages of bereavement:

- alarm
- numbness
- pining for the deceased – illusions or hallucinations of the deceased may occur
- depression
- recovery and reorganization.

MORBID GRIEF REACTIONS

Lindemann described the following morbid grief reactions:

- delay of reaction
- distorted reactions.

Distorted reactions were subclassified into:

- overactivity without a sense of loss
- the acquisition of symptoms belonging to the last illness of the deceased
- a recognized medical disease
- alteration in relationship to friends and relatives
- furious hostility against specific persons
- loss of affectivity
- a lasting loss of patterns of social interaction
- activities attaining a colouring detrimental to social and economic existence
- agitated depression.

DIFFERENTIATING BETWEEN BEREAVEMENT AND A DEPRESSIVE EPISODE

The diagnosis of Major Depressive Disorder in DSM-IV-TR is generally not given unless the symptoms are still present 2 months after the loss. However, the presence of certain symptoms that are not characteristic of a normal grief reaction may be helpful in differentiating bereavement from a Major Depressive Episode:

- guilt about things other than actions taken or not taken by the survivor at the time of the death
- thoughts of death other than the survivor feeling that he or she would be better off dead or should have died with the deceased person
- morbid preoccupation with worthlessness
- marked psychomotor retardation
- prolonged and marked functional impairment
- hallucinatory experiences other than thinking that he or she hears the voice of, or transiently sees the image of, the deceased person.

Freud (1917/1957) differentiated between normal grief and the depressive response by the presence of shame and guilt in the latter. Yearning for the lost object was considered to be part of the normal response to loss. It was overcome gradually as the mental representation was decathected.

NORMAL AGEING

Physical aspects

Health
In general, most elderly people in Western countries enjoy good health, in spite of the changes that occur in body systems with increasing age.

Cerebral changes
Blessed et al. (1968) found no histological evidence of dementia in the brains of 28 non-demented individuals. Evidence of cerebral atrophy was absent or slight in the majority, and

brain mass and ventricular size did not differ significantly from those of younger adults (Tomlinson *et al.*, 1968).

Social aspects

Stereotyping
Old age is generally a stigmatized period. For instance, people are complimented for looking younger than their chronological age.

Empty–nest syndrome
Prior to the onset of old age, parents usually witness their children leaving home, particularly in Western countries. The difficulties some parents encounter on being left on their own have been described as the empty-nest syndrome.

Ego integrity versus despair

This is Erikson's eighth and final stage of psychosocial development, occurring in old age.

Ego integrity
Successful resolution of the psychosocial crisis of this age leads to an integrated view of one's life, its meaning, its achievements (both for the self and others, including future generations), and the ways in which difficulties were coped with. There is an acceptance of one's mortality, a feeling that one's life has been lived in a satisfactory way, and a readiness to face death.

Despair
The alternative is despair, both on reflection of how life has been lived and the way in which others have been treated, and also on looking to the future and the sense of transience that is felt on facing the end of life. Rather than having a sense of contentment and completion, there is despair at the prospect of death.

Cognitive aspects

Prior to the late 1960s, it was generally believed that the normal ageing brain degenerates and that this is accompanied by intellectual deterioration. By the 1970s this view had been challenged on the basis of new research. Thus Schaie (1974) wrote:

> The presumed universal decline in adult intelligence is at best a methodological artifact and at worst a popular misunderstanding of the relation between individual development and socio-cultural change ... the major finding ... in the area of intellectual functioning is the demolishing of [the belief in] serious intellectual decrement in the aged.

Although the elderly do not generally perform as well as younger subjects on cognitive tasks dependent on processing speed, old age is not necessarily associated with a large decline in intellectual ability (Durkin, 1995). Reasons for this include:

* Different abilities contribute to intellectual behaviour, so that a reduction in one (e.g. processing speed) may be compensated for by an increase in another (such as experience-based judgement).

- Cross-sectional comparisons of different age groups may confound age differences with cohort effects.
- Changes in performance with age may be offset by practice.
- Crystallized intelligence (the ability to store and manipulate learned information) increases through adulthood and often remains high into old age.

DEATH AND DYING

Definitions

- *Timely death*. This refers to the situation in which the expected life expectancy is approximately equal to the actual length of time lived.
- *Untimely death*. This refers to the situation in which the actual length of time lived is significantly less than the expected life expectancy, as a result of one of the following:
  - premature death at a young age
  - sudden unexpected death
  - violent/accidental death.
- *Unintended death*. This refers to the situation in which death is unintended, usually occurring as a result of pathological processes or trauma.
- *Intended death*. This refers to the situation in which death is intended by the deceased, who played a part in his or her suicide.
- *Subintended death*. This refers to the situation in which the deceased may have manifested an unconscious desire to bring about his or her death, for example by facilitating the onset of death through psychoactive substance abuse.

Impending death

If it is believed that one's death is near, an individual may pass through the following five stages that are similar to those recognized as occurring in the terminally ill (Kübler-Ross, 1969):

- *Shock and denial*. The diagnosis may be disbelieved and another opinion sought. This first stage may never be passed.
- *Anger*. The person may be angry and wonder why this has happened to him/her.
- *Bargaining*. The person may, for example, try to negotiate with God.
- *Depression*. The symptomatology of a depressive episode is manifested.
- *Acceptance*. The person may finally come to terms with his or her mortality and understand the inevitability of death.

BIBLIOGRAPHY

Aiosa-Karpas, C.J., Karpas, R., Pelcovitz, D. *et al.* 1991: Gender identification and sex role attribution in sexually abused adolescent females. *Journal of the American Academy of Child and Adolescent Psychiatry* 30:266–271.
Allen LS, Gorski RA 1992: Sexual orientation and the size of the anterior commisure in the human brain. *Proceedings of the National Academy of Sciences* 85:7199–7202.

Bailey, J.M. & Pillard, R.C. 1991: A genetic study of male sexual orientation. *Archives of General Psychiatry* 48:1089–1096.

Bates, J.E. 1989: Concepts and measures of temperament. In Kohnstamm, G.A., Bates, J.E. & Rothbart, M.K. (eds) *Temperament in Childhood*. New York: John Wiley.

Bates, J.E., Wachs, T.D. & Van den Bos, G.R. 1995: Trends in research on temperament. *Psychiatric Services* 46:661–663.

Baumrind, D. 1967: Child care practices anteceding three patterns of pre-school behavior. *Genetic Psychology Monographs* 75:43–88.

Bell, D.C. & Bell, L.G. 1983: Parental validation and support in the development of adolescent daughters. In Grotevant, H.D. (ed.) *Adolescent Development in the Family*. San Francisco: Jossey Bass.

Bell, R.Q. 1968: A reinterpretation of the direction of effects in studies of socialization. *Psychological Review* 75:81–95.

Berscheid, E. & Walster, E. 1974: Physical attractiveness. In Berkowitz, L. (ed.) *Advances in Experimental Social Psychology*. New York: Academic Press.

Blessed, G., Tomlinson, B.E. & Roth, M. 1968: The association between quantitative measures of dementia and of senile change in the cerebral grey matter of elderly subjects. *British Journal of Psychiatry* 114:797–811.

Block, J. & Haan, N. 1971: *Lives Through Time*. Berkeley, CA: Bancroft Books.

Buss, D.M. *et al*. 1990: International preferences in selecting mates: a study of 37 cultures. *Journal of Cross-Cultural Psychology* 21:5–47.

Caspi, A. & Silva, P.A. 1995: Temperamental qualities at age three predict personality traits in young adulthood: longitudinal evidence from a birth cohort. *Child Development* 66:486–498.

Chess, S. & Thomas, A. 1984: *Origins and Evolution of Behavior Disorders: From Infancy to Early Adult Life*. New York: Brunner/Mazel.

Cosentino, C.E., Meyer-Bahlburg, H.F.I., Nat, D.R. *et al*. 1995: Sexual behavior problems and psychopathology symptoms in sexually abused girls. *Journal of the American Academy of Child and Adolescent Psychiatry* 34:1033–1042.

Dorner, G. 1986: Hormone-dependent brain development and preventative medicine. *Monographs in Neural Sciences* 12:17–27.

Dorner, G. 1989: Hormone-dependent brain development and neuroendocrine prophylaxis. *Experimental and Clinical Endocrinology* 94:4–22.

Durkin, K. 1995: *Developmental Social Psychology*. Cambridge, MA: Blackwell.

Elmer, E. & Gregg, C.S. 1967: Developmental characteristics of abused children. *Pediatrics* 40:596–602.

Erikson, E. 1959: *Growth and Crises of the Healthy Personality*. New York: International Universities Press.

Eshelman, J.R. 1985: One should marry a person of the same religion, race, ethnicity, and social class. In Feldman, H. & Feldman, M. (eds) *Current Controversies in Marriage and the Family*. Newbury Park, CA: Sage.

Finkelhor, D. 1984: *Child Sexual Abuse: New Theory and Research*. New York: Free Press.

Freud, A. 1936/1946: *The Ego and the Mechanisms of Defence* (trans. Baines, C). New York: International Universities Press.

Freud, S. 1917/1957: Mourning and melancholia. In *Standard Edition of the Complete Psychological Works of Sigmund Freud*, vol 14 (trans./ed. Strachey, J.). London: Hogarth.

Freud, S. 1926/1959: Inhibitions, symptoms and anxiety. In *Standard Edition of the Complete Psychological Works of Sigmund Freud*, vol. 20 (trans./ed. Strachey, J.). London: Hogarth.

Friedrich, W. & Reams, R. 1987: Course of psychological symptoms in sexually abused young children. *Psychotherapy* 24:160–171.

Gaensbauer, T. & Sands, K. 1979: Regulation of emotional expression in infants from two contrasting environments. *Journal of the American Academy of Child Psychiatry* 21:167–171.

George, C. & Main, M. 1979: Social interactions and young abused children: approach, avoidance, and aggression. *Child Development* 50:306–319.

Goodwin, J. 1985: Post-traumatic symptoms in incest victims. In Eth, S. & Pynoos, R.S. (eds) *Post-Traumatic Stress Disorder in Children*. Washington, DC: American Psychiatric Press.

Gooren, L., Fliers, E. & Courtney, K. 1990: Biological determinants of sexual orientation. *Annual Review of Sex Research* 1:175–196.

Gowers, S.G. (ed.) 2001: *Adolescent Psychiatry in Clinical Practice*. London: Arnold.

Graham, P. 1991: *Child Psychiatry: A Developmental Approach*, 2nd edn. Oxford: Oxford University Press.

Green, A.H. 1978: Psychiatric treatment of abused children. *Journal of the American Academy of Child Psychiatry* 17:356–371.

Green, A.H. 1985: Children traumatized by physical abuse. In Eth, S. & Pynoos, R.S. (eds) *Post-Traumatic Stress Disorder in Children*. Washington, DC: American Psychiatric Press.

Green, A.H., Voeller, K., Gaines, R. *et al.* 1981: Neurological impairment in battered children. *Child Abuse and Neglect* 5:129–134.

Gunnar, M.R. 1994: Psychoendocrine studies of temperament and stress in early childhood: expanding current models. In Bates, J.E. & Wachs, T.D. (eds) *Temperament: Individual Differences at the Interface of Biology and Behavior*. Washington, DC: American Psychological Association.

Hamer, D.H., Hu, S., Magnuson, V.L., Hu, N. & Pattatucci, A.M. 1993: A linkage between DNA markers on the X chromosome and male sexual orientation. *Science* 261:321–327.

Hatfield, E. & Traupmann, J. 1981: Intimate relationships: a perspective from equity theory. In Duck, S. & Gilmour, R. (eds) *Personal Relationships*, vol. 1. New York: Academic Press.

Herman, J. 1981: *Father–Daughter Incest*. Cambridge, MA: Harvard University Press.

Herman, J., Perry, J.C. & van der Kolk, B. 1989: Childhood trauma in borderline personality disorder. *American Journal of Psychiatry* 146:490–495.

Hetherington, E.M. & Clingempeel, W.G. 1992: Coping with marital transitions: a family systems perspective. *Monographs of the Society of Research into Child Development* 57 (serial no. 227).

Homans, G.C. 1961: *Social Behavior: Its Elementary Forms*. New York: Harcourt Brace.

Huston, T.L. 1973: Ambiguity of acceptance, social desirability and dating choice. *Journal of Experimental Social Psychology* 9:32.

King, M-C 1993: Human genetics: sexual orientation and the X [news and views]. *Nature* 364:288–289.

Kluft, R. 1985: *Childhood Antecedents of Multiple Personality*. Washington, DC: American Psychiatric Press.

Kübler-Ross, E. 1969: *On Death and Dying*. New York: Macmillan.

LeVay, S. 1991: A difference in hypothalamic structure between heterosexual and homosexual men. *Science* 253:1034–1037.

McCarty, L. 1986: Mother–child incest: characteristics of the offender. *Child Welfare* 65:447–458.

Maccoby, E.E. & Martin, J.A. 1983: Socialization in the context of the family: parent–child interaction. In Mussen, P.H. (ed.) *Handbook of Child Psychology. Vol. IV: Socialization, Personality, and Social Development*. New York: John Wiley.

Marks, I. 1987: The development of normal fear: a review. *Journal of Child Psychology and Psychiatry* 28:667–698.

Martin, H.P. 1972: The child and his development. In Kempe, C.H. & Helfer, R.E. (eds) *Helping the Battered Child and His Family*. Philadelphia: Lippincott.

Newcomb, T. 1956: The prediction of interpersonal attraction. *American Psychologist* 11:575.

Oates, K. 1986: *Child Abuse and Neglect: What Happens Eventually?* New York: Brunner/Mazel.

Offer, B. & Offer, J.B. 1975: *From Teenage to Young Manhood: A Psychological Study*. New York: Basic Books.

Oppenheimer, R., Howells, K., Palmer, L. *et al.* 1985: Adverse sexual experiences in childhood and clinical eating disorders: a preliminary description. *Journal of Psychosomatic Research* 19:157–161.

Perusse, D., Neale, M.C., Heath, A.C. & Eaves, L.J. 1994: Human parental behavior: evidence for genetic influence and potential implication for gene–culture transmission. *Behavioral Genetics* 24:327–335.

Plomin, R., Reiss, D., Hetherington, E.M. & Howe, G.W. 1994: Nature and nurture: genetic contributions to measures of the family environment. *Developmental Psychology* 30:32–43.

Putnam, F. 1985: Dissociation as a response to extreme trauma. In Kluft, R. (ed) *Childhood Antecedents of Multiple Personality Disorder.* Washington, DC: American Psychiatric Press.

Schaie, K.W. 1974: Translations in gerontology – from lab to life. Intellectual functioning. *American Psychologist* 29:802–807.

Schechter, M.D. & Roberge, L. 1976: Sexual exploitation. In Helfer, R.E. & Kempe, C.H. (eds) *Child Abuse and Neglect: The Family and the Community.* Cambridge, MA: Ballinger.

Seghorn, T.K., Prentky, R.A. & Boucher, R.J. 1987: Child sexual abuse in the lives of sexually aggressive offenders. *Journal of the American Academy of Child and Adolescent Psychiatry* 26:262–267.

Sgroi, S. 1982: *Handbook of Clinical Intervention in Child Sexual Abuse.* Lexington, MA: Lexington Books.

Steele, B.F. 1983: The effect of abuse and neglect on psychological development. In Call, J.D., Galenson, E. & Tyson, R.L. (eds) *Frontiers of Infant Psychiatry.* New York: Basic Books.

Thomas, A. & Chess, S. 1977: *Temperament and Development.* New York: Brunner/Mazel.

Tomlinson, B.E., Blessed, G. & Roth, M. 1968: Observations on the brains of non-demented old people. *Journal of the Neurological Sciences* 7:331–356.

Yates, A. 1982: Children eroticized by incest. *American Journal of Psychiatry* 139:482–485.

Zuckerman, M. 1991: *Psychobiology of Personality.* New York: Cambridge University Press.

5

Psychological assessment

PRINCIPLES OF MEASUREMENT

INTERVIEWS

Sources of error include:

- *Response set*. This is a tendency always to agree or to disagree with the questions asked.
- *Bias towards the centre*. This is a tendency always to avoid extreme responses. As a result, there is an excess choice of middle responses.
- *Extreme responding*. This is the opposite tendency of selecting extreme responses.
- *Social desirability*. This is the choice of responses that the subject believes the interviewer desires. It may be reduced through the inclusion of lie scales or the forced-choice technique.
- *Defensiveness*. The subject avoids giving too much self-related information.
- *Halo effect*. The observer allows his/her preconception to influence the responses.
- *Hawthorne effect*. The interviewer alters the situation by his or her presence.

SELF-PREDICTIONS

This is a direct method of measuring behaviour in which the subject is asked to give his or her own prediction concerning the behaviour under question. It can be combined with self-recording.

PSYCHOPHYSIOLOGICAL TECHNIQUES

These involve the direct use of physiological measurements in assessing behaviour.

NATURALISTIC OBSERVATIONS

These involve the assessment of behaviour as it occurs with minimum interference by the observer. In time-sampling techniques, the subject is observed during given time intervals at given times of the day or night.

Naturalistic observations are used in the functional analysis of problem behaviours. This method is sometimes referred to as ABC (Antecedents, Behaviours, Consequences).

SCALING

This refers to the conversion of raw data into types of scores more readily understood, for example ranks, (per)centiles and standardized scores.

NORM-REFERENCING

A norm is an average, common or standard performance under specified conditions. A test may be standardized to this norm.

CRITERION-REFERENCING

A criterion is a set of scores against which the success of a predictive test can be compared.

INTELLIGENCE

- *Aptitude* is the raw or potential ability of an individual.
- *Attainment* is the result of learning.

Components of intelligence

Charles Spearman, who discovered factor analysis, put forward the notion that all individuals possess, to varying extents, general abilities; this general intelligence factor is known as *g*. The main determinant of intelligence test scores was held to be *g* by Spearman.

A separate component of intelligence comprised specific abilities, known as *s*. Different intelligence subtests were held to index different *s* factors.

Overall, a person would be considered bright (high *g* factor) or not-so-bright (low *g* factor), but the person's actual overall intelligence would be calculated as follows:

Intelligence = *g* + (sum of the magnitudes of the various *s* factors)

For example, arithmetic performance would be a function of *g* plus the individual's aptitude for arithmetic (specific *s*).

Louis Thurstone (1938) criticized Spearman's *g*, and instead suggested that intelligence consisted of several primary abilities. On the basis of the factor analysis of a large database of intelligence test scores, he found the following seven primary abilities (Thurstone & Thurstone, 1963):

Verbal comprehension
Word fluency
Number
Space
Memory
Perceptual speed
Reasoning.

Mental age scale

The concept of the mental age (MA) was devised by Binet as the average intellectual ability, as measured by the level of problem-solving and reasoning. The scale was devised such that the average range of scores corresponds to the chronological age (CA).

For children with a higher than average level of intelligence, MA > CA. In contrast, for children with a lower than average level of intelligence, MA < CA.

The Stanford–Binet test can be applied to each year, up to the age of 15 years. Its reliability and validity are acceptable.

Intelligence quotient (IQ)

This is the ratio of the mental age to the chronological age, expressed as a percentage:

$$IQ = (MA/CA) \times 100$$

By convention, intelligence has a normal distribution with a mean of 100 and a standard deviation of 15.

There is a natural decline in intellectual ability with age. Performance IQ falls off with age more quickly than verbal IQ: the verbal–performance discrepancy. This decline is taken into account when raw scores are converted into IQ equivalents. Thus, although raw abilities decline with age, measured IQ remains constant.

Weschler intelligence scales

WECHSLER ADULT INTELLIGENCE SCALE (WAIS)

This well-standardized test gives both a verbal IQ and a performance IQ, and consists of 11 subtests, divided into six verbal subtests and five performance subtests.

Verbal subtests
The only one of these six subtests which is timed is the arithmetic subtest.

Information: 29 questions
Comprehension: 16 items including the interpretation of proverbs
Arithmetic: 14 mental arithmetic problems
Similarities: 14 pairs of items for which the subject is asked to state in what way each pair is alike
Digit span: lists of three to nine digits which must be remembered in the forward direction and lists of two to eight digits which must be remembered backwards
Vocabulary: the subject is asked to give the meaning of 35 words.

Performance subtests
All five of these subtests are timed.

Picture completion: 20 incomplete pictures are presented to the subject who is asked to state the important part missing from each one
Block design: the subject is asked to reproduce designs with red and white blocks
Picture arrangement: the subject is asked to arrange 10 sets of cartoon pictures so that their sequence makes sense

Object assembly: four jigsaw-type puzzles have to be assembled correctly

Digit symbol: symbols need to be matched to digits as rapidly as possible, using a given code.

The verbal and performance scores are added together to produce a full-scale IQ. The WAIS has a relatively high reliability and validity.

WESCHLER INTELLIGENCE SCALE FOR CHILDREN – REVISED (WISC-R)

This is a modified version of the WAIS for children between the ages of 5 and 15 years.

WESCHLER PRESCHOOL AND PRIMARY SCALE OF INTELLIGENCE (WPPSI)

This is a modified version of the WAIS for children between the ages of 4 and 6½ years.

Group ability tests

Unlike the above, these can be used by one examiner to assess the intellectual ability and aptitude of a group of people. An example is the Armed Services Vocational Aptitude Battery (ASVAB).

Nature–nurture

Potential intelligence (aptitude) is inherited, but environmental factors influence the fulfilment of potential (attainment).

Cultural influences

Tests of attainment can give rise to discrepant results when applied to people from different cultures. It is thought that tests measuring aptitude are less prone to such influences.

TECHNIQUES USED IN NEUROPSYCHOLOGICAL ASSESSMENT

Comprehensive test batteries

Halstead–Reitan Neuropsychological Test Battery

This comprehensive test battery can detect damage to the brain, and whether such damage is:

- lateralized – and if so, to which hemisphere it is lateralized
- associated with an acute or chronic disorder
- focal or diffuse.

The core test procedures of the Halstead–Reitan Neuropsychological Test Battery include:

- Halstead's Category Test – testing for learning, cognitive flexibility, and the ability to form abstract concepts
- Critical Flicker Frequency Test – measures the minimum frequency of light flickers that is perceived as a fused non-flickering light stimulus

- Trail Making Test – see below
- Tactual Performance Test – measures the level of tactual perception, manual dexterity and coordination, motor speed, and spatial memory
- Seashore Rhythm Test – assesses the ability to discriminate non-verbal auditory stimuli
- Speech Sounds Perception Test – assesses the ability to discriminate verbal auditory stimuli
- Finger Oscillation Test – measures motor speed in both the dominant and the non-dominant hands.

Ancillary procedures of the Halstead–Reitan Neuropsychological Test Battery include:

- Halstead–Wepman Aphasia Screening Test – a screening test for:
  - reading skills
  - writing skills
  - arithmetical skills
  - expressive language abilities
  - receptive language abilities
  - constructional apraxia
  - the ability to distinguish left from right
- Sensory–Perceptual Examination – tests for sensory and perceptual abilities
- WAIS-R – see above
- MMPI – see below and Chapter 1.

Luria–Nebraska Neuropsychological Battery
This battery is comparable to the Halstead–Reitan Neuropsychological Battery.

Language tests

Boston Naming Test
In this language test, the subject is asked to name 60 line drawings (Kaplan *et al.*, 1983).

Graded Naming Test
In this language test, the subject is asked to name 30 line drawings (McKenna & Warrington, 1983).

Token Test
A number of tokens, such as differently coloured rectangles and circular discs, are used in this test. The subject is asked to carry out progressively more complicated verbal instructions using these tokens (De Renzi & Vignolo, 1962). The Token Test is sensitive to minor impairment in language comprehension, and performance tends to be more impaired in aphasia than in people who are non-asphasic.

Speed and Capacity of Language Processing Test
This test (Baddeley *et al.*, 1992) consists of two parts. The first part is the Speed of Comprehension Test, in which the subject is asked to decide, as quickly as possible, whether each of a series of statements is true/sensible or false/not sensible (silly). The second part is the Spot-the-Word Test, in which 60 pairings of words with non-words are presented and the subject must decide which of each pair, in turn, is a real word. The Spot-the-Word Test controls for poor verbal skills and has been found to give a robust estimate of verbal intelligence and therefore premorbid intelligence. (In this respect, it is rather like the NART.)

Perception tests

Bender–Gestalt Test/Bender Visual Motor Gestalt Test
The subject is asked to copy nine designs (Bender, 1938, 1946).

Visual Object and Space Perception Battery
This battery tests visual perception (Warrington & James, 1991) and consists of the following nine tests:

    Screening test for visual impairment
    Incomplete letters
    Silhouettes
    Object decision
    Progressive silhouettes
    Dot counting
    Position discrimination
    Number location
    Cube analysis.

The last four of these tests are concerned with spatial perception.

Behavioural Inattention Test
This battery tests for unilateral visual neglect (*Wilson et al.*, 1987). The first six tests deal with visual neglect in the usual way:

    Line crossing
    Letter cancellation
    Star cancellation
    Figure copying and shape copying
    Line bisection
    Free drawing (clock; person; butterfly).

These are followed by nine behavioural tests:

    Picture scanning
    Telephone dialling
    Menu reading
    Article reading
    Clock face: telling the time and setting the time
    Coin sorting
    Address copying and sentence copying
    Map navigation
    Card sorting.

These nine behavioural tests include tasks that are activities of daily living and so help in rehabilitation assessments.

Memory tests

Benton Visual Retention Test
In this visual recall test, designs on cards are each presented to the subject for 10 seconds, after each of which the subject attempts to recall and draw each design (Benton, 1955, 1963). In order to

exclude visuoperceptual problems, the subject can also be asked separately to copy the designs with the cards on display. It may be used to test for brain damage and early cognitive decline.

Graham–Kendall Memory for Designs Test
This is another visual recall test in which the subject is asked to draw from immediate recall designs that are presented for five seconds each (Graham & Kendall, 1960).

Rey–Osterrieth Test
In this visual memory test, the subject is presented with a complex design. The subject is asked to copy this design and then, 40 minutes later, without previous notification that this will occur, the subject is asked to draw the same design again from memory (Rey, 1941; Osterrieth, 1944). Non-dominant temporal lobe damage can lead to impaired performance on this test, whereas domain temporal lobe damage tends not to (but is associated with verbal memory difficulties).

Paired associate learning tests
In these tests the subject is given paired associates to learn and then must respond appropriately (e.g. by stating the paired word) when the first, stimulus, words are given. Different forms of these tests, of varying difficulty, have been produced (e.g. Inglis, 1959; Isaacs & Walkey, 1964). These tests may be used to assess memory disorder in old age, independently of verbal intelligence.

Synonym Learning Test
This is a modified version of the Walton–Black Modified Word Learning Test, specifically for use in the differential diagnosis of dementia from depression in the elderly (particularly if combined with the Digit Copying Test). In the Synonym Learning Test, 10 words with which the subject is not familiar are first identified and then the subject is asked to learn their meanings (Kendrick et al., 1965).

Object Learning Test
This test has similar aims to those of the Synonym Learning Test, but is less stressful to take for elderly people. As with the Synonym Learning Test, the results of the Object Learning Test combined with those of the Digit Copying Test can aid in the differential diagnosis of dementia from depression in the elderly. In the Object Learning Test, the subject is exposed to drawings of familiar items on sections of cards, and asked to recall them (Kendrick et al., 1979).

Rey Auditory Verbal Learning Test
This is a word list learning test involving five presentations of a list containing 15 words, which the subject is asked to recall. The same then occurs with a second list of 15 words. Finally, the subject is asked to recall words from the first list, both immediately after completing the second recall task (involving the second list) and some time later (say, after 30 minutes). Information is obtained about immediate recall, the learning curve, primacy and recency effects, and learning strategies used.

California Verbal Learning Test
This is a word list learning test involving 16 words from four known categories. As with the Rey Auditory Verbal Learning Test, the California Verbal Learning Test gives information about immediate recall, the learning curve, and learning strategies used.

WMS-R
The Wechsler Memory Scale (revised) or WMS-R is a memory test battery that contains the following subtests (Wechsler, 1987):

Information and orientation questions
Mental control
Figural memory
Logical memory
Visual paired associates
Verbal paired associates
Visual reproduction
Digit span
Visual memory span
Delayed recall.

The mental control subtest tests for minor brain damage. The delayed recall is recall after 30 minutes for the contents of the following subtests:

Logical memory
Visual paired associates
Verbal paired associates
Visual reproduction.

Rivermead Behavioural Memory Test

This is another memory test battery (Wilson, 1987; Wilson *et al.*, 1991). It lays emphasis on tests that are related to skills required in daily living. The subtests of the Rivermead Behavioural Memory Test include:

Orientation: for time, date and place
Name recall: of a forename and surname associated with a given photograph
Picture recognition
Face recognition
Story recall: immediate recall and recall after a quarter of an hour
Route memory
Prospective memory.

Adult Memory and Information Processing Battery

This is also a memory test battery (Coughlan & Hollows, 1985). It contains the following four memory subtests:

Short story recall
Figure copy and recall
List learning
Design learning.

The Adult Memory and Information Processing Battery also contains the following two information-processing tests:

Number cancellation
Digit cancellation.

The norms used in this battery are age-stratified.

Intelligence tests

WAIS and similar tests

The intelligence tests based on the WAIS are considered in the previous section of this chapter.

NART

The National Adult Reading Test or NART (Nelson & McKenna, 1975; Nelson, 1982) is a reading test consisting of phonetically irregular words which have to be read aloud by the subject. If a person suffers deterioration in intellectual abilities, the person's premorbid vocabulary may remain less affected (or unaffected). The NART can therefore be used to estimate the premorbid IQ.

Raven's Progressive Matrices

This test of non-verbal intelligence consists of a series of printed designs from each of which a part is missing (Raven, 1958, 1982). The subject is required correctly to choose the missing part for each design from the alternatives offered. The test requires the perception of relations between abstract items.

Executive function (frontal lobe) tests

Stroop

There exist several types of Stroop test. A typical Stroop test involves giving a subject a card containing columns of colour names, printed in black on white, and asking the person to read aloud as many of the words as possible in two minutes. The words might be in columns, as follows:

RED	GREEN	BLUE	GREEN
BLUE	TAN	RED	GREEN
...	...	...	...

The correct answer to this part of the test, with the subject reading across rows, would be 'Red, green, blue, green, blue, tan, red, green, …'. The score is the total number of words correctly named in the two-minute period. This part of the test checks that the person is capable of following the directions and of reading such words (in the given print size, etc.) aloud. In the second part of the test, a similar card of columns of words is presented to the subject and the same instructions of reading out what the words say is given. This time, however, the words are not in black, but instead are printed in different colours. These colours are those described by some of the words, but such that no given word is printed in its own colour. For example, GREEN may be printed in blue the first time it occurs, and then in red the second time. (In each case, the correct answer is 'green'.) Again, the score is the total number of words correctly named in the two-minute period. Finally, a card constructed in a similar way to that used for the second part of the test is again presented to the subject, and this time he/she is asked to name the colour in which each word is printed, and to ignore the actual colour names printed. This is the Stroop interference test. For instance, if GREEN is printed in blue the first time it occurs, and then in red the second time, then the correct answers for these two occasions would be 'blue' and 'red', and not 'green' and 'green'.

This tests the (Stroop) interference that may occur between reading words and naming colours (Stroop, 1935; Trenerry et al., 1989; Lezak, 1995). Left (dominant) frontal lobe lesions are associated with poor performance on the Stroop test. The anterior cingulate cortex is particularly involved in carrying out this test (Pardo et al., 1990). However, activation of the anterior cingulate cortex does not invariably accompany the interference task. Another region of the brain that appears to be associated with this task is the left inferior precentral sulcus (at the border between the inferior frontal gyrus, the pars opercularis, and the ventral premotor area); this region appears to be involved with the mediation of competing articulatory demands during the interference condition of the Stroop test (Mead et al., 2002).

Verbal fluency

A typical verbal fluency test involves asking the subject to articulate as many words as possible, during two-minute intervals, starting with the letters F, A and S, in turn. Proper nouns (such as the name Forsythe) and derivatives such as plurals and different verb endings are not allowed to count together with the root words. For instance, one cannot count both 'font' and 'fonts', or 'float' and 'floated' and 'floating'. The score is the total number of allowable words achieved. Verbal fluency is impaired in left (dominant) frontal lobe lesions.

Tower of London Test

The Tower of London Test (Shallice, 1982) is based on the Tower of Hanoi game and test planning. The subject is asked to move coloured discs of varying size between three columns, either using a model or via a computer program (preferably with a touch screen), in order to achieve a given result. Left frontal lobe lesions are associated with poor performance on this test.

Wisconsin Card Sort Test

The Wisconsin Card Sort Test consists of a number of cards (64 in the original; 24 in the Modified Wisconsin Card Sort Test) which contain different shapes (circles, crosses, stars and triangles). Other variables include the number of shapes on a card, and the colour of the shapes on a given card (there are four possible colours for each card). Following the presentation of index cards, the subject has to sort the remaining cards corresponding to the index cards. Subjects are not given the variable(s) by means of which this sorting should occur, but are told if they are right or wrong each time. For instance, the first indexing variable might be colour. After a certain number of consecutive correct responses, the rule suddenly changes, without the subject being warned in advance. These days this test is more conveniently administered via a computer program, preferably using a touch screen. The Wisconsin Card Sort Test picks up perseverative errors (such as continuing for too long to sort cards by number, well after the indexing rule has changed to colour) and non-perseverative errors. Poor performance on this task is particularly associated with dysfunction of the left dorsolateral (pre-) frontal cortex.

Cognitive Estimates Test

In the absence of a reduction of intelligence quotient, some frontal lobe damaged people may give outrageously incorrect cognitive estimates of commonly known phenomena. For instance, asked to estimate the length of an adult elephant, such a person might venture a reply of 100 yards. This abnormality is exploited in the Cognitive Estimates Test, in which the subject is asked to give a series of cognitive estimates, such as estimating the height of the average man.

Six Elements Test

This is a strategy application test that attempts to uncover evidence of the organizational difficulty that may occur as a result of frontal lobe damage. The subject is asked to carry out six different tasks (in two groups of three) during a quarter of an hour. In order to maximize his or her score, the subject needs adequately to plan and schedule these tasks, while also monitoring the time that has elapsed.

Multiple Errands Task

This is another strategy application test that attempts to uncover evidence of the organizational difficulty that may occur as a result of frontal lobe damage. It is rather more difficult than the Six Elements Test. The subject is asked to carry out multiple errands, usually in an unfamiliar shopping centre.

Trail Making Test

There are two parts to this test (Trail A and Trail B). In the first part, a piece of paper is presented to the subject. On the paper are a number (say, 25) of circles, each labelled with a different number (from 1 to 25, say). The subject is asked to draw a trail, as quickly as possible, that passes through all the circles, starting with the lowest numbered one (say, 1) and ending with the highest number (25, say). In the second part of the test (Trail B), both numbers and letters are contained in the circles, and this time the subject is asked to draw a trail, as quickly as possible, that passes through all the circles, starting with the lowest numbered one (say, 1) and then passing to the circle with the lowest letter (A, say) and continuing to alternate between number and letter in increasing order, ending with the highest number and highest letter. So the two trails should be between circles labelled as follows:

Trail A: $1 \rightarrow 2 \rightarrow 3 \rightarrow 4 \rightarrow \ldots$
Trail B: $1 \rightarrow A \rightarrow 2 \rightarrow B \rightarrow 3 \rightarrow C \rightarrow \ldots$

The Trail Making Test tests the following abilities:

Sequencing
Cognitive flexibility
Visual scanning
Spatial analysis
Motor control
Alertness
Concentration.

Difficulties with cognitive flexibility or with complex conceptual tracking may manifest as much longer times being required for Trail B than would be expected from the Trail A time score.

Personality tests

Personality inventories have been considered in Chapter 1. Here, psychometric methods of assessing personality are summarized.

Objective tests

The items presented have limited responses. Objective tests include:

- 16PF (Sixteen Personality Factor Questionnaire) – see Chapter 1.
- MMPI (Minnesota Multiphasic Personality Inventory) – see Chapter 1.
- CPI (California Psychological Inventory) – see Chapter 1.
- EPQ (Eysenck Personality Questionnaire) – This contains 90 items in true/false format. Subjects are rated on the following dimensions: extraversion, introversion, and neuroticism.
- HDHQ (Hostility and Direction of Hostility Questionnaire) – This is used to measure relationships that could be affected by personality status.

In general, because of evidence that mental state markedly affects scoring of questionnaires, they have been replaced by interview schedules and other observer ratings.

Projective tests

The presented items have no one correct answer, instead taking the form of ambiguous stimuli, upon which the subject projects his or her personality. Their reliability and validity have not been established. Examples include the:

- Rorschach Inkblot Test
- Thematic Apperception Test (TAT)
- Sentence Completion Test (SCT).

Dementia tests and related tests

MMSE

The Mini-Mental State Examination or MMSE (Folstein *et al.*, 1975) is a brief test that can be routinely used rapidly to detect possible dementia, to estimate the severity of cognitive impairment, and to follow the course of cognitive changes over time. It can be used to differentiate between delirium and dementia (Anthony *et al.*, 1982). The combination of cognitive testing and an informant questionnaire has not been found to result in any advantage over the use of the MMSE alone in screening for dementia (Knafelc *et al.*, 2003). The MMSE includes the following assessments:

Orientation
Attention: serial subtraction or spelling a word (such as 'WORLD' backwards)
Immediate recall
Short-term memory
Naming common objects
Following simple verbal commands
Following simple written commands
Writing a sentence spontaneously
Copying a figure.

The total score that may be achieved is 30. Age and MMSE scores appear to be inversely related, from a median of 29 for Americans aged between 18 and 24 years to a median of 25 in those aged over 80 years. A total MMSE score of less than 24 tends to be considered as indicating cognitive impairment, in the absence of any other cause for such a low score (such as no more than four years of schooling, or learning disability).

CANTAB

The Cambridge Neuropsychological Test Automated Battery or CANTAB is an automated computerized battery that offers sensitive and specific cognitive assessment, preferably using a touch screen. The standard CANTAB consists of the following 13 computerized tasks:

- *Motor screening.* This screening task is administered before the other tasks and introduces the subject to the touch screen and checks that the subject can touch this properly and that he or she can hear, comprehend and follow instructions appropriately.
- *Big/little circle.* This tests that a subject can follow an explicit instructional rule and that he or she can then reverse this rule.
- *Delayed matching to sample.*
- *ID/ED shift.* This tests the ability to attend to specific attributes of compound stimuli and then to shift that attention as required.
- *Matching to sample visual search.* This is a speed/accuracy trade-off visual search task.
- *Paired associates learning.* This delayed response procedure tests list memory and then list learning (or visuospatial conditional learning).
- *Pattern recognition memory.*
- *Rapid visual information processing.* This tests vigilance (sustained attention) and working memory.
- *Reaction time.*

- *Spatial recognition memory.*
- *Spatial span.* This tests spatial memory span.
- *Spatial working memory.* This tests both spatial working memory and strategy performance.
- *Stockings of Cambridge.* This has replaced the Tower of London test in earlier versions of CANTAB, and is somewhat similar to the Tower of London Test described above.

Gresham Ward Questionnaire
In the Gresham Ward Questionnaire (Post, 1965) questions are asked that cover the following abilities:

Orientation in time
Orientation in place
Memory for past personal events
Memory for recent personal events
General information
Topographical orientation.

Blessed's Dementia Scale
This questionnaire (Blessed *et al.*, 1968) is administered to a relative or friend of the subject who is asked to answer the questions on the basis of performance over the previous six months. There are three sets of questions. The first set deals with activities of daily living such as:

Coping with small sums of money
Remembering a short list of items such as a shopping list
Finding their way indoors
Finding their way around familiar streets
Grasping situations or explanations
Recall of recent events
Tendency to dwell in the past.

The second set of questions deals with further activities of daily living including:

Ability to feed oneself
Ability to dress oneself
Level of incontinence, if any.

The third set of questions is concerned with changes in:

Personality
Interest
Drive.

Information–Memory–Concentration Test
This is a relatively straightforward set of questions that may be tried even by those with medium to severe levels of dementia.

GMS
The Geriatric Mental State Schedule or GMS is a semi-structured interview that assesses the subject's mental state.

CAMDEX
The Cambridge Examination for Mental Disorders of the Elderly or CAMDEX is an interview schedule consisting of three sections (Roth *et al.*, 1986, 1988):

- A structured clinical interview with the person is conducted to obtain systematic information about the present state, past history and family history.
- A range of objective cognitive tests are administered which constitute a mini-neuropsychological battery, known as the CAMCOG.
- A structured interview with a relative or other informant is conducted to obtain independent information about the respondent's present state, past history and family history.

The assessment also includes a brief physical and neurological examination, and recording the results of investigations.

Nurse-rated scales

- Crichton Geriatric Behaviour Rating Scale is a retrospective nursing-rated assessment.
- Clifton Assessment Schedule is another nursing-rated assessment.
- Stockton Geriatric Rating Scale is also a nursing-rated assessment.

PBE

The Present Behavioural Examination or PBE involves interviewing carers and rates psycho-pathological and behavioural changes in dementia.

MOUSEPAD

The Manchester and Oxford Universities Scale for the Psychopathological Assessment of Dementia or MOUSEPAD also involves interviewing carers and rates psychopathological and behavioural changes in dementia.

SCAG

The Sandoz Clinical Assessment: Geriatric or SCAG consists of 18 symptom areas and an overall global assessment, each being rated on an eight-point scale (from 0 = not present, to 7 = severe) (Shader *et al.*, 1974):

Mood depression	Emotional lability
Confusion	Fatigue
Mental alertness	Self-care
Motivation initiative	Appetite
Irritability	Dizziness
Hostility	Anxiety
Bothersome	Impairment of recent memory
Indifference to surroundings	Disorientation
Unsociability	Overall impression of the person.
Uncooperativeness	

Vineland Social Maturity Scale

The Vineland Social Maturity Scale consists of 117 items that assess different aspects of social maturity and social ability. Although it can be used for the assessment of dementia, the Vineland Social Maturity Scale is primarily designed to be used in the assessment of childhood development and learning disability.

PADL

The Performance Test of Activities of Daily Living or PADL is a simple performance test that assesses the self-care capacity of the subject by asking him or her to carry out certain essential activities of daily living.

BIBLIOGRAPHY

Anthony, J.C., Le Resche, L., Niaz, U., Von Korf, M.R. & Folstein, M.F. 1982: Limits of the 'Mini-Mental State' as a screening test for dementia and delirium among hospital patients. *Psychological Medicine* 12:397–408.

Baddeley, A., Emslie, H. & Nimmo-Smith, I. 1992 *The Speed and Capacity of Language Processing Test*. Bury St Edmunds: Thames Valley Test Co.

Bender, L. 1938: *A Visual Motor Gestalt Test and its Clinical Uses*. New York: American Orthopsychiatric Association.

Bender, L. 1946: *Instructions for the Use of Visual Motor Gestalt Test*. New York: American Orthopsychiatric Association.

Benton, A.L. 1955: *The Revised Visual Retention Test: Clinical and Experimental Applications*. New York: The Psychological Corp.

Benton, A.L. 1963: *The Revised Visual Retention Test: Clinical and Experimental Applications*. New York: The Psychological Corp.

Blessed, G., Tomlinson, B.E. & Roth, M. 1968: The association between quantitative measures of dementia and of senile change in the cerebral grey matter of elderly subjects. *British Journal of Psychiatry* 114:797–811.

Coughlan, A.K. & Hollows, S.E. 1985: *The Adult Memory and Information Processing Battery*. Leeds: A.K. Coughlan, Psychology Department, St James University Hospital.

De Renzi, E. & Vignolo, L.A. 1962: The token test: a sensitive test to detect receptive disturbances in aphasics. *Brain* 85:665–678.

Folstein, M.F., Folstein, S.E. & McHugh, P.R. 1975: 'Mini-mental state': a practical method for grading the cognitive state of patients for the clinician. *Journal of Psychiatric Research* 12:189–198.

Graham, F.K. & Kendall, B.S. 1960: Memory-for-designs test: revised general manual. *Perceptual and Motor Skills* 11:147–188.

Inglis, J. 1959: A paired-associate learning test for use with elderly psychiatric patients. *Journal of Mental Science* 105:440–443.

Isaacs, B. & Walkey, F.A. 1964: A simplified paired-associate test for elderly hospital patients. *British Journal of Psychiatry* 110:80–83.

Kaplan, E., Goodglass, H. & Weintraub, S. 1983: *Boston Naming Test*. Philadelphia: Lea & Febiger.

Kendrick, D.C., Parboosingh, R.-C. & Post, F. 1965: A synonym learning test for use with elderly psychiatric subjects: a validation study. *British Journal of Social and Clinical Psychology* 4:63–71.

Kendrick, D.C., Gibson, A.J. & Moyes, I.C.A. 1979: The revised Kendrick battery: clinical studies. *British Journal of Social and Clinical Psychology* 18:329–340.

Knafelc, R., Lo Giudice, D., Harrigan, S. *et al.* 2003: The combination of cognitive testing and an informant questionnaire in screening for dementia. *Age and Ageing* 32:541–547.

Lezak, M.D. 1995: *Neuropsychological Assessment*, 3rd edn. New York: Oxford University Press.

McKenna, P. & Warrington, E.K. 1983: *Graded Naming Test*. Windsor: NFER–Nelson.

Mead, L.A., Mayer, A.R., Bobholz, J.A. *et al.* 2002: Neural basis of the Stroop interference task: response competition or selective attention? *Journal of International Neuropsychological Society* 8:735–742.

Nelson, H.E. 1982: *The National Adult Reading Test Manual*. Windsor: NFER–Nelson.

Nelson, H.E. & McKenna, P. 1975: The use of current reading ability in the assessment of dementia. *British Journal of Social and Clinical Psychology* 14:259–267.

Osterrieth, P.-A. 1944: Le test depression copie d'une figure complexe: contribution à l'étude de la perception et de la mémoire. *Archives de Psychologie* 30:206–353.

Pardo, J.V., Pardo, P.J., Janer, K.W. & Raichle, M.E. 1990: The anterior cingulate cortex mediates processing selection in the Stroop attention of conflict paradigm. *Proceedings of the National Academy of Sciencesof the USA* 87:256–259.

Post, F. 1965: *The Clinical Psychiatry of Late Life*. Oxford: Pergamon.

Raven, J.C. 1958: *Guide to using the Mill Hill Vocabulary Scale and the Progressive Matrices Scales*. London: H.K. Lewis.

Raven, J.C. 1982: *Revised Manual for Raven's Progressive Matrices and Vocabulary Scale*. Windsor: NFER–Nelson.

Rey, A. 1941: L'examen psychologique dans les cas d'encéphalopathie traumatique. *Archives de Pathologie* 28:286–340.

Roth, M., Huppert, F.A., Tym, E. & Mountjoy, C.Q. 1988: *CAMDEX. The Cambridge Examination for Mental Disorders of the Elderly*. Cambridge: Cambridge University Press.

Roth, M., Tym, E., Mountjoy, C.Q. *et al.* 1986: CAMDEX: a standardised instrument for the diagnosis of mental disorder in the elderly with special reference to the early detection of dementia. *British Journal of Psychiatry* 149:698–709.

Shader, R.I., Harmatz, J.S. & Salzman, C. 1974: A new scale for clinical assessment in geriatric populations: Sandoz Clinical Assessment – Geriatric (SCAG). *Journal of the American Geriatrics Society* 22:107–113.

Shallice, T. 1982: Specific impairments of planning. In Broadbent, D.E. & Weiskrantz, L. (eds) *The Neuropsychology of Cognitive Function*. London: Royal Society.

Stroop, J.R. 1935: Studies of interference in serial verbal reactions. *Journal of Experimental Psychology* 18:643–662.

Thurstone, L.L. 1938: *Primary Mental Abilities*. Chicago: University of Chicago Press.

Thurstone, L.L. & Thurstone, T.G. 1963: *SRA Primary Abilities*. Chicago: Science Research Associates.

Trenerry, M.R., Crossan, B., Deboe, J. & Leber, W.R. 1989: *Stroop Neuropsychological Screening Test Manual*. Florida: Psychological Assessment Resources Inc.

Warrington, E.K. & James, M. 1991: *The Visual Object and Space Perception Battery*. Bury St Edmunds: Thames Valley Test Co.

Wechsler, D. 1987: *Wechsler Memory Scale – Revised Manual*. San Antonio, TX: The Psychological Corp.

Wilson, B.A. 1987: *Rehabilitation of Memory*. New York: Guildford Press.

Wilson, B.A., Cockburn, J. & Baddeley, A. 1991: *The Rivermead Behavioural Memory Test*, 2nd edn. Bury St Edmunds: Thames Valley Test Co.

Wilson, B.A., Cockburn, J. & Halligan, P. 1987: *Behavioural Inattention Test*. Fareham: Thames Valley Test Co.

6

Principles of evaluation and psychometrics

BASIC CONCEPTS

Qualitative data

Qualitative variables refer to attributes that can be categorized such that the categories do not have a numerical relationship with each other; e.g. eye colour.

Quantitative data

Quantitative variables refer to numerically represented data. These can be of the following types:

- *discrete* quantitative variables which can take on only known fixed values; e.g. the number of new patients seen each week in a psychiatric outpatient department
- *continuous* quantitative variables which can take on any value in a defined range; e.g. the height of psychiatric inpatients.

Scales of measurement

Table 6.1 summarizes the properties of different types of measurement scale.

Table 6.1   *Types of measurement scale*

Property	Nominal	Ordinal	Interval	Ratio
Categories mutually exclusive	√	√	√	√
Categories logically ordered		√	√	√
Equal distance between adjacent categories			√	√
True zero point				√

Reproduced with permission from Puri, B.K. 1996: *Statistics for the Health Sciences.* London: W.B. Saunders.

Sampling methods

Simple random sampling

A simple random sample is one chosen from a given population such that every possible sample of the same size has the same probability of being chosen.

Systematic sampling
This type of sampling saves time and effort. Common examples include:

- *Periodic sampling.* Every nth member of the population is chosen. This may not always lead to a random choice because of an unforeseen underlying pattern.
- *Using random numbers.* Using random numbers can be a better method than periodic sampling for ensuring random choice. Random numbers, obtained, for example, from a computer program, a scientific calculator with a (pseudo)random number generator, or a table of random numbers, can be used to choose every nth member of the population.
- *Stratified random sampling.* A given population is stratified before random samples are chosen from each stratum. This can be useful when studying a disease that varies with respect to sex and age, for example.

Frequency distributions

Frequency distribution
This is a systematic way of arranging data, with frequencies being given for categories of a qualitative or quantitative variable. For continuous quantitative variables the categories should be contiguous and mutually exclusive, and are known as class intervals.

Frequency table
This is a frequency distribution arranged in the form of a table, with the first column giving contiguous mutually exclusive values (which may be class intervals) of a variable and the adjoining column giving the corresponding frequencies.

Relative frequency
The relative frequency of a category/class interval/variable is the proportion of the total frequency corresponding to that category/class interval/variable:

Relative frequency = (frequency of category)/(total frequency)

Cumulative frequency
The cumulative frequency of a given value of a variable is the total frequency up to that value.

Cumulative frequency table
This is a cumulative frequency distribution arranged in the form of a table, with the first column giving contiguous mutually exclusive values (which may be class intervals) of a variable and the adjoining column giving the corresponding cumulative frequencies.

Cumulative relative frequency
The cumulative relative frequency of a given value of a variable is the total relative frequency up to that value.

Cumulative relative frequency table
This is a cumulative relative frequency distribution arranged in the form of a table, with the first column giving contiguous mutually exclusive values (which may be class intervals) of a variable and the adjoining column giving the corresponding cumulative relative frequencies.

Discrete probability distributions

Bernoulli trial
This is a trial or experiment having two and only two alternative outcomes.

Bernoulli distribution
This is the probability distribution for a discrete binary variable (range = 0, 1), which is a special case of the binomial distribution $B(1, p)$, where p is the probability of 'success':

> Mean = p
> Variance = $p(1 - p)$

Binomial distribution
The binomial distribution, $B(n, p)$, is the probability distribution for a discrete finite variable (range = 0, 1, 2, ..., n):

> Mean = np
> Variance = $np(1 - p)$

Poisson distribution
The Poisson distribution, Poisson (μ), is the probability distribution for a discrete infinite variable (range = 0, 1, 2, ...), where $\mu = np$:

> Mean = μ
> Variance = μ

The Poisson distribution can be used in situations in which the following criteria are fulfilled:

- Events occur randomly in time or space (length, area or volume).
- The events are independent (i.e. the outcome of any given event does not affect the outcome of any other).
- Two or more events cannot take place simultaneously.
- The mean number of events per given unit of time or space is constant.

Continuous probability distributions

Normal distribution
The normal distribution, $N(\mu, \sigma^2)$, is the probability distribution for a continuous variable (range = 3):

> Mean = μ
> Variance = σ^2

Properties of the normal distribution probability density function (p.d.f.) curve include:

- It is unimodal.
- It is continuous.
- It is symmetrical about its mean.
- Its mean, median and mode are all equal.
- The area under the curve is one.
- The curve tends to zero as the variable moves in either direction from the mean.

The interval one standard deviation either side of the mean of the p.d.f. of a normal distribution encloses 68.27% of the total area under the curve.

The interval two standard deviations either side of the mean of the p.d.f. of a normal distribution encloses 95.45% of the total area under the curve.

The interval three standard deviations either side of the mean of the p.d.f. of a normal distribution encloses 99.73% of the total area under the curve.

If $X \sim N(\mu, \sigma^2)$, then the standard normal variate Z is given by:

$$Z = (X - \mu)/\sigma$$

For $Z \sim N(0, 1)$:

Mean $= 0$
Variance $= 1$

The cumulative distribution function, $P(Z < z)$, is given by $\phi(z)$.

For $N(\mu, \sigma^2)$, the two-tailed 5% points are given by:

$$\mu - 1.96\sigma \quad \text{and} \quad \mu + 1.96\sigma$$

t distribution

When $n < 30$, the t distribution, $t(v)$ or t_v, is used in making inferences about the mean of a normal population when its variance is unknown. The t distribution is symmetrical about the mean but has longer tails than the normal distribution.

v is the number of degrees of freedom, and is given by:

$$v = n - 1$$

For $n \geq 30$, $t(v) \approx N(0, 1)$.

χ^2 distribution

The chi-squared distribution with v degrees of freedom, $\chi^2(v)$, is obtained from the sum of the squares of v independent variables, Z_1 to Z_v, where each $Z \sim N(0, 1)$:

If $W = \Sigma Z_i^2$, where $i = 1$ to v, and $Z_i \sim N(0, 1)$,
then $W \sim \chi^2(v)$

The chi-squared distribution is asymmetrical.

F distribution

The F distribution is related to the χ^2 distribution and is asymmetrical. A given F distribution is described in terms of v_1 and v_2, each of which gives a number of degrees of freedom. This is usually abbreviated to $F(v_1, v_2)$.

Summary statistics: measures of location

Measures of central tendency

The (arithmetic) mean (or average) of a sample with n items $(x_1, x_2, x_3, \ldots, x_n)$, $\bar{x}$, is given by:

$$\bar{x} = (\Sigma x)/n$$

The population mean, μ, of a population of size N is given by:

$$\mu = (\Sigma x)/N$$

The arithmetic mean is suitable for use with data measured on at least an interval scale. A major disadvantage is that it can be unduly influenced by an extreme value.

The *median* is the middle value of a set of observations ranked in order. If the number of observations is odd:

Median = middle value

If the number of observations is even:

Median = arithmetic mean of the two middle values

The median is suitable for use with data measured on at least an ordinal scale. It gives a better measure of central tendency than the mean for skewed (asymmetrical) distributions.

The *mode* of a distribution is the value of the observation occurring most frequently. The category/interval occurring most frequently is the modal category. It can be used with all measurement scales.

Quantiles

Quantiles are cut-off points that split a continuous distribution into equal groups.

- The *median* splits a distribution into two equal parts.
- The two *tertiles* split the distribution into three equal parts.
- The three *quartiles* split the distribution into four equal parts.
- The four *quintiles* split the distribution into five equal parts.
- The nine *deciles* split the distribution into 10 equal parts.
- The 99 *percentiles* split the distribution into 100 equal parts.

The kth quantile of n observations ranked in increasing order from the first to the nth is calculated by interpolating between the two observations adjacent to the qth, where q is given by:

$$q = k(n+1)/Q$$

where Q is the number of groups into which the quantiles divide the distribution.

Summary statistics: measures of dispersion

Range

The range is the difference between the smallest and largest values in a distribution:

Range = (largest value) − (smallest value)

It can be used with data that are measured on at least an interval scale.

Measures relating to quantiles

These are the most commonly used measures relating to quantiles:

- The *interquartile* range is the difference between the third and first quartiles.
- The *semi-quartile* range is half the interquartile range.
- The 10 to 90 *percentile* range is the difference between the 90th and 10th (per)centiles, or equivalently, between the ninth and first deciles.
- The *interdecile* range is the difference between the 90th and 10th (per)centiles, or equivalently, between the ninth and first deciles.

The median and interquartile or 10 to 90 percentile range can be more useful summary statistics than the mean and standard deviation for skewed distributions.

Standard deviation

The standard deviation of a distribution is based on deviations from the mean and has the same units as the original observations.

For a population of size N and mean μ, the population standard deviation, σ, is given by:

Population standard deviation, $\sigma = \sqrt{\{[\Sigma(x-\mu)^2]/N\}}$

For a sample of size n and mean $\bar{x}$, the sample standard deviation, s, is given by:

Sample standard deviation, $s = \sqrt{\{[\Sigma(x-\bar{x})^2]/(n-1)\}}$

The standard deviation can be used for data measured on at least an interval scale.

Variance

The variance is the square of the standard deviation and has units that are the square of those of the observations.

For a population of size N and mean μ, the population variance, σ^2, is given by:

Population variance, $\sigma^2 = [\Sigma(x-\mu)^2]/N$

For a sample of size n and mean $\bar{x}$, the sample variance, s^2, is given by:

Sample variance, $s^2 = [\Sigma(x-\bar{x})^2]/(n-1)$

The variance can be used for data measured on at least an interval scale.

Graphs

The graph of a function f is the set of points $(x, f(x))$.

DRAWING GRAPHS

A properly drawn graph should have the following properties:

- clearly labelled axes
- the independent variable represented (usually) on the horizontal axis
- a clear heading/caption or reference in the accompanying text
- the units for both axes clearly stated
- the scales given for both axes.

The scales may be, for example:

- linear
- logarithmic
- broken (which can be represented by a break in the axis).

LINEAR RELATIONSHIPS

If the graph of variable y against variable x is a straight line, these variables are related by the equation:

$y = mx + c$

in which m and c are constants: m is the gradient of the line, and c is the intercept of the line on the vertical axis (y-axis).

Power law relationship

If the graph of y against x is a straight line, where $y = \log Y$ and $x = \log X$ (the logarithm is to any base, so long as it is the same one in both cases), then variables X and Y are related by the equation:

$$Y = CX^m$$

in which m and C are constants such that m is the gradient of the line, and $\log C$ is the intercept of the line on the vertical axis (y-axis).

EXPONENTIAL RELATIONSHIPS

If the graph of y against x is a straight line, where $y = \ln Y$ and $x = X$ ($\ln Y$ is the logarithm of Y to base e, that is, $\log_e Y$), then variables X and Y are related by the equation:

$$Y = Ce^{mx}$$

in which m and C are constants such that m is the gradient of the line, and $\ln C$ is the intercept of the line on the vertical axis (y-axis).

This exponential relationship also holds if:

- e is replaced by 10
- $\ln Y$ is replaced by $\log_{10} Y$
- $\ln C$ is replaced by $\log_{10} C$.

OTHER RELATIONSHIPS INVOLVING EXPRESSIONS

If the graph of y against x is a straight line, where $y = g(Y)$ and $x = f(X)$ ($f(X)$ is an expression involving X, and $g(Y)$ is an expression involving Y), then variables X and Y are related by the equation:

$$g(Y) = m\, f(X) + c$$

in which m and c are constants: m is the gradient of the line, and c is the intercept of the line on the vertical axis (y-axis).

Outliers

Outliers are extreme values.

Measures of central tendency

Outliers can exert an extreme effect on the arithmetic mean, particularly when the total number of values is small. The median is less affected in such a case and may therefore be preferred.

Measures of dispersion

Outliers exert an extreme effect on the range. Measures relating to quantiles are less affected in such a case and may therefore be preferred. Since it takes into account all the values in a distribution, the standard deviation (or variance) may be affected by outliers, although less so than the range.

Correlation and linear regression

Outliers may exert an extreme effect on the results of correlation and linear regression. In such cases it may be necessary to consider excluding outliers from the calculations.

Stem-and-leaf plots

Stem-and-leaf plots can be used to represent a continuous variable. Their advantage over histograms is that they allow the representation of all the individual data. The stems consist of a vertical column of numbers on the left-hand side of the plot. The leaves are numbers to the right of the stems, which may, for example, represent tenths. All the individual data can then be derived by combining the individual leaves with their corresponding stems, while the shape of the overall plot indicates the shape of the distribution. They are particularly easy to represent in computer printouts. For instance, the distribution 13.5, 13.7, 14.5, 14.6, 14.6, 14.7, 15.2, 15.9 and 16.4 (arbitrary units) may be represented as the following stem-and-leaf plot:

```
13  5 7
14  5 6 6 7
15  2 9
16  4
```

Boxplots (box-and-whisker plots)

Boxplots can be used to represent a continuous variable. A boxplot consists of a box whose longer sides are placed vertically, with vertical lines (whiskers) extending vertically. It has the following features:

- The upper boundary of the box is the upper (third) quartile.
- The lower boundary of the box is the lower (first) quartile.
- The length of the box is the interquartile range.
- A thick horizontal line inside the box is the median (second quartile).
- The lower whisker extends to the smallest observation, excluding outliers.
- The upper whisker extends to the largest observation, excluding outliers.
- Outliers are indicated by the symbol O.

The above arrangement is sometimes represented horizontally (the whole plot being rotated through $-\pi/2$) if more convenient. Boxplots can be useful for comparing two or more sets of observations diagrammatically, before or in addition to more formal statistical analyses.

Scattergrams (scatter diagrams or dot graphs)

Scattergrams can be used to represent two continuous variables. Two orthogonal axes divide two-dimensional space into a coordinate system, in which each pair of observations is plotted. The two variables can then be compared diagrammatically, before or in addition to more formal statistical analyses.

DESCRIPTIVE AND INFERENTIAL STATISTICS

DESCRIPTIVE STATISTICS

Descriptive statistics are ways of organizing and describing data. Examples include:

- diagrams
- graphical representations
- numerical representations
- tables.

INFERENTIAL STATISTICS

Inferential statistics allow conclusions to be inferred from data. An example is inferring a likely range of values for the population mean from the sample mean.

Hypothesis testing: significance tests

A value or range of values for an unknown population parameter is hypothesized. A study/ experiment is then carried out and the value of the observed random variable is used to test whether or not the hypothesis should be rejected.

Null hypothesis
The initial hypothesis is the null hypothesis, H_0, usually representing no change:

$$H_0: \theta = \theta_0$$

where τ is the unknown parameter and θ_0 is its hypothesized value.

Alternative hypothesis
The alternative hypothesis, H_1, may, for example, be one of the following types:

$$H_1: \theta \neq \theta_0$$
$$H_1: \theta > \theta_0$$
$$H_1: \theta < \theta_0$$
$$H_1: \theta = \theta_1$$

Simple and composite hypotheses

- A simple hypothesis is one involving a single value for the population parameter.
- A composite hypothesis is one involving more than one value for the population parameter.

One-sided significance test
A one-sided significance test is a hypothesis test involving a composite alternative hypothesis of the following types:

$$H_1: \theta > \theta_0$$
$$H_1: \theta < \theta_0$$

Two-sided significance test

A two-sided significance test is a hypothesis test involving a composite alternative hypothesis of the following type:

$H_1: \theta \neq \theta_0$

Critical region and value

- The critical region is the region of the range of the random variable X such that if the observed value x falls in it, the null hypothesis, H_0, is rejected.
- The critical value(s) is (are) the value(s) of the test statistic expected from the null hypothesis, H_0, that define the boundary (boundaries) of the critical region.

Significance level

The significance level, α, is the size of the critical region and represents the following probability:

$\alpha = P(\text{type I error})$

where a type I error is the error of wrongly rejecting H_0 when it is true.

Steps in carrying out a significance/hypothesis test

Hypothesis testing is carried out as follows:

1 Formulate H_0.
2 Formulate H_1.
3 Specify α.
4 Decide on the study/experiment to be carried out.
5 Calculate the test statistic:

Test statistic = (appropriate statistic *minus* hypothesized parameter)/(standard error of statistic).

6 From the sampling distribution of the test statistic, create the test criterion for testing H_0 versus H_1.
7 Carry out the study/experiment.
8 Calculate the value of the test statistic from the sample data.
9 Calculate the value of the difference, d, between the value of the test statistic from the sample and that expected under H_0 (the critical value(s), defining the critical range).
10 If $P(d) < \alpha$, the result is statistically significant at the level of α (the 'p value') and H_0 is rejected.
11 If $P(d) \geq \alpha$, the result is not statistically significant at the level of α and H_0 cannot be rejected.
12 If H_0 is composite, the hypothesis test is designed so that the critical region size is the maximum value of the probability of rejecting H_0 when it is true.

Estimation: confidence intervals

From sample statistics, confidence statements can be made about the corresponding unknown parameters, by constructing confidence intervals. A confidence interval can be two-sided or one-sided; two-sided confidence intervals need not necessarily be symmetrical (central).

If a $100(1 - \alpha)\%$ confidence interval from a statistic (or statistics) is calculated, this implies that if the study were repeated with other random samples taken from the same parent population and further $100(1 - \alpha)\%$ confidence intervals similarly individually calculated, the overall proportion of these confidence intervals which included the corresponding population parameter(s) would tend to $100(1 - \alpha)\%$.

The two-sided central confidence interval for the unknown parameter θ of a distribution with confidence level $(1 - \alpha)$ can be derived from the random interval of the type:

$$(\theta_-(X), \theta_+(X))$$

By substituting the observation x for X, the realization of the random interval, $(\theta_-(x), \theta_+(x))$, is the two-sided central confidence interval for θ, in which:

- $\theta_-(x)$ is the lower confidence limit (confidence bound) for theta;
- $\theta_+(x)$ is the upper confidence limit (confidence bound) for theta.

Advantages of confidence intervals over p values

There has been a recent move away from simply quoting p values in psychiatric research to giving instead, or additionally, the corresponding confidence intervals. Advantages of estimation over hypothesis testing include:

- Testing the null hypothesis is often inappropriate for psychiatric research; for example it may reverse an investigator's idea (for instance that a new treatment will be more effective than a current one) and substitute instead the notion of no effect or no difference.
- A hypothesis test evaluates the probability of the observed study result, or a more extreme result, occurring if the null hypothesis were in fact true.
- Proper understanding of a study result is obscured in hypothesis testing by transforming it on to a remote scale constrained from zero to one.
- Obtaining a low p value, particularly $p < 0.05$, is widely interpreted as implying merit and leads to the findings being deemed important and publishable, whereas this status is often denied study results which have not achieved this arbitrary level.
- The p value on its own implies nothing about the magnitude of any difference between treatments.
- The p value on its own implies nothing even about the direction of any difference between treatments.
- This over-emphasis on hypothesis testing and the use of p values to dichotomize results into significant and non-significant has detracted from more useful procedures for interpreting the results of psychiatric research.
- Levels of significance are often quoted alone in the abstracts and texts of published papers without mentioning actual values, proportions, and so on, or their differences.
- Confidence intervals do not carry with them the pseudo-scientific hypothesis testing language of significance tests.
- Estimation and confidence intervals give a plausible range of values for the unknown parameter.
- Inadequate sample size is indicated by the relatively large width of the corresponding confidence interval.

SPECIFIC TESTS

t-test

The *t*-test is used for testing the null hypothesis that two population means are equal when the variable being investigated has a normal distribution in each population and the population variances are equal; that is, the *t*-test is a parametric test.

Independent-samples t-test

This procedure tests the null hypothesis that the data are a sample from a population in which the mean of a test variable is equal in two independent (unrelated) groups of cases.

Assuming equal population variances (which can be checked using Levene's test), the standard error of the difference between two means, $\bar{x}_1$ and $\bar{x}_2$, of two independent samples (taken from the same parent population) of respective sizes n_1 and n_2, and respective standard deviations s_1 and s_2, ($s_1 \approx s_2$) is given by:

Standard error of difference $= s\sqrt{[1/n_1 + 1/n_2]}$

where the pooled standard deviation s is given by:

$s = \sqrt{\{[(n_1 - 1)s_1^2 + (n_2 - 1)s_2^2]/(n_1 + n_2 - 2)\}}$

If the population variances cannot be assumed to be equal, then the standard error is given by:

Standard error of difference $= \sqrt{[s_1^2/n_1 + s_2^2/n_2]}$

Paired-samples t-test

This procedure tests the null hypothesis that two population means are equal when the observations for the two groups can be paired in some way. Pairing (a repeated-measures or within-subjects design) is used to make the two groups as similar as possible, allowing differences observed between the two groups to be attributed more readily to the variable of interest.

For n pairs, the appropriate standard error is given by:

Standard error of differences of paried observations $= s_d/\sqrt{n}$

where s_d is the standard deviation of the differences of the paired observations.

Chi-squared test

The chi-squared (χ^2) test is a non-parametric test that can be used to compare independent qualitative and discrete quantitative variables presented in the form of contingency tables containing the data frequencies.

Null hypothesis

For a given contingency table, under H_0:

Expected value of a cell $=$ (row total)(column total)/(sum of cells).

Calculation of chi-squared

The value of χ^2 for a contingency table is calculated from:

$\chi^2 = \Sigma[(O - E)^2/E]$

where O is the observed value and E is the expected value.

In order to use the χ^2 distribution, the number of degrees of freedom of a contingency table, v, is given by:

$v = (r - 1)(k - 1)$

where r is the number of rows and k is the number of columns.

2 × 2 contingency table

A 2 × 2 contingency table has one degree of freedom (see Table 6.2).

Table 6.2   *Observed values in a 2 × 2 contingency table*

	–	–	Total
–	a	y	$a + y$
–	b	z	$b + z$
Total	$a + b$	$y + z$	$a + b + y + z$

Reproduced with permission from Puri, B.K. 1996: *Statistics for the Health Sciences.* London: W.B. Saunders.

For a 2 × 2 contingency table, the following formula can be used to calculate ψ^2:

$$\chi^2 = (az - by)^2(a + b + y + z)/[(a + b)(y + z)(a + y)(b + z)]$$

Small expected values

For a contingency table with more than one degree of freedom, the following criteria (Cochran, 1954) should be fulfilled for the test to be valid:

- each expected value ≥ 1
- in at least 80% of cases, expected value >5.

For a 2 × 2 contingency table, all the expected values need to be at least 5 in order to use the above formula; therefore the overall total must be at least 20. If the total is less than 20, Fisher's exact probability test can be used. If $20 \leq$ total < 100, then a better fit with the continuous χ^2 distribution is provided by using Yates' continuity correction:

$$\chi^2_{\text{corrected}} = \{|az - by| - \tfrac{1}{2}(a + b + y + z)\}^2(a + b + y + z)/[(a + b)(y + z)(a + y)(b + z)]$$

Goodness-of-fit

The χ^2 test can be used to test how well an observed distribution fits a given distribution, such as the normal distribution. This can be applied to both discrete and continuous data and tests the hypothesis that a sample derives from a particular model.

Fisher's exact probability test

This test determines exact probabilities for 2 × 2 contingency tables. With the nomenclature of Table 6.2, the formula used is:

Exact probability of table $= (a + y)! \, (b + z)! \, (a + b)! \, (y + z)!/[(a + b + y + z)! \, a! \, b! \, y! \, z!]$

In order to test H_0, in addition to calculating the probability of the given table, the probabilities also have to be calculated of more extreme tables occurring by chance.

Mann–Whitney U test

This is a non-parametric alternative to the independent-samples t-test. The test statistic, U, is the smaller of U_1 and U_2:

$$U_1 = n_1 n_2 + \tfrac{1}{2} n_1 (n_1 + 1) - R_1$$
$$U_2 = n_1 n_2 + \tfrac{1}{2} n_2 (n_2 + 1) - R_2$$

where

n_1 = number of observations in the first group
n_2 = number of observations in the second group
R_1 = sum of the ranks assigned to the first group
R_2 = sum of the ranks assigned to the second group.

For $n_1 \geq 8$ and $n_2 \geq 8$, $U \approx N(\mu, \sigma^2)$, where:

$$\mu = n_1 n_2 / 2$$
$$\sigma^2 = n_1 n_2 (n_1 + n_2 + 1)/12$$

Confidence intervals

CONFIDENCE INTERVAL FOR THE DIFFERENCE BETWEEN TWO MEANS

The $100(1 - \alpha)\%$ confidence interval for the difference between two means is given by:

difference $- t_{1-\alpha/2}$ (standard error of difference)
to difference $+ t_{1-\alpha/2}$ (standard error of difference).

CONFIDENCE INTERVAL FOR THE DIFFERENCE BETWEEN TWO PROPORTIONS

For large sample sizes and population proportions not too close to 0 or 1, the $100(1 - \alpha)\%$ confidence interval for the difference between two proportions is given by:

difference $- z_{1-\alpha/2}$ (standard error of difference)
to difference $+ z_{1-\alpha/2}$ (standard error of difference).

where the standard error of the difference is given by:

Standard error of difference $= \sqrt{[\hat{p}_1 (1 - \hat{p}_1)/n_1 + \hat{p}_2 (1 - \hat{p}_2)/n_2]}$

with

$\hat{p}_1$ = sample estimate of first proportion
$\hat{p}_2$ = sample estimate of second proportion
n_1 = sample size of the first group
n_2 = sample size of the second group.

CONFIDENCE INTERVAL FOR THE DIFFERENCE BETWEEN TWO MEDIANS

For the following confidence intervals to be valid, the assumption is made that the two distributions whose possible difference is being estimated have the same shape but may differ in location.

Two unpaired samples
In order to determine the $100(1 - \alpha)\%$ confidence interval for the difference between two medians, the value of K must first be calculated from:

$$K = n_1 n_2 / 2 - z_{1-\alpha/2} \sqrt{[n_1 n_2 (n_1 + n_2 + 1)/12]}$$

where n_1 and n_2 are the sample sizes (both greater than 25), and K is rounded up to the nearest integer. The total number of possible differences is equal to $n_1 n_2$.

The $100(1 - \alpha)\%$ confidence interval for the median of these differences is from the Kth smallest to the Kth largest of the $n_1 n_2$ differences ($K \in Z^+$).

If n_1 and/or n_2 is less than or equal to 25, then tables based on the value of the corresponding Mann–Whitney test statistic can be used.

Two paired samples

In this case the value of K is calculated from:

$$K = n(n+1)/4 - z_{1-\alpha/2} \sqrt{[n(n+1)(2n+1)/24]}$$

where n (>50) is the the number of paired cases, and K is rounded up to the nearest integer.

The total number of possible means of two differences (including differences with themselves) is equal to $n(n+1)/2$.

The $100(1 - \alpha)\%$ confidence interval for the median of these mean differences is from the Kth smallest to the Kth largest of the $n(n+1)/2$ mean differences ($K \in Z^+$).

If $n \leq 50$, then tables based on the value of the corresponding Mann–Whitney test statistic can be used.

CLINICAL TRIALS

Clinical trials are planned experiments carried out on humans to assess the effectiveness of different forms of treatment.

CLASSIFICATION

The following classification of clinical trials is used by the pharmaceutical industry:

Phase I trial: clinical pharmacology and toxicity
Phase II trial: initial clinical investigation
Phase III trial: full-scale treatment evaluation
Phase IV trial: postmarketing surveillance.

Advantages of randomized trials

In a randomized trial all the subjects have the same probability of receiving each of the different forms of treatment being compared. The advantages of such randomization include:

- The effects of concomitant variables are distributed in a random manner between the comparison groups. These variables may be unknown.
- The allocation of subjects is not carried out in a subjective manner influenced by the biases of the investigators.
- Statistical tests used to analyse the results are on a firm foundation as they are based on what is expected to occur in random samples from parent populations having specified characteristics.

The gold standard of clinical trials is the randomized double-blind controlled trial in which:

- allocation of treatments to subjects is randomized

- each subject does not know which treatment has been received by him/her
- the investigator(s) do not know the treatment allocation before the end of the trial.

Disadvantages of non-randomized trials

Non-randomized trials may have concurrent or historical (that is, non-concurrent) controls. Both types of non-randomized trials have associated disadvantages in comparison with randomized trials.

Concurrent controls
It is not usually possible to confirm that the different treatment groups are comparable. Volunteer bias may also occur, with volunteers faring better than those who refuse to participate in a trial.

Historical controls
Here the control group consists of a group previously given an older/alternative treatment. This group is compared with suitable subjects receiving a new treatment being tested. Disadvantages of using historical controls include:

- It cannot be assumed that everything apart from the new treatment being tested has remained unchanged over time.
- The monitoring and care of current subjects receiving the new treatment are likely to be greater than those of the historical controls.
- The efficacy of the new treatment is likely to be over-estimated.
- The findings of such a trial may be not be widely accepted because of the lack of randomization.

MORE COMPLEX METHODS

FACTOR ANALYSIS

Factor analysis is an attempt to express a set of multivariate data as a linear function of unobserved, underlying dimensions, or (common) factors together with error terms (specific factors). The common factors associated with each observed variable have individual loadings.

PRINCIPAL-COMPONENTS ANALYSIS

Principal-components analysis is used to produce uncorrelated linear combinations of the observed variables of a multivariate dataset. The first component has maximum variance. Successive components account for progressively smaller parts of the total variance. Each component is uncorrelated with preceding components. A plot of the variance of each principal component against the principal-component number is known as a scree plot.

CORRESPONDENCE ANALYSIS

A correspondence analysis is similar to a principal-components analysis but is applied to contingency tables. It allows a two-dimensional contingency table to be presented as a two-dimensional graph in which one set of coordinates represents the rows of the table and the other set represents the columns. Rather than partitioning the total variance, as in principal-components analysis, there is a partition of the value of χ^2 for the contingency table.

DISCRIMINANT ANALYSIS

This is a method of classification applied to a multivariate dataset. Independent variables used to discriminate among the groups are known as discriminating variables. The discriminant function is a linear function of discriminating variables which maximizes the distance (or separation) between groups.

CLUSTER ANALYSIS

This is also a method of classification applied to a multivariate dataset which derives homogeneous groups or clusters of cases based on their values for the variable set. Hierarchical methods can be applied to the clusters.

MULTIVARIATE REGRESSION ANALYSIS

In this method a linear multivariate regression equation is fitted to a multivariate dataset. The multiple-regression coefficient is the maximum correlation between the dependent variable and multiple non-random independent variables, using a least-squares method.

PATH ANALYSIS

A series of multiple-regression analyses are used to allow hypotheses of causality between variables to be modelled and tested. A path diagram allows these variables and their hypothetical relationships to be represented graphically. It shows arrows between the variables, with regression coefficients (known as path coefficients) associated with these arrows. Chi-squared tests are used to test the model.

CANONICAL CORRELATION ANALYSIS

This is an extended form of multivariate regression in which the number of dependent variables is no longer confined to one. The maximum correlation between the set of independent variables and the set of dependent variables is known as the canonical correlation and gives information about interrelationships among the variables.

PROBLEMS OF MEASUREMENT IN PSYCHIATRY

AIMS OF MEASUREMENT

The main aims of measurement in psychiatry are:

- to help in the diagnostic process or in other forms of categorization
- to measure symptomatology ± its change.

PROBLEMS OF MEASUREMENT

Problems in measurement in psychiatry include:

- defining caseness
- assessment of behaviour

- assessment of cognitive performance
- assessment of mood
- assessment of delusions and hallucinations
- assessment of personality
- assessment of psychophysiological functioning
- assessing the degree to which an individual suffers from a psychiatric/psychological disorder.

Measurement methods

A range of measurement methods can be employed in psychiatric/psychological assessments. Examples include:

- observer rated scales: structured and semistructured standardized psychiatric interview schedules
- screening instruments
- behavioural observation studies
- self-predictions
- self-recording (e.g. diaries)
- self-rating scales for the assessment of mood
- self-rating scales for the assessment of personality
- psychophysiological techniques
- naturalistic observations
- psychometric measurements (e.g. of intelligence and personality).

Latent traits (constructs)

Psychological concepts such as attitude and intelligence are considered to be latent traits or hypothetical constructs that are believed to exist. Although not directly observable, constructs can be used to explain phenomena which can be observed and to make predictions. In the development and use of psychometric tests, in particular, factor analysis may be used to identify factors, corresponding to latent traits or hypothetical constructs, that may account for correlations observed between the scores on tests or subtests by a large sample of subjects.

Reliability

The reliability of a test or measuring instrument describes the level of agreement between repeated measurements. It can be expressed as the ratio of the variance of the true scores to the variance of the observed scores:

$$\text{Reliability} = \sigma_t^2/(\sigma_t^2 + \sigma_e^2)$$

where σ_t^2 is the true score variance, and σ_e^2 is the measurement error variance.

With this definition, the range of values that the reliability can take is given by:

$$0 \leq \text{reliability} \leq 1.$$

A low value, close to zero, implies low reliability, while a high value, close to one, implies high reliability.

TYPES OF RELIABILITY

- *Inter-rater reliability.* This describes the level of agreement between assessments of the same material made by two or more assessors at roughly the same time.
- *Intra-rater reliability.* This describes the level of agreement between assessments made by two or more assessors of the same material presented at two or more times.
- *Test–retest reliability.* This describes the level of agreement between assessments of the same material made under similar circumstances but at two different times.
- *Alternative-forms reliability.* This describes the level of agreement between assessments of the same material by two supposedly similar forms of the test or measuring instrument made either at the same time or immediately consecutively.
- *Split-half reliability.* This describes the level of agreement between assessments by two halves of a split test or measuring instrument of the same material made under similar circumstances. Since some tests or measuring instruments contain different sections measuring different aspects, in such cases it may be appropriate to create the halves by using alternative questions, thereby maintaining the balance of each half.

Statistical tests of reliability

PERCENTAGE AGREEMENT

Measuring the percentage agreement is the simplest but most unsatisfactory method of assessing the reliability, since it does not take into account agreement between observers owing to chance.

PRODUCT–MOMENT CORRELATION COEFFICIENT

The product–moment correlation coefficient, r, may give spuriously high results, particularly if there is chance agreement of many values. It may even give the maximum value of 1 for the agreement between two raters, even if they do not agree at all – if, for example, one of the raters consistently rates scores on the test or measuring instrument at twice the values rated by the other rater.

KAPPA STATISTIC

The kappa statistic (or coefficient), κ, is a measure of agreement in which allowance is made for chance agreement. It is most appropriate when different categories of measurement are being recorded and is calculated from the following formula:

$$\kappa = (P_o - P_c)/(1 - P_c)$$

where P_c is the chance agreement, and P_o is the observed proportion of agreement.
The range of values that κ can take is:

- $\kappa = 1$: complete agreement
- $0 < \kappa < 1$: observed agreement > chance agreement
- $\kappa = 0$: observed agreement = chance agreement
- $\kappa < 0$: observed agreement < chance agreement.

The weighted kappa, κ_w, is a version of κ that takes into account differences in the seriousness of disagreements (represented by the weightings).

INTRA–CLASS CORRELATION COEFFICIENT

The intra-class correlation coefficient, r_i, is more appropriate than κ or r if agreement is being measured for several items that can be regarded as part of a continuum or dimension. For two raters the value of r_i is derived from the corresponding value of r:

$$r_i = \{[\Sigma(s_1^2 + s_2^2) - (s_1 - s_2)^2]r - (\bar{x}_1 - \bar{x}_2)^2/2\}/\{(s_1^2 + s_2^2) + (\bar{x}_1 - \bar{x}_2)^2/2\}$$

where

r = product–moment correlation coefficient between the scores of the two raters
s_1 = standard deviation of the scores for the first rater
s_2 = standard deviation of the scores for the second rater
$\bar{x}_1$ = mean of the scores for the first rater
$\bar{x}_2$ = mean of the scores for the second rater.

It follows that:

If $\bar{x}_1 = \bar{x}_2$ and $s_1 = s_2$
then $r_i = r$;
else $r_i < r$

For more than two raters, the value of r_i is derived from the corresponding two-way ANOVA for (raters × subjects):

$$r_i = n_s(s_{ms} - e_{ms})/\{n_s s_{ms} + n_t r_{ms} + (n_s n_r - n_s - n_r)e_{ms}\}$$

where

n_r = number of raters
n_s = number of subjects
e_{ms} = error mean square
r_{ms} = raters mean square
s_{ms} = subjects mean square.

CRONBACH'S ALPHA

Cronbach's alpha, α, gives a measure of the average correlation between all the items when assessing split-half reliability. It thereby indicates the internal consistency of the test or measuring instrument.

Validity

The validity of a test or measuring instrument is the term used to describe whether it measures what it purports to measure.

TYPES OF VALIDITY

- *Face validity*. This is the subjective judgement as to whether a test or measuring instrument appears on the surface to measure the feature in question. In spite of its name it is not strictly a type of validity.
- *Content validity*. This examines whether the specific measurements aimed for by the test or measuring instrument are assessing the content of the measurement in question.

- *Predictive validity*. This determines the extent of agreement between a present measurement and one in the future.
- *Concurrent validity*. This compares the measure being assessed with an external valid yardstick at the same time.
- *Criterion validity*. This refers to predictive and concurrent validity together.
- *Incremental validity*. This indicates whether the measurement being assessed is superior to other measurements in approaching true validity.
- *Cross-validity*. Cross-validation of a test or measuring instrument is used to determine whether, after having its criterion validity established for one sample, it maintains criterion validity when applied to another sample.
- *Convergent validity*. Convergent validity is established when measures expected to be correlated, since they measure the same phenomena, are indeed found to be associated.
- *Divergent validity*. Divergent validity is established when measures discriminate successfully between other measures of unrelated constructs.
- *Construct validity*. Construct validity is determined by establishing both convergent and divergent validity, and is closely connected with the theoretical rationale underpinning the test or measuring instrument. It involves showing the power of the hypothetical construct(s) or latent traits both to explain observations and to make predictions.

Type I error

A type I error is the error of wrongly rejecting hypothesis H_0 when it is true. As mentioned above, the probability of making a type I error is denoted by α, the significance level:

$$\alpha = P(\text{type I error})$$

Type II error

A type II error is the error of wrongly accepting hypothesis H_0 when it is false. The probability of making a type II error is denoted by β:

$$\beta = P(\text{type II error})$$

Power

The power of a test is the probability that hypothesis H_0 is rejected when it is indeed false. It is related to β, the probability of making a type II error, in the following way:

$$\text{Power} = 1 - \beta$$

Sensitivity

The sensitivity of a test or measuring instrument is the proportion of positive results/cases correctly identified:

Sensitivity = (true positive)/(true positive *plus* false negative).

This ratio needs to be multiplied by 100 if the sensitivity is to be given as a percentage.

Specificity

The specificity of a test or measuring instrument is the proportion of negative results/cases correctly identified:

Specificity = (true negative)/(true negative *plus* false positive).

This ratio needs to be multiplied by 100 if the sensitivity is to be given as a percentage.

Predictive values

The predictive value of a *positive* result from a research measure is the proportion of the positive results that is true positive:

Predictive value of a positive result = (true positive)/(true positive *plus* false positive).

The predictive value of a *negative* result from a research measure is the proportion of the negative results that is true negative:

Predictive value of a negative result = (true negative)/(true negative *plus* false negative).

Biases

- *Selection bias.* This occurs when a characteristic associated with the variable(s) of interest leads to higher or lower participation in the research study, such as an epidemiological cross-sectional survey.
- *Observer bias.* In epidemiological studies, observer bias occurs when the researcher has clues about whether the subject is in the case or comparison group, leading to a biased assessment. This is particularly likely in studies involving retrospective assessments.
- *Recall bias.* In epidemiological studies, recall bias occurs when there is a difference in knowledge between the subjects in the case and in the comparison groups, leading to a biased recall. For example, in case–control studies the knowledge on the part of subjects (or, in the case of childhood disorders, their parents) as to whether or not they have a given disorder may bias their recall of exposure to putative risk factors.
- *Information bias.* Information bias includes both observer bias and recall bias.
- *Confounding bias.* In epidemiological studies, confounding bias occurs when the actual, but unexamined, underlying cause of the disorder being researched is associated with both the suspected risk factor and the disorder.

META-ANALYSIS, SURVIVAL ANALYSIS AND LOGISTIC REGRESSION

Meta-analysis

The term 'meta-analysis' is used to describe the process of evaluating and statistically combining results from two or more existing independent randomized clinical trials addressing similar questions in order to give an overall assessment.

DIFFICULTIES

The following are some difficulties associated with meta-analysis:

- There may be publication bias – trials showing a statistically significant difference are more likely to be published than those not finding a statistically significant result.
- Researchers finding 'non-significant' results may be less likely formally to write up their results for publication.
- One must arrive at selection criteria to determine which studies to include and which not to include in the meta-analysis.
- The different centres in which the different clinical trials have taken place may differ with respect to important variables in such a way as seriously to question the validity of combining their data.
- If the meta-analysis is of clinical trials carried out on widely differing population groups, to whom can the results of the meta-analysis properly be applied?

Survival analysis

This is a collection of statistical analysis techniques that can be applied to situations in which the time to a given event, such as death, illness onset or recovery, is measured, but not all individuals necessarily have to have reached this event during the overall time interval studied.

Survival function
The survival function, $S(t)$, is given by:

$$S(t) = P(t_s > t)$$

where t is time and t_s is the survival time. The survival function is also given by:

$$S(t) = 1 \ minus \ \text{cumulative distribution function of } t_s.$$

Survival curve
This is a plot of $S(t)$ (on the ordinate) versus t (on the abscissa). Instead of being drawn as continuous curves, sometimes survival curves are drawn in a stepwise fashion, with the steps occurring between estimated cumulative survival probabilities.

Hazard function
This measures the likelihood of an individual experiencing a given event, such as death, illness onset or recovery, as a function of time.

Logistic regression

This is a regression model used to predict the probability of a dichotomous variable, such as better/not better at the end of the treatment period, on the basis of a set of independent variables, x_1 to x_n:

$$P(\text{event}) = 1/\{1 + \exp[-(\alpha_0 + \alpha_1 x_1 + \ldots + \alpha_n x_n)]\}$$

where the coefficients α_0 to α_n are estimated using a maximum-likelihood method.

BIBLIOGRAPHY

Altman, D.G. 1991: *Practical Statistics for Medical Research*. London: Chapman & Hall.

Bryman, A. & Cramer, D. 1994: *Quantitative Data Analysis for Social Scientists*, revised edn. London: Routledge.

Cochran, W.G. 1954: Some methods for strengthening the common χ^2-test. *Biometrics* 10:417–451.

Coolican, H. 1994: *Research Methods and Statistics in Psychology*, 2nd edn. London: Hodder & Stoughton.

Dunn, G. & Everitt, B. 1995: *Clinical Biostatistics: An Introduction to Evidence-based Medicine*. London: Arnold.

Everitt, B. & Hay, D. 1992: *Talking About Statistics: A Psychologist's Guide to Design and Analysis*. London: Arnold.

Puri, B.K. 1996: *Statistics for the Health Sciences*. London: W.B. Saunders.

Puri, B.K. 2002: *SPSS in Practice: An Illustrated Guide*, 2nd edn. London: Arnold.

7

Social sciences

DESCRIPTIVE TERMS

Social class

A social class is a segment of the population sharing a broadly similar type and level of resources, with a broadly similar style of living and some shared perception of its common condition.

Determinants
The determinants of social class include:

- education
- financial status
- occupation
- type of residence
- geographical area of residence
- leisure activities.

Occupational classification
In British psychiatry, the following occupationally based classification given by the Office of Population Censuses and Surveys has traditionally been used:

Social class I: professional, higher managerial, landowners
Social class II: intermediate
Social class III: skilled, manual, clerical
Social class IV: semi-skilled
Social class V: unskilled
Social class 0: unemployed, students.

Members of the same household are assigned to the social class of the head of the household.

Socioeconomic status

The socioeconomic status of an individual is his or her position in the social hierarchy. It is related to social class and may increase, for example through educational achievement, or decrease, for example through unemployment or mental illness.

Relevance to psychiatric disorder and health care delivery

Psychiatric disorder

The incidence and prevalence of many psychiatric disorders have been found to vary with social class. In particular, the following disorders are more likely to be diagnosed in the lower social classes:

* schizophrenia
* alcohol dependence
* organic psychosis
* depressive episodes in women
* parasuicide/deliberate self-harm
* personality disorder.

The following disorders are more likely to be diagnosed in the upper social classes:

* anorexia nervosa in females
* bulimia nervosa in females
* bipolar mood disorder.

Relationship between social class and psychiatric disorder

The existence of a relationship between social class and a given psychiatric disorder does not necessarily imply causation, from social class to the disorder. In general, the following are possible explanations of such a relationship:

* *Downward social drift.* For example, the increased representation of schizophrenia in lower social classes may be partly a result of social drift.
* *Environmental stress.* Lower social class is associated with adverse life situations, material deprivation and the lower self-esteem that manual jobs entail. Women in lower social classes are more likely to experience severe life events and vulnerability factors.
* *Differential labelling.* For example, it may be that some people in Britain of Afro-Caribbean origin are more likely to be detained under mental health legislation and diagnosed as suffering from schizophrenia (although this may in fact reflect genuine differences in prevalence and incidence rates).
* *Differential treatment.* For example, there is a difference in the type of psychiatric treatment likely to be received by those from different social classes (see below).

Health care delivery

Those with a psychiatric disorder who are from lower social classes are more likely to:

* be admitted to hospital as psychiatric in-patients
* remain as psychiatric in-patients for longer
* receive physical treatments (e.g. electroconvulsive therapy).

Those with a psychiatric disorder who are from upper social classes are more likely to:

- spend a shorter period of time as psychiatric in-patients
- be treated as psychiatric out-patients without in-patient admission
- receive psychological treatments (e.g. individual psychotherapy).

Pathways to psychiatric care

Goldberg and Huxley (1980) described the existence of filters to psychiatric care, each of which depends on:

- social factors (e.g. such as age, sex, ethnic background, socioeconomic status)
- service organization and provision (e.g. time and location of clinics, length of waiting list)
- aspects of the disorder itself (e.g. its severity and chronicity).

These filters include:

- the decision to consult the general practitioner
- recognition of the disorder by the general practitioner
- the decision by the general practitioner as to whether or not to refer the patient to a specialist.

The Black Report on socioeconomic inequalities in health

According to the Black Report of 1980, which explored the difference in health and mortality in Britain between the social classes, when compared with individuals in social class I, individuals in social class V:

- have twice the neonatal mortality
- are twice as likely to die before retirement
- have an increased rate of almost all diseases.

Explanations

The following explanations for the relationship between social class and illness found in the Black Report on socioeconomic inequalities in health have been suggested:

- *Artefactual*. The health inequalities found are artificial.
- *Natural and social selection*. Good health is associated with an improvement in social class while poor health is associated with social drift downwards.
- *Materialist/structural*. Poor health is primarily a function of material deprivation. Inequalities in wealth and income distribution are associated with inequalities in health.
- *Cultural/behavioural*. Certain unhealthy behaviour patterns are more common in lower social classes (e.g. smoking, unhealthy diets), leading to health inequalities.

Changes after 10 years

A decade after the publication of the Black Report, Smith *et al.* (1990) reported the following:

- Social class differences in mortality had widened.
- Better measures of socioeconomic position showed greater inequalities in mortality.
- Inequalities in health had been found in all countries that collect relevant data.
- Measurement artefacts and social selection did not account for mortality differences.
- Social class differences existed for health during life as well as for the length of life.
- Trends in income distribution suggested a further likely widening of mortality differences.

HISTORICAL SOCIOLOGICAL THEORIES

Max Weber

Max Weber was born in Erfurt in Prussia in 1864, and died in Munich, Germany, in 1920.

Bureaucracy

Weber studied bureaucracy, starting with his 1908 studies on *Economies of Antiquity*. He started by outlining the development of modern forms of administration, and put forward the notion that states in which the political machinery was centred around officialdom formed the basis of modern bureaucratic structures. (He considered that ancient societies were not bureaucratic in the same way.) He suggested that there existed the following types of bureaucracy:

- religious communities
- states
- economies
- the judiciary
- the modern agency
- the military.

Rationalization

Rationalization was the term used to denote the way in which nature, society and the actions of individuals were oriented towards planning, technical procedures and rational actions.

Religion

According to Weber, social change can be caused by religious belief. He suggested that change can both cause and be caused by ideas. His thesis of *The Protestant Ethic and the Spirit of Capitalism* related capitalism to Protestantism. He had noted that, in his native Germany, there was a positive association between success in capitalist ventures and being of the Protestant faith or background. This association was caused, according to Weber, by the consequences of Puritan theology (as a reaction to the severity of Calvinism). For example, the combination of the work ethic (based on the Fourth Commandment), the belief that gain of wealth was a sign of being blessed, and an ascetic unwillingness of Puritans to enjoy the fruits of such labour themselves, would lead overall to yet further accumulation of capital.

Karl Marx

Karl Heinrich Marx was born in Trier in Prussia in 1818, and died in London, England, in 1883.

Communism

After he and his wife (newly wed) moved to Paris in 1843, Marx became a communist, authoring *Economic and Philosophic Manuscripts of 1844* (which was not published for about a century). In collaboration with Engels, he co-authored *The German Ideology* in 1845/6 (published in 1932), in which it was argued that historically nation states and societies generally had developed in such a way that the interests of the economically dominant class were favoured. (Such arguments might account for the difficulty that Marx and Engels encountered in trying to find a publisher for this work.) Some of the unpublished ideas contained in this work were summarized by Marx and Engels in their 1848 pamphlet *The Communist Manifesto*. Here, they also argued that all history had fundamentally been a history of class struggle.

Crime

Marx argued that powerful entities, such as corporations, could influence the definition of crime. Thus, while white collar crime was deemed punishable, acts by more privileged members of society, such as fraud and tax evasion, might go unpunished. Furthermore, corporate crimes might be carried out in order to increase company profits, even if they involved engaging in activities that may harm people (for instance, not paying heed to laws on health and safety, or disposing of toxic waste inappropriately).

Religion

Arguing that religion was 'an opiate of the masses', Marx held that religion came from the oppressed but benefited those at the top in society. He thought that organized religion:

- helped to anaesthetize the pain caused by oppression
- promised a reward in heaven or the after-life for those who endured oppression in their current lives
- provided justification for the current social order, including the position in this that a believer found themselves in
- promised that good behaviour would be rewarded
- suggested to the population that the current problems on the planet would be solved through divine intervention.

Emile Durkheim

Emile Durkheim was born in Epinal in France in 1858, and died in Paris, France, in 1917.

Anomie

Durkheim introduced the term 'anomie' to refer to social disconnectedness or a lack of social norms, which may be caused by a change in an individual's relationship with his or her social group, in which norms for conduct are absent, weak or conflicting. Two types of anomie may be distinguished (Boulton, 1998):

- *Acute anomie.* This is caused by a sudden change or crisis that leaves the individual in an unfamiliar situation.
- *Chronic anomie.* This refers to circumstances in which the rules of a social group have become unclear to the individual or do not provide the means of meeting his or her aspirations.

Causes of acute anomie include:

- migration
- bereavement
- work redundancy.

Causes of chronic anomie include:

- homelessness
- long-term unemployment.

Widespread anomie may lead to a breakdown in social order. Durkheim considered that science (in particular, social science), educational reform, and religion were ways of avoiding this.

Suicide

In his 1897 work *Suicide*, Durkheim suggested that there appeared to be an inverse relationship between, on the one hand, how integrated individuals were in their society and culture, and, on the other hand, the rate of suicide. A major cause of suicide, then, could be seen in terms of social forces. According to Durkheim there were, in fact, three types of suicide:

- *Altruistic suicide.* This results from social integration in a culture that accepts suicide as a way of expiating shame or blame.
- *Egoistic suicide.* This results in the context of the individual being socially further distanced from social norms and restraints, such that meaning is questioned.
- *Anomic suicide.* This also results in the context of the individual being socially further distanced from social norms and restraints, in which anomie exists.

Michel Foucault

Michel Foucault was born in Poitiers in France in 1926, and died in Paris, France, in 1984.

Principles of exclusion

In books such as his 1975 work *Discipline and Punish: The Birth of the Prison*, Foucault put forward his thesis that society uses institutions to carry out social exclusion. Such institutions included, he argued, the following:

- asylums
- hospitals
- prisons.

With regard to mental illness, Foucault argued that one of the principles of exclusion that society uses to define itself is the distinction between sanity and insanity.

Sexuality

Foucault made a study of the history of sexuality from ancient times. This was published in his 1976 to 1984 three-volume work *History of Sexuality*.

Talcott Parsons

Talcott Parsons was born in Colorado Springs in the USA in 1902, and died in Munich, Germany, in 1979. Aspects of his contribution to sociological theories are given elsewhere in this chapter.

Erving Goffman

Erving Goffman was born in Canada in 1922, and died in Philadelphia, USA, in 1982. Aspects of his contribution to sociological theories are given elsewhere in this chapter.

Jürgen Habermas

Jürgen Habermas was born in 1929 in Düsseldorf, Germany. In his two-volume magnus opus, *The Theory of Communicative Action*, Habermas built on the sociological theories of Max Weber, George

Herbert Mead, Emile Durkheim and Talcott Parsons to suggest reasoning capacities, besides traditional cognitive–instrumental reasoning, which carry out subjective and inter-subjective functions within the framework of societal interactions. He has gone on to defend modern society and civil society.

SOCIAL ROLES OF DOCTORS AND ILLNESS

SOCIAL ROLE

The social role of an individual in society is the pattern of behaviour in given social situations expected of that person in relation to his or her social status. It consists of:

- obligations – behaviours towards others expected of the individual
- rights – behaviours from others expected in return for obligations.

SOCIAL ROLE OF DOCTORS

In the model proposed by Parsons (1951), the role of the doctor includes:

- defining illness
- legitimizing illness
- imposing an illness diagnosis if necessary
- offering appropriate help.

Doctors therefore control access to the 'sick role' and they and patients have reciprocal obligations and rights.

The sick role

The sick role was defined by Parsons (1951) as the role given by society to a sick individual, and was considered to carry rights or privileges and obligations.

Rights (privileges)
According to Parsons, the sick role carries the following two rights for the sick individual:

- exemption from blame for the illness
- exemption from normal responsibilities while sick, such as the need to go to work.

Obligations
The sick individual has the following obligations:

- the wish to recover as soon as possible, including seeking appropriate help from the doctor
- cooperation with medical investigations and acceptance of medical advice and treatment.

Illness behaviour

Illness behaviour is a set of stages describing the behaviour adopted by sick individuals (Mechanic, 1978). It describes the way in which individuals respond to somatic symptoms and signs and the conditions under which they come to view them as abnormal. Illness behaviour therefore involves the manner in which individuals:

- monitor their bodies
- define and interpret their symptoms and signs
- take remedial action
- utilize sources of help.

Stages of illness behaviour
Illness behaviour includes the following stages:

The person is initially well.
Symptoms of the illness begin to be experienced.
The opinion of immediate social contacts is sought.
Contact is made with a doctor (or doctors).
The illness is legitimized by the doctor(s).
The individual adopts the sick role.
On recovery (or death), the dependent stage of the sick role is given up.
A rehabilitation stage is entered if the individual recovers.

Determinants of illness behaviour
The determinants of illness behaviour, according to Mechanic (1978), are:

- the visibility, recognizability or perceptual salience of deviant signs and symptoms
- the extent to which symptoms are seen as being serious
- the extent to which symptoms disrupt the family, work, and other social activities
- the frequency of appearance of deviant signs or symptoms, their persistence, and the frequency of recurrence
- the tolerance threshold of exposed deviant signs and symptoms
- available information, knowledge and cultural understanding of exposed deviant signs and symptoms
- basic needs leading to denial
- the competition between needs and illness responses
- competing interpretations assigned to recognized symptoms
- the availability and physical proximity of treatment resources and the costs in terms of time, money, effort and stigma.

FAMILY LIFE IN RELATION TO MAJOR MENTAL ILLNESS

Family life is guided by the explicit and implicit relationship rules that prescribe and limit the behaviour of members of the family and provide expectations within the family with respect to the roles, actions and consequences of individuals.

Elements of family functioning

Elements of family functioning of importance in relation to major mental illness (after Dare, 1985) include:

- *interactional patterns*: family members and relationships, communication patterns, hierarchical structure, control/authority systems, relationship with the outside world
- *sociocultural context of the family*: socioeconomic status, social mobility, migration status
- *location of the family in the life cycle*: number of transitions, adaptation requirements
- *inter-generational structure*: experiences of parents as children, influences of grandparents and extended family
- *family significance*: the significance of symptoms of mental illness for the family
- *family problem-solving skills*: family style, previous experience.

Schizophrenia

Historically, the following types of family dysfunction were at various times believed to be a cause of schizophrenia:

- schizophrenogenic mother
- double-bind
- marital skew and marital schism
- abnormal family communications.

These theories are now out of favour, but there is evidence for the more recent theory relating to the effects of expressed emotion with respect to relapse in schizophrenia.

Schizophrenogenic mother
This concept was put forward by Fromm-Reichman in 1948. Schizophrenia was said to be a consequence of an inadequate relationship between the future sufferer from schizophrenia, as a child, and his or her mother. Characteristics of the schizophrenogenic mother were said to include her being:

- rejecting
- aloof
- overly protective
- overtly hostile.

Double-bind
This concept was put forward by Bateson and colleagues in 1956. The parents communicated with the child (the future sufferer from schizophrenia) in abnormal ways leading to feelings of ambivalence and ambiguity, with messages that were typically:

- vague
- ambiguous
- confusing.

Schizophrenia developed as a result of exposure to such double-bind situations.

Marital skew and marital schism
This concept was put forward by Lidz and colleagues in 1957:

- *marital skew*: dominant and eccentric mother; passive and dependent father
- *marital schism*: parental conflict, argument, and hostility leading to divided loyalties to mother and father on the part of the child (the future sufferer from schizophrenia).

Abnormal family communications

This concept was put forward by Wynne and colleagues in 1958 and suggested that disordered communication took place between the parents of schizophrenics.

Expressed emotion

In an outcome study of 200 patients, mainly with schizophrenia, Brown *et al.* (1958) found that those discharged to their families had a poor outcome, with the highest relapse rate occurring in those families having close and frequent contact with the patients.

Subsequent follow-up studies have confirmed the association of high expressed emotion in families, characterized by the frequent, intense expression of emotion and a pushy and critical attitude by relatives to the patient, with an increased relapse rate in family members with schizophrenia.

In assessing expressed emotion, the five relevant scales of the Camberwell Family Interview (CFI) are:

- *critical comments*: indicating unambiguous dislike or disapproval
- *hostility*: expressed towards the person rather than his or her behaviour
- *emotional over-involvement*: exaggerated self-sacrificing or over-protective concern
- *warmth*: based on sympathy, affection and empathy
- *positive remarks*: expressing praise or approval of the patient.

The first three of these are associated with high expressed emotion and predict relapse (Vaughn & Leff, 1976), as shown in Table 7.1.

Table 7.1 *Effects of expressed emotion on the relapse rates of treated and untreated patients with schizophrenia in the 9 months following discharge*

	Relapse rate in 9 months following discharge
Antipsychotic medication, low expressed emotion family	12%
Antipsychotic medication, high expressed emotion family, <35 hours/week face-to-face contact	42%
No antipsychotic medication, high expressed emotion family, >35 hours/week face-to-face contact	92%

Mood disorders

Expressed emotion

As with schizophrenia, high expressed emotion at home is associated with an increased risk of relapse of depression.

Vulnerability factors

Two of the four vulnerability factors found by Brown and Harris to make women more susceptible to suffer from depression following life events (see below) were:

- lack of a confiding relationship
- having three or more children under the age of 15 years at home.

Problem drinking and alcohol dependence

Family life often suffers as a result of excessive alcohol consumption, with the breakdown of relationships, marriages and families being common. This may result from the following consequences of excessive alcohol consumption:

- mood changes
- personality deterioration
- verbal abuse
- physical violence
- psychosexual disorders
- pathological jealousy
- associated gambling
- associated abuse of other psychoactive substances.

Learning disability/mental retardation

Psychological processes that may occur in families with an impaired or disabled member (after Bicknell, 1983) include:

- shock → panic → denial
- denial → shopping around
- denial → over-protection/rejection
- grief → projection of grief
- guilt
- anger
- bargaining → late rejection
- acceptance → infantilization
- ego-centred work → 'other'-centred work
- over-identification.

LIFE EVENTS

Definition
Life events are sudden changes, which may be positive or negative, in an individual's social life which disrupt its normal course.

Life-change scale
Table 7.2 gives some life-change values for life events in the Holmes and Rahe Social Readjustment Rating Scale (after Holmes & Rahe, 1967).

The full Holmes and Rahe Social Readjustment Rating Scale introduced in 1967 consists of a self-report questionnaire containing 43 classes of life event.

Aetiology of psychiatric disorders

In order to demonstrate that life events have an aetiological role in a given psychiatric disorder, the following criteria should be fulfilled:

Table 7.2 *Some life-change values for life events in the Holmes & Rahe Social Readjustment Rating Scale*

Life event	Life-change value
Death of spouse	100
Divorce	73
Marital separation	65
Gaol term	63
Death of close family member	63
Personal injury or illness	53
Marriage	50
Being sacked from job	47
Retirement	45
Marital reconciliation	45
Pregnancy	40
Birth of child	39
Death of close friend	37
Child leaving home for good	29
Problems with in-laws	29
Problems with boss	23
Change in sleeping habits	16
Change in eating habits	15
Minor legal violation	11

- The occurrence of life events should correlate with onset of the disorder.
- The life events should precede the onset of the disorder and not the other way round.
- A hypothetical construct should exist with confounded variables excluded.
- The relationship between life events and the psychiatric disorder should be found to occur in different populations and at different times.

Difficulties in the evaluation of life events

There are methodological problems in the evaluation of life events:

- Assessments tend to be retrospective, which can lead to difficulties such as:
  - biased recall
  - fall-off in recall with time
  - retrospective contamination
  - effort after meaning.
- Causation and association need to be separated.
- There is contextual evaluation.
- There is subjective evaluation.

A widely used instrument for current research into life events and psychiatric disorder is the Life Events and Difficulties Schedule (LEDS) of Brown and Harris (1978, 1989) which has the following features:

- semi-structured interview schedule
- 38 areas probed
- detailed narratives collected about events, including their circumstances

- high reliability
- high validity.

Clinical significance

Depression
Many studies have found a relationship between life events and the onset of depression. In the 6–12 months prior to the onset, compared with normal controls, patients have a three- to five-fold greater chance of having suffered at least one life event with major negative long-term implications (involving threat or loss). However, most people who experience adverse life events do not develop depression; as mentioned above, Brown and Harris (1978) identified four vulnerability factors that make women more susceptible to suffer from depression following life events:

- loss of mother before the age of 11 years
- not working outside the home
- a lack of a confiding relationship
- having three or more children under the age of 15 years at home.

Schizophrenia
The evidence tends to suggest that independent life events are more likely to occur prior to relapse rather than prior to first onset of schizophrenia (Brown & Birley, 1968; Tennant, 1985).

Anxiety
There is some evidence that life events are more likely to occur prior to anxiety (Finlay-Jones & Brown, 1981; Miller & Ingham, 1985). From their study of life events occurring in the year before the onset of three types of cases of psychiatric disorder of recent onset (depression, anxiety, and mixed depression/anxiety) in young women, and normal controls, Finlay-Jones and Brown (1981) argued that a life event involving severe loss was a causal agent in the onset of depression, and life events involving severe danger were a causal agent in the onset of anxiety states. Cases of mixed depression/anxiety were more likely to report both a severe loss and a severe danger before onset.

Mania
In general, the results of life-event studies of mania are conflicting.

Parasuicide/deliberate self–harm
There is strong evidence that threatening life events are more common prior to self-poisoning attempts (e.g. Morgan *et al.*, 1975; Farmer & Creed, 1989).

Functional disorders
Threatening life events have been found to be more likely to precede functional disorders presenting physically such as abdominal pain without an organic cause (Creed, 1981; Craig & Brown, 1984) and menorrhagia (Harris, 1989).

RESIDENTIAL INSTITUTIONS

SOCIAL INSTITUTIONS: DEFINITION AND EXAMPLES

A social institution is an established and sanctioned form of relationship between social beings. Examples of social institutions include:

- the family
- political parties
- religious groups.

TOTAL INSTITUTIONS: DEFINITION AND EXAMPLES

A total institution is an organization in which a large number of like-situated individuals, cut off from the wider society for an appreciable period of time, together lead an enclosed formally administered round of life (Goffman, 1961). Examples of total institutions include:

- older large psychiatric hospitals
- prisons
- monasteries
- large ships.

GOFFMAN

From his study of the large St Elizabeth's Hospital in Washington, DC, Goffman (1961) was one of the first to suggest that institutions may be harmful. Concepts introduced by Goffman include:

- *The total institution.*
- *Binary management.* The daily lives of patients were highly regulated by staff who appeared to live in a different world to the patients.
- *Binary living.*
- *Batch living.* Whereas normally life consists of a balance between work, home life and leisure time, these three distinct entities did not exist in the total institution studied.
- *Institutional perspective.* The existence of an institutional perspective leads to the assumption that there exists an overall rational plan.
- *Mortification process.* This is the process whereby an individual becomes an inhabitant of a total institution.
- *Betrayal funnel.* This is the start of the mortification process through which relatives, via doctors, send the individual into a psychiatric hospital.
- *Role-stripping.* The patient is processed through the admissions procedure, which would also usually include being physically stripped naked for the purposes of a physical examination.
- *Patient/inmate role.* Patients or inmates could be considered to be metaphorically baptized into this role through the admissions procedure, which would usually include bathing before being given institutional clothing.
- *Moral career.* There are gradual changes in perception of patients about themselves and others, occurring as a result of institutionalization.

Reactions to the mortification process

According to Goffman, patients were said to show various possible reactions to the mortification process, including:

- withdrawal
- open rebellion
- colonization – the patient pretends to show acceptance
- conversion
- institutionalization – actual acceptance both outwardly and inwardly.

INSTITUTIONAL NEUROSIS

Barton (1959) used the term 'institutional neurosis' to describe a syndrome he considered to be caused by institutions in which the individual shows:

- apathy
- inability to plan for the future
- submissiveness
- withdrawal
- low self-esteem.

SECONDARY AND PRIMARY HANDICAPS

Wing (1967, 1978) used the term 'secondary handicap' to include both institutional neurosis and similar features occurring in individuals living outside total institutions.

- *Primary handicap.* This may be psychiatric illness, somatic illness, or social difficulties that the individual has to contend with.
- *Secondary handicap.* This results from the unfortunate way in which other people may react to the primary handicap, both inside and outside total institutions.

THE THREE MENTAL HOSPITALS STUDY

Wing and Brown (1961, 1970) carried out an important comparative study in the 1960s of three British mental hospitals (Netherne Hospital, South London; Severalls Hospital, Essex; and Mapperley Hospital, Nottingham). These hospitals were chosen because they had different social conditions but otherwise were similar in that they had patients with schizophrenia who suffered illnesses of similar severity, similar catchment area populations, and all such patients were accepted for admission. Thus it was hoped to test the hypothesis that social environment could influence schizophrenic symptoms and behaviour. A strong association was found between poverty of the social environment and severity of 'clinical poverty', the latter consisting of:

- blunted affect
- poverty of speech
- social withdrawal.

ETHNIC MINORITIES, ADAPTATION AND MENTAL HEALTH

PREVALENCE OF SCHIZOPHRENIA

In Britain, there is a higher rate of diagnosis of schizophrenia in Afro-Caribbean and Irish populations, compared with the indigenous population, and a lower rate in those of South Asian origin.

Causes of different prevalence rates

There are various explanations of the differing prevalence rates of schizophrenia in ethnic minorities in Britain:

- Those who migrate from their countries of origin have a greater likelihood of having schizophrenia or a predisposition for schizophrenia (social selection). However, there is a reduced rate in Asians and an increased rate in second-generation Afro-Caribbeans.
- Migration is associated with increased stress leading to an increased precipitation of schizophrenia in those with an underlying predisposition. However, there is a reduced rate in Asians and an increased rate in second-generation Afro-Caribbeans.
- Discrimination and deprivation lead to an increased rate of schizophrenia, or an increased precipitation of schizophrenia in those with an underlying predisposition (social causation). However, there is a reduced rate in Asians.
- Schizophrenia is over-diagnosed in Afro-Caribbeans.

DEPRESSION AND ANXIETY

Those from ethnic minorities may not tell their doctor they feel depressed or anxious. For example:

- Afro-Caribbean men when depressed may instead complain of erectile dysfunction or reduced libido.
- South Asians may somatize depression and/or anxiety.

PROFESSIONS

CHARACTERISTICS OF PROFESSIONS

The characteristics of professional status include:

- the possession of practical skills based on theoretical knowledge aquired over an extended period of formal training/education
- assessments of competence carried out by the profession
- belonging to an organization
- recognition by the state of the professional organization
- adherence to a code of conduct
- providing altruistic service
- the possession of a monopoly of practice in a particular field.

PROFESSIONAL GROUPS INVOLVED IN PATIENT CARE

Long-established professions in health care services include doctors, pharmacists and dentists. Newer 'semi-professions' or 'sub-professions' include:

- psychiatric nurses
- clinical psychologists
- non-medically trained psychotherapists
- occupational therapists.

'Semi-professions' or 'sub-professions' may increase their 'professionalization' over time, for instance by increasing the length of training and training requirements. Conversely, professional groups involved in patient care may decrease their 'professionalization' over time, for instance by going on strike even if this adversely affects patient care.

BIBLIOGRAPHY

Barton, W.R. 1959: *Institutional Neurosis*. Bristol: Wright.

Bicknell, J. 1983: The psychopathology of handicap. *British Journal of Medical Psychology* 56:167–178.

Boulton, M. 1998: Sociology. In Puri, B.K. & Tyrer, P.J. (eds) *Sciences Basic to Psychiatry*, 2nd edn. Edinburgh: Churchill Livingstone.

Brown, G.W. & Birley, J.L. 1968: Crises and life changes and the onset of schizophrenia. *Journal of Health and Social Behaviour* 9:203–214.

Brown, G.W. & Harris, T.O. (eds) 1978: *Social Origins of Depression: A Study of Psychiatric Disorder in Women*. London: Tavistock.

Brown, G.W. & Harris, T.O. (eds) 1989: *Life Events and Illness*. New York: Guilford Press.

Brown, G.W., Carstairs, G.M. & Topping, G.C. 1958: The posthospital adjustment of chronic mental patients. *Lancet* 2:658–659.

Craig, T.K.J. & Brown, G.W. 1984: Goal frustration and life events in the etiology of painful gastrointestinal disorder. *Journal of Psychosomatic Research* 28:411–421.

Creed, F. 1981: Life events and appendicectomy. *Lancet* 1:1381–1385.

Creed, F. 1992: Life-events. In Weller, M. & Eysenck, M. (eds) *The Scientific Basis of Psychiatry*, 2nd edn. London: W.B. Saunders.

Dare, C. 1985: Family Therapy. In Rutter, M. & Hersov, L. (eds) *Child and Adolescent Psychiatry: Modern Approaches*. Oxford: Blackwell Scientific.

Farmer, R. & Creed, F. 1989: Life events and hostility in self-poisoning. *British Journal of Psychiatry* 154:390–395.

Finlay-Jones, R. & Brown, G.W. 1981: Types of stressful life event and the onset of anxiety and depressive disorders. *Psychological Medicine* 11:803–815.

Goffman, E. 1961: *Asylums: Essays on the Social Situation of Mental Patients and Other Inmates*. New York: Doubleday.

Goldberg, D. & Huxley, P. 1980: *Mental Illness in the Community: The Pathways to Psychiatric Care*. London: Tavistock.

Harris, T.O. 1989: Disorders of menstruation. In Brown, G.W. & Harris, T.O. (eds) *Life Events and Illness*. New York: Guildford Press.

Holmes, T.H. & Rahe, R.H. 1967: The Social Readjustment Rating Scale. *Journal of Psychosomatic Research* 11:213–217.

Jones, K. 1993: Social sciences in relation to psychiatry. In Kendall, R.E. & Zealley, A.K. (eds) *Companion to Psychiatric Studies*, 5th edn. Edinburgh: Churchill Livingstone.

Mechanic, D. 1978: *Medical Sociology*, 2nd edn. Glencoe: Free Press.

Miller, P.M. & Ingham, J.G. 1985: Dimensions of experience and symptomatology. *Journal of Psychosomatic Research* 29:475–488.

Morgan, H.G., Burns-Cox, C.J., Pocock, H. *et al.* 1975: Deliberate self-harm: clinical and socio-economic characteristics of 368 patients. *British Journal of Psychiatry* 127:564–574.

Parsons, T. 1951: *The Social System*. Glencoe: Free Press.

Scrambler, G. (ed.) 1991: *Sociology as Applied to Medicine*, 3rd edn. London: Baillière Tindall.

Smith, G.D., Bartley, M. & Blane, D. 1990: The Black Report on socioeconomic inequalities in health 10 years on. *British Medical Journal* 301:373–377.

Tantum, D. & Birchwood, M. (eds) 1994: *Psychiatry and the Social Sciences*. London: Gaskell.

Tennant, C.C. 1985: Stress and schizophrenia: a review. *Integrative Psychiatry* 3:248–261.

Vaughn, C.E. & Leff, J.P. 1976: The influence of family and social factors on the course of schizophrenic illness. *British Journal of Psychiatry* 129:125–137.

Wing, J.K. 1967: Social treatment, rehabilitation and management. In Coppen, A. & Walker, A. (eds) *Recent Developments in Schizophrenia*. British Journal of Psychiatry Special Publication no. 1.

Wing, J.K. 1978: *Schizophrenia: Towards A New Synthesis.* London: Academic Press.

Wing, J.K. & Brown, G.W. 1961: Social treatment of chronic schizophrenia: a comparative survey of three mental hospitals. *Journal of Mental Science* 107:847–861.

Wing, J.K. & Brown, G.W. 1970: *Institutionalism and Schizophrenia: A Comparative Study of Three Mental Hospitals 1960–1968.* London: Cambridge University Press.

8

Descriptive psychopathology

DISORDERS OF GENERAL BEHAVIOUR

UNDER–ACTIVITY

Stupor

The key features of stupor, when the term is used in its psychiatric sense, include:

- mutism
- immobility
- occasional periods of excitement and over-activity.

Stupor is seen in:

- catatonic stupor
- depressive stupor
- manic stupor
- epilepsy
- hysteria.

In neurology the term 'stupor' refers to a person who responds to pain and loud sounds, and may exhibit brief monosyllabic utterances and some spontaneous motor activity takes place.

Depressive retardation

This is a lesser form of psychomotor retardation occurring in depression which, in its extreme form, merges with depressive stupor.

Obsessional slowness

This may occur secondary to repeated doubts and compulsive rituals.

OVER–ACTIVITY

Psychomotor agitation

A person with psychomotor agitation manifests:

- excessive over-activity, which is usually unproductive
- restlessness.

Hyperkinesis
In hyperkinesis, which may be seen in children and adolescents, the following features occur:

- over-activity
- distractibility
- impulsivity
- excitability.

Somnambulism (sleep walking)
A complex sequence of behaviours is carried out by a person who rises from sleep and is not fully aware of his or her surroundings.

Compulsion (compulsive ritual)
This is a repetitive and stereotyped seemingly purposeful behaviour. It is the motor component of an obsessional thought. Examples of compulsions include:

- *checking rituals*
- *cleaning rituals*
- *counting rituals*
- *dipsomania*: a compulsion to drink alcohol
- *dressing rituals*
- *kleptomania*: a compulsion to steal
- *nymphomania*: a compulsive need in the female to engage in sexual intercourse
- *polydipsia*: a compulsion to drink water
- *satyriasis*: a compulsive need in the male to engage in sexual intercourse
- *trichotillomania*: a compulsion to pull out one's hair.

ABNORMAL POSTURE AND MOVEMENTS

Particularly in schizophrenia, but sometimes also in other disorders such as some learning disabilities, the following abnormal movements may occur: ambitendency, echopraxia, mannerisms, negativism, posturing, stereotypies and waxy flexibility.

- *Ambitendency*. The person makes a series of tentative incomplete movements when expected to carry out a voluntary action.
- *Echopraxia*. This refers to the automatic imitation by the person of another person's movements. It occurs even when the person is asked not to.
- *Mannerisms*. These are repeated involuntary movements that appear to be goal directed.
- *Negativism*. This is a motiveless resistance to commands and to attempts to be moved.
- *Posturing*. The person adopts an inappropriate or bizarre bodily posture continuously for a long time.
- *Stereotypies*. These are repeated regular fixed patterns of movement (or speech) which are not goal directed.
- *Waxy flexibility* (cerea flexibilitas). There is a feeling of plastic resistance resembling the bending of a soft wax rod as the examiner moves part of the person's body; that body part then remains 'moulded' by the examiner in the new position.

- *Tics.* These are repeated irregular movements involving a muscle group and may be seen following encephalitis, in Huntington's disease and in Gilles de la Tourette's syndrome, for example.
- *Parkinsonism.* The features of parkinsonism include:
  - a resting tremor
  - cogwheel rigidity
  - postural abnormalities
  - a festinant gait.

DISORDERS OF SPEECH

DISORDERS OF RATE, QUANTITY AND ARTICULATION

- *Dysarthria.* This is difficulty in the articulation of speech.
- *Dysprosody.* This is speech with the loss of its normal melody.
- *Logorrhoea* (volubility). The speech is fluent and rambling with the use of many words.
- *Mutism.* This is the complete loss of speech.
- *Poverty of speech.* There is a restricted amount of speech. If the person replies to questions, he or she may do so with monosyllabic answers.
- *Pressure of speech.* There is an increase in both the quantity and rate of speech, which is difficult to interrupt.
- *Stammering.* The flow of speech is broken by pauses and the repetition of parts of words.

DISORDERS OF THE FORM OF SPEECH

- *Circumstantiality.* Thinking appears slow with the incorporation of unnecessary trivial details. The goal of thought is finally reached, however.
- *Echolalia.* This is the automatic imitation by the person of another person's speech. It occurs even when the person does not understand the speech (which may be in another language, for example).
- *Flight of ideas.* The speech consists of a stream of accelerated thoughts with abrupt changes from topic to topic and no central direction. The connections between the thoughts may be based on:
  - chance relationships
  - clang associations
  - distracting stimuli
  - verbal associations (e.g. alliteration and assonance).
- *Neologism.* This is a new word constructed by the person or an everyday word used in a special way by the person.
- *Passing by the point* (vorbeigehen). The answers to questions, although clearly incorrect, demonstrate that the questions are understood. For example, when asked 'What colour is grass?', the person may reply 'Blue'. It is seen in the Ganser syndrome, first described in criminals awaiting trial.
- *Perseveration.* In perseveration (of both speech and movement) mental operations are continued beyond the point at which they are relevant. Particular types of perseveration of speech are:
  - *palilalia*: the person repeats a word with increasing frequency
  - *logoclonia*: the person repeats the last syllable of the last word.

- *Thought blocking*. There is a sudden interruption in the train of thought, before it is completed, leaving a 'blank'. After a period of silence, the person cannot recall what he or she had been saying or had been thinking of saying.

DISORDERS (LOOSENING) OF ASSOCIATION (FORMAL THOUGHT DISORDER)

These occur particularly in schizophrenia and may be considered to be a schizophrenic language disorder. Examples include knight's-move thinking, in which there are odd tangential associations between ideas, leading to disruptions in the smooth continuity of the speech, and schizophasia, also called 'word salad' or 'speech confusion', in which the speech is an incoherent and incomprehensible mixture of words and phrases. Schneider described the following features of formal thought disorder:

- *derailment*: the thought derails onto a subsidiary thought
- *drivelling*: there is a disordered intermixture of the constituent parts of one complex thought
- *fusion*: heterogeneous elements of thought are interwoven with each other
- *omission*: a thought or part of a thought is senselessly omitted
- *substitution*: a major thought is substituted by a subsidiary thought.

DISORDERS OF EMOTION

DISORDERS OF AFFECT

Affect is a pattern of observable behaviours which is the expression of a subjectively experienced feeling state (emotion), and is variable over time, in response to changing emotional states (DSM-IV-TR).

- *Blunted affect*. In a person with a blunted affect the externalized feeling tone is severely reduced.
- *Flat affect*. This consists of a total or almost total absence of signs of expression of affect.
- *Inappropriate affect*. This is an affect that is inappropriate to the thought or speech it accompanies.
- *Labile affect*. A person with a labile affect has a labile externalized feeling tone which is not related to environmental stimuli.

DISORDERS OF MOOD

Mood is a pervasive and sustained emotion which, in the extreme, markedly colours the person's perception of the world (DSM-IV-TR).

- *Dysphoria*. This is an unpleasant mood.
- *Depression*. This is a low or depressed mood. It may be accompanied by anhedonia, in which the ability to enjoy pleasurable activities is lost. In normal grief or mourning, the sadness is appropriate to the loss.
- *Elation*. This is an elevated mood or exaggerated feeling of well-being that is pathological. It is seen in mania.
- *Euphoria*. This is a personal and subjective feeling of unconcern and contentment, usually seen after taking opiates or as a late sequel to head injury.
- *Irritability*. This is a liability to outbursts or a state of reduced control over aggressive impulses towards others. It may be a personality trait or may accompany anxiety. It also occurs in premenstrual syndrome.

- *Apathy*. There is a loss of emotional tone and the ability to feel pleasure, associated with detachment or indifference.
- *Alexithymia*. This is difficulty in the awareness of or description of one's emotions.

DISORDERS RELATED TO ANXIETY

- *Anxiety*. This is a feeling of apprehension, tension or uneasiness owing to the anticipation of an external or internal danger. Types of anxiety include:
    - *phobic anxiety*: the focus of the anxiety is avoided (phobias are a disorder of thought content)
    - *free-floating anxiety*: the anxiety is pervasive and unfocused.
- *panic attacks*: anxiety is experienced in acute, episodic, intense attacks and may be accompanied by physiological symptoms.
- *Fear*. This is anxiety caused by a realistic danger that is recognized at a conscious level.
- *Agitation*. There is excessive motor activity associated with a feeling of inner tension.
- *Tension*. There is an unpleasant increase in psychomotor activity.

DISORDERS OF THOUGHT CONTENT

PREOCCUPATIONS

- *Hypochondriasis*. This is a preoccupation with a fear of having a serious illness which is not based on real organic pathology but instead on an unrealistic interpretation of physical signs or sensations as being abnormal.
- *Monomania*. This is a pathological preoccupation with a single object.
- *Egomania*. This is a pathological preoccupation with oneself.

OBSESSIONS

Obsessions are repetitive senseless thoughts which are recognized as irrational by the person and which are unsuccessfully resisted. Themes include:

- aggression
- dirt and contamination
- fear of causing harm
- religious
- sexual.

PHOBIAS

A phobia is a persistent irrational fear of an activity, object or situation leading to avoidance. The fear is out of proportion to the real danger and cannot be reasoned away, being out of voluntary control. Some types of phobia are:

- *Acrophobia* is a fear of heights.
- *Agoraphobia* literally means a fear of the market place. It is a syndrome with a generalized high anxiety level anxiety about, or avoidance of, places or situations from which escape might be difficult, or embarrassing, or in which help may not be available in the event of having a panic

attack or panic-like symptoms. Objects of fear may include crowds, open and closed spaces, shopping, social situations, and travelling by public transport.

- *Algophobia* is a fear of pain.
- *Claustrophobia* is a fear of closed spaces.
- *Social phobia* is a fear of personal interactions in a public setting, such as public speaking, eating in public, and meeting people.
- *Specific (simple) phobia* is a fear of discrete objects (e.g. snakes) or situations.
- *Xenophobia* is a fear of strangers.
- *Zoophobia* is a fear of animals.
- *Phobias of internal stimuli.* These include obsessive phobias and illness phobias, which overlap with hypochondriasis.

ABNORMAL BELIEFS AND INTERPRETATIONS OF EVENTS

OVER-VALUED IDEAS

An overvalued idea is an unreasonable and sustained intense preoccupation maintained with less than delusional intensity; that is, the person is able to acknowledge the possibility that the belief may not be true. The idea or belief held is demonstrably false and is not one that is normally held by others of the person's subculture. There is a marked associated emotional investment.

DELUSIONS

A delusion is a false belief based on incorrect inference about external reality that is firmly sustained despite what almost everyone else believes and despite what constitutes incontrovertible and obvious proof or evidence to the contrary. The belief is not one ordinarily accepted by other members of the person's culture or subculture (e.g. it is not an article of religious faith). When a false belief involves a value judgement, it is regarded as a delusion only when the judgement is so extreme as to defy credibility (DSM-IV-TR).

- *Mood-congruent delusion.* The content of the delusion is appropriate to the mood of the person.
- *Mood-incongruent delusion.* The content of the delusion is not appropriate to the mood of the person.
- *Primary delusion.* A delusion that arises fully formed without any discernible connection with previous events. It may be preceded by a delusional mood in which the person is aware of something strange and threatening happening.
- *Bizarre delusion.* A delusion involving a phenomenon that the person's culture would regard as totally implausible.
- *Delusional jealousy* (pathological jealousy; Othello syndrome; delusion of infidelity). A delusion that one's sexual partner is unfaithful.
- *Delusion of being controlled.* Feelings, impulses, thoughts, or actions of the person are experienced as being under the control of some external force rather than under his or her own control.
- *Delusion of doubles* (l'illusion de sosies). A delusion that a person known to the person has been replaced by a double. It is seen in Capgras' syndrome.
- *Delusion of poverty.* A delusion that one is in poverty.
- *Delusion of reference.* The theme is that events, objects or other people in one's immediate

environment have a particular and unusual significance. These delusions are usually of a negative or pejorative nature, but also may be grandiose in content (DSM-IV). When similar thoughts are held with less than delusional intensity they are ideas of reference.

- *Delusion of self-accusation*. A delusion of one's own guilt.
- *Erotomania* (de Clérambault's syndrome). A delusion that another person, usually of higher status, is deeply in love with the individual.
- *Grandiose delusion*. A delusion of inflated worth, power, knowledge, identity, or special relationship to a deity or famous person.
- *Persecutory (querulant) delusion*. The central theme is that one (or someone to whom one is close) is being attacked, harassed, cheated, persecuted, or conspired against (DSM-IV-TR).
- *Somatic delusion*. A delusion whose main content pertains to the appearance or functioning of one's body (DSM-IV-TR).

PASSIVITY PHENOMENON

This is a delusional belief that an external agency is controlling aspects of the self which are normally entirely under one's own control. Passivity phenomena include the following:

- *Thought alienation*. The person believes that his or her thoughts are under the control of an outside agency or that others are participating in his or her thinking; it includes:
  - *thought insertion*: the delusion that certain of one's thoughts are not one's own, but rather are inserted into one's mind by an external agency
  - *thought withdrawal*: the delusion that one's thoughts are being removed from one's mind by an external agency
  - *thought broadcasting*: the delusion that one's thoughts are being broadcast out loud so that they can be perceived by others.
- *Made feelings*. This is the delusional belief that one's own free will has been removed and that an external agency is controlling one's feelings.
- *Made impulses*. This is the delusional belief that one's own free will has been removed and that an external agency is controlling one's impulses.
- *Made actions*. This is the delusional belief that one's own free will has been removed and that an external agency is controlling one's actions.
- *Somatic passivity*. This is the delusional belief that one is a passive recipient of somatic or bodily sensations from an external agency.

DELUSIONAL PERCEPTION

In a delusional perception the person attaches a new and delusional significance to a familiar real perception without any logical reason.

ABNORMAL EXPERIENCES

SENSORY DISTORTIONS

- *Hyperaesthesias*. These are changes in sensory perception in which there is an increased intensity of sensation. *Hyperacusis* is an increased sensitivity to sounds.
- *Hypoaesthesias*. These are changes in sensory perception in which there is a decreased intensity of sensation. *Hypoacusis* is a decreased sensitivity to sounds.

- *Changes in quality*. Changes in quality of sensations occur particularly with visual stimuli, giving rise to visual distortions. Colourings of visual perceptions include:
  - *chloropsia* – green
  - *erythropsia* – red
  - *xanthopsia* – yellow.
- *Dysmegalopsia*. Changes in spatial form include:
  - *macropsia*: objects are seen larger or nearer than is actually the case
  - *micropsia*: objects are seen smaller or farther away than is actually the case.

SENSORY DECEPTIONS

Illusions
An illusion is a false perception of a real external stimulus.

Hallucinations
A hallucination is a false sensory perception in the absence of a real external stimulus. A hallucination is perceived as being located in objective space and as having the same realistic qualities as normal perceptions. It is not subject to conscious manipulation and only indicates a psychotic disturbance when there is also impaired reality testing. Hallucinations can be mood congruent or mood incongruent. Types of hallucination include:

- *auditory*
- *autoscopy* (phantom mirror image): the person sees himself or herself and knows that it is he or she
- *extracampine*: the hallucination occurs outside the person's sensory field
- *functional*: the stimulus causing the hallucination is experienced in addition to the hallucination itself
- *gustatory*
- *hallucinosis*: hallucinations (usually auditory) occur in clear consciousness
- *hypnagogic*: the hallucination (usually visual or auditory) occurs while falling asleep
- *hypnopompic*: the hallucination (usually visual or auditory) occurs while waking from sleep
- *olfactory*
- *reflex*: a stimulus in one sensory field leads to a hallucination in another sensory field
- *somatic*: somatic hallucinations include:
  - *tactile* (haptic) hallucinations: superficial and usually involving sensations on or just under the skin in the absence of a real stimulus; these include the sensation of insects crawling under the skin (*formication*)
  - *visceral* hallucinations of deep sensations
- *trailing phenomenon*: moving objects are seen as a series of discrete discontinuous images
- *visual*.

Pseudo-hallucinations
A pseudo-hallucination is a form of imagery arising in the subjective inner space of the mind. It lacks the substantiality of normal perceptions and occupies subjective space rather than objective space. It is not subject to conscious manipulation. An *eidetic image* is a vivid and detailed reproduction of a previous perception. In *pareidolia*, vivid imagery occurs without conscious effort while looking at a poorly structured background.

DISORDERS OF SELF-AWARENESS (EGO DISORDERS)

These include disturbances of:

- awareness of self-activity, including:
  - *depersonalization*: one feels that one is altered or not real in some way
  - *derealization*: the surroundings do not seem real
- the immediate awareness of self-unity
- the continuity of self
- the boundaries of the self.

COGNITIVE DISORDERS

DISORIENTATION

This is a disturbance of orientation in time, place or person.

DISORDERS OF ATTENTION

- *Distractibility.* A distractible subject's attention is drawn too frequently to unimportant or irrelevant external stimuli.
- *Selective inattention.* In selective inattention, anxiety-provoking stimuli are blocked out.

DISORDERS OF MEMORY

- *Amnesia.* This is the inability to recall past experiences.
- *Hypermnesia.* In hypermnesia the degree of retention and recall is exaggerated.
- *Paramnesia.* A paramnesia is a distorted recall leading to falsification of memory. Paramnesias include:
  - *confabulation*: gaps in memory are unconsciously filled with false memories
  - *déjà vu*: the subject feels that the current situation has been seen or experienced before
  - *déjà entendu*: the illusion of auditory recognition
  - *déjà pensé*: the illusion of recognition of a new thought
  - *jamais vu*: the illusion of failure to recognize a familiar situation
  - *retrospective falsification*: false details are added to the recollection of an otherwise real memory.

DISORDERS OF INTELLIGENCE

- *Learning disability* (mental retardation). Learning difficulty or mental retardation is classified by DSM-IV-TR and ICD-10 according to the intelligence quotient (IQ) of the subject:
  - $50 \leq IQ \leq 70$ ($50 \leq IQ \leq 69$ in ICD-10): mild mental retardation
  - $35 \leq IQ \leq 49$: moderate mental retardation
  - $20 \leq IQ \leq 34$: severe mental retardation
  - $IQ < 20$: profound mental retardation.
- *Dementia.* This is a global organic impairment of intellectual functioning without impairment of consciousness.
- *Pseudo-dementia.* This resembles dementia clinically, but is not organic in origin.

DISORDERS OF CONSCIOUSNESS

Levels of consciousness

The neurological terms used to describe progressively more unconscious levels are as follows:

- *Somnolence* (drowsiness). A subject who is drowsy or somnolent can be awoken by mild stimuli and will be able to speak comprehensibly, albeit perhaps for only a little while before falling asleep again.
- *Stupor.* A stuporose person responds to pain and loud sounds. Brief monosyllabic utterances and some spontaneous motor activity may occur.
- *Semi-coma.* A semi-comatose person will withdraw from the source of pain but spontaneous motor activity does not take place.
- *Deep coma.* No response can be elicited and there is no response to deep pain nor is there any spontaneous movement. Tendon, pupillary and corneal reflexes are usually absent.
- *Death.*

Clouding of consciousness

The person is drowsy and does not react completely to stimuli. There is disturbance of attention, concentration, memory, orientation and thinking.

Delirium

The person is bewildered, disoriented and restless. There may be associated fear and hallucinations. Variations include:

- *oneiroid state*: a dream-like state in a person who is not asleep
- *torpor*: the person is drowsy and easily falls asleep
- *twilight state*: a prolonged oneiroid state of disturbed consciousness with hallucinations.

Fugue

This is a state of wandering from the usual surroundings in which there is also loss of memory.

APHASIAS

- *Receptive (sensory) aphasia* (Wernicke's fluent aphasia). Difficulty is experienced in comprehending the meaning of words. Types include:
    - *agnosic alexia*: words can be seen but cannot be read
    - *pure word deafness*: words that are heard cannot be comprehended
    - *visual asymbolia*: words can be transcribed but cannot be read.
- *Intermediate aphasia.* Types of intermediate aphasia include:
    - *central (syntactical) aphasia*: there is difficulty in arranging words in their proper sequence
    - *nominal aphasia*: there is difficulty in naming objects.
- *Expressive (motor) aphasia* (Broca's nonfluent aphasia). This refers to difficulty in expressing thoughts in words while comprehension remains.
- *Global aphasia.* Both receptive aphasia and expressive aphasia are present at the same time.
- *Jargon aphasia*: The person utters incoherent meaningless neologistic speech.

APRAXIAS AND AGNOSIAS

APRAXIAS

Apraxia is an inability to perform purposive volitional acts, which does not result from paresis, incoordination, sensory loss or involuntary movements. It may be considered to be the motor equivalent of agnosia.

- *Constructional apraxia.* There is difficulty in constructing objects or copying drawings. This is closely associated with visuospatial agnosia, with some authorities treating the two as being essentially the same.
- *Dressing apraxia.* There is difficulty in putting on one's clothes correctly.
- *Ideomotor apraxia.* There is difficulty in carrying out progressively more difficult tasks, for example involving touching parts of the face with specified fingers.
- *Ideational apraxia.* There is difficulty in carrying out a coordinated sequence of actions.

AGNOSIAS AND DISORDERS OF BODY IMAGE

Agnosia is an inability to interpret and recognize the significance of sensory information, which does not result from impairment of the sensory pathways, mental deterioration, disorders of consciousness and attention, or, in the case of an object, a lack of familiarity with the object.

- *Visuospatial agnosia.* See 'constructional apraxia' above.
- *Visual (object) agnosia.* A familiar object, which can be seen though not recognized by sight, can be recognized through another modality such as touch or hearing.
- *Prosopagnosia.* This is an inability to recognize faces. In the *mirror sign*, which may occur in advanced Alzheimer's disease, a person may misidentify his or her own mirrored reflection.
- *Agnosia for colours.* The person is unable correctly to name colours, although colour sense is still present.
- *Simultanagnosia.* The person is unable to recognize the overall meaning of a picture whereas its individual details are understood.
- *Agraphognosia or agraphaesthesia.* The person is unable to identify, with closed eyes, numbers or letters traced on his or her palm.
- *Anosognosia.* There is a lack of awareness of disease, particularly of hemiplegia (most often following a right parietal lesion).
- *Coenestopathic state.* There is a localized distortion of body awareness.
- *Autotopagnosia.* This is an inability to name, recognize or point on command to parts of the body.
- *Astereognosia.* Objects cannot be recognized by palpation.
- *Finger agnosia.* The person is unable to recognize individual fingers, be they his or her own or those of another person.
- *Topographical disorientation.* This can be tested by using a locomotor map-reading task in which the person is asked to trace out a given route by foot.
- *Distorted awareness of size and shape.* For example, a limb may be felt to be growing larger.
- *Hemisomatognosis or hemidepersonalization.* The person feels that a limb (which in fact is present) is missing.
- *Phantom limb.* The continued awareness occurs of the presence of a limb that has been removed.
- *Reduplication phenomenon.* The person feels that part or all of the body has been duplicated.

BIBLIOGRAPHY

Hamilton, M. (ed.) 1985: *Fish's Clinical Psychopathology*, 2nd edn. Bristol: Wright.

Institute of Psychiatry 1973: *Notes on Eliciting and Recording Clinical Information.* Oxford: Oxford University Press.

Leff, J.P. & Isaacs, A.D. 1990: *Psychiatric Examination in Clinical Practice*, 3rd edn. Oxford: Blackwell Scientific.

Sims, A.C.P. 1985: *Symptoms in the Mind.* London: Baillière Tindall.

9

Psychoanalytic theories

SIGMUND FREUD (1856–1939)

EARLY INFLUENCES

Those who had an important early influence on Freud, and his pre-psychoanalytic theories, included:

- Helmholz and Brücke – the physicochemical basis of brain function; concepts of energy and conservation; the Helmholtz School of Medicine
- Meynert – neuroanatomy and behaviour
- Charcot – hysteria and hypnosis.

Freud also gained important ideas from the writings of:

- Darwin – the theory of evolution by natural selection
- Hughlings Jackson – the relationship of brain structure and function.

PROTO-PSYCHOANALYTIC PHASE (1887 TO *c.* 1897)

Studies on hysteria

In 1895, Josef Breuer and Sigmund Freud published *Studies on Hysteria*. This included the case of Anna O. (Bertha Pappenheim) who had been treated by Breuer for hysterical symptomatology, including limb paralysis, associated with her father's illness. The development of hysteria in general was considered to take the following course:

1. The cause consisted of real experiences, which were usually traumatic.
2. The (traumatic) event(s) gave rise to painful/unpleasant memories and represented ideas incompatible with conscious belief structures.
3. These memories and ideas were then repressed.
4. However, the powerful affects associated with them gave rise to somatic hysterical manifestations, sometimes including re-enactments of the (traumatic) event(s).
5. In consciousness there remain mnemonic symbolic representations of the event(s).

6   Bringing the event(s) to consciousness leads to a discharge or release of the associated affects ('psychic pus') and resolution of the hysterical symptomatology (*abreaction*).

Technical development
The techniques employed by Freud progressed gradually through the following major phases:

* The use of *hypnosis*.
* *The concentration method*. The patient, lying on a couch with eyes closed, was asked leading questions, and Freud would press his hands on the patient's forehead.
* *Free association*. The patient, with open eyes but lying on a couch, was encouraged to articulate, without censorship, all thoughts that came to mind.

Project for a Scientific Psychology
This was mostly written by Freud in 1895, and published after his death, in 1950. It consists essentially of an attempt to link psychological processes with neurophysiology.

TOPOGRAPHICAL MODEL OF THE MIND

This was set out in Freud's *The Interpretation of Dreams* (1900) and developed during the following two decades until its eventual replacement by the structural model. In this model the mind is considered to consist of the following three parts: the unconscious, the preconscious and the conscious.

The unconscious
This contains memories, ideas and affects that are repressed. Characteristic features include:

* outside awareness
* operating system – *primary process* thinking
* motivating principle – the pleasure principle
* access – access to its repressed contents is difficult, occurring when the censor gives way, for instance by becoming:
  * relaxed (e.g. in dreaming)
  * fooled (e.g. in jokes)
  * overpowered (e.g. in neurotic symptomatology)
* system position:
  * no negation
  * timelessness (reference to time is bound up in unconsciousness)
  * image-oriented
  * connotative
  * symbolic
  * non-linear.

The preconscious
This part of the mind develops during childhood and serves to maintain repression and censorship. Characteristic features include:

* outside awareness
* operating system – *secondary process* thinking
* motivating principle – the reality principle
* access – access can occur through focused attention
* system position:

- bound by time
- word-oriented
- denotative
- linear.

The conscious

The conscious can be considered to be an attention sensory organ. Characteristic features include:

- within awareness
- operating system – *secondary process* thinking
- motivating principle – the reality principle
- access – easy
- system position:
  - bound by time
  - word-oriented
  - declarative
  - linear.

Censorship

Freud described the censorship process in the following way:

> Let us compare the system of the unconscious to a large entrance hall, in which the mental impulses jostle one another like separate individuals. Adjoining this entrance hall there is a second narrow room, a kind of drawing room, in which consciousness also resides but on the threshold between these two rooms a watchman performs his function; he examines the different mental impulses, acts as a censor, and will not admit them into the drawing room if they displease him. It does not make much difference if the watchman turns away from a particular impulse at the threshold itself or if he pushes it back across the threshold after it has entered the drawing room. If they have already pushed their way forward to the threshold and have been turned back by the watchman then they are inadmissible to the consciousness; we speak of them as *repressed* but even the impulses which the watchman has allowed to cross the threshold are not on that account necessarily conscious as well; they can only become so if they succeed in catching the eye of consciousness. They are therefore justified in calling the second room the system of the *preconscious*.

Primary process

This is the operating system of the unconscious. Its attributes include:

- *displacement*: an apparently insignificant idea is invested with all the psychical depth of meaning and intensity originally attributed to another idea
- *condensation*: all the meanings and several chains of association converge on to a single idea standing at their point of intersection
- *symbolization*: symbols are used rather than words.

Characteristics of primary process thinking include (Sklar, 1989):

- *timelessness*: the concept of time only develops after a period in the mind of a child in connection to conscious reality (e.g. periodicity or chaos of feeding)
- *disregard of reality* of the conscious world
- *psychical reality*: memories of a real event and of imagined experience are not distinguished; abstract symbols are treated concretely
- *absence of contradiction*: opposites have a psychic equivalence
- *absence of negation*.

Secondary process
This is the operating system of the preconscious and the conscious.

- *Time* flows forward linearly.
- *Reality* is regarded – the content and logical basis of ideas is important.
- *Verbal word-presentations* are used.
- *Contradictions* are recognized and should not exist.

Pleasure principle
This is the motivating principle of primary process. It is mainly inborn. Pain/'unpleasure' is avoided and pleasure is sought through tension discharge. This leads to:

- wish fulfilment
- the discharge of instinctual drives.

Reality principle
This is the motivating principle of secondary process. It is the result of external reality. It leads to:

- delayed gratification.

DREAMING

In his *The Interpretation of Dreams* (1900), Freud referred to dreams as 'the Royal Road to the Unconscious'.

Dream composition
Dreams were considered to be composed of:

- *day residue*: memories of the waking hours before the dream that are particularly emotionally charged
- *nocturnal stimuli*: external stimuli (e.g. noise, moisture, touch), and internal stimuli (e.g. pain, urinary bladder distension)
- *unconscious wishes*
- *latent dream*: the day residue, nocturnal stimuli and unconscious wishes.

Dream work
This refers to the process whereby the latent dream is converted into the manifest dream. Operations that contribute to dream work can include:

- *displacement*
- *condensation*
- *symbolization*
- *secondary elaboration* (secondary revision) – the process of revising and/or elaborating the dream after awakening in order to make it more consistent with the rules of secondary process.

STRUCTURAL MODEL OF THE MIND

This was set out in Freud's *The Ego and the Id* (1923) and replaced the topographical model. In this model the mind is considered to consist of the following three parts:

- the *id*
- the *ego*
- the *superego*.

The id

Most of the id is unconscious. It contains primordial energy reserves derived from instinctual drives. Its aim is to maximize pleasure by fulfilling these drives.

The ego

According to Freud, the principal characteristics of the ego are as follows:

> In consequence of the preestablished connection between sense and perception and muscular action, the ego has voluntary movement at its command. It has the task of self-preservation. As regards external events, it performs that task by becoming aware of stimuli by storing up experiences about them (in the memory), by avoiding excessively strong stimuli (through adaptation), and finally by learning to bring about expedient changes in the external world to its own advantage (through activity). As regards internal events in relation to the id, it performs that task by gaining control over the demands of the instinct, by deciding whether they are to be allowed satisfaction, by postponing that satisfaction to times and circumstances favourable in the external world, or by suppressing their excitations entirely. It is guided in its activity by consideration of the tension produced by stimuli, whether these tensions are present in it or introduced into it.

Although much of the ego is conscious, most of its activity occurs without consciousness. Owing to its direct access to perception, reality testing takes place in the ego. However, the ego can be said to serve the following 'three harsh masters':

- the superego
- reality
- the id.

The superego

The superego is concerned with issues of morality. It develops initially as a result of the imposition of parental restraint. Although more of the superego is conscious than is the case for the id, most of its activity occurs without consciousness.

Relationship between the id, ego and superego

Freud described this relationship in the following way:

> We were justified; in dividing the ego from the id ... [But] the ego is identical with the id, and is merely a specially differentiated part of it. ... if a real split has occurred between the two, the weakness of the ego becomes apparent. But if the ego remains bound up with the id and indistinguishable from it, then it displays its strength. The same is true of the relation between the ego and the super-ego. In many situations the two are merged; and as a rule we can only distinguish one from the other when there is a tension or conflict between them. In repression the decisive fact is that the ego is an organization and the id is not. The ego is, indeed, the organized portion of the id. We should be quite wrong if we pictured the ego and the id as two opposing camps ...

RESISTANCE

This is everything, in words and actions of the analysand, that obstructs him or her gaining access to the unconscious. It can be used in psychoanalysis as a means to reach the repressed; indeed the forces at work in resistance and repression are the same.

TRANSFERENCE

Sklar (1989) described the important features of the transference:

The transference is an unconscious process in which the patient transfers to the therapist feelings, emotions and attitudes that were experienced and/or desired in the patient's childhood, usually in relation to parents and siblings. It can be a passionate demand for love and hate in past relationships between the child and the adult. This is a complex field that includes the unconscious splitting of the therapist into masculine and feminine and locating unconscious affect and thinking of the 'child' part of the patient in relation to the maternal and paternal aspects of the therapist (i.e. oedipal transference). Furthermore, the direction of such a transference can be both positive and negative. Thus, Freud encountered transference in many variations and certainly also in its hidden form, transformed by resistance. The therapist's transference represents on the one hand the most powerful ally but, on the other, in terms of transference's resistance, a therapeutic difficulty.

COUNTERTRANSFERENCE

Sklar (1989) described the important features of the countertransference:

The countertransference is the therapist's own feelings, emotions and attitudes to his patient. In the treatment mode, the therapist needs to screen out those that are mediated only by the therapist, and take note of those generated in the therapist from emotional contact with the patient. The latter can be an interesting aspect of the patient, e.g. the therapist may have the feelings of the patient as child in relation to the patient enacting the parent. Thus, in the reverse transference, an aspect of the patient is located in the therapist as a communication.

INSTINCTUAL DRIVES

Freud used the German word *Trieb* to refer to an instinctual drive. Unfortunately, this has often been translated into the word 'instinct', a concept different from a 'drive'. Important instinctual drives identified by Freud were:

- *libido*: sexual 'instinct' and energy of the eros
- *eros*: life preservation 'instinct'
- *thanatos*: death 'instinct'.

PSYCHOSEXUAL DEVELOPMENT

The stages of psychosexual development identified by Freud were the oral, anal, phallic, latency and genital phases.

- *Oral phase* – from birth to around 15–18 months of age. Erotogenic pleasure is derived from sucking. In addition to the mother's breast, the infant has a desire to place other objects in his or her mouth.
- *Anal phase* – from around 15–18 months to 30–36 months of age. Erotogenic pleasure is derived from stimulation of the anal mucosa, initially through faecal excretion, and later also through faecal retention.
- *Phallic phase* – from around 3 years of age to around the end of the fifth year. Boys pass through the *Oedipal complex*. Girls develop penis envy and pass through the *Electra complex*.
- *Latency stage* – from around 5–6 years to the onset of puberty. The sexual drive remains relatively latent during this period.
- *Genital stage* – from the onset of puberty to young adulthood. A strong resurgence in the sexual drive takes place. Successful resolution of conflicts from this and previous psychosexual stages leads to a mature, well-integrated adult identity.

CARL JUNG (1875–1961)

Jung founded the psychoanalytic school of analytic psychology. Jung was originally an important member of Sigmund Freud's inner circle and indeed at one time his designated successor.

DIFFERENCES BETWEEN JUNGIAN AND FREUDIAN THEORY

Jung came to different conclusions to Freud on a number of issues, including the following:

- *Libido theory.* Jung did not believe that libido was confined to being sexual, but considered the libido as being the unitary force of every manifestation of psychic energy.
- *Nature of the unconscious.* Jung believed in the *collective unconscious*, later referred to as the *objective psyche*, which he considered contained latent memories of our cultural, racial and phylogenetic past. In Jungian theory the objective psyche gives rise to consciousness.
- *Causality.* Rather than explaining present events in terms of Freudian psychic determinism, Jungian theory employs:
  - *causality*: offers an explanation in terms of the past
  - *teleology*: offers an explanation in terms of the future potential
  - *synchronicity*: offers an explanation in terms of causation at the boundary of the physical world with the psychical ('mystic') world.
- *Dreaming.* Jungian theory views the contents of dreams within a phylogenetic framework in which archetypes may be projected on to others.

ARCHETYPES

The archetypes of the objective psyche are energy-field configurations manifesting themselves as representational images having universal symbolic meaning and typical emotional and behavioural patterns. Five important types of archetype are identified in Jungian theory:

- *Anima.* This is the feminine prototype within each person.
- *Animus.* This is the masculine prototype within each person.
- *Persona.* This is the outward mask covering the individual's personality and allowing social demands to be balanced with internal needs. Both a public and a private persona may be possessed by a person. The persona may be represented in terms of clothing in dreams.
- *Shadow.* This represents repressed animal instincts arising from phylogenetic development and in dreams manifests itself as another person of the same sex.
- *Self.* This is a central archetype holding together conscious and unconscious aspects, including future potential, archetypes and complexes.

COMPLEXES

Complexes surround archetypes and can be defined as feeling-toned ideas. They develop from an interaction of personal experiences and archetypal models.

MENTAL OPERATIONS

Jungian theory postulates four operations of the mind: feeling, intuition, sensation and thinking.

- *Feeling.* This allows feelings:
  - anger and joy
  - love and loss

- pleasure and pain.
Judgements regarding good and evil also use this operation.
- *Intuition.* This is perception through unconscious processes.
- *Sensation.* This allows the acquisition of factual data.
- *Thinking.* This is composed of logic and reasoning. It is verbal and ideational.

EXTROVERSION AND INTROVERSION

- *Extroversion.* The individual's concerns and mental operations are directed to the objective reality in the external world.
- *Introversion.* The individual's concerns and mental operations are directed to the subjective reality of the inner world.

INDIVIDUATION

This is the process of personality growth leading to the development of a unique realization of what one intrinsically is.

MELANIE KLEIN (1882–1960)

Klein, who lacked any formal higher education and never developed a full theory of development, was a controversial figure in the British Psycho-Analytical Society. When she began developing her theories, Sigmund Freud viewed her as potentially challenging the work in child analysis of his daughter, Anna Freud.

It is now known that Klein analysed her three children and wrote them up as disguised clinical cases. She proposed that the aim of child psychoanalysis was to 'cure' all children of their 'psychoses'.

DIFFERENCES BETWEEN KLEINIAN AND FREUDIAN THEORY

Among the important differences between the theories of Klein and Freud were the following.

Object relations
Klein believed that the infant was capable of object relations.

Paranoid–schizoid position
Rejecting the critical importance of autoeroticism for the infant, Klein believed instead that the *paranoid position* – later, under the influence of Fairburn, renamed the *paranoid–schizoid position* – developed as a result of frustration during the first year of life with pleasurable contact with objects such as the *good breast*. The paranoid–schizoid position, characterized by isolation and persecutory fears, developed as a result of the infant viewing the world as part objects, using the following defence mechanisms:

- introjection (internalization)
- projective identification
- splitting.

Objects viewed by the infant as good are believed to be introjected, while those viewed as bad are split or projected.

Aggression
A strong emphasis was placed on aggression, occurring particularly during the paranoid–schizoid position.

Depressive position
This is said to develop by the age of 6 months when the child no longer views the world in terms of part objects but realizes that objects are whole, and the world is not perfect.

Development of the ego and superego
The ego and a primitive superego are present, according to Klein, during the first year of life.

EARLY DEVELOPMENT

The stages of development during the first year were considered to include, in chronological order:

- *oral frustration*
- *oral envy* (of parental 'oral' sex) and *oral sadism*, leading to Oedipal impulses
- a longing for the *oral incorporation of father's penis*, by *aggressive desires* to bring about the destruction of mother's body (which contains father's penis)
- *castration anxiety* in boys and fear of destruction of her own body in girls
- emergence of the *primitive superego*
- *introjection* of pain-causing objects
- development of a *cruel superego*
- *ejection of the superego*.

ANALYTIC PLAY TECHNIQUE

The analysis of children's play was considered to be the homologue, for children, of the free association technique and dream interpretation for adults.

DONALD WINNICOTT (1897–1971)

Winnicott was a British paediatrician who became a psychoanalyst. He was a contemporary of Anna Freud and Melanie Klein, between whom he at one time tried to mediate. He made important contributions to object relations theory and his reputation has grown steadily since his death.

THE MOTHER–BABY DYAD

Winnicott believed it was wrong to consider the baby in isolation, noting that there was:

> ... no such thing as an infant (apart from the maternal provision).

COUNTERTRANSFERANCE

Objective countertransference
Winnicott broadened the understanding of the countertransference from that of Freud, speaking of the *objective* countertransference. The objectivity derived from his belief that the counter-transference was an understandable and normal reaction to the personality and behaviour of the analysand.

Countertransference hate

Winnicott normalized the existence of countertransference hate. He gave reasons why a mother hates her infant (male or female) even from the start of their relationship. He then drew an analogy from this mother–infant dyad to the therapist–patient relationship. Winnicott suggested that the countertransference hate should be articulated to the analysand at the end of therapy, but most analysts would tend not to go this far.

MOTHERHOOD

- *Good-enough mother*. The good-enough mother is a mother who responds to her baby's communications and meets his or her needs within an optimal zone of frustration and gratification.
- *Pathological mother*. This is a mother who imposes her own needs over those of her baby, causing her baby to create a *false self* in order to protect his or her *true self*.
- *Capacity to be alone*. Good parenting by the mother, allowing her child to become increasingly autonomous while at the same time being dependent on her, results in the child being able to be himself or herself in the presence of his/her mother, and vice versa. This was termed the 'capacity to be alone' in the presence of another.

TRANSITIONAL OBJECT

This is an object, which is neither oneself nor another person (including mother), which is selected by an infant at between 4 and 18 months of age for self-soothing and anxiety-reduction. Examples include a blanket or toy that helps the infant go to sleep. It helps during the process of separation–individuation. In adults, transitional phenomena that may allow us to cope with loneliness and separation can include music, religion and scientific creativity.

OTHER CONCEPTS

Other important concepts associated with Winnicott include:

- *the holding environment*: a therapeutic ambiance or setting allowing the patient to experience safety, and so facilitating psychotherapy
- *the potential space*: an area of experiencing identified as existing between the baby and the object; it subsequently underlies all play, imagination, dreams and the interdependence of transference and countertransference
- *the squiggle game*: a play therapy technique
- *at-one-ment*
- *primary maternal preoccupation*
- *regression to dependence*
- *going on being*
- *impingement*
- *object usage*.

THE PSYCHODYNAMIC THEORY OF DEFENCE MECHANISMS

- *Repression*. The basic defence, repression is the pushing away (*Verdrangung*) of unacceptable ideas, affects, emotions, memories and drives, relegating them to the unconscious. When it is successful, no trace remains in consciousness but some affective excitation does remain.

- *Reaction formation.* This is a psychological attitude diametrically opposed to an oppressed wish and constituting a reaction against it. It is often seen in patients with obsessive–compulsive disorder.
- *Isolation.* Thoughts/affects/behaviour are isolated so that their links with other thoughts or memories are broken. It is often seen in patients with obsessive–compulsive disorder.
- *Undoing* (what has been done). An attempt is made to negate or atone for forbidden thoughts, affects or memories. This defence mechanism is seen, for example, in the compulsion of magic in patients with obsessive–compulsive disorder.
- *Projection.* Unacceptable qualities, feelings, thoughts or wishes are projected on to another person or thing. This is often seen in paranoid patients.
- *Projective identification.* The subject not only sees the other as possessing aspects of the self which have been repressed, but constrains the other to take on those aspects. It is a primitive form of projection.
- *Identification.* Attributes of others are taken into oneself.
- *Introjection.* In phantasy, the subject transposes objects and their qualities from the external world into himself or herself.
- *Incorporation.* Another's characteristics are taken on.
- *Turning against the self.* An impulse meant to be expressed to another is turned against oneself.
- *Reversal into the opposite.* The polarity of an impulse is reversed in the transition from activity to passivity.
- *Rationalization.* An attempt to explain in a logically consistent or ethically acceptable way, ideas, thoughts and feelings whose true motive is not perceived. It operates in everyday life as well as in delusional symptoms.
- *Sublimation.* A process that utilizes the force of a sexual instinct in drives, affects and memories in order to motivate creative activities having no apparent connection with sexuality.
- *Idealization.* The object's qualities are elevated to the point of perfection.
- *Regression.* Transition, at times of stress and threat, to moods of expression and functioning that are on a lower level of complexity, so that one returns to an earlier level of maturational functioning.
- *Denial.* The external reality of an unwanted or unpleasant piece of information is denied.
- *Splitting.* 'Good' objects, affects and memories are divided from 'bad' ones. This is often seen in patients with borderline personality disorder.
- *Distortion.* External reality is reshaped to suit inner needs.
- *Acting out.* Unconscious emotional conflicts or feelings are expressed directly in actions without the person being consciously aware of their meanings.
- *Displacement.* Emotions, ideas or wishes are transferred from their original object to a more acceptable substitute.
- *Intellectualization.* Excessive abstract thinking occurs in order to avoid conflicts or disturbing feelings.

BIBLIOGRAPHY

Freud, A. 1936: *The Ego and the Mechanisms of Defence.* London: Hogarth.

Freud, S. 1953/1966: *The Standard Edition of the Complete Psychological Works of Sigmund Freud,* vols 1–24. London: Hogarth.

Hall, C.S. 1956: *A Primer of Freudian Psychology.* London: George Allen & Unwin.

Jung, C.G. 1961: *Memories, Dreams, Reflections.* New York: Random House.

Jung, C.G. 1964: *Man and His Symbols.* New York: Doubleday.

Klein, M. 1948: *Contributions to Psycho-Analysis, 1921–1945.* London: Hogarth.

Klein, M. 1949: *The Psycho-Analysis of Children*, 3rd edn. London: Hogarth.

Ogden, T.H. 1992: The dialectically constituted/decentred subject of psychoanalysis: II. The contributions of Klein and Winnicott. *International Journal of Psycho-Analysis* 73:613–626.

Segal, H. 1980: *Melanie Klein.* New York: Viking.

Sklar, J. 1989: Dynamic psychopathology. In Puri, B.K. & Sklar, J.: *Examination Notes for the MRCPsych Part I.* London: Butterworth–Heinemann.

Winnicott, D.W. 1949: Hate in the Counter-Transference. *International Journal of Psycho-Analysis* 30:69–74.

Winnicott, D.W. 1958: *Collected Papers: Through Paediatrics to Psycho-Analysis.* New York: Basic Books.

Winnicott, D.W. 1965: *The Maturational Processes and the Facilitating Environment.* New York: International Universities Press.

Winnicott, D.W. 1971: *Playing and Reality.* New York: International Universities Press.

10

Neuroanatomy

ORGANIZATION OF THE NERVOUS SYSTEM

STRUCTURAL ORGANIZATION

The nervous system can be divided structurally into:

- the central nervous system (CNS)
- the peripheral nervous system (PNS).

The CNS consists of:

- the brain
- the spinal cord.

It is well protected by the skull and vertebral column and the meninges (layers of connective tissue membrane):

- the dura mater – outermost layer
- the arachnoid mater – middle layer
- the pia mater – inner layer.

Cerebrospinal fluid (CSF) in the subarachnoid space offers further protection of the CNS.
The PNS consists of:

- the cranial nerves
- the spinal nerves
- other neuronal processes and cell bodies lying outside the CNS.

The PNS is not as well protected as the CNS.

FUNCTIONAL ORGANIZATION

The nervous system can be divided functionally into:

- the somatic nervous system, concerned primarily with the innervation of voluntary structures

- the autonomic nervous system, concerned primarily with the innervation of involuntary structures.

  The autonomic nervous system is subdivided into two parts:

- the sympathetic
- the parasympathetic.

DEVELOPMENTAL ORGANIZATION

During ontogeny, the midline neural tube differentiates into the following vesicles:

- *Prosencephalon*. This differentiates into the telencephalon.
- *Telencephalon*. This gives rise to the cerebral hemispheres and contains the:
  - pallium
  - rhinencephalon
  - corpus striatum
  - medullary centre.
- *Diencephalon*. This consists of the:
  - thalamus
  - subthalamus
  - hypothalamus
  - epithalamus – consisting of the habenular nucleus and pineal gland.
- *Mesencephalon*. This consists of the:
  - tectum – consisting of the corpora quadrigemina, made up of the
    superior colliculi
    inferior colliculi
  - basis pedunculi
  - tegmentum – containing
    the red nucleus
    fibre tracts
    grey matter surrounding the cerebral aqueduct.
- *Rhombencephalon*. This differentiates into the:
  - metencephalon – consisting of the
    pons
    oral part of the medulla oblongata
    cerebellum
  - myelencephalon – the caudal part of the medulla oblongata.

Figure 10.1 shows the main ontological divisions at an early stage and at a later stage of neurodevelopment.

TYPES OF NERVOUS SYSTEM CELL

Neurones

Classification by morphology
On a morphological basis, neurones can be classified as:

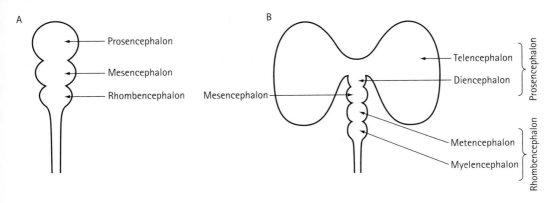

Figure 10.1   *Ontological development of the cerebral vesicles. A: At an early stage. B: At a later stage.*

- unipolar – the perikaryon has one neurite
- bipolar – the perikaryon has two neurites
- multipolar – each neurone has one axon and more than one dendrite.

Classification by size
An alternative classification is on the basis of size:

- Golgi type I – long axon
- Golgi type II – short axon terminating near the parent cell
- amacrine – no axon.

Neuroglia

Neuroglia, or interstitial cells, outnumber neurones five- to ten-fold.

- *Central nervous system.* The main types of neuroglia in the CNS are:
  - astrocytes
  - oligodendrocytes
  - microglia
  - ependyma.
- *Peripheral nervous system.* The main types of neuroglia in the PNS are:
  - Schwann cells
  - satellite cells.
- *Astrocytes.* There are two types of astrocytes or astroglia:
  - fibrous astrocytes
  - protoplasmic astrocytes.
  - They are multipolar and their functions include:
    - structural support of neurones
    - phagocytosis
    - forming CNS neuroglial scar tissue
    - contributing to the blood–brain barrier.

- *Oligodendrocytes.* The functions of oligodendrocytes or oligodendroglia include:
  - CNS myelin sheath formation
  - phagocytosis.
- *Microglia.* These are the smallest neuroglial cells and are most abundant in the grey matter. Their functions include acting as scavenger cells at sites of CNS injury.
- *Ependymal cells.* These line the cavities of the CNS. Their functions include aiding the flow of CSF (cilial beating). Types of ependymal cell include:
  - choroidal epithelial cells – cover the surfaces of the choroidal plexi
  - ependymocytes – line the central canal of the spinal cord and ventricles
  - tanycytes – line the floor of the third ventricle over the hypothalamic median eminence.
- *Schwann cells.* In addition to being part of myelinated peripheral nerves, Schwann cells encircle some unmyelinated peripheral nerve axons. Their functions include:
  - PNS myelin sheath formation
  - neurilemma formation.
- *Satellite cells.* Satellite cells, or capsular cells, are found in:
  - sensory ganglia
  - autonomic ganglia.

  Their functions include neuronal support in sensory and autonomic ganglia.

FRONTAL LOBES

FRONTAL OPERCULUM

This consists of areas 44, 45 and 47.

- *Broca's area.* This is the core of the frontal operculum on the dominant (usually left) side, and consists of areas 44 and 45. A lesion in this region can lead to expressive (motor) aphasia (Broca's nonfluent aphasia).
- *Right side.* Lesions in the non-dominant frontal operculum can lead to dysprosody.

SUPERIOR MESIAL REGION

This contains:

- *supplementary motor area* (SMA, the mesial part of area 6)
- *anterior cingulate cortex* (area 24).

Lesions of the left or right superior mesial region can lead to akinetic mutism.

INFERIOR MESIAL REGION

This consists of:

- *orbital cortex* (including areas 11, 12 and 32)
- *basal forebrain.*

Lesions of the orbital cortex (either side) can lead to a form of acquired sociopathy.
The basal forebrain includes the following nuclei:

- diagonal band of Broca
- nucleus accumbens

- septal nuclei
- substantia innominata.

Lesions of the basal forebrain (either side) can lead to amnesia (retrograde and anterograde) and confabulation.

DORSOLATERAL PREFRONTAL CORTEX

The dorsolateral prefrontal cortex (DLPFC) contains areas 8, 9, 10 and 46. Lesions in this region can lead to abnormalities in cognitive executive functions, impairment of verbal (left) or non-verbal (right) intellectual functions, memory impairments affecting recency and frequency judgements, poor organization, poor planning, poor abstraction, and disturbances in motor programming. Left-sided lesions may cause impaired verbal fluency, while right lesions may cause impaired non-verbal (design) fluency.

TEMPORAL LOBES

SUPERIOR TEMPORAL GYRUS

The posterior part of the superior temporal gyrus, area 22, forms (on the left) Wernicke's area. Lesions in this region can lead to a receptive (sensory) aphasia (Wernicke's fluent aphasia).

POSTERIOR INFEROLATERAL REGION

This consists of:

- posterior portion of the *middle temporal gyrus* (part of area 37)
- posterior portion of the *inferior temporal gyrus* (part of area 37)
- posterior portion of the *fourth temporal gyrus* (part of area 37).

Lesions in this region, and in the adjoining occipitotemporal junction, can lead to prosopagnosia and impaired object recognition.

ANTERIOR INFEROLATERAL REGION

This consists of:

- anterior portion of the *middle temporal gyrus* (part of area 21)
- anterior portion of the *inferior temporal gyrus* (part of area 20)
- anterior portion of the *fourth temporal gyrus* (part of area 20)
- *temporal pole* (area 38).

Lesions in the left side can lead to anomia and defects in accessing the reference lexicon. Lesions in the right side can lead to an inability to name facial expressions. Retrograde anmesia may result from bilateral lesions.

MESIAL TEMPORAL REGION

This consists of:

- *parahippocampal gyrus* (areas 27 and 28)

- *amygdala*
- *entorhinal cortex*
- *hippocampus.*

Left-sided lesions can lead to anterograde amnesia affecting verbal information, while right-sided lesions can lead to anterograde amnesia affecting non-verbal information. Bilateral lesions can lead to verbal and non-verbal anterograde amnesia.

PARIETAL LOBES

TEMPOROPARIETAL JUNCTION

The posterior part of the inferior parietal lobule together with the posterior part of the superior temporal gyrus (Wernicke's area) form the greater Wernicke's area. Left-sided lesions can lead to a receptive (sensory) aphasia (Wernicke's fluent aphasia), while right-sided lesions can lead to phonagnosia (impairment in the ability to recognize familiar voices) and amusia (impaired ability to recognize and process music).

INFERIOR PARIETAL LOBULE

This consists of:

- *angular gyrus* (area 39)
- *supramarginal gyrus* (area 40).

Lesions on the left can lead to conduction aphasia and tactile agnosia. Lesions on the right can lead to anosognosia, neglect, tactile agnosia and anosodiaphoria (impaired concern with respect to neurological deficits).

OCCIPITAL LOBES

The occipital lobe contains:

- *primary visual cortex* (area 17)
- *visual association cortices* (areas 18 and 19).

Lesions of the dorsal region (superior to the calcarine fissure) and adjoining parietal region (areas 7 and 39) can lead to partial (unilateral lesions) or a full-blown (bilateral lesions) Balint's syndrome, consisting of:

- simultanagnosia
- ocular apraxia or psychic gaze paralysis
- optic ataxia.

Bilateral dorsal lesions can also lead to astereopsis and impaired visual motion perception. Lesions of the left ventral region (inferior to the calcarine fissure) can lead to contralateral (right) acquired (central) hemiachromatopsia (impaired visual colour perception) and acquired (pure) dyslexia. Lesions of the right ventral region can lead to contralateral (left) acquired (central) hemiachromatopsia and apperceptive visual agnosia. Bilateral lesions can lead to acquired (central) hemiachromatopsia affecting the whole visual field, associative visual agnosia, and prosopagnosia.

BASAL GANGLIA

COMPONENTS

Authorities differ on the components of the basal ganglia. According to Snell (1987) the basal ganglia consist of the:

- corpus striatum
  - caudate nucleus
  - lentiform nucleus
- amygdala (amygdaloid nucleus or amygdaloid body)
- claustrum.

The lentiform nucleus consists of the:

- globus pallidus
- putamen.

Some of these structures are shown in the diagrammatic sketch of Figure 10.2.

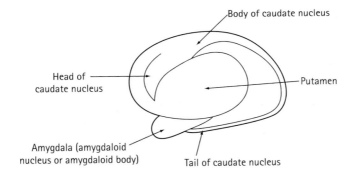

Figure 10.2   *Sketch of the basal ganglia of the left adult cerebral hemisphere.*

CONNECTIONS OF THE LENTIFORM NUCLEUS

Afferents

Afferents to the putamen come from the:

- caudate nucleus
- cerebral cortex.

Afferents to the globus pallidus come from the:

- caudate nucleus
- putamen
- substantia nigra.

Efferents

- Efferents from the putamen pass to the globus pallidus.
- Efferents from the globus pallidus pass to the:
  - hypothalamus

- reticular formation
- substantia nigra
- subthalamus
- ventroanterior nucleus of the thalamus
- ventrolateral nucleus of the thalamus.

FRONTAL–SUBCORTICAL CIRCUITS

Alexander *et al.* (1986) have identified five parallel frontal–subcortical circuits which together form one of the main organizational networks of the brain and are central to brain–behaviour relationships. They connect specific regions of the frontal cortex with the basal ganglia and the thalamus in circuits that mediate:

- motor activity
- eye movements
- behaviour.

The overall structure of each circuit is as follows:

> frontal lobe cortex → caudate nucleus → globus pallidus/substantia nigra → thalamus → frontal lobe cortex

Circuits

- *Motor circuit*. This originates in the SMA and subserves motor function.
- *Oculomotor circuit*. This originates in the frontal eye fields and subserves eye movements.
- *Dorsolateral prefrontal circuit*. This originates in the DLPFC and subserves executive cognitive functions.
- *Lateral orbitofrontal circuit*. This originates in the lateral orbital cortex and subserves personality.
- *Anterior cingulate circuit*. This originates in the anterior cingulate cortex and subserves motivation.

LIMBIC SYSTEM

LIMBIC LOBE

This was described by Broca in 1878 as an arrangement of cortical structures around the diencephalon, forming a border on the medial side of each cerebral hemisphere between the neocortex and the remainder of the brain.

- *Cortical areas*. Cortical areas of the limbic lobe form the limbic cortex and include the:
  - cingulate gyrus
  - parahippocampal gyrus
  - subcallosal gyrus.
- *Nuclei*. Subcortical nuclei that are part of the limbic lobe include the:
  - amygdaloid nucleus
  - septal nucleus.

COMPONENTS

There is disagreement as to precisely which structures form part of the modern definition of the limbic system. A good guide is provided by both Snell (1987) and Trimble (1981).

Cortical areas
Cortical areas that are generally considered to be part of the limbic system nowadays include the:

- cingulate gyrus
- gyrus fasciolaris
- hippocampal formation:
  - dendate gyrus
  - hippocampus
  - parahippocampal gyrus
- indusium griseum
- olfactory tubercle
- paraterminal gyrus (precommissural septum)
- prepiriform cortex
- secondary olfactory area (entorhinal area)
- subcollosal gyrus
- subiculum.

Nuclei
Subcortical nuclear groups that are generally considered to be part of the limbic system nowadays include the:

- amygdala (amygdaloid nucleus)
- anterior thalamic nucleus
- dorsal tegmental nucleus
- epithalamic nucleus
- habenula
- hypothalamic nuclei
- mammillary bodies
- raphe nucleus
- septal nucleus (septal area)
- superior central nucleus
- ventral tegmental area.

Connecting pathways
Connecting pathways of the limbic system include the:

- anterior commissure
- cingulum
- dorsal longitudinal fasciculus
- fornix
- lateral longitudinal striae
- mammillotegmental tract
- mammillothalamic tract
- medial forebrain bundle
- medial longitudinal striae
- stria terminalis
- stria medullaris thalami.

INTERNAL ANATOMY OF THE TEMPORAL LOBES

HIPPOCAMPAL FORMATION

The hippocampal formation consists of the:

- dendate gyrus
- hippocampus
- parahippocampal gyrus.

DENDATE GYRUS

This gyrus lies between the hippocampal fimbria and the parahippocampal gyrus. Anteriorly, it is continuous with the uncus. Posteriorly, it is continuous with the indusium griseum. Histologically, it is made up of the following three layers:

- molecular layer (outer)
- granular layer
- polymorphic layer (inner).

HIPPOCAMPUS

This grey matter structure lies mainly in the floor of the inferior horn of the lateral ventricle. Anteriorly, it forms the pes hippocampus. Posteriorly, it ends inferior to the splenium of the corpus callosum. Axons from each alveus converge medially to form the fimbria and crus of the fornix. Histologically, the hippocampus is made up of the following three layers:

- molecular layer (outer)
- pyramidal layer
- polymorphic layer (inner).

Afferent connections of the hippocampus include fibres that originate from the:

- cingulate gyrus
- dendate gyrus
- hippocampus (the opposite one)
- indusium griseum
- parahippocampal gyrus
- secondary olfactory area (entorhinal area)
- septal nucleus (septal area).

PARAHIPPOCAMPAL GYRUS

This gyrus is separated from the remaining cerebral cortex by the collateral sulcus. Anteriorly, it is continuous with the uncus. The subiculum of the parahippocampal gyrus allows the passage of nerve fibres from the secondary olfactory cortex (entorhinal area) to the dendate gyrus.

AMYGDALA

The amygdala is also known as the amygdaloid nucleus, body or complex. It is continuous with the tail of the caudate nucleus, lying anterior and superior to the tip of the inferior horn of the lateral ventricle.

Afferent connections

Afferent connections received by the amygdala include the:

- amygdala (the opposite one, via the anterior commissure)
- dopaminergic brain stem nuclei
- frontal association area
- lateral olfactory stria
- noradrenergic brainstem nuclei
- septal nucleus (septal area)
- serotonergic brainstem nuclei
- temporal association area
- uncus.

Efferent connections

Parts of the brain to which efferent connections pass from the amygdala include the:

- hypothalamus (via the stria terminalis)
- septal nucleus (septal area) (via the stria terminalis)
- corpus striatum
- frontal association area
- lateral olfactory stria
- temporal association area
- thalamus.

MAJOR WHITE MATTER PATHWAYS

CORPUS CALLOSUM

This is the largest set of inter-hemispheric connecting fibres. It lies inferior to the longitudinal fissure and superior to the diencephalon. It connects homologous neocortical areas.

The main divisions of the corpus callosum (rostral first) are the:

- rostrum
- genu
- body
- splenium.

These are shown in the diagrammatic sketch of the corpus callosum of Figure 10.3, which also shows some adjacent structures.

FORNIX

This is the major efferent subcortical white matter tract of the hippocampus. The two crura of the fornix, each formed from axons from the alveus of the hippocampus, converge inferior to the corpus callosum and form the body of the fornix. The body of the fornix is connected anteriorly with the inferior surface of the corpus callosum via the septum pellucidum. The body of the fornix then divides into the two columns of the fornix.

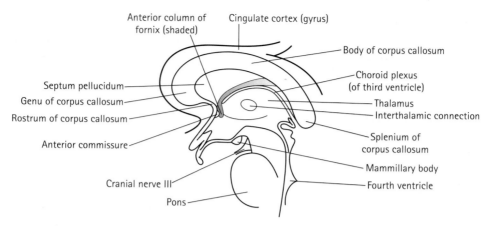

Figure 10.3 *Sketch of the corpus callosum in a midsagittal section of the adult human brain. The adjacent cingulate cortex and septum pellucidum are also indicated. Note that the rostral direction is towards the left.*

Destination of fibres in the fornix

The efferent connections of the hippocampus, via the fornix, include the:

- anterior hypothalamus
- anterior nucleus of the thalamus
- habenular nucleus
- lateral preoptic area
- mammillary body (medial nucleus)
- septal nucleus (septal area)
- tegmentum of the mesencephalon.

PAPEZ CIRCUIT

This is the concept introduced by Papez, in 1937, of a supposed limbic-system reverberating circuit constituting the neuronal mechanism of emotion. It consisted of the:

- hippocampus
- hypothalamus
- anterior nucleus of the thalamus
- cingulate gyrus.

The postulated circuit was as follows:

hippocampus → (via the fornix)
→ mammillary bodies of the hypothalamus → (via a synaptic connection)
→ anterior nucleus of the thalamus → (the neuroimpulse then radiates up)
→ cingulate gyrus → (via the cingulum)
→ hippocampus.

ARCUATE BUNDLE

This is a specific group of association fibres arranged in a curved shape running parallel to the cortical surface which, on the dominant (usually left) side, connects the more rostral Broca's area with Wernicke's area.

ANTERIOR COMMISSURE

This small nerve fibre bundle crosses the midline in the lamina terminalis and connects homologous areas of the neocortex and paleocortex. Parts of the limbic system in the two cerebral hemispheres that are connected via the anterior commissure include the:

- amygdala
- hippocampus
- parahippocampal gyrus.

CRANIAL NERVES

I: OLFACTORY NERVE

This contains the central processes of the olfactory receptors, which pass from the olfactory mucosa, through the cribriform plate of the ethmoid, to synapse with the olfactory bulb mitral cells. Axons then pass in the olfactory tract to the primary olfactory cortex (also known as the periamygdaloid and prepiriform areas) via the lateral olfactory striae.

II: OPTIC NERVE

This contains retinal ganglion cell axons which pass to the optic chiasma. At the optic chiasma:

- Medial retinal fibres, containing temporal visual field information, pass to the contralateral optic tract.
- Lateral retinal fibres, containing nasal visual field information, pass to the ipsilateral optic tract.

Most optic tract fibres synapse in the thalamic lateral geniculate body, while a minority (concerned with pupillary and ocular reflexes) pass directly to the pretectal nucleus and superior colliculi, bypassing the lateral geniculate body. From the lateral geniculate body the optic radiation passes, via the retrolenticular part of the internal capsule, to the visual cortex.

III: OCULOMOTOR NERVE

This nerve has two motor nuclei:

- The main oculomotor nucleus (also known as the somatic efferent nucleus) supplies all the extrinsic ocular muscles with the exception of the superior oblique and lateral rectus.
- The accessory parasympathetic nucleus (also known as the Edinger–Westphal nucleus) sends preganglionic parasympathetic fibres to the constrictor pupillae and ciliary muscles.

IV: TROCHLEAR NERVE

This supplies one extrinsic ocular muscle, namely the superior oblique.

V: TRIGEMINAL NERVE

This is the largest cranial nerve.

Nuclei of the trigeminal nerve

The trigeminal nerve has four nuclei:

- main sensory nucleus
- spinal nucleus
- mesencephalic nucleus
- motor nucleus.

Sensory components of the trigeminal nerve

The main divisions and branches of the trigeminal nerve, which together constitute the main sensory innervation of most of the head and face, are as follows:

- *Ophthalmic nerve or division*
    - *frontal nerve*: innervates, via the supraorbital and supratrochlear branches, the
        upper eyelid
        scalp (anterior to the lamboid suture)
    - *lacrimal nerve*: innervates the
        lacrimal gland
        lateral conjunctiva
        upper eyelid
    - *nasociliary nerve*: innervates the
        eyeball
        medial lower eyelid
        nasal skin
        nasal mucosa.
- *Maxillary nerve or division*
    - *infraorbital nerve*: innervates the
        skin of the cheek
    - *superior alveolar nerve*: innervates the
        upper teeth
    - *zygomatic nerve*: innervates the
        skin of the temple (via the zygomaticotemporal branch)
        skin of the cheek (via the zygomaticofacial branch).
    - Branches from the sphenopalatine ganglion include the
        greater palantine nerve
        lesser palantine nerve
        long sphenopalatine nerve
        nasal branches
        pharyngeal branches
        short sphenopalatine nerve.
- *Mandibular nerve or division*
    - *auriculotemporal nerve*: innervates the
        skin of the temple
        auricle division
    - *buccal nerve*: innervates the
        skin of the cheek
        mucous membrane of the cheek
    - *inferior alveolar nerve*: innervates the
        lower teeth
        lower lip

skin of the chin
- *lingual nerve*: innervates the
  anterior two-thirds of the tongue
  mucous membrane of the mouth.

Motor component of the trigeminal nerve
The motor component of the trigeminal nerve supplies the:

- muscles of mastication
- anterior belly of the digastric
- mylohyoid
- tensor tympani
- tensor veli palatini.

VI: ABDUCENT NERVE

This supplies one extrinsic ocular muscle, namely the lateral rectus.

VII: FACIAL NERVE

The facial nerve has three nuclei:

- main motor nucleus
- parasympathetic nuclei
- sensory nucleus (the superior part of the tractus solitarius nucleus).

Main motor nucleus
This supplies the:

- muscles of facial expression
- auricular muscles
- posterior belly of the digastric
- stapedius
- stylohyoid.

Corticonuclear fibres from the contralateral cerebral hemisphere are received by the part of the main motor nucleus supplying the lower face muscles. Corticonuclear fibres from both cerebral hemispheres are received by the part of the main motor nucleus supplying the upper face muscles.

Parasympathetic nuclei
These include:

- *lacrimal nucleus*: supplies the
  - lacrimal gland
- *superior salivary nucleus*: supplies the
  - nasal gland
  - palatine gland
  - sublingual gland
  - submandibular gland.

Sensory nucleus
This receives taste fibres, via the geniculate ganglion, from the:

- anterior two-thirds of the tongue
- floor of the mouth
- hard palate
- soft palate.

Chorda tympani

This is a branch of the facial nerve given off before it passes through the stylomastoid foramen. The chorda tympani joins the lingual branch of the mandibular division of the trigeminal nerve.

VIII: VESTIBULOCOCHLEAR NERVE

This nerve consists of the following two parts:

- *Cochlear nerve* – concerned with hearing. Its fibres are the central processes of the cochlear spiral ganglion cells, terminating in the anterior and posterior cochlear nuclei.
- *Vestibular nerve* – concerned with the maintenance of equilibrium. Its fibres are the central processes of vestibular ganglion neurones, terminating in the lateral, medial, superior and inferior vestibular nuclei.

IX: GLOSSOPHARYNGEAL NERVE

The glossopharyngeal nerve has three nuclei:

- main motor nucleus
- parasympathetic nucleus (the inferior salivary nucleus)
- sensory nucleus (part of the tractus solitarius nucleus).

Main motor nucleus

This supplies the stylopharyngeus. Corticonuclear fibres from both cerebral hemispheres are received by the main motor nucleus.

Parasympathetic nucleus

This receives inputs from the:

- hypothalamus
- olfactory system
- tractus solitarius nucleus
- trigeminal sensory nucleus.

Preganglionic fibres reach the otic ganglion via the tympanic plexus and the lesser petrosal nerve. Postganglionic fibres supply the parotid gland by means of the auriculotemporal branch of the mandibular nerve.

Sensory nucleus

This receives taste information from the posterior of the tongue.

X: VAGUS NERVE

The vagus nerve has three nuclei:

- main motor nucleus
- parasympathetic nucleus (the dorsal nucleus)
- sensory nucleus (the inferior part of the tractus solitarius nucleus).

Main motor nucleus

This supplies the:

- intrinsic muscles of the larynx
- constrictor muscles of the pharynx.

Corticonuclear fibres from both cerebral hemispheres are received by the main motor nucleus.

Parasympathetic nucleus

This receives inputs from the:

- hypothalamus
- glossopharyngeal nerve
- heart
- lower respiratory tract
- gastrointestinal tract, as far as the transverse colon.

It supplies the:

- involuntary muscle of the heart
- lower respiratory tract
- gastrointestinal tract, as far as the distal one-third of the transverse colon.

Sensory nucleus

This receives taste information from the inferior ganglion of the vagus nerve.

XI: ACCESSORY NERVE

This nerve consists of two parts:

- *Cranial root.* This supplies, via the vagus nerve, muscles of the:
    - larynx
    - pharynx
    - soft palate.
- *Spinal root.* This supplies the:
    - sternocleidomastoid
    - trapezius.

XII: HYPOGLOSSAL NERVE

This supplies the:

- intrinsic muscles of the tongue
- styloglossus
- hyoglossus
- genioglossus.

SPINAL CORD

DIVISIONS

From rostral to caudal, the spinal cord is divided into the following five parts:

- cervical – 8 pairs of spinal nerves
- thoracic – 12 pairs of spinal nerves
- lumbar – 5 pairs of spinal nerves
- sacral – 5 pairs of spinal nerves
- coccygeal – 1 pair of spinal nerves.

ASCENDING WHITE COLUMN TRACTS

- *Anterior.* The ascending anterior white column tracts include the anterior spinothalamic tract, which carries light touch and pressure sensations.
- *Lateral.* The ascending lateral white column tracts include the:
  - anterior and posterior spinocerebellar tracts, which carry proprioceptive, pressure and touch sensations
  - lateral spinothalamic tract, which carries pain and temperature sensations
  - spino-olivary tract, which carries proprioceptive and cutaneous sensations
  - spinotectal tract, which is involved with spinovisual reflexes.
- *Posterior.* The ascending posterior white column tracts include the:
  - fasciculus cuneatus, which carries discriminative touch and proprioceptive sensations
  - fasciculus gracilis, which carries vibration sensations.

DESCENDING WHITE COLUMN TRACTS

- *Anterior.* The descending anterior white column tracts include the:
  - anterior corticospinal tract, which is involved with voluntary movement
  - reticulospinal fibres, which are involved with motor function
  - vestibulospinal tract, which is involved with muscle tone control
  - tectospinal tract, which is involved with a head-turning reflex and movement of the upper limbs in response to acoustic, cutaneous and visual stimuli.
- *Lateral.* The descending lateral white column tracts include the:
  - lateral corticospinal tract, which is involved with voluntary movement
  - rubrospinal tract, which is involved with muscular activity
  - lateral reticulospinal tract, which is involved with muscular activity
  - descending autonomic fibres, which are involved with visceral function control
  - olivospinal tract – (?) involved with muscular activity.

MAJOR NEUROCHEMICAL PATHWAYS

NIGROSTRIATAL DOPAMINERGIC PATHWAY

The presynaptic components of this pathway are formed by:

- A8 dopaminergic neurones – located in the reticular formation of the mesencephalon
- A9 dopaminergic neurones – located in the pars compacta of the substantia nigra.

Their axons pass, via the medial forebrain bundle, to terminate mostly in the:

- caudate nucleus
- putamen

- amygdala.

This pathway is concerned with sensorimotor coordination.

MESOLIMBIC–MESOCORTICAL DOPAMINERGIC PATHWAY

This pathway originates in A10 dopaminergic neurones, located in the ventral tegmental area of the mesencephalon. Their axons pass, via the medial forebrain bundle, to terminate mostly in the:

- nucleus accumbens
- olfactory tubercle
- bed nucleus of the stria terminalis
- lateral septum
- cingulate cortex
- entorhinal cortex
- medial prefrontal cortex.

ASCENDING NORADRENERGIC PATHWAY FROM THE LOCUS COERULEUS

The main noradrenergic nucleus is the locus coeruleus, located in the dorsal pons. At least five noradrenergic tracts arise from it:

- Three ascend, via the medial forebrain bundle, to supply mainly the:
  - ipsilateral cerebral cortex
  - thalamus
  - hypothalamus
  - limbic system
  - olfactory bulb.
- The fourth, via the superior cerebellar peduncle, supplies the cerebellar cortex.
- The fifth descends in the mesencephalon and spinal cord.

BASAL FOREBRAIN CHOLINERGIC PATHWAY

Cholinergic neurons of this pathway originate in the basal forebrain, including:

- Ch4 cholinergic neurones – located in the nucleus basalis of Meynert
- Ch2 and Ch3 cholinergic neurones – located in the diagonal band nucleus (of Broca)
- Ch1 cholinergic neurones – located in the medial septal nucleus.

Their main innervation is as follows:

- Ch4: cerebral cortex, amygdala and corpus striatum
- Ch1: hippocampal formation
- Ch2: hippocampal formation
- Ch3: olfactory bulb.

(Note that most of the cholinergic innervation of the corpus striatum is intrinsic and not from this pathway.)

BRAINSTEM CHOLINERGIC PATHWAY

Cholinergic neurons of this pathway originate in the brainstem, including:

- Ch5 cholinergic neurones – located in the pedunculopontine nucleus
- Ch6 cholinergic neurones – located in the laterodorsal tegmental nucleus.

Their (Ch5 and Ch6) main innervation is to the:

- thalamus
- cerebral cortex
- basal forebrain
- corpus striatum
- globus pallidus
- subthalamic nucleus
- substantia nigra.

Ch5 neurones are more closely interconnected with extrapyramidal structures, while Ch6 neurones send more projections to nuclei of the limbic system and to medial prefrontal cortex.

GLUTAMATE SYSTEM

Neurones using glutamate, an excitatory neurotransmitter, include:

- cerebral cortical pyramidal cells
- hippocampal pyramidal cells
- primary sensory afferents
- cerebellar granule cells
- cerebellar climbing fibres.

The cerebral cortex contains abundant NMDA (N-methyl-D-aspartate) receptors, which serve an integral role in corticocortical and corticofugal glutamatergic neurotransmission.

ASCENDING SEROTONIN SYSTEM

During embryogenesis, two groups of serotonergic neurones develop:

- a superior group – located at the boundary between the mesencephalon and the pons
- an inferior group – located from the pons caudally to the cervical spinal cord.

The superior group gives rise to the superior raphe nuclei and is largely responsible for the origin of ascending serotonergic fibres projecting to the forebrain. The main superior raphe nuclei are the:

- caudal linear nucleus (the most rostral)
- dorsal raphe nucleus
- median raphe nucleus
- supralemniscal nucleus.

Ascending fibres pass from the superior raphe nuclei, via pathways such as the dorsal raphe cortical tract (the largest pathway in primates) and the medial forebrain bundle (the largest pathway in the rat), to innervate the forebrain. Particularly important destinations include the:

- suprachiasmatic nucleus
- substantia nigra
- limbic system
- periventricular regions
- primary sensory areas of the cerebral cortex
- association areas of the cerebral cortex.

BIBLIOGRAPHY

Alexander, G.E., DeLong, M.R. & Strick, P.L. 1986: Parallel organisation of functionally segregated circuits linking basal ganglia and cortex. *Annual Review of Neuroscience* 9:357–381.

Heimer, L. 1995: *The Human Brain and Spinal Cord*. Berlin: Springer.

Puri, B.K. & Tyrer, P.J. 2004: *Sciences Basic to Psychiatry*, 3rd edn. Edinburgh: Churchill Livingstone.

Snell, R.S. 1987: *Clinical Neuroanatomy for Medical Students*, 2nd edn. Boston: Little, Brown.

Trimble, M.R. 1996: *Neuropsychiatry*, 2nd edn. Chichester: John Wiley.

11

Neuropathology

DEMENTIAS

Alzheimer's disease

Macroscopic neuropathology
Macroscopic changes in Alzheimer's disease include:

- global brain atrophy
- ventricular enlargement
- sulcal widening.

The atrophy is usually most marked in the frontal and temporal lobes.

Histopathology
Histological changes in the cerebral cortex in Alzheimer's disease include:

- neuronal loss
- shrinking of dendritic branching
- reactive astrocytosis
- neurofibrillary tangles
- neuritic plaques (senile plaques).

There is a positive correlation between the number of neurofibrillary tangles and neuritic plaques, on the one hand, and, on the other, the degree of cognitive impairment.

Histological changes seen commonly in the hippocampus include:

- granulovacuolar degeneration
- Hirano bodies
- neurofibrillary tangles
- neuritic plaques (senile plaques).

Ultrastructural pathology

Neuritic plaques contain a core made of amyloid. This consists of 8-nm extracellular filaments made up mainly of the β-peptide, Aβ or β/A4. Scattered deposits of amyloid β protein in the brain in Alzheimer's disease have been found to localize to activated microglia.

Aβ or β/A4 is derived from the β-amyloid precursor protein (APP).

Neurochemical pathology

Neurochemical changes that have been reported in Alzheimer's disease include:

- ↓acetylcholinesterase
- ↓choline acetyltransferase
- ↓GABA
- ↓noradrenaline.

Pick's disease

Pick's disease is one histological type of frontotemporal dementia.

Macroscopic neuropathology

Macroscopic changes in Pick's disease include:

- selective asymmetrical atrophy of the anterior temporal lobes and frontal lobes
- knife-blade gyri
- ventricular enlargement.

Histopathology

Histological changes in Pick's disease include:

- Pick's bodies
- neuronal loss
- reactive astrocytosis.

These changes may be seen in the:

- cerebral cortex
- basal ganglia
- locus coeruleus
- substantia nigra.

Ultrastructural pathology

Pick's bodies consist of:

- straight neurofilaments
- paired helical filaments
- endoplasmic reticulum.

Multi-infarct dementia

ICD-10 classes multi-infarct dementia under vascular dementia.

Macroscopic neuropathology

Macroscopic changes in multi-infarct dementia include:

- multiple cerebral infarcts
- local or general brain atrophy
- ventricular enlargement
- arteriosclerotic changes in major arteries.

Clinically, the following relationships have been found usually to hold approximately for the total volume of the infarcts:

- 50 mL < volume ≤ 100 mL: cognitive impairment
- volume > 100 mL: dementia.

Histopathology

Histological changes include those of infarction and ischaemia.

Lewy body disease

The generic term 'dementia with Lewy bodies' was proposed at the first International Workshop on Lewy Body Dementia in 1995. It was described in 1923 by Friedrich Lewy in a large proportion of his patients suffering from paralysis agitans which had coincident plaques and neurofibrillary tangles. Lewy body dementia includes the following types of dementia:

- diffuse Lewy body disease
- senile dementia of Lewy body type
- Lewy body variant of Alzheimer's disease.

Histopathology

Histological changes in the brain in dementia caused by Lewy body disease include:

- Lewy bodies
- neuronal loss
- neurofibrillary tangles
- neuritic plaques (senile plaques).

Compared with Parkinson's disease, in which Lewy bodies are also found, in dementia caused by Lewy body disease the density of Lewy bodies is much higher in the:

- cingulate gyrus
- parahippocampal gyrus
- temporal cortex.

Ultrastructural pathology

Lewy bodies contain:

- protein neurofilaments
- granular material
- dense core vesicles
- microtubule assembly protein
- ubiquitin
- tau protein.

Creutzfeldt–Jakob disease

Creutzfeldt–Jakob disease (CJD) is transmitted by infection with a prion. In addition to the brain changes mentioned below, CJD disease is also associated with degeneration in spinal cord long descending tracts. It has an incubation period of many years. Infection may be transmitted from surgical specimens, from postmortem preparations (such as corneal grafts) and from human pituitary glands; the latter have been used to produce human somatotropin for clinical use. In 1995 in Britain a new variant of Creutzfeldt–Jakob disease (nvCJD) was reported which, it has been suggested, may be linked to transmission, possibly via the food chain, from the neuropathologically related disorder bovine spongiform encephalopathy (BSE).

Macroscopic neuropathology
There may be little or no gross atrophy of the cerebral cortex evident in rapidly developing cases. In those surviving the longest, changes seen may include:

- selective cerebellar atrophy
- generalized cerebral atrophy
- ventricular enlargement.

Histopathology
Histological changes in the brain in dementia caused by Creutzfeldt–Jakob disease include:

- status spongiosus
- neuronal degeneration without inflammation
- astrocytic proliferation.

Punch–drunk syndrome

This is also known as post-traumatic dementia or boxing encephalopathy.

Macroscopic neuropathology
Typical macroscopic changes include:

- cerebral atrophy
- ventricular enlargement
- perforation of the septum pellucidum
- thinning of the corpus callosum.

Histopathology
Histological changes in the brain in punch-drunk syndrome include:

- neuronal loss
- neurofibrillary tangles.

CEREBRAL TUMOURS

The main types of cerebral tumours, listed in order of relative frequency, are:

- gliomas

- metastases
- meningeal tumours
- pituitary adenomas
- neurilemmomas
- haemangioblastomas
- medulloblastomas.

Gliomas
These are tumours derived from glial cells and their precursors, and include:

- astrocytomas – derived from astrocytes
- oligodendrocytomas – derived from oligodendrocytes
- ependymomas – derived from ependymal cells.

Metastases
Cerebral metastases derive particularly from primary neoplasia in the lung, breast, kidney, colon, ovary, prostate and thyroid.

Meningeal tumours
These include:

- meningiomas
- meningeal sarcomas (very rare)
- primary malignant melanomas derived from pia-arachnoid melanocytes (very rare).

Pituitary adenomas
These include, in approximate order of relative frequency (commonest first):

- sparsely granulated PRL (prolactin/lactotrophin/mamotrophin) cell adenomas
- oncocytomas
- null cell adenomas
- gonadotroph cell adenomas
- corticotroph cell adenomas
- densely granulated GH (growth hormone/somatotrophin) cell adenomas
- sparsely granulated GH cell adenomas
- mixed (GH cell–PRL cell) adenomas
- silent 'corticotroph' adenomas, subtype 2
- unclassified adenomas
- acidophil stem cell adenomas
- silent 'corticotroph' adenomas, subtype 1
- silent 'corticotroph' adenomas, subtype 3
- mammosomatotroph cell adenomas
- thyrotroph cell adenomas
- densely granulated GH cell adenomas.

Neurilemmomas
These are also known as schwannomas. They are derived from Schwann cells and include acoustic neuromas.

Haemangioblastomas
These are derived from blood vessels.

Medulloblastomas

These cerebellar tumours are embryonal tumours.

SCHIZOPHRENIA

Gross neuropathology

- *Brain mass.* There is a slight but significant reduction in brain mass in schizophrenia, compared with controls and allowing for differences in height, body mass, sex and year of birth (Brown *et al.*, 1986; Pakkenburg, 1987; Bruton *et al.*, 1990).
- *Brain length.* Bruton *et al.* (1990) found a significant reduction in the maximum anteroposterior length of formalin-fixed cerebral hemispheres in schizophrenia, compared with age- and sex-matched normal controls. Both hemispheres were shorter in schizophrenia compared with the controls.
- *Cerebral volumes.* In the postmortem brains of patients with schizophrenia, compared with age- and sex-matched controls, Pakkenburg (1987) found a significant reduction in the volumes of the:
  - cerebral hemispheres
  - cerebral cortex
  - central grey matter.
  - The volumes of the white matter did not differ significantly.
- *Hippocampus and parahippocampal gyrus.* Altshuler *et al.* (1990) studied the area and shape of the anterior hippocampus and parahippocampal gyrus in postmortem brains from schizophrenic, non-schizophrenic suicide, and non-psychiatric controls. No significant differences were found in hippocampal area, but the parahippocampal gyrus was significantly smaller in the schizophrenic group compared with the control group.

  Bogerts *et al.* (1990) also studied postmortem brains of schizophrenic patients and control subjects. Compared with the controls, in the schizophrenic group the hippocampal formation was significantly smaller in the right and left hemispheres. The reduction in hippocampal volume in the male schizophrenics was greater than in the female schizophrenics.
- *Ventricular volume.* Ventricular enlargement has been found in a number of postmortem studies of schizophrenic brains (e.g. Brown *et al.*, 1986; Pakkenburg, 1987; Bruton *et al.*, 1990). The ventricular enlargement particularly affects the temporal horn (Crow *et al.*, 1989), indicating temporal lobe neuropathology.
- *Temporal lobe.* The majority of postmortem studies have found a reduction in temporal lobe volume in schizophrenia. While the grey matter is reduced in volume, particularly at the level of the amygdala and anterior hippocampus, the volume of the white matter tends not to be reduced.

Morphometric studies

Temporal lobe

Pyramidal cell disorientation in the hippocampus has been reported by Kovelman and Scheibel (1984) and by Conrad *et al.* (1991), although this failed to be found by Altshuler *et al.* (1987).

Jeste and Lohr (1989) found that schizophrenic patients had a significantly lower pyramidal cell density than normal controls in the left CA4 hippocampal region.

Cytoarchitectural abnormalities have been reported in the entorhinal cortex in schizophrenia (Arnold *et al.*, 1991). These changes, which suggest disturbed development, included:

- aberrant invaginations of the surface
- disruption of cortical layers
- heterotopic displacement of neurons
- paucity of neurons in superficial layers.

Arnold *et al.* (1995) found that schizophrenic postmortem brains had a smaller neurone size in the hippocampal regions of:

- the subiculum
- CA1
- layer II of the entorhinal cortex.

It is of note that the subiculum, CA1, and the entorhinal cortex are the major subfields of the hippocampal region that maintain the afferent and efferent connections of the hippocampus with widespread cortical and subcortical targets. It was therefore concluded that the smaller size of neurones in these subfields may reflect the presence of structural or functional impairments that disrupt these connections, which in turn could have behavioural sequelae.

Reduced hippocampal mossy cell fibre staining has also been reported by Goldsmith and Joyce (1995).

Akbarian *et al.* (1993a) found a distorted distribution of nicotinamide–adenine dinucleotide phosphate–diaphorase (NADPH–d) neurones in the hippocampal formation and in the neocortex of the lateral temporal lobe, consistent with anomalous cortical development in the lateral temporal lobe.

Other cortical areas

Compared with control brains, Benes *et al.* (1986) found significantly lower neuronal density in the following cortical regions in schizophrenic brains:

- prefrontal cortex: layer VI
- anterior cingulate cortex: layer V
- primary motor cortex: layer III.

The glial density also tended to be lower throughout most layers of all three above regions. However, there were no differences in the neurone/glia ratios or neuronal size between the two groups. These results suggest the occurrence of a dysplastic process rather than degeneration in schizophrenia.

Benes *et al.* (1987) confirmed the presence of greater numbers of long, vertical, associative axons in the anterior cingulate cortex of schizophrenic patients relative to control subjects. On the basis of this finding they suggested that there might be an increase of associative inputs into the anterior cingulate cortex in schizophrenia.

Akbarian *et al.* (1993b) found a distorted distribution of NADPH–d neurones in the dorsolateral prefrontal area of schizophrenic postmortem brains, consistent with anomalous cortical development in this region.

Akbarian *et al.* (1995) have also found that the prefrontal cortex of schizophrenics shows reduced expression for glutamic acid decarboxylase (GAD) in the absence of significant cell loss, suggesting an activity-dependent down-regulation of neurotransmitter gene expression.

Other brain regions

The results of studies of the corpus callosum and cerebellum have yielded inconsistent results.

Synaptic pathology

Synaptic vesicles
Soustek (1989) found clusters of large numbers of synaptic vesicles in presynaptic knobs in the cerebral cortex of schizophrenic postmortem brains but not in brains from control subjects.

Synaptophysin
Synaptophysin is a presynaptic vesicle protein the distribution and abundance of which provides a synaptic marker which can be reliably measured in postmortem brains.

Eastwood *et al.* (1995) found that in schizophrenic brains, compared with controls, synaptophysin mRNA was reduced bilaterally in:

- CA4
- CA3
- the subiculum
- the parahippocampal gyrus.

(The effect of antipsychotic medication was discounted as a separate rat study showed no effect of haloperidol treatment on hippocampal synaptophysin mRNA.) Furthermore, Eastwood and Harrison (1995) found decreased synaptophysin in the medial temporal lobe in schizophrenia, compared with controls, using immunoautoradiography. Significant reductions were found in the:

- dentate gyrus
- subiculum
- parahippocampal gyrus.

Gliosis

Almost all recent quantitative studies investigating the regions of greatest structural differences in schizophrenic patients have not shown significant gliosis (e.g. Jellinger, 1985; Roberts *et al.*, 1987; Bruton *et al.*, 1990). This negative finding is consistent with either of the following possibilities:

1 The structural change in schizophrenic brains results from an embryonic insult prior to the third trimester (since the developing brain does not show reactive gliosis until approximately the third trimester).
2 A neuropathological process occurs at or after the third trimester but does not usually initiate a glial reaction.

AUTISM

Histological changes

Bauman and Kemper (1985) studied the brain of a 29-year-old autistic man and found, compared with the brain of an age- and sex-matched normal control, abnormalities in the:

- hippocampus
- subiculum
- entorhinal cortex
- septal nuclei

- mammillary body
- amygdala (selected nuclei)
- neocerebellar cortex
- roof nuclei of the cerebellum
- inferior olivary nucleus.

Neuropathological studies suggest that the microscropic neuroanatomical abnormalities in autism begin early in gestation, probably in the second trimester (Bauman, 1991).

Cerebellar pathology

Both neuropathological and structural neuroimaging studies have indicated that hypoplastia of the cerebellar vermis as well as hypoplasia of the cerebellar hemispheres occurs in some subjects with autism.

Reduced Purkinje cell count

Ritvo *et al.* (1986) compared the cerebellums of four autistic subjects with those of three comparison subjects without central nervous system pathology and one with phenytoin toxicity. Total Purkinje cell counts were found to be significantly lower in the cerebellar hemisphere and vermis of each autistic subject than in the comparison subjects.

Neocerebellar abnormality

In their study of subjects with autism, Courchesne *et al.* (1988) measured the size of the cerebellar vermis using magnetic resonance imaging and compared these with its size in controls. The neocerebellar vermal lobules VI and VII were found to be significantly smaller in autism. This appeared to be a result of developmental hypoplasia rather than shrinkage or deterioration after full development had been achieved. In contrast, the adjacent vermal lobules I to V, which are ontogenetically, developmentally and anatomically distinct from lobules VI and VII, were found to be of normal size. Maldevelopment of the vermal neocerebellum had occurred in both retarded and nonretarded patients with autism. The authors suggested that this localized maldevelopment might serve as a temporal marker to identify the events that damage the brain in autism, as well as other neural structures that might be concomitantly damaged. They concluded that the neocerebellar abnormality may:

- directly impair cognitive functions that may be attributable to the neocerebellum
- indirectly affect – through its connections to the brain stem, hypothalamus and thalamus – the development and functioning of one or more systems involved in cognitive, sensory, autonomic and motor activities
- occur concomitantly with damage to other neural sites the dysfunction of which directly underlies the cognitive deficits in autism.

MOVEMENT DISORDERS

Parkinson's disease

Idiopathic Parkinson's disease is characterized by a loss of dopaminergic neurones in the substantia nigra.

Macroscopic neuropathology

Macroscopic changes in idiopathic Parkinson's disease include:

- depigmentation of the substantia nigra, particularly the zona compacta
- depigmentation of the locus coeruleus.

Diffuse cortical atrophy may take place.

Histopathology

Histological changes in idiopathic Parkinson's disease include:

- neuronal loss
- reactive astrocytosis
- the presence of Lewy bodies in the:
    - substantia nigra
    - dorsal motor nucleus of the vagus
    - hypothalamus
    - nucleus basalis of Meynert
    - locus coeruleus
    - Edinger–Westphal nucleus
    - raphe nuclei
    - cerebral cortex
    - olfactory bulb
- the presence of melanin-containing macrophages.

Neurochemical pathology

Neurochemical changes in idiopathic Parkinson's disease include reduced inhibitory dopaminergic action of the nigrostriatal pathway on striatal cholinergic neurones.

Huntington's disease (chorea)

Huntington's disease (or chorea) results from a mutation of the protein huntingtin and is characterized by a selective loss of discrete neuronal populations in the brain with progressive degeneration of efferent neurones of the neostriatum and sparing of dopaminergic afferents, resulting in progressive atrophy of the neostriatum.

Macroscopic neuropathology

Macroscopic changes in Huntington's disease include:

- small brain with reduced mass
- marked atrophy of the corpus striatum, particularly the caudate nucleus
- marked atrophy of the cerebral cortex, particularly the frontal lobe gyri (the parietal lobe is less often affected)
- dilatation of the lateral and third ventricles.

Histopathology

Histological changes in Huntington's disease include:

- neuronal loss in the cerebral cortex, particularly the frontal cortex
- neuronal loss in the corpus striatum, particularly neurones using as neurotransmitters

- GABA and enkephalin
- GABA and substance P
- astrocytosis in affected regions.

In the affected regions there is relative sparing of the following neuronal populations:

- diaphorase-positive neurones containing nitric oxide synthase (NOS)
- large cholinesterase-positive neurones.

Neurochemical pathology
Neurochemical changes that have been reported in Huntington's disease include:

- ↓GABA
- ↓glutamic acid decarboxylase
- ↓acetylcholine
- ↓substance P
- ↑somatostatin
- ↓corticotrophin-releasing factor (CRF)
- dopamine hypersensitivity.

Evidence has recently been put forward suggesting that phospholipid-related signal transduction in advanced Huntington's disease is impaired (Puri, 2001).

Tardive dyskinesia

Tardive dyskinesia is a syndrome of potentially irreversible involuntary hyperkinetic dyskinesias that may occur during long-term treatment with antipsychotic (neuroleptic) medication. The most important hypotheses concerning the neurochemical pathology of tardive dyskinesia are:

- dopamine hypersensitivity
- free-radical induced neurotoxicity
- GABA insufficiency
- noradrenergic dysfunction.

Dopamine hypersensitivity hypothesis
According to this hypothesis the following sequence of events takes place:

> long-term treatment with antipsychotic (neuroleptic) medication
> →chronic dopamine receptor blockade
> →dopamine D2 receptor hypersensitivity in the nigrostriatal pathway
> →tardive dyskinesia.

Evidence in favour of this hypothesis includes:

- studies of denervation-induced hypersensitivity in muscles
- animal experiments in which, following discontinuation of antipsychotic drugs, acute dopamine agonist challenges led to increased oral stereotyped behaviour
- animal experiments in which repeated antipsychotic treatment may have led to increased brain dopamine D2 receptors.

There are some problems with the hypothesis:

- There are differences in the chronology of onset of symptoms between humans and animal models.

- There is only limited support for dopamine hypersensitivity from postantipsychotic dopamine turnover experiments in monkeys.
- Postmortem human brain tissue studies have not shown significant differences in D2 receptor binding between schizophrenic patients with tardive dyskinesia and schizophrenic patients without tardive dyskinesia.
- Blood biochemical assays have not shown consistent significant differences between patients with tardive dyskinesia and patients without tardive dyskinesia with respect to:
  - prolactin
  - somatotrophin.
- No consistent significant differences have been shown between patients with tardive dyskinesia and patients without tardive dyskinesia with respect to:
  - plasma homovanillic acid
  - urinary homovanillic acid
  - CSF homovanillic acid.
- Dopamine agonists do not strikingly exacerbate tardive dyskinesia.
- Dopamine antagonist antipsychotics may sometimes worsen tardive dyskinesia.

A modification of this hypothesis includes a role for dopamine D_1 receptors, but many of the above problems also apply again. Moreover, postmortem human brain tissue studies have not shown significant differences in D_1 receptor binding between schizophrenic patients with tardive dyskinesia and schizophrenic patients without tardive dyskinesia.

Free-radical induced neurotoxicity
According to this hypothesis the following sequence of events takes place:

long-term treatment with antipsychotic (neuroleptic) medication
→increased catecholamine turnover
→free-radical byproducts
→membrane lipid peroxidation in the basal ganglia (the basal ganglia have a high oxidative metabolism)
→tardive dyskinesia.

Evidence in favour of this hypothesis includes:

- α-tocopherol (vitamin E) being of benefit in rodent models of antipsychotic induced dyskinesia
- some studies showing increased blood or CSF levels of lipid peroxidation byproducts in patients with tardive dyskinesia compared with those without tardive dyskinesia.

One problem with this hypothesis is that vitamin E treatment of tardive dyskinesia in general does not lead to major clinical improvement.

GABA insufficiency
According to one version of this hypothesis, the following sequence of events takes place:

long-term treatment with antipsychotic (neuroleptic) medication
→destruction of GABAergic neurones in the striatum
→decreased feedback inhibition
→tardive dyskinesia.

According to another version, the sequence of events is:

long-term treatment with antipsychotic (neuroleptic) medication
→decreased GABAergic neuronal activity in the pars reticulata of the substantia nigra
→decreased inhibition of involuntary movements
→tardive dyskinesia.

The following is evidence in favour of these hypotheses:

- It has been shown that striatonigral GABAergic neurones feed back on dopaminergic nigrostriatal neurones to reduce their activity.
- Antipsychotic-treated dyskinetic monkeys have been found to have a decrease in glutamic acid decarboxylase, compared with similarly treated monkeys without tardive dyskinesia, in the:
  - substantia nigra
  - globus pallidus
  - subthalamic nucleus.
- Patients with tardive dyskinesia have been found on postmortem to have a significant decrease in glutamic acid decarboxylase activity, compared with patients without tardive dyskinesia, in the subthalamic nucleus.
- The following GABAergic agonists have generally shown promise as potential therapeutic agents:
  - benzodiazepines
  - baclofen
  - gamma–vinyl GABA

There are some problems with the hypothesis:

- Rodent models of tardive dyskinesia do not show consistent GABA function changes with antipsychotic treatment.
- It has not so far proved possible effectively to treat tardive dyskinesia with GABAergic drugs.

Noradrenergic dysfunction

According to this hypothesis, noradrenergic over-activity contributes to the pathophysiology of tardive dyskinesia. Evidence in favour of this hypotheses includes:

- Patients with tardive dyskinesia have been found to have significantly greater dopamine β-hydroxylase activity than those without tardive dyskinesia.
- platelet ^{3}H-dihydroergocryptine-α_2 adrenergic receptor binding and CSF noradrenaline have been found to be significantly correlated with the severity of tardive dyskinesia.

One problem with the hypothesis is that it has not so far proved possible effectively to treat tardive dyskinesia with noradrenergic drugs.

BIBLIOGRAPHY

Akbarian, S., Vinuela, A., Kim, J.J. et al. 1993a: Distorted distribution of nicotinamide–adenine dinucleotide phosphate–diaphorase neurons in temporal lobe of schizophrenics implies anomalous cortical development. Archives of General Psychiatry 50:178–187.

Akbarian, S., Bunney, W.E., Potkin, S.G. et al. 1993b: Altered distribution of nicotinamide–adenine dinucleotide phosphate–diaphorase cells in frontal lobe of schizophrenics implies disturbances of cortical development. Archives of General Psychiatry 50:169–177.

Akbarian, S., Kim, J.J., Potkin, S.G. et al. 1995: Gene expression for glutamic acid decarboxylase is reduced without loss of neurons in prefrontal cortex of schizophrenics. Archives of General Psychiatry 52:258–266.

Altshuler, L.L., Conrad, A., Kovelman, J.A. & Scheibel, A. 1987: Hippocampal pyramidal cell orientation in schizophrenia: a controlled neurohistologic study of the Yakovlev collection. Archives of General Psychiatry 44:1094–1098.

Altshuler, L.L., Casanova, M.F., Goldberg, T.E. & Kleinman, J.E. 1990: The hippocampus and parahippocampus in schizophrenia, suicide, and control brains. Archives of General Psychiatry 47:1029–1034.

Arnold, S.E., Hyman, B.T., Van Hoesen, G.W. & Damasio, A.R. 1991: Some cytoarchitectural abnormalities of the entorhinal cortex in schizophrenia. *Archives of General Psychiatry* 48:625–632.

Arnold, S.E., Franz, B.R., Gur, R.C. *et al.* 1995: Smaller neuron size in schizophrenia in hippocampal subfields that mediate cortical–hippocampal interactions. *American Journal of Psychiatry* 152:738–748.

Bauman, M.L. 1991: Microscopic neuroanatomic abnormalities in autism. *Pediatrics* 87:791–796.

Bauman, M. & Kemper, T.L. 1985: Histoanatomic observations of brain in early infantile autism. *Neurology* 35:866–874.

Benes, F.M., Davidson, J. & Bird, E.D. 1986: Quantitative cytoarchitectural studies of the cerebral cortex of schizophrenics. *Archives of General Psychiatry* 43:31–35.

Benes, F.M., Majocha, R., Bird, E.D. & Marotta, C.A. 1987: Increased vertical axon numbers in cingulate cortex of schizophrenics. *Archives of General Psychiatry* 44:1017–1021.

Bogerts, B., Falkai, P., Haupts, M. *et al.* 1990: Postmortem volume measurements of limbic system and basal ganglia structures in chronic schizophrenics: initial results from a new brain collection. *Schizophrenia Research* 3:295–301.

Brown, R., Colter, N., Corsellis, J.A. *et al.* 1986: Postmortem evidence of structural brain changes in schizophrenia: differences in brain weight, temporal horn area, and parahippocampal gyrus compared with affective disorder. *Archives of General Psychiatry* 43:36–42.

Bruton, C.J., Crow, T.J., Frith, C.D. *et al.* 1990: Schizophrenia and the brain: a prospective clinico-neuropathological study. *Psychological Medicine* 20: 285–304.

Conrad, A.J., Abebe, T., Austin, R., Forsythe, S. & Scheibel, A.B. 1991: Hippocampal pyramidal cell disarray in schizophrenia as a bilateral phenomenon. *Archives of General Psychiatry* 48:413–417.

Courchesne, E., Yeung Courchesne, R., Press, G.A., Hesselink, J.R. & Jerningan, T.L. 1988: Hypoplasia of cerebellar vermal lobules VI and VII in autism. *New England Journal of Medicine* 318:1349–1354.

Crow, T.J., Ball, J., Bloom, S.R. *et al.* 1989: Schizophrenia as an anomaly of development of cerebral asymmetry: a postmortem study and a proposal concerning the genetic basis of the disease. *Archives of General Psychiatry* 46:1145–1150.

Eastwood, S.L. & Harrison, P.J. 1995: Decreased synaptophysin in the medial temporal lobe in schizophrenia demonstrated using immunoautoradiography. *Neuroscience* 69:339–343.

Eastwood, S.L., Burnet, P.W. & Harrison, P.J. 1995: Altered synaptophysin expression as a marker of synaptic pathology in schizophrenia. *Neuroscience* 66:309–319.

Goldsmith, S.K. & Joyce, J.N. 1995: Alterations in hippocampal mossy fiber pathway in schizophrenia and Alzheimer's disease. *Biological Psychiatry* 37:122–126.

Jellinger, K. 1985: Neuromorphological background of pathochemical studies in major psychoses. In Beckman, H. (ed.) *Pathochemical Markers in Major Psychoses*. Heidelberg: Springer Verlag, 1–23.

Jeste, D.V. & Lohr, J.B. 1989: Hippocampal pathologic findings in schizophrenia: a morphometric study. *Archives of General Psychiatry* 46:1019–1024.

Kovelman, J.A. & Scheibel, A.B. 1984: A neurohistological correlate of schizophrenia. *Biological Psychiatry* 19:1601–1621.

Pakkenberg, B. 1987: Postmortem study of chronic schizophrenic brains. *British Journal of Psychiatry* 151:744–752.

Puri, B.K. 2001: Impaired phospholipid-related signal transduction in advanced Huntington's disease. *Experimental Physiology* 86:683–685.

Ritvo, E.R., Freeman, B.J., Scheibel, A.B. *et al.* 1986: Lower Purkinje cell counts in the cerebella of four autistic subjects: initial findings of the UCLA/NSAC autopsy research report. *American Journal of Psychiatry* 143:862–866.

Roberts, G.W., Colter, N., Lofthouse, R., Johnstone, E.C. & Crow, T.J. 1987: Is there gliosis in schizophrenia? Investigation of the temporal lobe. *Biological Psychiatry* 22:1459–1468.

Soustek, Z. 1989: Ultrastructure of cortical synapses in the brain of schizophrenics. *Zentralblatt für Allgemeine Patholic und Pathologische Anatomie* 135:25–32.

12

Neuroimaging techniques

X-RAY

X-ray radiography is a form of structural imaging.

NEUROPSYCHIATRIC APPLICATIONS

The main use nowadays of skull radiography is in the assessment of trauma. It may also be useful in the detection of intracranial expanding lesions.

CT

CT is X-ray computerized tomography or computed tomography. It was previously known as computerized axial tomography (CAT). CT is a form of structural imaging. The basis of CT is as follows:

1 X-ray beams are passed through a given tissue plane in different directions.
2 Scintillation counters record the emerging X-rays.
3 A computer reconstructs the emerging X-ray data.
4 Radiodensity maps are produced.

This procedure is repeated for successive adjacent planes, thereby building up an image of, for example, the whole brain.

NEUROPSYCHIATRIC APPLICATIONS

Where available, CT and MRI (see below) have largely replaced skull radiography. Clinical uses of CT include the detection of:

- shifts of intracranial structures
- intracranial expanding lesions
- cerebral infarction
- cerebral oedema
- cerebral atrophy and ventricular dilatation
- atrophy of other structures
- demyelination changes and other causes of radiodensity change.

It is also widely used in neuropsychiatric research.

PET

PET is positron emission tomography. It is a form of functional imaging. The basis of PET neuroimaging is as follows:

1 A positron-emitting radioisotope or radiolabelled ligand is introduced into the cerebral circulation. Routes commonly used are:
   - intravenous administration (the radioactive substance is in solution)
   - by inhalation (the radioactive substance is in gaseous form).
2 Then:
   - → blood flow ± cerebral tissue binding in the brain
   - → emission of positrons
   - → positron–electron interactions
   - → dual γ photon emissions
   - → detection of γ photons
   - → computer reconstruction of emerging γ photon data.
3 Slice images are produced of the distribution of the radioisotopes in the brain.

The positron-emitting radioisotopes used can be produced in small cyclotrons.

NEUROPSYCHIATRIC APPLICATIONS

PET neuroimaging can give information about:

- metabolic changes
- regional cerebral blood flow (rCBF)
- ligand binding.

Clinical applications of PET include:

- cerebrovascular disease
- Alzheimer's disease
- epilepsy, prior to neurosurgery
- head injury.

Some measurements made by PET, for example the study of regional cerebral blood flow, are likely to be increasingly replaced by functional magnetic resonance imaging (fMRI), since the latter does not require the use of radioactive isotopes. On the other hand, fMRI is not a suitable replacement for PET for ligand binding studies.

SPECT

SPECT is single-photon emission computerized tomography. It is also known as SPET (single-photon emission tomography). It is a form of functional imaging. The basis of SPECT neuroimaging is as follows:

1   A radioisotope or radiolabelled ligand is introduced into the cerebral circulation. Routes commonly used are:
      intravenous administration (the radioactive substance is in solution)
      by inhalation (the radioactive substance is in gaseous form).
2   Then:
      → blood flow ± cerebral tissue binding in the brain
      → single γ photon emissions
      → detection of γ photons
      → computer reconstruction of emerging γ photon data.
3   Slice images are produced of the distribution of the radioisotopes in the brain.

NEUROPSYCHIATRIC APPLICATIONS

SPECT neuroimaging can give information about:

- regional cerebral blood flow (rCBF)
- ligand binding.

It is also of use in conditions in which the onset of the symptomatology being studied (e.g. epileptic seizures, auditory hallucinations) may occur at a time when the patient is not in or near a scanner; a suitable radioligand (e.g. 99m-technetium hexamethylpropylene amine oxime – HMPAO) can be administered at the material time and the patient scanned afterwards.

Clinical applications of SPECT include Alzheimer's disease.

The resolution of SPECT is generally poorer than that of PET, and both are likely to be increasingly replaced by fMRI. However, fMRI is not a suitable replacement for SPECT for ligand studies or for the type of study mentioned above in which the onset of the symptomatology being studied may occur at a time when the subject is not in or near a scanner.

MRI

MRI is magnetic resonance imaging. It was previously referred to as nuclear magnetic resonance (NMR). *In vivo* NMR is now taken to include MRI, MRA (magnetic resonance angiography), MRS (magnetic resonance spectroscopy), and fMRI. In addition, it is possible to carry out *in vitro* NMR studies of tissues at higher magnetic field strengths (say, over 11 teslas) than are currently allowed for human subjects.

MRI and MRA are forms of structural imaging. MRS and fMRI are types of functional imaging. The basis of MRI is as follows:

1   The patient is placed in a strong static magnetic field.
2   Then:
   - → alignment of proton spin axes
   - → pulses of radio-frequency waves at specified frequencies are administered

- • → this additional energy is absorbed
- • → some protons jump to a higher quantum level
- • → radiowaves are emitted when these protons return to the lower quantum level
- • → the radio-frequency (RF) wave frequencies are measured
- • → precession in each voxel is determined and T_1 (longitudinal relaxation time) and T_2 (transverse relaxation time) calculated
- • → proton density, T_1, T_2 pixel intensities.

3 Anatomical magnetic resonance images are produced.

The data are actually collected in the temporal domain, and need to be converted into the frequency domain using Fourier transformation.

In some circumstances it may be useful to administer a paramagnetic contrast enhancing agent such as gadolinium DTPA.

NEUROPSYCHIATRIC APPLICATIONS

MRI is useful in most clinical and research studies requiring high-resolution neuroanatomical imaging.

BIBLIOGRAPHY

Bydder, G.M. 1983: Clinical aspects of NMR imaging. In Steiner, R. (ed.) *Recent Advances in Radiology and Medical Imaging*. Edinburgh: Churchill Livingstone, 15–33.

Costa, D.C. & Ell, P.J. 1991: *Brain Blood Flow in Neurology and Psychiatry*. Edinburgh: Churchill Livingstone.

Costa, D.C., Morgan, G.F. & Lassen, N.A. 1993: *New Trends in Nuclear Neurology and Psychiatry*. London: John Libbey.

Gadian, D.G. 1995: *NMR and its Applications to Living Systems*, 2nd edn. Oxford: Oxford University Press.

Ketonen, L.M. & Berg, M.J. 1996: *Clinical Neuroradiology*. London: Arnold.

Puri, B.K. 2000: MRI and MRS in neuropsychiatry. In Young, I.R., Grant, D.M. & Harris, R.K. (eds) *Methods in Biomedical Magnetic Resonance Imaging and Spectroscopy*. New York: John Wiley.

13

Neurophysiology

PHYSIOLOGY OF NEURONES, SYNAPSES AND RECEPTORS

Neurones

Resting membrane ion permeabilities
The comparative permeabilities to different ions of the resting neuronal membrane are as follows:

- K^+ (potassium ions) – relatively permeable
- Na^+ (sodium ions) – relatively impermeable
- Cl^- (chloride ions) – freely permeable
- organic anions – relatively impermeable.

Resting membrane potential
There is a negative resting membrane potential of around -70 mV. It is maintained by the sodium pump, which actively transports Na^+ out of the cell and K^+ into the cell. Energy for this process is provided by ATP.

Changes in membrane ion permeabilities
The neuronal membrane ion permeabilities may change in response to stimulation:

- *Depolarization*. The membrane potential increases; that is, it becomes less negative. This *increases* the probability of an action potential being generated.
- *Hyperpolarization*. The membrane potential decreases; that is, it becomes more negative. This *decreases* the probability of an action potential being generated.

Action potential
Neuronal stimulation leads to local depolarization.

If degree of depolarization > (a critical threshold) $\rightarrow$ nerve impulse or action potential.

During an action potential, the membrane potential rapidly becomes positive, before returning to become negative. This is caused by an increase first in Na^+ permeability, allowing the inflow of Na^+, and then in K^+ permeability (with a rapid reduction in Na^+ permeability at the same time), causing an outflow of K^+ and thereby restoring the negative membrane potential. The sodium pump then restores the original ionic concentrations.

- *Propagation of action potential.* An action potential is propagated by the depolarization spreading laterally to adjacent parts of the neurone.
- *All-or-none phenomenon.* The passage of an action potential along a neurone is an all-or-none phenomenon.
- *Absolute refractory period.* This is the period during which the active part of the neuronal membrane has a reversed polarity so that conduction or initiation of another action potential is not possible in it.
- *Relative refractory period.* This is the period of repolarization after an action potential, during which hyperpolarization occurs, making it more difficult for stimulation to allow the membrane potential to reach the critical threshold.
- *Conduction in unmyelinated fibres.* The greater the diameter of the fibre the faster is the rate of transmission.
- *Conduction in myelinated fibres.* The action potential appears to jump from one node of Ranvier to the next, skipping the intervening myelinated parts. This rapid form of conduction is known as saltatory conduction.

Synapses

Synapses may be found between:

- two neurones
- motoneurones and muscle cells
- sensory neurones and sensory receptors.

A *synaptic cleft* is the gap at a synapse between the membrane of a presynaptic fibre and that of the postsynaptic fibre.

There are two types of synapse:

- *Chemical.* This is the more common type, in which a chemical neurotransmitter is stored in presynaptic vesicles.
- *Electrical.* These are faster than chemical synapses, with direct membrane-to-membrane connection via gap junctions.

Synaptic transmission

At chemical synapses the following events take place during synaptic transmission:

1   An action potential arrives at the presynaptic membrane.
2   There is influx of Ca^{2+} (calcium ions).
3   Presynaptic vesicles fuse to the presynaptic membrane.
4   Neurotransmitter is released into the synaptic cleft.
5   There is passage of neurotransmitter across the synaptic cleft.
6   Neurotransmitter binds to postsynaptic receptors.
7   There are ion permeability changes in the postsynaptic membrane.
8   There is postsynaptic depolarization or hyperpolarization (depending on the type of neurotransmitter).

Excitatory postsynaptic potentials

Excitatory postsynaptic potentials, or EPSPs, occur in the postsynaptic membrane (because of depolarization) following release of an excitatory neurotransmitter from the presynaptic neurone at central excitatory synapses.

Inhibitory postsynaptic potentials

Inhibitory postsynaptic potentials, or IPSPs, occur in the postsynaptic membrane (because of hyperpolarization) following release of an inhibitory neurotransmitter from the presynaptic neurone at central inhibitory synapses.

Summation

One EPSP on its own is not usually sufficient to initiate an action potential. However, temporal and/or spatial summation may allow the degree of depolarization to reach the critical threshold. IPSPs, on summating with EPSPs, counter the effect of the latter.

Sensory receptors

The main types of sensory receptor in humans are:

- mechanoreceptors
- thermoreceptors
- light receptors
- nociceptors
- chemoreceptors.

Adaptation

In response to a continuous prolonged appropriate stimulus, most sensory receptors exhibit adaptation:

- phasic receptors – the receptor firing stops
- tonic receptors – the receptor firing frequency falls to a low maintained level.

PITUITARY HORMONES

Anterior pituitary hormones

Table 13.1 shows the anterior pituitary hormones and their corresponding hypothalamic releasing factors (hormones) and release-inhibiting factors (hormones).

ACTH

This is a single-chain peptide which stimulates the production of the steroid hormone cortisol by the adrenal glands.

FSH

Follicle-stimulating hormone consists of two peptide chains, α and β. FSH stimulates the gonads (ovaries and testes).

Table 13.1 *The anterior pluitary hormones and their corresponding hypothalamic releasing factors (hormones) and release-inhibiting factors (hormones)*

Anterior pituitary hormone	Hypothalamic releasing factor (hormone) and/or release–inhibiting factor (hormone)
Corticotropin (adrenocorticotrophic hormone, ACTH)	Corticotropin releasing factor (hormone) (CRF or CRH)
Follicle-stimulating hormone (FSH)	Gonadotropin releasing factor (hormone) (GnRF or GnRH)
Luteinizing hormone (LH)	Gonadotropin releasing factor (hormone) (GnRF or GnRH)
Melanocyte-stimulating hormone (MSH)	MSH release inhibitory factor (MIH)
Prolactin	Prolactin releasing factor (PRF) Prolactin release inhibitory factor (PIF) (dopamine)
Somatotropin (growth hormone, GH)	Growth hormone releasing factor (hormone) (GRF or GRH; somatocrinin) Growth hormone release inhibitory factor (somatostatin)
Thyrotropin (thyroid–stimulating hormone, TSH)	Thyrotropin releasing factor (hormone) (TRF or TRH)

- *In males*, FSH stimulates seminiferous tubule Sertoli cells to promote the growth of spermatozoa and also stimulates the release of inhibin A (the α subunit) and inhibin B (the β subunit). (In turn, inhibin causes a negative feedback on the secretion of FSH by the anterior pituitary gland.)
- *In females*, FSH stimulates the development of follicles. It also stimulates the activity of aromatose, which in turn stimulates the conversion of ovarian androgens into oestrogens. As in males, FSH stimulates the release of inhibin (from stromal cells of the ovary), which in turn causes a negative feedback on the secretion of FSH by the anterior pituitary gland.

LH

Luteinizing hormone consists of two peptide chains, α and β; the α chain of LH is the same as that of FSH. LH stimulates the gonads (ovaries and testes).

- *In males*, LH stimulates the testicular Leydig cells to produce testosterone.
- *In females*, LH stimulates the ovaries to produce androgens. In menstruating females, a surge of LH mid-cycle induces ovulation.

MSH

Melanocyte-stimulating hormone does not appear to be found in the human anterior pituitary. Its functions in relation to pigmentation appear to have been taken over by ACTH and β-lipotrophin.

Prolactin

Prolactin is a single-chain peptide hormone that acts on the mammary glands to stimulate the secretion of milk (normally during lactation). It also inhibits activity of the testes and ovaries.

GH

Growth hormone is a peptide hormone that stimulates the hepatic secretion of IGF-1 (insulin-like growth factor-1; previously termed somatomedin C). In turn, binding of IGF-1 to widespread IGF-BP (IGF-binding proteins) leads to the stimulation of anabolism (by stimulating the retention of calcium, phosphorus and nitrogen, thereby promoting growth in bones, for example) and stimulating the widespread biosynthesis of protein and collagen. Another important action of IGF-1 is in terms of opposing the action of insulin.

TSH

Thyroid-stimulating hormone consists of two peptide chains, α and β; the α chain of TSH is the same as that of LH (and of FSH). TSH stimulates the synthesis by the thyroid gland of the thyroid hormones T_4 and T_3. TSH also stimulates the release of T_4 and T_3 from the thyroid gland. (In turn, T_3 exerts a negative feedback control on the secretion of TRH and TSH.)

Posterior pituitary hormones

The hypothalamus is responsible for the neurosecretion of the two posterior pituitary hormones:

- arginine vasopressin (argipressin or antidiuretic hormone; AVP or ADH)
- oxytocin.

Note that, strictly speaking, these are actually hypothalamic hormones rather than pituitary hormones, as they are synthesized in the supraoptic and paraventricular nuclei of the anterior hypothalamus, and then transported to and stored in the posterior pituitary gland.

AVP or ADH

Arginine vasopressin or antidiuretic hormone is a nonapeptide that acts on the distal convoluted tubule and collecting ducts of the renal nephron to exert an antidiuretic effect.

Oxytocin

Oxytocin is a nonapeptide that stimulates contraction of the uterine myometrium during parturition (and perhaps during sexual intercourse), and, postpartum, stimulates the ejection of milk from the mammary glands during lactation. In rats, it has been found that centrally administered oxytocin has a satiety action (in both males and females). Oxytocin also has a natriuretic action in both males and females.

INTEGRATED BEHAVIOURS

Regulatory behaviour

A regulatory behaviour is one that is controlled by a homeostatic mechanism. Examples include behaviours related to hunger (feeding) and thirst (drinking).

In contrast, a non-regulatory behaviour is one that is not controlled by a homeostatic mechanism. Examples include sexual behaviour and parenting behaviour.

Pain

The neural pathway for pain is as follows.

Pain detection by receptors (for example, nociceptors in the skin)
$\rightarrow$ dorsal-root ganglion neurones to spinal cord
$\rightarrow$ ventral spinothalamic tract
$\rightarrow$ medial lemniscus
$\rightarrow$ ventrolateral thalamus
$\rightarrow$ primary somatosensory cortex.

According to the gate theory of pain, gates in the spinal cord, involving activity in spinal cord interneurones, can modify the perception of pain. These gates may also exist in the brainstem and even the cerebral cortex. This theory may explain why shifting attention away from the source of pain to something else may help reduce the severity of the pain that the subject is conscious of.

Hormonal substances, such as endorphins, may also influence the perception of pain. For example, during times of war, a soldier at the front may hardly feel any pain initially following a traumatic bodily injury such as the loss of part of a limb. In contrast, the same injury incurred in civilian life during peacetime may cause the same person to scream out in agony.

Motor function

At its simplest, motor activity involves the following pathway:

> Activity in the motor cortex (primary motor cortex – precentral gyrus, Brodmann area 4)
> → ipsilateral corticospinal tract
> → pyramidal decussation
> → ipsilateral (mainly) ventral corticospinal tract (moves midline muscles) and contralateral (mainly) lateral corticospinal tract (moves limb muscles).

Arousal

Further details regarding sleep and arousal are given later in this chapter. Here, we consider the changes in thalamocortical systems that occur in sleep and arousal. Basically, the hypothalamus appears to contain neuronal circuits that mediate homeostatic sleep mechanisms.

One important subcortical circuit involved is as follows. Output from the ventrolateral preoptic area, suprachiasmatic nucleus, and tuberomammillary nucleus of the hypothalamus synchronizes the non-rapid-eye-movement/rapid-eye-movement (NREM–REM) sleep cycle mechanisms of the pontine brainstem. The parts of the latter that appear to be particularly involved are the:

- locus coeruleus
- raphe nuclei
- dorsolateral tegmental nucleus
- pedunculo pontine tegmental nucleus.

A second subcortical system of importance involves output from the ventrolateral preoptic area, suprachiasmatic nucleus, and tuberomammillary nucleus of the hypothalamus to the thalamus, and thence to the cerebral cortex.

Sexual behaviour

This is a non-regulatory form of behaviour with complex control mechanisms.

Sex hormones have an important effect on the brain. In male fetuses, during development testosterone masculinizes the brain. This is the *organizing effect* of the hormone. This effect is particularly noteworthy in the hypothalamic preoptic area; this area is much larger in males following exposure to testosterone.

In the adult brain, sex hormones have an *activating effect*. In male adults, testosterone acts on the amygdala to stimulate the motivation to carry out sexual activity. Testosterone also acts on the hypothalamus to stimulate copulatory behaviour. In particular, stimulation of the medial preoptic area, in the presence of circulating testosterone, induces copulatory behaviour in primates.

(Destruction of the medial preoptic area in male monkeys, in which testosterone is circulating, is associated with an abolition of mating; but masturbation in the presence of out-of-reach females has been noted.) In female adults, ovarian hormones also appear to act on the amygdala to stimulate the motivation to carry out sexual activity. In infrahuman quadrapedal mammals, the action of ovarian hormones on the ventromedial hypothalamus stimulates lordosis (arching of the back, staying still with the back side elevated – a position that is receptive for copulatory behaviour).

Humans are aware of the importance of cognitive influences on sexual behaviour. The influence of the cerebral cortex in this context is clearly important but complex. For instance, while frontal lobe lesions are often associated with a loss of sexual inhibition, loss of libido may also occur in some cases.

Hunger

Feeding is a regulatory behaviour that particularly involves inputs from the following systems:

* digestive system (including insulin) and satiety signals
* hypothalamus
* cognition.

Insulin
The most important hormone which affects caloric homeostasis is insulin. When hungry, first the smell and then the taste of a meal causes signals to be sent in the following way:

Smell of food ± taste of food
$\rightarrow$ aroma and taste signals
$\rightarrow$ cerebral cortex
$\rightarrow$ hypothalamus
$\rightarrow$ dorsal motor nucleus of the vagus nerve (cranial nerve X)
$\rightarrow$ vagal cholinergic fibres
$\rightarrow$ pancreas
$\rightarrow$ insulin secretion from pancreatic B cells.

This is known as the *cephalic phase* of insulin secretion.

Entry of food into the stomach and duodenum leads to a further secretion of insulin; this is the *gastrointestinal phase* of insulin secretion.

Breakdown products from digested food enter the bloodstream and directly act on the pancreas, further stimulating the secretion of insulin. This is known as the *substrate phase* of insulin secretion.

Satiety signals
Gastric distension, for example following the ingestion of food, gives rise to satiety signals along the following pathway:

Food ingestion
$\rightarrow$ gastric distension
$\rightarrow$ stimulation of gastric wall stretch receptors
$\rightarrow$ vagal nerve transmission
$\rightarrow$ nucleus of tractus solitarius and area postrema (in the brainstem)
$\rightarrow$ hypothalamus
$\rightarrow$ cerebral cortex
$\rightarrow$ perception of gastric distension.

There exist other systems that also provide feedback to the brain from the alimentary canal. For example, as the ingested (and partially digested) food reaches the intestines, many different peptides are released. Just one of these, CCK (cholecystokinin), can stimulate vagal afferents carrying pyloric gastric stretch receptor signals to the brainstem, thereby providing synergy with the satiety signal system outlined above. Moreover, infrahuman mammalian experiments have demonstrated the satiety action of CCK directly infused into the hypothalamus. Another neuropeptide that may affect hunger is oxytocin, intracerebroventricular injection of which decreases food intake in rats.

Caloric intake also has a direct satiety effect, although the precise mechanism by which this occurs is not clear at the time of writing.

Satiety signals are also given rise to by postgastric actions of ingested food. One mechanism involved is undoubtedly related to the liver.

The hormone leptin (or Ob protein), biosynthesized in adipose tissue, has a circulating plasma concentration that is positively correlated with overall adiposity. Leptin has a satiety action when experimentally directly infused into cerebral ventricles, and hypothalamic leptin receptors have been identified.

Hypothalamus

Rodent experiments from the 1950s onwards have suggested these facts:

- The ventrolateral hypothalamus (VLH) contains a hunger centre; bilateral damage to this area causes aphagia in rats.
- The ventromedial hypothalamus (VMH) contains a satiety centre; damage to this area may cause hyperphagia in rats.

This is known as the *dual-centre hypothesis*. More recent evidence has suggested that this simple hypothesis is, in fact, incorrect. The true reason why bilateral ventromedial hypothalamic damage leads to hyperphagia is related to:

- an increase in parasympathetic tone
- an increase in vagal reflexes (and therefore an increased rate of gastric emptying)
- a reduction in sympathetic tone
- a resetting of a hypothetical homeostatic set point
- an increase in the accumulation of stored fat
- a reduction in satiety duration following feeding.

Opposite effects occur following bilateral ventrolateral hypothalamus damage.

The neuropeptide NPY (neuropeptide Y) appears to act on the paraventricular nucleus to increase food intake.

Cognitive factors

As with sexual behaviour, cognitive factors are clearly of importance in the integrated behaviour of hunger and feeding. The ability of people to fast, for example, shows that cognitive activity can override satiety signalling and any putative hypothalamic factors.

The amygdala is thought to play some role in hunger and feeding. It is known, for example, that damage to the amygdala is associated with the abolition of taste-aversion learning and also with a change in the types of food that are preferred.

Damage to the inferior prefrontal cortex often appears to be associated with reduced food intake. This may, however, be at least partly related to the fact that this part of the cerebral cortex receives olfactory signals, so that damage to the cortex may reduce the ability to respond to the aroma and taste of food.

Thirst

Drinking is a regulatory behaviour. There are two types of homeostatic mechanisms that are of relevance, and that give rise to two different types of thirst. They are:

- osmotic homeostasis (related to osmotic thirst)
- volume homeostasis (related to hypovolaemic thirst).

Osmotic thirst

Osmotic thirst occurs when the concentrations of solutes in body fluids such as the plasma become too high. This may occur as a result of a rise in concentration of one or more solutes (for example, following sodium loading after eating a meal rich in sodium salts such as sodium chloride and monosodium glutamate). It may also occur as a result of water deprivation (dehydration) or the copious loss of dilute fluids such as sweat. Under any of these circumstances, the osmotic homeostatic mechanism requires that water be drunk.

Before the behaviour associated with osmotic thirst kicks in, the body relies on its large posterior pituitary stores of AVP (arginine vasopressin) to try to rectify the osmolality of the extracellular and intracellular fluid compartments. The mechanism appears to involve the following pathway.

> Increase in solutes/water deprivation/dehydration/loss of dilute fluid
> → raised extracellular fluid osmolality (and therefore also raised intracellular fluid osmolality via osmosis)
> → stimulation of osmoreceptor cells in the organ of the lamina terminalis, subfornical organ, median preoptic nucleus, and magnocellular neurones in the supraoptic nucleus and paraventricular nucleus
> → projections from the organ of the lamina terminalis to the median preoptic nucleus, and to the magnocellular AVP-secreting cells of the supraoptic nucleus and paraventricular nucleus further stimulate these other brain regions
> → secretion of AVP from the posterior pituitary
> → stimulation of AVP V_2 renal receptors
> → increased water permeability of distal convoluted tubules and collecting ducts of nephrons
> → increased water retention, increased urinary osmolality, and reduced urinary volume
> → restoration of extracellular fluid osmolality.

At the time of writing, the neural pathways in the forebrain that are related to thirst have not been clearly identified.

Another mechanism involved in osmotic homeostasis and osmotic thirst is the increased urinary excretion of sodium ions as a result of the actions of ANP (atrial natriuretic peptide) and oxytocin. ANP is released from the cardiac atria in response to increased atrial distension, in turn caused by hyperosmolality of the extracellular fluid. The release of oxytocin from the posterior pituitary has been mentioned earlier in this chapter.

Hypovolaemic thirst

Hypovolaemic thirst occurs when the total volume of body fluids such as the plasma becomes too low. This may occur as a result of blood loss, for example. The hypovolaemic homeostatic mechanism requires that fluids that contain solutes be drunk; if only pure water were drunk, then hypo-osmolality would result. In experiments, hypovolaemic rats that are given a choice of pure water or concentrated sodium chloride solution have been observed to drink enough of each in order to be imbibing isotonic levels overall.

One mechanism involved is the following:

Blood loss of greater than 10% of normal blood volume
→ detection by stretch receptors in veins that enter the cardiac right atrium; larger blood volume decreases are also detected by stretch receptors in the aortic arch and carotid sinus
→ vagal nerve transmission
→ nucleus of tractus solitarius (in the medulla oblongata)
→ supra-optic nucleus and paraventricular nucleus of hypothalamus (including via a noradrenergic pathway from ventrolateral medulla A_1 cells)
→ secretion of AVP from the posterior pituitary
→ stimulation of AVP V_2 renal receptors
→ increased water permeability of distal convoluted tubules and collecting ducts of nephrons
→ increased water retention, increased urinary osmolality, and reduced urinary volume
→ reverses hypovolaemia.

Another mechanism that also operates starts with the kidneys, as follows.:

Hypovolaemia
→ reduced renal perfusion pressure and reduced delivery of sodium ions to the distal tubule of the nephron
→ renal secretion of renin
→ catalyzes the conversion of hepatic angiotensinogen into angiotensin I
→ conversion into angiotensin II (catalyzed by angiotensin-converting enzyme from the lungs)
→ vasoconstriction and stimulation of adrenal secretion of aldosterone
→ aldosterone stimulates renal conservation of sodium ions
→ reverses hypovolaemia.

Angiotensin II also acts as a neurotransmitter in the brain in the following way:

Angiotensin II (A II)
→ binding to AII receptors in the subfornical organ (which does not have a blood–brain barrier)
→ supra-optic nucleus and paraventricular nucleus
→ secretion of AVP from the posterior pituitary
→ stimulation of AVP V_2 renal receptors
→ increased water permeability of distal convoluted tubules and collecting ducts of nephrons
→ increased water retention, increased urinary osmolality, and reduced urinary volume
→ reverses hypovolaemia.

The central action of angiotensin II also stimulates thirst.

AROUSAL AND SLEEP

Sleep architecture

Sleep is divided into the following two phases:

- *rapid-eye-movement* (REM) sleep, during which the eyes undergo rapid movements and there is a high level of brain activity

- *non-REM* sleep, during which there is reduced neuronal activity.

Stages of sleep

The following stages normally occur during normal non-REM sleep:

stage 0 – quiet wakefulness and shut eyes; EEG: alpha activity
stage 1 – falling asleep; EEG: low amplitude, ↓ alpha activity, low-voltage theta activity
stage 2 – light sleep; EEG: 2–7 Hz, occasional sleep spindles and K complexes
stage 3 – deep sleep; ↑ delta activity (20–50%)
stage 4 – deep sleep; ↑↑ delta activity (>50%).

Stage 3 + stage 4 = slow-wave sleep (SWS).

Physiological correlates of sleep

REM sleep

Features of REM sleep include:

- ↑ recall of dreaming if awoken during REM sleep
- ↑ complexity of dreams
- ↑ sympathetic activity
- transient runs of conjugate ocular movements
- maximal loss of muscle tone
- ↑ heart rate
- ↑ systolic blood pressure
- ↑ respiratory rate
- ↑ cerebral blood flow
- occasional myoclonic jerks
- penile erection or ↑ vaginal blood flow
- ↑ protein synthesis (rat brain).

Non–REM sleep

Features of non-REM sleep include:

- ↓ recall of dreaming if awoken during REM sleep
- ↓ complexity of dreams
- ↑ parasympathetic activity
- upward ocular deviation with few or no movements
- abolition of tendon reflexes
- ↓ heart rate
- ↓ systolic blood pressure
- ↓ respiratory rate
- ↓ cerebral blood flow
- penis not usually erect.

Causes of the sleeping–waking cycle

There are two main theories accounting for the sleeping–waking cycle:

- monoaminergic (or biochemical, two-stage, Jouvet's) model
- cellular (or Hobson's) model.

Monoaminergic model
In this model:

- non-REM sleep is associated with serotonergic neuronal activity – raphe complex
- REM sleep is associated with noradrenergic neuronal activity – locus coeruleus.

Cellular model
In this model three groups of central neurones are of importance. These groups, and their corresponding neurotransmitters, are the:

- pontine gigantocellular tegmental fields (nucleus reticularis pontis caudalis) – acetylcholine
- dorsal raphe nuclei – serotonin
- locus coeruleus – noradrenaline.

THE ELECTROENCEPHALOGRAM (EEG)

CONVENTIONAL RECORDING TECHNIQUES

The conventional EEG recording involves placing electrodes on the scalp, and is therefore non-invasive. The positions of the electrodes is usually according to the International 10–20 System, which entails measurements from the following scalp landmarks:

- the nasion
- the inion
- the right auricular depression
- the left auricular depression.

In this system, proportions of scalp distances are 10% or 20%, and midline electrodes are denoted by the subscript z.

In *ambulatory* electroencephalography the output is stored on a suitable portable recorder.

SPECIALIZED RECORDING TECHNIQUES

- *Nasopharyngeal leads.* Electrodes are positioned in the superior part of the nasopharynx. This method can be used to obtain recordings from the inferior and medial temporal lobe.
- *Sphenoidal electrodes.* Electrodes are inserted between the mandibular coronoid notch and the zygoma. This method can be used to obtain recordings from the inferior temporal lobe.
- *Electrocorticography.* Electrodes are placed directly on the surface of the brain.
- *Depth electroencephalography.* Electrodes are placed inside the brain.

Normal EEG rhythms

Classification according to frequency band
Normal EEG rhythms are classified according to frequency as follows:

- delta: frequency <4 Hz

- theta: 4 Hz ≤ frequency < 8 Hz
- alpha: 8 Hz ≤ frequency < 13 Hz
- beta: frequency ≥ 13 Hz.

Lambda activity

Lambda activity occurs over the occipital region in subjects with their eyes open. It is related to ocular movements during visual attention.

Mu activity

Mu activity occurs over the motor cortex. It is related to motor activity and is abolished by movement of the contralateral limb.

Spikes and waves

- *Spikes.* These are transient high peaks that last less than 80 ms.
- *Sharp waves.* These are conspicuous sharply defined wave formations that rise rapidly, fall more slowly, and last more than 80 ms.

The effect of drugs

- *Antidepressants.* In general, antidepressants cause increased delta activity.
- *Antipsychotics.* In general, antipsychotic drugs cause:
  decreased beta activity
  increased low-frequency delta activity and/or increased theta activity.
- *Anxiolytics.* In general, anxiolytics, including barbiturates and benzodiazepines, cause:
  increased beta activity
  decreased alpha activity (sometimes).
- *Lithium.* Therapeutic levels of lithium lead to only small EEG effects which are likely to be missed on visual analysis of routine recordings.

BIBLIOGRAPHY

Carpenter, R.H.S. 2002: *Neurophysiology*, 4th edn. London: Arnold.

Emslie-Smith, D., Paterson, C.R., Scratcherd, T. & Read, N.W. (eds) 1988: *Textbook of Physiology*, 11th edn. Edinburgh: Churchill Livingstone.

Guyton, A.C. & Hall, J.E. 2000: *Textbook of Medical Physiology*, 10th edn. Philadelphia: W.B. Saunders.

Puri, B.K. & Tyrer, P.J. 2004: *Sciences Basic to Psychiatry*, 3rd edn. Edinburgh: Churchill Livingstone.

Stein, J.F. 1982: *An Introduction to Neurophysiology*. Oxford: Blackwell.

14

Neurochemistry

TRANSMITTER SYNTHESIS, STORAGE AND RELEASE

TRANSMITTER SYNTHESIS

The synthesis of the neurotransmitters noradrenaline, serotonin, dopamine, GABA and acetylcholine is considered later in this chapter.

TRANSMITTER STORAGE

The transmitter at a synaptic cleft is stored in presynaptic vesicles. Each vesicle contains one quantum, usually corresponding to several thousand molecules, of transmitter.

TRANSMITTER RELEASE

Transmitter release from synaptic vesicles takes place by exocytosis in a process controlled by Ca^{2+} influx. Because the number of vesicles released is an integer, transmitter release is essentially quantal in nature. The Ca^{2+} enters via voltage-dependent ion channels. Importantly, Na^+ influx and/or K^+ efflux are not needed for transmitter release. Ca^{2+} influences or regulates:

- the probability of vesicular transmitter release
- vesicular fusion
- the transport of synaptic vesicles to the presynaptic active zone of exocytosis
- post-tetanic potentiation
- tonic depolarization of the presynaptic neurone.

ION CHANNELS

Ion channels are now classified into families on the basis of genetic sequence homology and, usually, pore-lining α subunit topology. The main families are as follows:

- 6-TM
- 2-TM
- 4-TM or 8-TM
- ionotropic glutamate receptors
- nicotinic ACh and related receptors
- intracellular calcium ion channels
- chloride ion channels.

THE 6–TM FAMILY

These are voltage-gated ion channels which each contain six transmembrane segments (hence their name). Members of this family include the following ion channels:

- voltage-gated sodium channels
- voltage-gated calcium channels
- voltage-gated potassium channels
- calcium-activated potassium channels
- hyperpolarization-activated cation channels involved in rhythmic activities
- cyclic nucleotide-gated cation channels involved in sensory transduction
- vanilloid receptors involved in sensory transduction.

THE 2–TM FAMILY

These ion channels each have two transmembrane segments in each pore-lining subunit. They include:

- Kir (inwardly rectifying potassium ion channels)
- amiloride-sensitive epithelial sodium ion channel
- the P_{2X} ATP receptor
- the Phe-Met-Arg-Phe-amide-activated sodium ion channel.

THE 4–TM OR 8–TM FAMILY

These are two-pore potassium ion channels. They are leak channels that partly help bring about the resting membrane potential of cells.

IONOTROPIC GLUTAMATE RECEPTORS

These ligand-gated channels have a pore-lining domain that is similar to that of the Kir α subunit, except that it is 'upside down'.

NICOTINIC ACh AND RELATED RECEPTORS

These receptors each contain five subunits. Members of this family include:

- nicotinic acetylcholine (ACh) receptor
- 5-HT_3 serotonergic receptor
- glycine receptor
- $GABA_A$ receptor.

INTRACELLULAR CALCIUM ION CHANNELS

Members of this family include:

- IP_3 inositol triphosphate receptors
- ryanodine receptors.

CHLORIDE ION CHANNELS

These have a widespread distribution.

RECEPTORS

STRUCTURE

In general, the receptors to which neurotransmitters bind are proteins located on the external surface of cell membranes. Until the 1980s receptors were classified and identified pharmacologically but not according to their structures. Since 1983, however, when the primary amino acid sequence of a receptor subunit of the nicotinic acetylcholine receptor was discovered, the DNA of an increasing number of receptor proteins have been sequenced, and hence their amino acid sequences discovered. This has led to a further clarification of receptor classification. It has also become evident that, as expected, for receptors of classical neurotransmitters the amino acids forming the binding site are on or close to the extracellular side of the receptor.

FUNCTION

The main function of a receptor is the molecular recognition of a signalling molecule, which in the case of neurotransmission is a neurotransmitter, leading in turn to signal transduction. A receptor generally responds to neurotransmitter binding in one of two ways:

- neurotransmitter binding $\rightarrow$ opening of transmembrane ion channel
- receptor–neurotransmitter $\rightarrow$ second-messenger system activation/inhibition.

G proteins

G proteins (named after their ability to bind guanosine triphosphate (GTP) and guanosine diphosphate (GDP)) are often involved in transmembrane signalling, linking receptors to intracellular effector systems. For neurotransmitter binding, the following types of G protein may be involved:

- Gs
- Gi
- Go
- Gq.

Second messengers

Two of the most important second messenger systems are:

- receptor-neurotransmitter complex $\rightarrow$ G protein binding to receptor–neurotransmitter complex $\rightarrow$ adenylate cyclase activation (or inhibition) $\rightarrow$ cyclic AMP (cAMP)
- neurotransmitter binding $\rightarrow$ hydrolysis of phosphatidylinositol biphosphate (a membrane

phospholipid) $\rightarrow$ diacylglycerol and IP_3 (inositol triphosphate); diacylglycerol activates protein kinase C, while IP_3 causes endoplasmic reticulum calcium release, in turn activating calmodulin-dependent protein kinase.

ADRENOCEPTORS

The adrenergic receptors are coupled to G proteins, via which they produce their physiological effects. At the time of writing, the main adrenergic receptors and their main effectors (via G protein α subunits) are believed to be:

- $\alpha_{1A} \rightarrow \uparrow Ca^{2+}$ (via Gi/Go)
- $\alpha_{1B} \rightarrow \uparrow IP_3$ (via Gq)
- $\alpha_{1C} \rightarrow \uparrow IP_3$ (via Gq)
- $\alpha_{1D} \rightarrow \uparrow IP_3$ (via Gq)
- α_{2A} (human)/α_{2D} (probably rat homologue) $\rightarrow \downarrow$ adenylyl cyclase, $\uparrow K^+$, $\downarrow Ca^{2+}$ (via Gi)
- $\alpha_{2B} \rightarrow \downarrow$ adenylate cyclase (via Gi)
- $\alpha_{2C} \rightarrow \downarrow$ adenylate cyclase (via Go)
- $\beta_1 \rightarrow \uparrow$ adenylate cyclase (via Gs)
- $\beta_2 \rightarrow \uparrow$ adenylate cyclase (via Gs).

The excitatory α_1 adrenoceptors are postsynaptic, while the inhibitory α_2 adrenoceptors are found as both presynaptic and postsynaptic receptors.

SEROTONERGIC RECEPTORS

The main serotonergic receptors, grouped according to their relative homologies, and their signalling systems, believed to exist at the time of writing, are as follows:

- $5\text{-}HT_{1A} \rightarrow \downarrow$ adenylate cyclase
- $5\text{-}HT_{1B} \rightarrow \downarrow$ adenylate cyclase
- $5\text{-}HT_{1D\alpha} \rightarrow \downarrow$ adenylate cyclase
- $5\text{-}HT_{1D\beta} \rightarrow \downarrow$ adenylate cyclase
- $5\text{-}HT_{1E} \rightarrow \downarrow$ adenylate cyclase
- $5\text{-}HT_{2A} \rightarrow \uparrow IP_3$
- $5\text{-}HT_{2B} \rightarrow \uparrow IP_3$
- $5\text{-}HT_{2C} \rightarrow \uparrow IP_3$
- $5\text{-}HT_3$ – ion channel
- $5\text{-}HT_{5A}$ – signalling system not known at the time of writing
- $5\text{-}HT_{5B}$ – signalling system not known at the time of writing
- $5\text{-}HT_6 \rightarrow \uparrow$ adenylate cyclase
- $5\text{-}HT_7 \rightarrow \uparrow$ adenylate cyclase.

DOPAMINERGIC RECEPTORS

The dopaminergic receptors are coupled to G proteins, via which they produce their physiological effects. At the time of writing, the main dopaminergic receptors and their main effectors (via G protein α subunits) are believed to be:

- $D_1 \rightarrow \uparrow$ adenylate cyclase (via Gs)
- $D_2 \rightarrow \downarrow$ adenylate cyclase, $\uparrow K^+$, $\downarrow Ca^{2+}$ (via Gi/Go)
- $D_3 \rightarrow \downarrow$ adenylate cyclase, $\uparrow K^+$, $\downarrow Ca^{2+}$ (via Gi/Go)

- $D_4 \rightarrow \downarrow$ adenylate cyclase, $\uparrow K^+$, $\downarrow Ca^{2+}$ (via Gi/Go)
- $D_5 \rightarrow \uparrow$ adenylate cyclase (via Gs).

GABA RECEPTORS

The GABA receptor superfamilies may be large, with multiple types of GABA subunits having been cloned. In general, there are two main types of receptor, the main effects of which are:

- $GABA_A \rightarrow \uparrow Cl^-$ (via a receptor-gated ion channel)
- $GABA_B \rightarrow \uparrow K^+ \pm Ca^{2+}$ effects (via G protein coupling).

CHOLINERGIC RECEPTORS

Cholinergic receptors transduce signals via coupling with G proteins. At the time of writing, the following types are recognized:

- nicotinic
- M1 (muscarinic)
- M2 (muscarinic)
- M3 (muscarinic)
- M4 (muscarinic)
- M5 (muscarinic).

GLUTAMATE RECEPTORS

The types of glutamate receptor recognized are:

- NMDA (*N*-methyl-D-aspartate) receptors
- AMPA (α-amino-3-hydroxy-5-methyl-4-isoxazole propionic acid) receptors
- KA (kainic acid) receptors
- mGluRs (metabotropic glutamate receptors) (= *trans*-ACPD receptors).

The first three classes are ionotropic glutamate receptors that are coupled directly to cation-specific ion channels.

NMDA receptors
At the time of writing, the NMDA receptor subtype is believed to include two families of subunits:

- NMDAR1 (= NR1)
- NMDAR2 (= NR2).

In turn, the following splice variants of NMDAR1 have been recognized:

- NMDAR1A (= NR1a)
- NMDAR1B (= NR1b)
- NMDAR1C (= NR1c)
- NMDAR1D (= NR1d)
- NMDAR1E (= NR1e)
- NMDAR1F (= NR1f)
- NMDAR1G (= NR1g).

Variants of NMDAR2 are modulatory subunits that form heteromeric channels but not homomeric channels.

AMPA receptors

AMPA receptors can be formed from one or any two of:

- GluR1
- GluR2
- GluR3
- GluR4.

KA receptors

KA receptors include:

- GluR5
- GluR6
- GluR7
- KA1
- KA2.

mGluRs

The mGluRs are coupled to G proteins, unlike the other classes of glutamate receptor. At the time of writing, the following subtypes have been cloned:

- mGluR1
- mGluR2
- mGluR3
- mGluR4
- mGluR5
- mGluR6.

These have been categorized into the following subgroups:

- subgroup I = mGluR1 and mGluR5
- subgroup II = mGluR2 and mGluR3
- subgroup III = mGluR4 and mGluR6.

The effector system for subgroup I involves stimulation of phospholipase C, while that for both subgroup II and subgroup III involves inhibition of adenylate cyclase.

CLASSICAL NEUROTRANSMITTERS

Noradrenaline

Biosynthesis

The primary biosynthetic pathway is:

tyrosine
$\rightarrow$ DOPA (3,4-dihydroxyphenylalanine)
$\rightarrow$ dopamine
$\rightarrow$ noradrenaline.

The corresponding enzymes are:

- tyrosine hydroxylase (acts on tyrosine)
- aromatic amino acid decarboxylase = DOPA decarboxylase (acts on DOPA)
- dopamine-β-hydroxylase (acts on dopamine).

Metabolism

The metabolic degradation of noradrenaline may begin with the action of either catechol-O-methyltransferase (COMT) or monoamine oxidase (MAO). The catabolic pathway starting with the action of COMT is as follows:

noradrenaline
$\rightarrow$ normetanephrine
$\rightarrow$ 3-methoxy-4-hydroxyphenylglycolaldehyde
$\rightarrow$ VMA (vanillyl mandelic acid) = 3-methoxy-4-hydroxymandelic acid.

The corresponding enzymes are:

- COMT (acts on noradrenaline)
- MAO (acts on normetanephrine)
- aldehyde dehydrogenase (acts on 3-methoxy-4-hydroxyphenylglycolaldehyde).

The catabolic pathway starting with the action of MAO has two major branches. The first branch is as follows:

noradrenaline
$\rightarrow$ 3,4-dihydroxyphenylglycolaldehyde
$\rightarrow$ 3,4-dihydroxymandelic acid
$\rightarrow$ VMA (vanillyl mandelic acid) = 3-methoxy-4-hydroxymandelic acid.

The corresponding enzymes are:

- MAO (acts on noradrenaline)
- aldehyde dehydrogenase (acts on 3,4-dihydroxyphenylglycolaldehyde)
- COMT (acts on 3,4-dihydroxymandelic acid).

The second branch is as follows:

noradrenaline
$\rightarrow$ 3,4-dihydroxyphenylglycolaldehyde
$\rightarrow$ 3,4-dihydroxyphenylglycol
$\rightarrow$ MHPG (3-methoxy-4-hydroxyphenylglycol).

The corresponding enzymes are:

- MAO (acts on noradrenaline)
- aldehyde reductase (acts on 3,4-dihydroxyphenylglycolaldehyde)
- COMT (acts on 3,4-dihydroxyphenylglycol).

Re-uptake

Following its release into the synaptic cleft, the main method of inactivation of noradrenaline is by means of re-uptake by presynaptic neurones.

Serotonin

Biosynthesis
The primary biosynthetic pathway is:

> tryptophan
> → 5-hydroxytryptophan
> → serotonin.

The corresponding enzymes are:

- tryptophan hydroxylase (acts on tryptophan)
- 5-hydroxytryptophan decarboxylase = amino acid decarboxylase) (acts on 5-hydroxytryptophan).

Metabolism
The metabolic degradation of serotonin is as follows:

> serotonin
> → 5-HIAA (5-hydroxyindoleacetic acid).

The enzyme catalyzing this is MAO_A (MAO type A).

Dopamine

Biosynthesis
The primary biosynthetic pathway is:

> tyrosine
> → DOPA (3,4-dihydroxyphenylalanine)
> → dopamine.

The corresponding enzymes are:

- tyrosine hydroxylase (acts on tyrosine)
- aromatic amino acid decarboxylase = DOPA decarboxylase (acts on DOPA).

Metabolism
The metabolic degradation of dopamine may begin with the action of either COMT or MAO. The catabolic pathway starting with the action of COMT is as follows:

> dopamine
> → 3-methoxytyramine
> → 3-methoxy-4-hydroxyphenylacetaldehyde
> → HVA (homovanillic acid).

The corresponding enzymes are:

- COMT (acts on dopamine)
- MAO (acts on 3-methoxytyramine)
- aldehyde dehydrogenase (acts on 3-methoxy-4-hydroxyphenylacetaldehyde).

(A less important pathway allows 3-methoxy-4-hydroxyphenylacetaldehyde to be metabolized to 3-methoxy-4-hydroxyphenylethanol via the action of aldehyde reductase.)

The catabolic pathway starting with the action of MAO is as follows:

dopamine
→ 3,4-dihydroxyphenylacetaldehyde
→ DOPAC (dihydroxyphenylacetic acid)
→ HVA.

The corresponding enzymes are:

- MAO (acts on dopamine)
- aldehyde dehydrogenase (acts on 3,4-dihydroxyphenylacetaldehyde)
- COMT (acts on DOPAC).

Re-uptake

Following its release into the synaptic cleft, the main method of inactivation of dopamine is by means of re-uptake by presynaptic neurones.

GABA

Biosynthesis

GABA is derived from glutamic acid via the action of GAD (glutamic acid decarboxylase).

Metabolism

The metabolic breakdown of GABA to glutamic acid and succinic semialdehyde involves the action of GABA transaminase (GABA-T).

Acetylcholine

Biosynthesis

Acetylcholine is derived from acetyl CoA and choline, in a reaction catalyzed by choline acetyltransferase.

Metabolism

After release into the synaptic cleft, acetylcholine is hydrolyzed by cholinesterase into choline and ethanoic (acetic) acid.

NEUROPEPTIDES

Some neurotransmitters consist of small proteins, or peptides. In this section, the following neuropeptide transmitters are considered: CRH, CCK and the endogenous opioid peptides.

CORTICOTROPHIN-RELEASING HORMONE

The cell bodies responsible for secreting corticotrophin-releasing factor or hormone (CRF or CRH) are located in the hypothalamic paraventricular nucleus. CRH is secreted from the hypothalamus into the hypothalamopituitary portal system and in turn regulates the release of POMC (pro-opiomelanocortin)-derived peptides, including corticotropin, from the adenohypophysis.

CHOLECYSTOKININ

Cholecystokinin (CCK), first located as gastrointestinal and pancreatic hormone, occurs in high concentrations in the central nervous system, particularly in the cerebral cortex, hypothalamus and limbic system. From a neuropsychiatric viewpoint, important cholecystokinin-like peptide fragments in the brain include CCK-tetrapeptide (CCK-4) and octapeptide (CCK-8).

ENDOGENOUS OPIOIDS

Endogenous opioids isolated from the central nervous system are derived from peptide precursor molecules:

- POMC → corticotropin, β-lipotropin
- proenkephalin → met-enkephalin, leu-enkephalin
- prodynorphin → dynorphin A, dynorphin B, α-neoendorphin.

The enkephalins met-enkephalin and leu-enkephalin are each pentapeptides.

BIBLIOGRAPHY

Carpenter, R.H.S. 2002: *Neurophysiology*, 4th edn. London: Arnold.

Emslie-Smith, D., Paterson, C.R., Scratcherd, T. & Read, N.W. (eds) 1988: *Textbook of Physiology*, 11th edn. Edinburgh: Churchill Livingstone.

Guyton, A.C. & Hall, J.E. 2000: *Textbook of Medical Physiology*, 10th edn. Philadelphia: W.B. Saunders.

Puri, B.K. & Tyrer, P.J. 2004: *Sciences Basic to Psychiatry*, 3rd edn. Edinburgh: Churchill Livingstone.

Stryer, L. 1995: *Biochemistry*, 4th edn. New York: W.H. Freeman.

15

General principles of psychopharmacology

HISTORICAL OVERVIEW

Antidepressants

Tricyclic antidepressants and MAOIs

Tricyclic antidepressants and monoamine oxidase inhibitors (MAOIs) were introduced between 1955 and 1958:

- *MAOIs.* These arose from the observation of elevated mood in patients with tuberculosis being treated with the MAOI iproniazid, and less toxic MAOIs were subsequently developed. Kline was one of the first to report the value of MAOI treatment in depression.
- *Tricyclic antidepressants.* Kuhn observed the antidepressant action of imipramine, while studying chlorpromazine-like agents.

SSRIs

The selective serotonin re-uptake inhibitors (SSRIs) were introduced in the late 1980s.

RIMA, SNRI, NARI and NaSSA

The reversible inhibitor of monoamine oxidase-A (RIMA), selective noradrenaline and serotonin re-uptake inhibitor (SNRI), selective noradrenaline re-uptake inhibitor (NARI) and noradrenergic and specific serotonergic antidepressant (NaSSA) were introduced in the 1990s.

Lithium

In 1886, Lange proposed the use of lithium for treating excited states. Lithium was introduced by Cade in 1949. Following his finding from animal experiments that lithium caused lethargy, Cade observed (in 1948) that it led to clinical improvement in a patient with mania.

Antipsychotics

Reserpine
Reserpine was introduced by Sen and Bose in 1931, and in 1953 Kline confirmed that it was a treatment for schizophrenia.

Typical antipsychotics
Important dates in the introduction of typical antipsychotics in psychiatric treatment in the twentieth century include:

- In 1950, chlorpromazine was synthesized by Charpentier, who was attempting to synthesize an antihistaminergic agent for anaesthetic use. Laborit then reported that chlorpromazine could induce an artificial hibernation.
- The efficacy of chlorpromazine in the treatment of psychosis was reported by Paraire and Sigwald in 1951, and by Delay and Deniker in 1952.
- In 1958, haloperidol was synthesized by Janssen.

Clozapine
Important dates in the introduction and, after 1988, the reintroduction of the atypical antipsychotic clozapine include:

- In 1958, clozapine was synthesized as an imipramine analogue. Its actions appeared to be closer to chlorpromazine than to imipramine.
- In 1961/2, the first clinical trial in schizophrenia (University Psychiatric Clinic, Bern) gave disappointing results. Low doses of clozapine were used.
- In 1966, Gross and Langner reported good results in chronic schizophrenia.
- From 1975, clozapine was withdrawn from general clinical use in some countries owing to cases of fatal agranulocytosis (including eight such deaths in Finland in 1975).
- In 1988, Kane and colleagues reported positive results from their multicentre double-blind study of clozapine versus chlorpromazine in treatment-resistant schizophrenia. Subsequent studies showed that social functioning also improved in response to clozapine.

Anxiolytics

Barbiturates
The first barbiturate, barbituric acid (malonylurea), was synthesized in 1864. The barbiturates were introduced in 1903.

Benzodiazepines
The benzodiazepine chlordiazepoxide was synthesized in the late 1950s by Sternbach (working for Roche) and introduced in 1960.

CLASSIFICATION

The examples given in each class of drug are not meant to be exhaustive.

Antipsychotics (neuroleptics)

TYPICAL ANTIPSYCHOTICS

In the following classification, note that the piperidine group of phenothiazines includes thioridazine, which is classed here as an atypical antipsychotic.

- phenothiazines – aliphatic
  - chlorpromazine
  - levomepromazine (methotrimeprazine)
  - promazine
- phenothiazines – piperazines
  - fluphenazine
  - trifluoperazine
  - perphenazine
  - prochlorperazine
- phenothiazines – piperidines
  - pipothiazine palmitate
  - pericyazine
- butyrophenones
  - haloperidol
  - droperidol
  - benperidol
  - trifluperidol
- thioxanthenes
  - flupentixol
  - zuclopenthixol
- diphenylbutylpiperidines
  - pimozide
  - fluspirilene.

ATYPICAL ANTIPSYCHOTICS

The atypical antipsychotics include:
- clozapine
- quetiapine
- risperidone
- sulpiride (a substituted benzamide; may also be categorized as a typical antipsychotic)
- amisulpride
- thioridazine (which may also be categorized as a typical antipsychotic)
- olanzapine
- sertindole (available only on a named-patient basis in the UK at the time of writing)
- zotepine
- aripiprazole (partial agonist at dopamine receptors).

Antimuscarinics (anticholinergics)

Antimuscarinic (anticholinergic) drugs used in the treatment of parkinsonism resulting from pharmacotherapy with antipsychotics include:

- procyclidine
- trihexyphenidyl/benzhexol
- benzatropine (benztropine)
- orphenadrine
- biperiden.

Prophylaxis of bipolar mood disorder

The drugs most commonly used in the prophylaxis of bipolar mood disorder are:

- lithium salts (carbonate and citrate)
- sodium valproate
- carbamazepine
- larnotrigine.

Antidepressants

TRICYCLIC ANTIDEPRESSANTS

Tricyclic antidepressants include:

- dibenzocycloheptanes
  - amitriptyline
  - nortriptyline
- iminodibenzyls
  - clomipramine
  - imipramine
  - trimipramine
- others
  - amoxapine
  - dosulepin/dothiepin
  - doxepin
  - lofepramine.

TRICYCLIC-RELATED ANTIDEPRESSANTS

Tricyclic-related antidepressants include:

- trazodone.

TETRACYCLIC ANTIDEPRESSANTS

Tetracyclic antidepressants include:

- maprotiline
- mianserin.

MAOIS

Monoamine oxidase inhibitors include:

- hydrazine compounds
  - phenelzine

- isocarboxazid
- non-hydrazine compounds
  - tranylcypromine.

SSRIs

Selective serotonin re-uptake inhibitors include:

- fluvoxamine
- fluoxetine
- sertraline
- paroxetine
- citalopram
- escitalopram.

RIMA

There is currently one reversible inhibitors of monoamine oxidase-A (RIMA) in clinical use:

- moclobemide.

SNRI

At the time of writing there is one serotonin noradrenaline re-uptake inhibitor (SNRI) in clinical use:

- venlafaxine.

NARI

The selective noradrenaline re-uptake inhibitor (NARI) in clinical use is:

- reboxetine.

NaSSA

The noradrenergic and specific serotonergic antidepressant (NaSSA) in clinical use is:

- mirtazapine.

Benzodiazepines

Long-acting benzodiazepines include:

- diazepam
- alprazolam
- chlordiazepoxide
- clorazepate
- flunitrazepam
- flurazepam
- nitrazepam.

Short-acting benzodiazepines include:

- lorazepam
- lormetazepam
- oxazepam
- temazepam.

Other anxiolytics

Non-benzodiazepine anxiolytics in clinical use include:

- azaspirodecanediones – buspirone
- β-adrenoceptor blocking drugs – e.g. propranolol.

Drugs used in alcohol dependence

The following drugs are used in alcohol dependence:

- acamprosate
- disulfiram
- benzodiazepines
- clomethiazole.

Drugs used in opioid dependence

The following drugs are used in opioid dependence:

- methadone
- lofexidine
- naltrexone
- buprenorphine.

Antiandrogens

At the time of writing, there is one antiandrogen used for psychiatric reasons:

- cyproterone acetate.

OPTIMIZING PATIENT COMPLIANCE

Factors that can help optimize patient compliance include:

- patient education
- setting reasonable expectations
- reducing the number of tablets to be taken
- reducing dosage frequency

- labelling medicine containers clearly
- parenteral/depot administration
- using alternative medication if there are troublesome side-effects
- involving family members.

It is particularly important to avoid polypharmacy, if possible, and to prescribe a simple, straightforward drug regimen for elderly patients. Containers used by the elderly should take into account the possibility that the patient may have arthritis, and may also be designed to allow the pharmacist to place the appropriate medication for each intake in clearly labelled boxes.

PLACEBO EFFECT

DEFINITION

A placebo refers to any therapy or component of therapy that is deliberately used for its non-specific, psychological or psychophysiological effect, or its presumed specific effect, but that is without specific activity for the condition being treated.

Mechanisms of the placebo effect

White *et al.* (1985) have proposed the following biopsychosocial model for the mechanisms of the placebo effect:

- homoestatic mechanisms
  - central nervous system function
  - autonomic nervous system function
  - peripheral nervous system function
  - endocrine function
  - immune function
- classical conditioning
- operant conditioning
- cognitive–affective–behavioural self-control
- hypnosis
- the doctor's attitude
- the patient's expectations
- transitional object phenomena.

Pill factors

The strength of the placebo effect varies with the physical form of the medication, including the size, type, colour and number of pills (Buckalew & Coffield, 1982; Blakwell *et al.*, 1972). For example, the relative placebo effect for the following physical forms has been found to be stronger:

- multiple pills > single pills
- larger pills > smaller pills
- capsules > tablets.

Examples of the relative potency of medication varying with pill colour include (Schapira, 1970):

- Anxiety symptoms responded better to green tablets.
- Depressive symptoms responded better to yellow tablets.

Controlling for the placebo effect

The above factors can be taken into account in clinical practice. In clinical trials it is important to control for the placebo effect, and this is achieved in the randomized double-blind placebo-controlled design (see Chapter 6).

PRESCRIBING FOR PSYCHIATRIC PATIENTS

Prescribing for psychiatric patients includes taking into consideration the following factors (Cookson *et al.*, 1993):

- the symptoms to be targeted in the short and long term
- age
- physical health
- circumstances
- drugs already being taken, including home remedies
- the effectiveness, or otherwise, of previous drug treatments
- personality
- lifestyle
- social setting
- the choice of actual drugs
    - dose size
    - dose schedule
- when to review outcome and who should help report it
- the role of the community psychiatry nurse and the GP in providing medication and monitoring progress.

BIBLIOGRAPHY

Blackwell, B., Bloomfield, S.S. & Buncher, C.R. 1972: Demonstration to medical students of placebo responses and nondrug factors. *Lancet* i:1279–1282.

Buckalew, L.W. & Coffield, K.E. 1982: An investigation of drug expectancy as a function of capsule color and size and preparation form. *Journal of Clinical Psychopharmacology* 2:245–248.

Cookson, J., Crammer, J. & Heine, B. 1993: *The Use of Drugs in Psychiatry*, 4th edn. London: Gaskell.

Healy, D. 2002: *Psychiatric Drugs Explained*, 3rd edn. Edinburgh: Churchill Livingstone.

Puri, B.K. 2005: *Drugs in Psychiatry*. Oxford: Oxford University Press.

Schapira, K., McClelland, H.A., Griffiths, N.R. *et al.* 1970: Study of the effects of tablet colour in the treatment of anxiety states. *British Medical Journal* 2:446–449.

Silverstone, T. & Turner, P. 1995: *Drug Treatment in Psychiatry*, 5th edn. London: Routledge.

White, L., Tursky, B. & Schwartz, G. (eds) 1985: *Placebo: Theory, Research, and Mechanisms*. New York: Guilford Press, 431–447.

16

Pharmacokinetics

ABSORPTION

Routes of administration

Enteral administration
Enteral administration routes employ the gastrointestinal tract, from which the drug is absorbed into the circulation. They include administration via the following routes:

- oral
- buccal
- sublingual
- rectal.

Parenteral administration
This includes administration via the following routes:

- intramuscular
- intravenous
- subcutaneous
- inhalational
- topical.

Rate of absorption

The rate of absorption of a drug from its site of administration depends on the following factors:

- the form of the drug
- the solubility of the drug, which is influenced by factors such as:
  - the pK_a of the drug
  - particle size

- the ambient pH
- the rate of blood flow through the tissue in which the drug is sited.

Oral administration

Mechanisms of absorption
The main mechanisms of absorption of drugs from the gastrointestinal tract are:

- passive diffusion
- pore filtration
- active transport.

Site of absorption
The main site of absorption of most psychotropic drugs (which tend to be lipophilic at a physiological pH) from the gastrointestinal tract is the small intestine.

Factors influencing absorption
Factors influencing absorption of drugs from the gastrointestinal tract include:

- gastric emptying
- gastric pH
- intestinal motility
- presence/absence of food: the presence of food delays gastric emptying
- intestinal microflora
- area of absorption
- blood flow.

The antimuscarinic actions of some psychotropic medication leads to delayed gastric emptying.

Rectal administration

Advantages
Advantages of rectal administration over the oral route include:

- It can be used if the patient cannot swallow (e.g. because of vomiting).
- Gastric factors are bypassed.
- It can be used for drugs that are irritant to the stomach.
- There is reduced first-pass metabolism.
- It can be useful in uncooperative patients.
- It can be used to administer diazepam during an epileptic seizure, for example in a patient with a learning difficulty.

Disadvantages
Disadvantages of rectal administration include:

- embarrassment
- presence of a variable amount of faecal matter, leading to an unpredictable rate of absorption
- local inflammation following frequent use of this route.

Intramuscular administration

Factors influencing absorption
The rate of absorption of drugs administered intramuscularly is increased in the following circumstances:

- lipid-soluble drugs
- drugs with a low relative molecular mass
- increased muscle blood flow (e.g. after physical exercise or during emotional excitement).

Disadvantages
Disadvantages of intramuscular administration include:

- pain
- usually unacceptable for self-administration
- risk of damage to structures such as nerves
- some drugs (e.g. paraldehyde) may cause sterile abscess formation
- reduced muscle blood flow (e.g. in cardiac failure), leading to reduced absorption
- tissue binding or precipitation from solution after intramuscular administration (e.g. for chlordiazepoxide, diazepam, phenytoin), leading to reduced absorption
- increased creatine phosphokinase occurs, which may interfere with diagnostic cardiac enzyme assays.

This route should not be used if the patient is receiving anticoagulant therapy.

Intravenous administration

Advantages
Advantages of intravenous administration include:

- rapid intravenous administration leading to rapid action – useful in emergency situations
- drug dose can be titrated against patient response
- large volumes can be administered slowly
- this route can be used for drugs that cannot be absorbed by other routes
- first-pass metabolism is by-passed.

Disadvantages
Disadvantages of intravenous administration include:

- adverse effects may occur rapidly
- dangerously high blood levels may be achieved
- it is difficult to recall the drug once administered
- risk of sepsis
- risk of thrombosis
- risk of air embolism
- risk of injection into tissues surrounding the vein, which may lead to necrosis
- risk of injection into an artery, which may lead to spasm
- cannot be used with insoluble drugs.

DISTRIBUTION

The rate and degree of distribution of psychotropic drugs between the lipid, protein and water components of the body are influenced by the:

- lipid solubility of the drug
- plasma protein binding
- volume of distribution
- blood–brain barrier
- placenta.

Lipid solubility

Increased lipid solubility is associated with increased volume of distribution. This is the case for most psychotropic drugs at physiological pH.

Plasma protein binding

Drugs circulate around the body partly bound to plasma proteins and partly free in the water phase of plasma. This plasma protein binding, which is reversible and competitive, acts as a reservoir for the drug. The main plasma binding protein for acidic drugs is albumin, while basic drugs, including many psychotropic drugs, can also bind to other plasma proteins such as lipoprotein and α_1-acid glycoprotein. The extent of plasma protein binding varies with a number of factors:

- plasma drug concentration
- plasma protein concentration – reduced in:
  - hepatic disease
  - renal disease
  - cardiac failure
  - malnutrition
  - carcinoma
  - surgery
  - burns
- drug interactions:
  - displacement
  - plasma protein tertiary structure change
- concentration of physiological substances (e.g. urea, bilirubin and free fatty acid).

Volume of distribution

This is a theoretical concept relating the mass of a drug in the body to the blood or plasma concentration:

> Volume of distribution = (mass of a drug in the body at a given time)/(concentration of the drug at that time in the blood or the plasma).

A higher volume of distribution in general corresponds to a shorter duration of drug action. Factors that may influence the volume of distribution include:

- drug lipid solubility: increased lipid solubility (e.g. most psychotropic drugs) is associated with an increased volume of distribution
- adipose tissue: weight gain (e.g. some psychotropic drugs) leads to increased adipose tissue which leads to an increased volume of distribution
- increasing age: reduced proportion of lean tissue leads to increased volume of distribution
- sex
- physical disease.

Blood–brain barrier and brain distribution

Components
Components of the blood–brain barrier include:

- tight junctions between adjacent cerebral capillary endothelial cells
- cerebral capillary basement membrane
- gliovascular membrane.

Drug lipid solubility
A high rate of penetration of the blood–brain barrier occurs for non-polar highly lipid soluble drugs, since the brain is a highly lipid organ. Most psychotropic drugs, being highly lipid soluble, can therefore easily cross the blood–brain barrier.

Infection
Infection may alter the normal functioning of the blood–brain barrier.

Receptors
The existence of specific brain receptors for many psychotropic drugs leads to psychotropic drug protein binding in the brain, thereby forming a central nervous system reservoir. This does not occur in the CSF, with its very low protein concentration.

Active transport
Active transport mechanisms are used to cross the blood–brain barrier by some physiological substances and drugs (e.g. levodopa).

Diffusion
Some small molecules diffuse readily into the brain and CSF from the cerebral circulation (e.g. lithium ions).

Placenta

Drugs may transfer into the fetal circulation from the maternal circulation across the placenta by means of:

- passive diffusion
- active transport
- pinocytosis.

Since drugs may cause teratogenesis during the first trimester, they should be avoided during this time if at all possible.

METABOLISM

While some highly water-soluble drugs (e.g. lithium) are excreted unchanged by the kidneys, others, such as most highly lipid-soluble psychotropic drugs, first undergo metabolism (biotransformation) to reduce their lipid solubility and make them more water-soluble, prior to renal excretion. Metabolism sometimes results in the production of pharmacologically active metabolites (e.g. amitriptyline → nortriptyline). Sites of metabolism include the:

- liver (the most important site of metabolism)
- kidney
- adrenal (suprarenal) cortex
- gastrointestinal tract
- lung
- placenta
- skin
- lymphocytes.

HEPATIC PHASE I METABOLISM (BIOTRANSFORMATION)

This leads to a change in the drug molecular structure by the following non-synthetic reactions:

- oxidation (the most common)
- hydrolysis
- reduction.

The most important type of oxidation reaction is that carried out by microsomal mixed-function oxidases, involving the cytochrome P450 isoenzymes.

HEPATIC PHASE II METABOLISM (BIOTRANSFORMATION)

This is a synthetic reaction involving conjugation between a parent-drug/drug-metabolite/endogenous-substance and a polar endogenous molecule/group. Examples of the latter include:

- glucuronic acid
- sulphate
- acetate
- glutathione
- glycine
- glutamine.

The resulting water-soluble conjugate can be excreted by the kidney if the relative molecular mass is less than about 300. If the relative molecular mass is higher, the conjugate can be excreted in the bile.

FIRST–PASS EFFECT

The first-pass effect (first-pass metabolism or presystemic elimination) is the metabolism undergone by an orally absorbed drug during its passage from the hepatic portal system through the liver before entering the systemic circulation. It varies between individuals and may be reduced by, for example, hepatic disease, food or drugs that increase hepatic blood flow.

ELIMINATION

Elimination (excretion) of drugs and drug metabolites can take place by means of the:

- kidney – the most important organ for such elimination
- bile and faeces
- lung
- saliva
- sweat
- sebum
- milk.

With the exception of pulmonary excretion, in general water-soluble polar drugs and drug metabolites are eliminated more readily by excretory organs than are highly lipid-soluble non-polar ones.

BIBLIOGRAPHY

Cookson, J., Crammer, J. & Heine, B. 1993: *The Use of Drugs in Psychiatry*, 4th edn. London: Gaskell.

King, D.J. 1995: *Seminars in Clinical Psychopharmacology*. London: Gaskell.

Puri, B.K. 2005: *Drugs in Psychiatry*. Oxford: Oxford University Press.

Silverstone, T. & Turner, P. 1995: *Drug Treatment in Psychiatry*, 5th edn. London: Routledge.

17

Pharmacodynamics

ANTIPSYCHOTICS

Typical antipsychotics

Many of the actions of chlorpromazine, the archetypal antipsychotic, are believed to result from antagonist action to the following neurotransmitters:

- dopamine
- acetylcholine – muscarinic receptors
- adrenaline/noradrenaline
- histamine.

Many of these actions also occur, to varying extents, with other typical antipsychotics.

ANTIDOPAMINERGIC ACTION

In general, typical antipsychotics are postulated to act clinically by causing postsynaptic blockade of dopamine D_2 receptors; their antagonism at these receptors is related to their clinical antipsychotic potencies. It is the antidopaminergic action on the mesolimbic–mesocortical pathway which is believed to be the effect required for this clinical action.

The antidopaminergic action on the tuberoinfundibular pathway causes hormonal side-effects. Hyperprolactinaemia, resulting from the fact that dopamine is a prolactin-inhibitory factor, causes:

- galactorrhoea
- gynaecomastia
- menstrual disturbances
- reduced sperm count
- reduced libido.

The antidopaminergic action on the nigrostriatal pathway causes extrapyramidal symptoms:

- parkinsonism
- dystonias

- akathisia
- tardive dyskinesia.

ANTIMUSCARINIC ACTION

The central antimuscarinic (anticholinergic) actions may cause:

- convulsions
- pyrexia.

    Peripheral antimuscarinic symptoms include:

- dry mouth
- blurred vision
- urinary retention
- constipation
- nasal congestion.

ANTIADRENERGIC ACTION

Antiadrenergic actions may cause:

- postural hypotension
- ejaculatory failure.

ANTIHISTAMINIC ACTION

Antihistaminic effects include drowsiness.

Atypical antipsychotics

The atypical antipsychotics have a greater action than do typical antipsychotics on receptors other than dopamine D_2 receptors. For example, clozapine, the archetypal atypical antipsychotic, has a higher potency of action than do typical antipsychotics on the following receptors:

- 5-HT_2
- D_4
- D_1
- muscarinic
- α-adrenergic.

DRUGS USED IN THE TREATMENT OF AFFECTIVE DISORDERS

LITHIUM

Lithium ions, Li^+, are monovalent cations that cause a number of effects, some of which may account for its therapeutic actions, including:

- $\uparrow$ intracellular Na^+
- $\downarrow$ Na,K-ATPase pump activity

- ↑ intracellular Ca^{2+} in erythrocytes in mania and depression
- ↑ erythrocyte choline
- ↑ erythrocyte phospholipid catabolism (via phospholipase D)
- ↓Ca^{2+} in platelets in bipolar disorder
- ↑ serotonergic neurotransmission
- ↓central 5-HT$_1$ and 5-HT$_2$ receptor density (demonstrated in the hippocampus)
- ↑dopamine turnover in hypothalamic–tuberoinfundibular dopaminergic neurones
- ↓ central dopamine synthesis (dose-dependent)
- normalization of low plasma and CSF levels of GABA in bipolar disorder
- ↑ GABAergic neurotransmission
- ↓ low-affinity GABA receptors in the corpus striatum and hypothalamus (chronic lithium administration)
- ↑ met-enkephalin and leu-enkephalin in the basal ganglia and nucleus accumbens
- ↑ dynorphin in the corpus striatum.

TRICYCLIC ANTIDEPRESSANTS

The most important postulated modes of action in the brain of tricyclic antidepressants in achieving therapeutic effects are:

- inhibition of re-uptake of noradrenaline
- inhibition of re-uptake of serotonin.

For this reason, tricyclic antidepressants are also known as monoamine re-uptake inhibitors, or MARIs. Peripherally, most tricyclic antidepressants also have an antimuscarinic action, which gives rise to peripheral antimuscarinic side-effects such as:

- dry mouth
- blurred vision
- drowsiness
- urinary retention
- constipation.

Postural hypotension occurs as a result of the antiadrenergic action.

SSRIs

The most important postulated mode of action in the brain of SSRIs (selective serotonin re-uptake inhibitors) in achieving therapeutic effects is:

- inhibition of re-uptake of serotonin.

Their relatively selective action on serotonin reuptake means that SSRIs are less likely than tricyclic antidepressants to cause antimuscarinic side-effects. They are, however, more likely to cause gastrointestinal side-effects such as nausea and vomiting.

MAOIs

The most important postulated mode of action in the brain of MAOIs (monoamine oxidase inhibitors) in achieving therapeutic effects is:

- irreversible inhibition of MAO-A and MAO-B.

In the central nervous system, MAO-A (monoamine oxidase type A) acts on:

- noradrenaline
- serotonin
- dopamine
- tyramine.

In the central nervous system, MAO-B (monoamine oxidase type B) acts on:

- dopamine
- tyramine
- phenylethylamine
- benzylamine.

The inhibition of peripheral pressor amines, particularly dietary tryramine, by MAOIs can lead to a hypertensive crisis when foodstuffs rich in tyramine are eaten (see Chapter 18).

RIMA

The most important postulated mode of action in the brain of the RIMA (reversible inhibitor of monoamine oxidase-A) in achieving therapeutic effects is:

- reversible inhibition of MAO-A.

SNRI

The most important postulated modes of action in the brain of the SNRI (serotonin noradrenaline re-uptake inhibitor) in achieving therapeutic effects are:

- inhibition of re-uptake of noradrenaline
- inhibition of re-uptake of serotonin.

NARI

The most important postulated mode of action in the brain of the NARI (selective noradrenaline re-uptake inhibitor) in achieving therapeutic effects is:

- selective inhibition of the re-uptake of noradrenaline.

NaSSA

The most important postulated modes of action in the brain of the NaSSA (noradrenergic and specific serotonergic antidepressant) in achieving therapeutic effects are:

- increased release of noradrenaline by antagonism of inhibitory presynaptic α_2-adrenoceptors
- increased release of serotonin by enhancement of a facilitatory noradrenergic input to serotonergic cell bodies
- increased release of serotonin by antagonism of inhibitory presynatpic α_2-adrenoceptors on serotonergic neuronal terminals.

ANXIOLYTICS AND HYPNOTICS

BENZODIAZEPINES

The most important postulated mode of action in the brain of benzodiazepines in achieving central therapeutic effects is:

- binding to $GABA_A$ receptors.

BUSPIRONE

The most important postulated mode of action in the brain of the azaspirodecanedione buspirone in achieving central therapeutic effects is:

- partial agonism at $5-HT_{1A}$ receptors.

BETA-ADRENOCEPTOR BLOCKING DRUGS

The most important postulated mode of action of the β-adrenoceptor blocking drugs in achieving anxiolytic effects is:

- antagonism at peripheral β-adrenoceptors.

ZOPICLONE

The cyclopyrrolone zopiclone is believed to achieve a central hypnotic effect by acting on the same receptors as do benzodiazepines.

ZOLPIDEM

The imidazopyridine zolpidem in believed to achieve a central hypnotic effect by acting on the same receptors as do benzodiazepines.

ANTI-EPILEPTIC AGENTS

CARBAMAZEPINE

Carbamazepine, which has a tricyclic antidepressant-like structure, may achieve its anticonvulsant effect on the basis of the following actions:

- binding to and inactivation of voltage-dependent Na^+ channels
- increased K^+ conductance
- partial agonism at the adenosine A_1 subclass of P_1 purinoceptors.

SODIUM VALPROATE

Sodium valproate may achieve its anticonvulsant effect on the basis of the following actions:

- increased GABA
  - ↓ GABA breakdown
  - ↑ GABA release

- ↓ GABA turnover
- ↑ GABA-B receptor density
- ↑ neuronal responsiveness to GABA
- reduced Na^+ influx
- increased K^+ conductance.

PHENYTOIN

The mechanism of anticonvulsant action of phenytoin is unknown, but may involve:

- membrane stabilization
  - Na^+ channel binding
  - Ca^{2+} channel binding
- benzodiazepine receptor binding
- GABA receptor function modulation.

PHENOBARBITONE

The actions of phenobarbitone may be similar to those given above for phenytoin.

GABAPENTIN

Gabapentin is believed to achieve its anticonvulsant effect by means of the following action:

- binding to a unique cerebral receptor site.

VIGABATRIN

Vigabatrin is believed to achieve its anticonvulsant effect by means of the following action:

- inhibition of GABA transaminase, leading to increased GABA release.

LAMOTRIGINE

Lamotrigine is believed to achieve its anticonvulsant effect by means of the following action:

- inhibition of glutamate release.

NEUROCHEMICAL EFFECTS OF ECT

NORADRENALINE

ECT probably leads to increased noradrenergic function. In particular, ECT acutely causes:

- increased cerebral noradrenaline activity
- increased cerebral tyrosine hydroxylase activity
- increased plasma catecholamines, particularly adrenaline.

Chronic ECS (electroconvulsive shock) leads to:

- reduced β-adrenergic receptor density.

The last effect may be a result of receptor down-regulation.

SEROTONIN

ECT probably leads to increased serotonergic function. In particular, ECT acutely causes:

- increased cerebral serotonin concentration.

Chronic ECS leads to:

- increased 5-HT$_2$ receptor density.

DOPAMINE

ECT probably leads to increased dopaminergic function. In particular, ECT acutely causes:

- increased cerebral dopamine concentration
- increased cerebral concentration of dopamine metabolites
- increased behavioural responsiveness to dopamine agonists.

In rat substantia nigra, repeated electroconvulsive shocks lead to:

- increased dopamine D$_1$ receptor density
- increased second-messenger potentiation at dopamine D$_1$ receptors.

GABA

ECT may cause a functional increase in GABAergic activity.

ACETYLCHOLINE

ECT probably leads to decreased central cholinergic function. In particular, ECT acutely causes:

- reduced cerebral acetylcholine concentration
- increased cerebral acetyltransferase activity
- increased cerebral acetylcholinesterase activity
- increased CSF acetylcholine concentration.

Chronic ECS leads to:

- reduced muscarinic cholinergic receptor density in the cerebral cortex
- reduced muscarinic cholinergic receptor density in the hippocampus
- reduced second-messenger response in the hippocampus.

ENDOGENOUS OPIOIDS

Chronic ECS leads to:

- increased cerebral met-enkephalin concentration and synthesis
- increased cerebral β-endorphin concentration and synthesis
- changes in opioid ligand binding.

ADENOSINE

Chronic ECS leads to:

- increased cerebral adenosine A$_1$ purinoceptor density.

BIBLIOGRAPHY

Bloom, F.E. & Kupfer, D.J. (eds) 1995: *Psychopharmacology: The Fourth Generation of Progress.* New York: Raven Press.

Cookson, J., Crammer, J. & Heine, B. 1993: *The Use of Drugs in Psychiatry,* 4th edn. London: Gaskell.

Healy, D. 2002: *Psychiatric Drugs Explained*, 3rd edn. Edinburgh: Churchill Livingstone.

King, D.J. 1995: *Seminars in Clinical Psychopharmacology.* London: Gaskell.

Puri, B.K. 2005: *Drugs in Psychiatry.* Oxford: Oxford University Press.

Silverstone. T. & Turner, P. 1995: *Drug Treatment in Psychiatry*, 5th edn. London: Routledge.

18

Adverse drug reactions

TYPES OF ADVERSE DRUG REACTIONS

CLASSIFICATION

Adverse drug reactions may be classified as:

- intolerance
- idiosyncratic reactions
- allergic reactions
- drug interactions.

CAUSAL RELATIONSHIP

The following criteria have been suggested as making it more likely that a causal connection exists between a drug and an alleged effect (Edwards, 1995):

- There is a close temporal relationship between the effect and the taking of the drug, or toxic levels of the drug or its active metabolites in body fluids have been demonstrated.
- The effect differs from manifestations of the disorder being treated.
- No other substances are being taken or withdrawn when the effect occurs.
- The reaction disappears when treatment is stopped.
- The effect reappears with a rechallenge test.

INTOLERANCE

In drug intolerance the adverse reactions are consistent with the known pharmacological actions of the drug. These adverse drug reactions may be dose-related.

IDIOSYNCRATIC REACTIONS

Idiosyncratic adverse drug reactions are reactions which are not characteristic or predictable and which are associated with an individual human difference not present in members of the general population.

ALLERGIC REACTIONS

Allergic reactions to drugs involve the body's immune system, with the drug interacting with a protein to form an immunogen which causes sensitization and the induction of an immune response. Criteria suggesting an allergic reaction include:

- There is a different time-course from that of the pharmacodynamic action; e.g:
  - there is delayed onset of the adverse drug reaction
  - the adverse drug reaction manifests only following repeated drug exposure.
- There may be no dose-related effect, with subtherapeutically small doses leading to sensitization or allergic reactions.
- There is a hypersensitivity reaction, unrelated to the pharmacological actions of the drug.

  Types of allergic reaction to drugs include:

- anaphylactic shock – type I hypersensitivity reaction
- haematological reactions – type II, III or IV hypersensitivity reaction; e.g.:
  - haemolytic anaemia
  - agranulocytosis
  - thrombocytopenia
- allergic liver damage – type II ± III hypersensitivity reaction
- skin rashes – type IV hypersensitivity reaction
- generalized autoimmune (systemic lupus erythamtosus-like) disease – type IV hypersensitivity reaction.

DRUG INTERACTIONS

Adverse drug reactions may result from interactions between different drugs. These may result from:

- pharmacokinetic interactions
- pharmacodynamic interactions.

Pharmacokinetic interactions

Pharmacokinetic interactions between drugs include:

- precipitation or inactivation following the mixing of drugs
- chelation
- changes in gastrointestinal tract motility
- changes in gastrointestinal tract pH
- drug displacement from binding sites
- enzyme induction
- enzyme inhibition
- competition for renal tubular transport
- changes in urinary pH, leading to changes in drug excretion.

Pharmacodynamic interactions

Pharmacodynamic interactions between drugs include:

- inhibition of drug uptake
- inhibition of drug transport
- interaction at receptors

- synergism
- changes in fluid and electrolyte balance.

PSYCHOTROPIC MEDICATION

Typical antipsychotics

In the previous chapter, the major categories of adverse drug reactions are given that are believed to be caused by antagonist action to the following neurotransmitters:

- dopamine
- acetylcholine – muscarinic receptors
- adrenaline/noradrenaline
- histamine.

Other important adverse drug reactions include:

- photosensitization
- hypothermia or pyrexia
- allergic (sensitivity) reactions
- neuroleptic malignant syndrome
- effects of chronic pharmacotherapy.

Photosensitization
Photosensitization is more common with chlorpromazine than with other typical antipsychotics.

Hypothermia or pyrexia
Interference with temperature regulation is a dose-related side-effect.

Allergic (sensitivity) reactions
Sensitivity reactions include:

- agranulocytosis
- leucopenia
- leucocytosis
- haemolytic anaemia.

Neuroleptic malignant syndrome
Neuroleptic malignant syndrome is characterized by:

- hyperthermia
- fluctuating level of consciousness
- muscular rigidity
- autonomic dysfunction:
  - tachycardia
  - labile blood pressure
  - pallor
  - sweating
  - urinary incontinence.

Laboratory investigations commonly, but not invariably, demonstrate:

- increased creatinine phosphokinase
- increased white blood count
- abnormal liver function tests.

Neuroleptic malignant syndrome requires urgent medical treatment.

Chronic pharmacotherapy

Long-term high-dose pharmacotherapy may cause ocular and skin changes, such as:

- opacity of the lens and/or cornea
- purplish pigmentation of the skin, conjunctiva, cornea and/or retina.

Atypical antipsychotics

CLOZAPINE

Clozapine may cause neutropenia and potentially fatal agranulocytosis, because of which regular haematological monitoring is required. Other side-effects of clozapine include hypersalivation, reduced convulsive threshold, impaired glucose tolerance, diabetes mellitus, constipation which may be severe, paralytic ileus, tachycardia (1:10), myocarditis, cardiomyopathy and side-effects common to chlorpromazine, including extrapyramidal symptoms.

OLANZAPINE

Olanzapine may cause:

- mild, transient antimuscarinic side-effects
- drowsiness
- speech difficulty
- exacerbation of Parkinson's disease
- akathisia
- asthenia
- increased appetite
- weight gain
- raised triglyceride levels
- oedema
- diabetes mellitus
- hyperprolactinaemia.

The last of these side-effects only rarely manifests clinically. Less commonly, olanzapine may also cause:

- blood dyscrasias
- bradycardia
- rash
- photosensitivity
- priapism
- hepatitis
- pancreatitis.

It may also cause an elevation in the level of creatine kinase.

RISPERIDONE

Risperidone may cause:

- insomnia
- agitation
- anxiety
- headache
- drowsiness
- impairment of concentration
- fatigue
- blurred vision
- constipation
- nausea and vomiting
- dyspepsia
- abdominal pain
- hyperprolactinaemia
- sexual dysfunction
- priapism
- urinary incontinence
- tachycardia
- hypertension
- rash
- rhinitis.

The hyperprolactinaemia caused by risperidone may manifest as:

- galactorrhoea
- menstrual disturbances
- amenorrhoea
- gynaecomastia.

The following side-effects have also been reported in connection with risperidone:

- cerebrovascular accidents
- neutropenia
- thrombocytopenia.

Rare side-effects of risperidone include:

- seizures
- hyponatraemia
- abnormal regulation of temperature
- oedema.

SERTINDOLE

This atypical antipsychotic was suspended in the UK following a number of cases of sudden deaths in patients that appeared to be related to the prolongation of the QT interval caused by sertindole. At the time of writing, sertindole has been reintroduced into the UK, but its use is restricted to a named-patient basis for use in patients who are enrolled in clinical studies and who are not tolerant of at least one other antipsychotic drug.

Antimuscarinic drugs

Antimuscarinic drugs used in parkinsonism may give rise to the following side-effects:

- antimuscarinic side-effects (see Chapter 17)
- worsening of tardive dyskinesia
- gastrointestinal tract disturbances
- hypersensitivity.

Lithium

Renal function
Since lithium ions are excreted mainly by the kidneys, renal function must be checked prior to commencing pharmacotherapy with lithium.

Plasma levels
The therapeutic index of lithium is low and therefore regular plasma lithium level monitoring is required.

Therapeutic index = (toxic dose)/(therapeutic dose).

The dose is adjusted to achieve a lithium level of 0.4–1.0 mmol/L for prophylactic purposes, with lower levels being used in the elderly.

Side–effects
Side-effects of lithium therapy include:

- fatigue
- drowsiness
- dry mouth
- a metallic taste
- polydipsia
- polyuria
- nausea
- vomiting
- weight gain
- diarrhoea
- fine tremor
- muscle weakness
- oedema.

Oedema should not be treated with diuretics since thiazide and loop diuretics reduce lithium excretion and can thereby cause lithium intoxication.

Intoxication
Signs of lithium intoxication include:

- mild drowsiness and sluggishness, leading to giddiness and ataxia
- lack of coordination
- blurred vision

- tinnitus
- anorexia
- dysarthria
- vomiting
- diarrhoea
- coarse tremor
- muscle weakness.

Concomitant use of NSAIDs, and any condition causing sodium depletion can lead to raised lithium levels and risk of lithium intoxication.

Severe overdosage
At lithium plasma levels of greater than 2 mmol/L, the following effects can occur:

- hyperreflexia and hyperextension of the limbs
- toxic psychoses
- convulsions
- syncope
- oliguria
- circulatory failure
- coma
- death.

Chronic therapy
Long-term treatment with lithium may give rise to:

- thyroid function disturbances:
  - goitre
  - hypothyroidism
- memory impairment
- nephrotoxicity
- cardiovascular changes:
  - T-wave flattening on the ECG
  - arrhythmias
- hyperparathyroidism, hypercalcemia.

Thyroid function tests are usually carried out routinely every 6 months in order to check for lithium-induced disturbances.

Withdrawal
Too rapid a withdrawal leads to an excess of manic relapses.

Pregnancy and lactation
Teratogenic in pregnancy. Avoid in lactation.

Carbamazepine

Since carbamazepine may lower the white blood count, regular monitoring of plasma carbamazepine levels should be carried out.

Tricyclic antidepressants

The psychopharmacological basis of important side-effects of tricyclic antidepressants is as follows:

- blockade of ACh muscarinic receptors
- blockade of histamine H_1 receptors
- blockade of α_1-adrenoceptors
- blockade of 5-HT$_{2/1c}$ serotonergic receptors
- membrane stabilization.

Blockade of muscarinic receptors
This leads to antimuscarinic side-effects (see Chapter 17).

Blockade of histamine H_1 receptors
This can lead to:

- weight gain
- drowsiness.

Blockade of α_1-adrenoceptors
This can lead to:

- drowsiness
- postural hypotension
- sexual dysfunction
- cognitive impairment.

Blockade of 5-HT$_{2/1c}$ receptors
This can lead to weight gain.

Membrane stabilization
Membrane stabilization can lead to:

- cardiotoxicity
- reduced seizure threshold.

Cardiovascular side-effects
These include:

- ECG changes
- arrhythmias
- postural hypotension
- tachycardia
- syncope.

Allergic and haematological reactions
These include:

- agranulocytosis
- leucopenia
- eosinophilia
- thrombocytopenia
- skin rash

- photosensitization
- facial oedema
- allergic cholestatic jaundice.

Endocrine side-effects

These include:

- testicular enlargement
- gynaecomastia
- galactorrhoea.

Others

Other side-effects include:

- tremor
- black tongue
- paralytic ileus
- sweating
- hyponatraemia (particularly in the elderly)
- neuroleptic malignant syndrome (very rare with tricyclic antidepressants)
- abnormal liver function tests
- movement disorders
- pyrexia
- (hypo)mania
- blood glucose changes.

SSRIs

Important side-effects that may occur with SSRIs include:

- dose-related gastrointestinal side-effects:
  - nausea
  - vomiting
  - diarrhoea
- headache
- restlessness
- sleep disturbance
- anxiety
- delayed orgasm.

MAOIs

DANGEROUS FOOD INTERACTIONS

As mentioned in Chapter 17, the inhibition of peripheral pressor amines, particularly dietary tryramine, by MAOIs can lead to a hypertensive crisis when foodstuffs rich in tyramine are eaten. Foods that should therefore be avoided when on treatment with MAOIs include:

- cheese (except cottage cheese and cream cheese)
- meat extracts and yeast extracts

- alcohol (particularly chianti, fortified wines and beer)
- non-fresh fish
- non-fresh meat
- non-fresh poultry
- offal
- avocado
- banana skins
- broad-bean pods
- caviar
- herring (pickled or smoked).

Dangerous drug interactions
Medicines that should be avoided by patients taking MAOIs include:

- indirectly acting sympathomimetic amines; e.g.:
  - amphetamine
  - fenfluramine
  - ephedrine
  - phenylpropanolamine
- cough mixtures containing sympathomimetics
- nasal decongestants containing sympathomimetics
- L-dopa
- pethidine
- tricyclic antidepressants.

Other side-effects
Other side-effects of MAOIs include:

- antimuscarinic actions
- hepatotoxicity
- appetite stimulation
- weight gain.

Tranylcypromine may cause dependency.

Benzodiazepines

An important side-effect of benzodiazepines is psychomotor impairment. If benzodiazepines are taken regularly for four weeks or more, dependence may develop, so that sudden cessation of intake may then lead to a withdrawal syndrome whose main features include:

- anxiety symptoms:
  - palpitations
  - tremor
  - panic
  - dizziness
  - nausea
  - sweating
  - other somatic symptoms
- low mood

- abnormal experiences:
  - depersonalization
  - derealization
  - hypersensitivity to sensations in all modalities
  - distorted perception of space
  - tinnitus
  - formication
  - a strange taste
- influenza-like symptoms
- psychiatric/neurological symptoms:
  - epileptic seizures
  - confusional states
  - psychotic episodes
- insomnia
- loss of appetite
- weight loss.

Buspirone

The main side-effects of buspirone are:

- dizziness
- headache
- excitement
- nausea.

Disulfiram

If alcohol is drunk while disulfiram is being taken regularly, acetaldehyde accumulates. Thus, ingesting even small amounts of alcohol then causes unpleasant systemic reactions, including:

- facial flushing
- headache
- palpitations
- tachycardia
- nausea
- vomiting.

Ingestion of large amounts of alcohol while being treated with disulfiram can lead to:

- air hunger
- arrhythmias
- severe hypotension.

Cyproterone acetate

Side-effects of this antiandrogen agent in males include:

- inhibition of spermatogenesis
- tiredness
- gynaecomastia
- weight gain
- improvement of existing acne vulgaris
- increased scalp hair growth
- female pattern of pubic hair growth.

Liver function tests should be carried out regularly owing to a theoretical risk to the liver. Dyspnoea may result from high-dose treatment.

OFFICIAL GUIDANCE

The official guidance in Britain on the use of antipsychotic drugs and benzodiazepines is given in this section. BNF is the abbreviation for the latest *British National Formulary*, a six-monthly publication of the British Medical Association and the Royal Pharmaceutical Society of Great Britain.

Antipsychotic doses above the BNF upper limit

The Royal College of Psychiatrists has published advice on the use of antipsychotic doses above the BNF upper limit. This advice is reproduced in the BNF.

Unless otherwise stated, doses in the BNF are licensed doses; any higher dose is therefore *unlicensed*.

1 Consider alternative approaches including adjuvant therapy and newer or atypical neuroleptics such as clozapine.
2 Bear in mind risk factors, including obesity. Particular caution is indicated in older patients, especially those aged over 70.
3 Consider the potential for drug interactions – published in an appendix to the BNF.
4 Carry out an ECG to exclude untoward abnormalities such as prolonged QT interval. Repeat ECG periodically and reduce dose if prolonged QT interval or other adverse abnormality develops.
5 Increase dose slowly and not more often than once weekly.
6 Carry out regular pulse, blood pressure and temperature checks. Ensure that the patient maintains adequate fluid intake.
7 Consider high-dose therapy to be for a limited period and review regularly; abandon if no improvement after 3 months (return to standard dosage).

Important note
When prescribing an antipsychotic for administration on an emergency basis, it must be borne in mind that the intramuscular dose should be *lower* than the corresponding oral dose (owing to absence of the first-pass effect), particularly if the patient is very active (increased blood flow to muscle considerably increases the rate of absorption). The prescription should specify the dose in the context of *each route* and should *not* imply that the same dose can be given by mouth or by intramuscular injection. The dose should be reviewed *daily*.

Benzodiazepines

In Britain, the Committee on Safety of Medicines (CSM) has issued the following advice with respect to the presciption of benzodiazepines:

1 Benzodiazepines are indicated for the short-term relief (2–4 weeks only) of anxiety that is severe, disabling or subjecting the individual to unacceptable distress, occurring alone or in association with insomnia or short-term psychosomatic, organic or psychotic illness.
2 The use of benzodiazepines to treat short-term 'mild' anxiety is inappropriate and unsuitable.
3 Benzodiazepines should be used to treat insomnia only when it is severe, disabling or subjecting the individual to extreme distress.

Prevention of adverse drug reactions

The BNF gives the following advice for preventing adverse drug reactions:

1 Never use any drug unless there is a good indication. If the patient is pregnant do not use a drug unless the need for it is imperative.
2 It is very important to recognize allergy and idiosyncrasy as causes of adverse drug reactions. Ask whether the patient has had previous reactions.
3 Ask whether the patient is already taking other drugs including self-medication. Remember that interactions may occur.
4 Age and hepatic or renal disease may alter the metabolism or excretion of drugs, so that much smaller doses may need to be prescribed. Pharmacogenetic factors may also be responsible for variations in the rate of metabolism, notably of isoniazid and the tricyclic antidepressants.
5 Prescribe as few drugs as possible and give very clear instructions to the elderly or any patient likely to misunderstand complicated instructions.
6 When possible use a familiar drug. With a new drug be particularly alert for adverse reactions or unexpected events.
7 If serious adverse reactions are liable to occur, warn the patient.

REPORTING

In Britain, the CSM holds an information database for adverse drug reactions. Doctors practising in Britain are asked to report adverse drug reactions to: Medicines and Healthcare Products Regulatory Agency, CSM, Freepost, London SW8 5BR (Tel: 0800 731 6789).

Yellow prepaid lettercards for reporting are available from the above address, by dialling a 24-hour Freefone service (Tel: 0800 731 6789), and from the back of the BNF book. Adverse drug reactions can also be reported via the Internet on the following website: www.mca.gov.uk/yellowcard.

ADROIT

ADROIT (Adverse Drug Reactions On-line Information Tracking) is an on-line service used in Britain to monitor adverse drug reactions.

Newer drugs
In the BNF these are indicated by the symbol ▼. The BNF advises that doctors are asked to report all suspected reactions.

Established drugs
The BNF advises that doctors are asked to report all serious suspected reactions. These include those that are fatal, life-threatening, disabling, incapacitating, or which result in or prolong hospitalization.

BIBLIOGRAPHY

Bloom, F.E. & Kupfer, D.J. (eds) 1995: *Psychopharmacology: The Fourth Generation of Progress.* New York: Raven Press.

British Medical Association & Royal Pharmaceutical Society of Great Britain. *British National Formulary.* London: BMA/RPSGB.

Cookson, J., Crammer, J. & Heine, B. 1993: *The Use of Drugs in Psychiatry,* 4th edn. London: Gaskell.

Edwards, J.G. 1995: Adverse reactions to and interactions with psychotropic drugs: mechanisms, methods of assessment, and medicolegal considerations. In Healy, D. 2002: *Psychiatric Drugs Explained,* 3rd edn. Edinburgh: Churchill Livingstone.

King, D.J. (ed.) *Seminars in Clinical Psychopharmacology.* London: Gaskell, 480–513.

Puri, B.K. 2005: *Drugs in Psychiatry.* Oxford: Oxford University Press.

19

Genetics

BASIC CONCEPTS

CHROMOSOMES

Number
In normal humans the genome is distributed on 46 chromosomes in each somatic cell nucleus:

- one pair of sex chromosomes
- 44 autosomes = 22 pairs of chromosomes.

Sex chromosomes
The sex chromosomes are the X and Y chromosomes:

- normal females: XX
- normal males: XY.

Karyotype
This is an arrangement of the chromosomal make-up of somatic cells that can be produced by carrying out the following procedures in turn:

- Arrest cell division at an appropriate stage.
- Disperse the chromosomes.
- Fix the chromosomes.
- Stain the chromosomes.
- Photograph the chromosomes.
- Identify the chromosomes.
- Arrange the chromosomes.

Centromere
This is the somewhat constricted region of each chromosome that is particularly evident during mitosis and meiosis.

Metacentric chromosomes

These are chromosomes with a centrally or almost centrally positioned centromere.

Acrocentric chromosomes

These are chromosomes in which the centromere is very near to one end.

Chromosomal map

The system agreed at the International Paris Conference in 1971 is as follows:

First position – a number (1 to 22) or letter (X or Y) that identifies the chromosome.
Second position – p (short arm of chromosome) or q (long arm of chromosome)
Third position (region) – a digit corresponding to a stretch of the chromosome lying between two relatively distinct morphological landmarks
Fourth position (band) – a digit corresponding to a band derived from the staining properties of the chromosome.

CELL DIVISION

Mitosis

This is the process of nuclear division allowing many somatic cells to undergo cell division via the following stages:

- interphase
- prophase
- metaphase
- anaphase
- telophase.

Meiosis

This process involves two stages of cell division and occurs in gametogenesis via the following stages:

- interphase
- prophase I
- metaphase I
- anaphase I
- telophase I
- prophase II
- metaphase II
- anaphase II
- telophase II.

Chromosomal division takes place once during meiosis, so that the resulting gametes are haploid. Recombination takes place duing prophase I.

GENE STRUCTURE

Genes, the biological units of heredity, consist of *codons* grouped into *exons* with intervening nucleotide sequences known as *introns*. The introns do not code for amino acids. Genes also contain nucleotide sequences at their beginning and end that allow transcription to take place accurately. Thus, starting from the 5′ end (upstream), a typical eukaryotic gene contains the following:

- upstream site regulating transcription
- promotor (TATA)
- transcription initiation site
- 5′ non-coding region
- exons
- introns
- 3′ non-coding region, containing a poly A addition site.

TRANSCRIPTION

This is the step in gene expression in which information from the DNA molecule is transcribed on to a primary RNA transcript. This is followed by splicing and nuclear transport, so that the information (minus that from introns) then exists in the cytoplasm of the cell on mRNA (messenger RNA).

TRANSLATION

Following transcription, splicing and nuclear transport, translation is the process in gene expression whereby mRNA acts as a template allowing the genetic code to be deciphered to allow the formation of a peptide chain. This process involves tRNA molecules.

PATTERNS OF INHERITANCE

In this section, R and S are dominant alleles, and r and s the corresponding recessive alleles.

Law of uniformity
Consider two homozygous parents with genotypes RR and rr, respectively. Mating (×) results in the next (F1) generation having the genotype shown:

Parents: RR × rr
F1:   Rr

Mendel's first law
This is also known as the law of segregation:

Parents: Rr × Rr
F1:   RR: Rr: rr = 1:2:1

Mendel's second law
This is also known as the law of independent assortment:

Parents: RRSS × rrss
F1:   RrSs
F2:   independent assortment of different alleles → RRSS, RRSs, …, rrss

Autosomal dominant inheritance
Autosomal dominant disorders result from the presence of an abnormal dominant allele causing the individual to manifest the abnormal phenotypic trait. Features of autosomal dominant transmission include:

- The phenotypic trait is present in all individuals carrying the dominant allele.
- The phenotypic trait does not skip generations – vertical transmission takes place.
- Males and females are affected.
- Male to male transmission can take place.
- Transmission is not solely dependent on parental consanguineous matings.
- If one parent is homozgyous for the abnormal dominant allele, all the members of F1 will manifest the abnormal phenotypic trait.

Variable expressivity can cause clinical features of autosomal dominant disorders to vary between affected individuals. This, together with reduced penetrance, may give the appearance that the disorder has skipped a generation. The sudden appearance of an autosomal dominant disorder may occur as a result of a new dominant mutation.

Autosomal recessive inheritance
Autosomal recessive disorders result from the presence of two abnormal recessive alleles causing the individual to manifest the abnormal phenotypic trait. Features of autosomal recessive transmission include:

- Heterozygous individuals are generally carriers who do not manifest the abnormal phenotypic trait.
- The rarer the disorder, the more likely it is that the parents are consanguineous.
- The disorder tends to miss generations but the affected individuals in a family tend to be found among siblings – horizontal transmission takes place.

X-linked recessive inheritance
In X-linked recessive disorders a recessive abnormal allele is carried on the X chromosome. All male (XY) offspring inheriting this allele manifest the abnormal phenotypic trait. Other features of X-linked recessive transmission include:

- Male to male transmission does not take place.
- Female heterozygotes are carriers.

X-linked dominant inheritance
In X-linked dominant disorders a dominant abnormal allele is carried on the X chromosome. If an affected male mates with an unaffected female, all the daughters and none of the sons are affected. If an unaffected male mates with an affected heterozygous female, half the daughters and half the sons, on average, are affected. Again, male to male transmission does not take place.

Anticipation
This refers to the occurrence of an autonomic dominant disorder at earlier ages of onset or with greater severity in the succeeding generations. In Huntington's disease it has been shown to be caused by expansions of unstable triplet repeat sequences.

Mosaicism
Abnormalities in mitosis can give rise to an abnormal cell line. Such mosaicism may affect somatic cells (somatic mosaicism) or germ cells (gonadal mosaicism).

Uniparental disomy
This refers to the phenomenon in which an individual inherits both homologues of a chromosome pair from the same parent.

Genomic imprinting

This refers to the phenomenon in which an allele is differentially expressed depending on whether it is maternally or paternally derived.

Mitochondrial inheritance

Since mtDNA (mitochondrial DNA) is essentially maternally inherited, mitochondrial inheritance may explain some cases of disorders that affect both males and females but that are transmitted through females only and not through males.

TRADITIONAL TECHNIQUES

Family studies

Methodology

The rates of illness in the first- and second-degree relatives of probands are compared with the corresponding rates in the general population. First-degree relatives have, on average, 50% of the genome in common with the proband, and include the biological:

- father
- mother
- brothers
- sisters
- children.

Second-degree relatives have, on average, 25% of the genome in common with the proband, and include the biological:

- grandfathers
- grandmothers
- uncles
- aunts
- nephews
- nieces
- grandsons
- granddaughters.

Difficulties

Difficulties (and possible solutions) with family studies applied to psychiatric disorders include:

- Psychiatric disorders need to be considered longitudinally. Lifetime expectancy rates or morbid risks can be used.
- At the time of the study some relatives may not have reached an age range during which the disorder manifests itself. Weinberg's age-correction method can be used.
- Genetic factors are not separated well from environmental factors. Twin and adoption studies can be used.

Twin studies

Methodology
The rates of illness in co-twins of monozygotic (MZ) and dizygotic (DZ) probands are compared. MZ twins share 100% of the genome, whereas DZ twins share, on average, 50% of their genome. The rate of concurrence of a disorder in the co-twin of a proband is the *concordance rate*:

Pairwise rate (as a percentage) = (number of concordant pairs of twins)/(total number of twin pairs) × 100%.

Probandwise rate (as a percentage) = (number of co-twins of probands in whom the disorder is concurrent)/(total number of co-twins) × 100%.

Difficulties
Difficulties (and possible solutions) with twin studies applied to psychiatric disorders include:

- Pairwise and probandwise concordance rates usually give different results. Take care to note the method used to determine the concordance rate.
- Zygosity was determined less accurately in older twin studies. Use modern, more accurate methods.
- Diagnostic variability occurred in older twin studies. Use more detailed modern diagnostic criteria.
- Sampling bias may occur. Use twin registers.
- Twins are at greater risk of central nervous system abnormalities resulting from birth injury or congenital abnormalities (risk to MZ twins > risk to DZ twins), which may introduce errors if central nervous system abnormalities contribute to the disorder being studied.
- Assortative mating may lead to a relative increase in the rate of illness in DZ twins compared with MZ twins.
- Age-correction techniques may introduce errors, so do not use them.
- The environment does not necessarily affect twins equally. Use adoption studies.

Adoption studies

Methodology
Individuals are studied who have been brought up by unrelated adoptive parents from an early age, instead of by their biological parents. Types of adoption studies include:

- adoptee studies
- adoptee family studies
- cross-fostering studies
- adoption studies involving monozygotic twins.

Difficulties
Difficulties with adoption studies applied to psychiatric disorders include:

- Few cases fulfil the criteria for adoption studies.
- Adoption studies take a long time to carry out.
- Information about the biological father may not be available.
- Adoption may cause indeterminate psychological sequelae for the adoptees.
- The process of adoption is unlikely to be random.
- In MZ twin studies it cannot be assumed that the environmental influences on each twin are more or less equivalent following adoption.

TECHNIQUES IN MOLECULAR GENETICS

Restriction enzymes

Restriction enzymes, also known as restriction endonucleases, cleave DNA only at locations containing specific nucleotide sequences. Different restriction enzymes target different nucleotide sequences, but a given restriction enzyme targets the same sequence.

Gene library

This is a set of cloned DNA fragments representing all the genes of an organism or of a given chromosome.

Molecular cloning

This technique can be used to create a gene library. It can be carried out by splicing a given stretch of (human) DNA, cleaved using a restriction enzyme, into a bacterial plasmid having at least one antibiotic resistance gene. After reintroduction of the resulting recombinant plasmid into bacteria, antibiotic selective pressure causes these bacteria to reproduce. Multiple recoverable copies of the original (human) DNA are contained in the resulting bacterial colonies.

Gene probes

These are lengths of DNA that are constructed so that they have a nucleotide sequence complementary, or almost complementary, to that of a given part of the genome, with which, therefore, they can hybridize under suitable conditions.

Oligonucleotide probes

These are small gene probes that can be used to detect single-base mutations.

Southern blotting

This is a technique that allows the transfer of DNA fragments from gel, where electrophoresis and DNA denaturation have taken place, to a nylon or nitrocellular filter. It involves overlaying the gel with the filter and in turn overlaying the filter with paper towels. A solution is then blotted through the gel to the paper towels. Autoradiography can then be used to identify the fragments of interest on the filter. The technique is named after its inventor, Edwin Southern.

Restriction fragment–length polymorphisms

Restriction fragment-length polymorphisms, or RFLPs, are polymorphisms at restriction enzyme cleavage sites that give rise to fragments of different lengths following restriction enzyme digestion. They can be used as DNA markers and are usually inherited in a simple Mendelian fashion.

Recombination

As mentioned above, recombination takes place during prophase I of meiosis. There is alignment and contact of homologous chromosome pairs during prophase I, allowing genetic information to cross over between adjacent chromatids. This process of crossover or recombination causes a change in the alleles carried by the chromatids at the end of the first meiotic division.

LINKAGE ANALYSIS

Genetic markers

A DNA polymorphism, such as a restriction fragment-length polymorphism, if linked to a given disease locus, can be used as a genetic marker in linkage analysis without its precise chromosomal location being known. Genetic markers can also be used in presymptomatic diagnosis and prenatal diagnosis.

Linkage
This is the phenomenon whereby two genes close to each other on the same chromosome are likely to be inherited together.

Linkage phases
For two alleles occurring at two linked loci in a double heterozygote, the following linkage phases can occur:

- coupling: the two alleles are on the same chromosome
- repulsion: the two alleles are on opposite chromosomes of a pair.

Recombinant fraction
This is a measure of how often the alleles at two loci are separated during meiotic recombination. Its value can vary from zero to 0.5.

Lod scores
The lod score for a given recombinant fraction is the logarithm to base 10 of the odds $P_1:P_2$, where P_1 is the probability of there being linkage for a given recombinant fraction, and P_2 is the probability of there being no measurable linkage. Thus the lod score gives a measure of the probability of two loci being linked. The lod score method was devised by Morton.

Maximum–likelihood score
This is the value of the recombinant fraction that gives the highest value for the lod score. It represents the best estimate that can be made for the recombinant fraction from the given available data.

CONDITIONS ASSOCIATED WITH CHROMOSOMAL ABNORMALITIES

Autosomal abnormalities

Down's syndrome
The causes of Down's syndrome are:

- Approximately 95% of cases result from trisomy 21 (47, +21) following non-disjunction during meiosis.
- Approximately 4% result from translocation involving chromosome 21; exchange of chromosomal substance may occur between chromosome 21 and:
  - chromosome 13
  - chromosome 14
  - chromosome 15
  - chromosome 21
  - chromosome 22.
- The remaining cases are mosaics.

Note that almost all subjects with Down's syndrome who live beyond the age of 40 years show evidence of Alzheimer's disease.

Edward's syndrome

This is caused by trisomy 18 (47, +18).

Patau syndrome

This is caused by trisomy 13 (47, +13).

Cri–du–chat syndrome

This partial aneusomy results from the partial deletion of the short arm of chromosome 5. Its characteristic kitten-like high-pitched cry has been localized to 5p15.3. Its other clinical features have been localized to 5p15.2, known as the cri-du-chat critical region of CDCCR.

Sex chromosome abnormalities

Klinefelter's syndrome

In this syndrome, phenotypic males possess more than one X chromosome per somatic cell nucleus. Genotypes include:

- 47,XXY (that is, one extra X chromosome per somatic cell nucleus); this is the most common genotype in Klinefelter's syndrome
- 48,XXXY
- 49,XXXXY
- 48,XXYY.

XYY syndrome

In this syndrome, phenotypic males have the genotype 47,XYY.

Triple X syndrome

In this syndrome, phenotypic males have the genotype 47,XYY.

Tetra–X syndrome

In this syndrome, also known as super-female syndrome, phenotypic females have the genotype 48,XXXX.

Turner syndrome

In this syndrome, phenotypic females have the genotype 45,X (= 45,XO).

PRINCIPAL INHERITED CONDITIONS ENCOUNTERED IN PSYCHIATRIC PRACTICE

Alzheimer's disease

The gene for APP (amyloid precursor protein) is located on the long arm of human chromosome 21 and is a member of a gene family which includes the amyloid precursor-like proteins (APLP) 1 and 2. This may explain the link between Alzheimer's disease and Down's syndrome (see above). The apolipoprotein E ε4 allele is common in Alzheimer's disease, while the ε2 allele is less common than would be expected by chance. It may be that the ε4 allele is associated with increased accumulation of β-amyloid protein, while the reverse is true for the ε2 allele.

Autosomal dominant disorders

HUNTINGTON'S DISEASE

Huntington's disease (chorea) is a progressive, inherited neurodegenerative disease which is characterized by autosomal dominant transmission and the emergence of abnormal involuntary movements and cognitive deterioration, with progression to dementia and death over 10–20 years. The *huntingtin* gene responsible is located on the short arm of chromosome 4; this genetic mutation consists of an increased number of CAG (cytosine–adenine–guanine) repeats. (The normal number of such repeats at this locus is between 11 and about 34.) The age of onset is strongly determined by the number of repeat units, but once symptoms develop, the rate of progression is relatively uninfluenced by CAG repeat length.

PHACOMATOSES

The phacomatoses (or phakomatoses), which exhibit neurocutaneous signs, include:

- tuberous sclerosis
- neurofibromatosis
- von Hippel–Lindau syndrome
- Sturge–Weber syndrome.

There are three main forms of tuberous sclerosis:

- TSC1 (tuberous sclerosis type 1), caused by a gene on chromosome 9
- TSC2 (tuberous sclerosis type 2), caused by a gene on chromosome 16
- TSC3 (tuberous sclerosis type 3), caused by a translocation that involves chromosome 12.

Neurofibromatosis is caused by an abnormality in the NF-1 gene (in the region 17q11.2).

EARLY–ONSET ALZHEIMER'S DISEASE

A minority of cases of Alzheimer's disease are inherited as an early-onset autosomal dominant disorder. The mutations concerned tend to be found on chromosome 14 or chromosome 21.

OTHER DISORDERS

Other disorders that can be inherited in an autosomal dominant manner include:
- acrocephalosyndactyly type I
- acrocallosal syndrome
- acrodysostosis
- De Barsey syndrome
- periodic paralyses.

Autosomal recessive disorders

DISORDERS OF PROTEIN METABOLISM

There are many disorders of protein metabolism that can be inherited in an autosomal recessive manner. They include:

- *Phenylketonuria* (incidence 1 in 12 000). A reduction in phenylalanine hydroxylase causes an increase in circulating phenylalanine. The Guthrie test is used to screen for this disorder.
- *Hartnup disorder or disease* (incidence 1 in 14 000). This is a renal-transport amino aciduria in which there is reduced absorption of neutral amino acids (including tryptophan) from the alimentary canal and renal tubules, causing reduced biosynthesis of nicotinic acid.
- *Histidinaemia* (incidence 1 in 18 000). This is a reduction in histidase causing an increased level of histidine in the blood and urine.
- *Homocystinuria* (incidence 1 in 50 000) This is a reduction in cystathionine β-synthase causing an increased level of homocystine in the blood and urine.
- *Maple-syrup urine disorder* (incidence 1 in 120 000). This is a reduction in oxo acid decarboxylase causing the presence of branched-chain amino acids (valine, leucine and isoleucine) in the blood and urine.
- *Carbamoyl phosphate sythetase deficiency* (or *hyperammonaemia*) (incidence <1 in 100 000). This is a urea cycle disorder in which hyperammonaemia occurs.
- *Argininosuccinate sythetase deficiency* (or *citrullinaemia*) (incidence <1 in 100 000). This is a urea cycle disorder in which there is increased citrulline in the blood and urine.
- *Argininosuccinate lyase deficiency* (or *argininosuccinic aciduria*) (incidence <1 in 100 000). This is a urea cycle disorder in which there is increased argininosuccinic acid in the blood and urine.
- *Arginase deficiency* (or *argininaemia*) (incidence <1 in 100 000). This is a urea cycle disorder in which there is increased arginine in the blood.
- *Cystathioninuria* (incidence of about 1 in 200 000). A reduction in γ-cystathioninase causes increased cystathionine in the blood and urine.

Further disorders are:

- cystinuria
- hydroxyprolinaemia
- hyperlysinaemia
- non-ketotic hyperglycinaemia
- ornithinaemia
- Stimmler syndrome
- type II tyrosinaemia
- Oast-house urine syndrome.

DISORDERS OF CARBOHYDRATE METABOLISM AND LYSOSOMAL STORAGE

These disorders can be inherited in an autosomal recessive manner. They include:

- *Gaucher's disease* (incidence of type I Gaucher's disease is between 1 in 600 and 1 in 2400 in Ashkenazi Jewish populations). This is a reduction in lysosomal cerebroside β-glucosidase causing an abnormal accumulation of glucosylceramide.
- *Tay–Sachs disease* (incidence 1 in 4000 in Ashkenazi Jewish populations). This is a G_{M2} gangliosidosis in which a reduction in lysosomal hexosaminidase A causes an abnormal accumulation of G_{M2} ganglioside.
- *Sanfilippo syndrome* (or *MPS type III*) (incidence 1 in 24 000). This is a mucopolysaccharidosis. Types A, B, C and D are recognized.
- *Hurler's syndrome* (or *MPS type I*) (incidence about 1 in 100 000). This is a mucopolysaccharidosis. A reduction in lysosomal α-L-iduronidase causes abnormal accumulation of dermatan sulfate and heparin sulfate.

- *Metachromatic leukodystrophy* (incidence about 1 in 100 000). This is a sulfatidosis (sulphatidosis).
- *Sandhoff disease* (incidence about 1 in 300 000). This is a G_{M2} gangliosidosis in which there is an abnormal accumulation of G_{M2} gangliosides and oligosaccharides.
- *Niemann–Pick disease* (types I and II; both are rare). Type I is caused by a reduction in lysosomal sphingomyelinase causing abnormal accumulation of sphingomyelin.
- *G_{M1} gangliosidoses* (types I, II and III; all are rare). Type I is the infantile type, type II is the juvenile type and type III is the adult type. In all three types there is a reduction in lysosomal β-galactosidase causing an abnormal accumulation of G_{M1} ganglioside.

Further disorders are:

- fucosidosis
- galactosaemia
- hereditary fructose intolerance
- Krabbe disease
- mannosidosis
- Pompe disease
- von Gierke disease.

OTHER DISORDERS

There are many other disorders inherited in an autosomal recessive manner. Many are rare or very rare. They include:

- Alexander disease
- cerebelloparenchymal disorders
- Coat disease
- Cockayne syndrome
- Cohen syndrome
- Friedrich's ataxia
- Laurence–Moon syndrome
- macrocephaly
- oculocerebral syndrome
- oculorenocerebellar syndrome
- Refsum disease
- Rubinstein syndrome
- Turcot syndrome
- Wilson disease (hepatolenticular degeneration).

X-linked dominant disorders

Disorders that can be inherited in an X-linked dominant manner include:

- ornithine transcarbamoylase (incidence of about 1 in 500 000) – a urea cycle disorder in which hyperammonaemia occurs
- Aicardi syndrome
- Coffin–Lowry syndrome
- Rett syndrome.

X-linked recessive disorders

Disorders that can be inherited in an X-linked recessive manner include:

- Hunter's syndrome (MPS type II) (incidence about 1 in 100 000) – a mucopolysaccharidosis in which there is a reduction in lysosomal iduronidate 2-sulfatase
- Lesch–Nyan syndrome (incidence about 1 in 100 000) – a reduction in hypoxanthine–guanine phosphoribosyltransferase causes increased synthesis of urate and hyperuricaemia
- cerebellar ataxia
- fragile X syndrome
- Lowe syndrome
- testicular feminization syndrome
- X-linked spastic paraplegia
- W syndrome.

BIBLIOGRAPHY

McGuffin, P., Owen, M.J., O'Donovan, M.C., Thapar, A. & Gottesman, I.I. 1994: *Seminars in Psychiatric Genetics.* London: Gaskell.
Puri, B.K. & Tyrer, P.J. 2004: *Sciences Basic to Psychiatry*, 3rd edn. Edinburgh: Churchill Livingstone.

20

Epidemiology

NOTE

This chapter may usefully be read in conjunction with Chapter 6, which deals with the principles of evaluation and psychometrics. In addition to topics that are epidemiological in nature, this chapter also includes a few related subjects that are of value in the analysis of trial data.

DISEASE FREQUENCY

INCIDENCE

The incidence of a disease is the rate of occurrence of new cases of the disease in a defined population over a given period of time. It is equal to the number of new cases over the given period of time divided by the total population at risk (see below) during the same period of time.

Units

The unit of incidence is T^{-1}; that is, $(\text{time})^{-1}$. For instance, Dunham (1965) gave the incidence of schizophrenia as:

$$0.00022 \ \text{year}^{-1}$$
$$= 0.00022 \ \text{per year}$$
$$= 0.22 \ \text{per } 1000 \ \text{per year}$$
$$= 22 \ \text{per } 100\,000 \ \text{per year, etc.}$$

PREVALENCE

The prevalence of a disease is the proportion of a defined population that has the disease at a given time.

- *Point prevalence.* This is the proportion of a defined population that has a given disease at a given point in time.
- *Period prevalence.* This is the proportion of a defined population that has a given disease during a given interval of time.

- *Lifetime prevalence.* This is the proportion of a defined population that has or has had a given disease (at any time during each individual's lifetime thus far) at a given point in time.
- *Birth defect rate.* This is the proportion of live births that has a given disease.
- *Disease rate at post mortem.* This is the proportion of bodies, on which post mortems are carried out, that has a given disease.

Units

Prevalence, being a proportion or ratio of two numbers, does not have units. A given prevalence value may, however, be multiplied by 100 to express it as a percentage. For example, according to Jablensky and Sartorius (1975), the annual prevalence of schizophrenia is:

$$0.002 \text{ to } 0.004$$
$$= 2 \text{ to } 4 \text{ per } 1000$$
$$= 0.2\text{--}0.4\%.$$

(Note that the annual prevalence is a type of period prevalence.)

POPULATION AT RISK

This is the population of individuals free of a given disease, who have not already had the disease by the time of the commencement of a given period of time, who are at risk of becoming new cases of the disease.

CHRONICITY

The chronicity of a disease is its average duration. It has the units of time.

STEADY–STATE RELATIONSHIP BETWEEN POINT PREVALENCE AND INCIDENCE

In the steady state, in which the incidence of a disease is constant over a given time period and the time between caseness onset and ending is constant, the following relationship holds:

$$P = ID$$

where P is the point prevalence, I is the incidence, and D is chronicity.

CASE IDENTIFICATION, CASE REGISTERS, MORTALITY AND MORBIDITY STATISTICS

CASE IDENTIFICATION

Caseness

An overall threshold is ideally defined in order to establish caseness: that is, to differentiate cases of a given psychiatric disorder from non-cases. Classification systems and screening can be used to help identify cases.

Classification

Classification systems that are useful in case identification are those that provide specific operational diagnostic criteria as guides for making each psychiatric diagnosis. A widely used example in psychiatry is that of DSM-IV-TR.

Screening

Screening, by means of psychiatric assessment instruments, can be used to identify cases. The instruments used should have good sensitivity and specificity:

Sensitivity = (true +ve)/[(true +ve) + (false −ve)]
Specificity = (true −ve)/[(true −ve) + (false +ve)]

In terms of the generalized diagnostic and test results shown in Table 20.1, the sensitivity and specificity are given by:

Sensitivity = $a/(a+c)$
Specificity = $d/(b+d)$.

Table 20.1   *Generalized diagnostic and test results*

Test result	True diagnosis	
	Positive	*Negative*
Positive	a	b
Negative	c	d

After Puri, B.K. 1998: Epidemiology. In Puri, B.K. & Tyrer, P.J. *Sciences Basic to Psychiatry*, 2nd edition. Edinburgh: Churchill Livingstone.

The predictive value of a positive test result (or positive predictive value) is the proportion of the positive results that is truly positive, while the predictive value of a negative test result (negative predictive value) is the proportion of the negative results that is truly negative. The efficiency of the test is the proportion of all the results that is true. In terms of the notation of Table 20.1, these are given by the following expressions:

Positive predictive value = $a/(a+b)$
Negative predictive value = $d/(c+d)$
Efficiency = $(a+d)/(a+b+c+d)$.

The sensitivity, specificity, predictive values and efficiency of a test are often expressed in terms of percentages, simply by multiplying the above formulae by 100.

Three further measures (which may also be expressed as percentages by multiplication by 100) that may be derived from Table 20.1 are:

Screen prevalence = $(a+b)/(a+b+c+d)$
Disease prevalence = $(a+c)/(a+b+c+d)$
Test accuracy = $(a+d)/(a+b+c+d)$.

Likelihood ratio

This is a function of both the sensitivity and the specificity of a test, and indexes how much the test result will change the odds of having a disease/disorder.

- The likelihood ratio for a *positive* result, LR+, is given by:

LR+ = sensitivity/(1 − specificity)

  - It indexes the increase in the odds of having a disease when the test result is positive.

- The likelihood ratio for a *negative* result, LR−, is given by:

  LR− = (1 − sensitivity)/specificity

  - It indexes the decrease in the odds of having a disease when the test result is negative.

Pre-test odds
The pre-test odds are a function of the prevalence of the disease and may be calculated as follows:

  Pre-test odds = prevalence/(1 − prevalence)

(Prevalence, in this context, is also sometimes known as the pre-test probability.)

Post-test odds
The post-test odds of a disease are the odds that a patient has a disease, and incorporate information relating to:

- disease prevalence
- the patient pool
- the likelihood ratio
- pre-test odds (that is, risk factors for the patient).

  The post-test odds are calculated as follows:

  Post-test odds = (pre-test odds) × (likelihood ratio)

CASE REGISTERS

Examples of case registers that have proved useful in epidemiological studies and psychiatric research generally include:

- Swedish and Danish twin registers
- psychiatric case registers, containing records of those who have been treated for psychiatric disorders in certain hospitals or catchment areas.

  Limitations of case registers include:

- The registered individuals may move out of the defined geographical area.
- The registers may not be kept up to date for other reasons.

MORTALITY STATISTICS

Mortality rate
This is the number of deaths in a defined population during a given period of time divided by the population size during that time period. This measure is also sometimes referred to as the 'crude mortality ratio' or CMR. It may be expressed as a percentage by multiplying the ratio by 100.

- *Standardized mortality rate.* This is the mortality rate adjusted to compensate for a confounder.
- *Age-standardized mortality rate.* This is the mortality rate adjusted to compensate for the confounding effect of age.
- *Standardized mortality ratio.* The standardized mortality ratio, or SMR, is the ratio of the observed standardized mortality rate, derived from the population being studied, to the expected standardized mortality rate, derived from a comparable standard population. It may be expressed as a percentage by multiplying the ratio by 100.

Life expectancy

This is a measure of the mean length of time that an individual can be expected to live based on the assumption that the mortality rates used remain constant. It is calculated from the ratio of the total time a hypothetical group of people is expected to live to the size of that group.

MORBIDITY RATE

This is the rate of occurrence of new non-fatal cases of a given disease in a defined population at risk during a given period of time.

- *Standardized morbidity rate.* This is the morbidity rate adjusted to compensate for a confounder.
- *Age-standardized morbidity rate.* This is the morbidity rate adjusted to compensate for the confounding effect of age.
- *Standardized morbidity ratio.* The standardized morbidity ratio is the ratio of the observed standardized morbidity rate, derived from the population being studied, to the expected standardized morbidity rate, derived from a comparable standard population. It may be expressed as a percentage by multiplying the ratio by 100.

MEASUREMENTS OF RISK

The terms described in this section can usefully be related to the 2 × 2 contingency table shown in Table 20.2, as used in analytical epidemiological studies. Similarly, they also apply to the critical appraisal of, for example, prospective cohort studies, such as the one shown in Table 20.3.

Table 20.2 *Generalized 2 × 2 contingency table used in analytical epidemiological studies*

Exposure to risk factor	Outcome		Total
	Disease	*No disease*	
Positive	a	b	$a + b$
Negative	c	d	$c + d$
Total	$a + c$	$b + d$	$a + b + c + d$

After Puri, B.K. 1998: Epidemiology. In Puri, B.K. & Tyrer, P.J. *Sciences Basic to Psychiatry,* 2nd edition. Edinburgh: Churchill Livingstone.

Table 20.3 *Generalized prospective cohort study results*

Group	Outcome		Total
	Positive	*Negative*	
Cohort	a	b	$a + b$
Control	c	d	$c + d$
Total	$a + c$	$b + d$	$a + b + c + d$

RELATIVE RISK

In terms of analytical epidemiological studies, the relative risk of a disease with respect to a given risk factor is the ratio of the incidence of the disease in people exposed to that risk factor to the incidence of the disease in people not exposed to that same risk factor. In Table 20.2, this equates to the ratio of $a/(a + b)$ to $c/(c + d)$.

In terms of prospective cohort studies, the relative risk is the ratio of the probability of a positive outcome in the cohort group (exposed) to the probability of a positive outcome in the control group (not exposed). In Table 20.3, this again equates to the ratio of $a/(a + b)$ to $c/(c + d)$.

Thus, in terms of both Tables 20.2 and 20.3:

Relative risk $= a(c + d)/[c/(a + b)]$

The relative risk does not have any units, being the ratio of two numbers, and it can take on any non-negative real value; that is, relative risk ≥ 0.

ATTRIBUTABLE RISK

This is the incidence of the disease in the group exposed to the risk factor of interest minus the incidence in the group not exposed to this risk factor. The attributable risk is also known as the 'risk difference' or the 'absolute excess risk'. In terms of Table 20.2:

Attributable risk
= risk difference
= absolute excess risk
= absolute risk increase
$= [a/(a + b) − [c/(c + d)]$

RELATIVE RISK INCREASE

This is the absolute risk increase as a proportion of the risk in the 'unexposed' group, and is given by:

Relative risk increase $= \{[a/(a + b)] − [c/(c + d)]\}/[c/(c + d)]$

ABSOLUTE RISK REDUCTION

This is another measure of the difference in the risk between the two groups being studied, but this time indexing the risk reduction following exposure to the index factor. In the notation of the tables of this section, it is given by:

Absolute risk reduction $= [c/(c + d)] − [a/(a + b)]$

RELATIVE RISK REDUCTION

This is the absolute risk reduction as a proportion of the risk in the 'unexposed' group, and is given by:

Relative risk reduction $= \{[c/(c + d)] − [a/(a + b)]\}/[c/(c + d)]$

NUMBER NEEDED TO TREAT

The number needed to treat (NNT) expresses the benefit of an active treatment over a placebo. It can be used in summarizing the results of a trial, and in individualized medical decision making. It takes the value of the nearest integer (or 'whole' number) equal to or higher than the following expression:

$1/\{[c/(c + d)] − [a/(a + b)]\}$

ODDS RATIO

If Table 20.3 is taken to refer to a retrospective study, in which the variable consists of exposure or non-exposure to a given factor, while the outcome consists of being in the disease group or the control group, the odds that subjects in the disease group were exposed to the factor are given by a/b. Similarly, the odds that subjects in the control group were exposed to the factor are given by c/d.

These results follow from the following definition:

Odds of an event taking place = (probability of that event)/(1 − probability of that event)

The odds ratio is the ratio of the odds that subjects in the disease group were exposed to the factor to the odds that subjects in the control group were exposed to the factor. In terms of Table 20.4, we have:

Odds ratio = $ad/(bc)$

Table 20.4 *Generalized retrospective (case–control) study results*

Outcome	Variable		Total
	Exposure	*No-exposure*	
Disease group	a	b	$a + b$
Control	c	d	$c + d$
Total	$a + c$	$b + d$	$a + b + c + d$

In the case of retrospective epidemiological studies (see Table 20.2), if the disease is relatively rare, we have:

$a \ll b \Leftrightarrow a + b \approx b$

and

$c \ll d \Leftrightarrow c + d \approx d$

Hence, in this case:

Relative risk $\approx ad/(bc)$ = odds ratio.

STUDY DESIGN

Hierarchy of research methods

Beginning with the type of research method generally considered to have the lowest credibility, and in increasing order of generally accepted strength of evidence, the types of research studies that are most often used are as follows:

- case reports
- case series
- cross-sectional studies
- retrospective studies
- prospective studies/trials

- randomized double-blind placebo-controlled clinical trials
- meta-analyses (or other systematic reviews) of randomized double-blind placebo-controlled clinical trials.

This hierarchical order should not necessarily be taken as being set in stone. For example, case reports involving the first use of an innovative treatment can be of great value.

Confounding

One of the most important confounding factors in studies is age, particularly, for example, in the calculation of morbidity and mortality rates in epidemiological studies. There are various methods that may be used to compensate for confounding variables. These include:

- standardization (e.g. age can be compensated for by means of age standardization)
- stratification
- randomization
- matching (in terms of the confounder(s)) of controls with patients/subjects/index cases
- restriction (to restrict entry into the study of subjects who are not affected by the confounder(s))
- mathematical and statistical modelling techniques.

BIBLIOGRAPHY

Dunham, H.W. 1965: *Community and Schizophrenia: An Epidemiological Analysis.* Detroit: Wayne State University Press.

Jablensky, A. & Sartorius, N. 1975: Culture and schizophrenia. *Psychological Medicine* 5:113–124.

Puri, B.K. & Tyrer, P.J. 2004: *Sciences Basic to Psychiatry*, 3rd edn. Edinburgh: Churchill Livingstone.

21

Medical ethics and principles of law

ADVOCACY

An advocate enters into a relationship with the patient, to speak on his or her behalf and to represent the patient's wishes or stand up for his or her rights. An advocate has no legal status – the patient should have an idea of personal preferences so that the advocate truly represents the patient's wishes.

APPOINTEESHIP

An appointee is someone authorized by the Department of Social Security to receive and administer benefits on behalf of someone else, who is not able to manage his or her affairs. It can be used solely to administer money derived from social security benefits, and cannot be used to administer any other income or assets. If benefits accumulate, application may need to be made to the Public Trust Office or the Court of Protection to gain access to the accumulated capital.

POWERS OF ATTORNEY

A power of attorney is a means whereby one person (the donor) gives legal authority to another person (the attorney) to manage his or her affairs. The donor has sole responsibility for the decision as to whether power of attorney is given, provided the donor fully understands the implications of what he or she is undertaking.

An ordinary power of attorney allows the attorney to deal with the donor's financial affairs generally, or it can be limited to specific matters. An ordinary power of attorney is automatically revoked by law when the donor loses his or her mental capacity to manage personal affairs.

An Enduring Power of Attorney allows a person to decide who should manage his or her affairs if the person becomes mentally incapable. This has been possible since 1985. An Enduring Power of Attorney continues in force after the donor has lost the mental capacity to manage his or her affairs, provided it is registered with the Public Trust Office. It is thus of use for people with early dementia who can set their affairs in order early in the illness provided the illness has not already progressed to a point where the person is unable to manage personal affairs. Once the donor is unable to manage personal affairs, the attorney must apply to the Public Trust Office for registration of the Enduring Power of Attorney to allow the attorney authority to continue to act.

COURT OF PROTECTION

This is an office of the Supreme Court. It exists to protect the property and affairs of persons who, through mental disorder, are incapable of managing personal financial affairs. The Court's powers are limited to dealing with the financial and legal affairs of the person concerned. Only one medical certificate is required, from a registered medical practitioner who has examined the patient. Guidance to medical practitioners accompanies the certificate of incapacity.

The Court appoints somebody to manage the patient's affairs on his or her behalf. This person is called the *receiver*. It may be a relative, friend, solicitor or other person. The receiver must keep accounts and spend the patient's money on things that will benefit the patient. The Court must give permission before the disposal of capital assets such as property.

TESTAMENTARY CAPACITY

To make a will, a person must be of *sound disposing mind*. This means that the person must:

- understand to whom he or she is giving personal property
- understand and recollect the extent of that personal property
- understand the nature and extent of the claims upon the person, both of those included and those excluded from the will.

A valid will is not invalidated by the subsequent impairment of testamentary capacity.

CAPACITY TO DRIVE

The responsibility for making the decision about whether or not a person should continue to drive is that of the Driver and Vehicle Licensing Authority (DVLA), with a doctor acting only as a source of information and advice. The driver has a duty to keep the DVLA informed of any condition that may impair the ability to drive. The doctor is responsible for advising the patient to inform the DVLA of a condition likely to make driving dangerous. If the patient fails to take this advice, the doctor may then contact the DVLA directly. Tables 21.1–3 summarize the advice of the DVLA to British doctors with respect to fitness to drive in patients with psychiatric disorders. In this table, two types of licence are referred to:

- *Group 1 licence.* A driver with a mobility allowance may drive from the age of 16 years. Licences are normally issued until age 70, unless restricted to a shorter duration for medical reasons. There is no upper age limit, but after the age of 70 licences are renewable every three years.
- *Group 2 licence.* These licences can be issued at the age of 21 years and are valid until the age of 45. They are then issued every five years to the age of 65 unless restricted to a shorter duration for medical reasons. From the age of 65, the licence is issued annually.

Table 21.1 *Advice of the DVLA to doctors with respect to fitness to drive in patients with psychiatric disorders*

Psychiatric disorder	Group 1 entitlement	Group 2 entitlement
Neurosis e.g. anxiety state/depression	DVLA need not be notified. Driving need not cease. Patients must be warned about the possible effects of medication which may affect fitness. However, serious psychoneurotic episodes affecting or likely to affect driving should be notified to DVLA and the person advised not to drive.	Driving should cease with serious acute mental illness from whatever cause. Driving may be permitted when the person is symptom-free and stable for a period of 6 months. Medication must not cause side-effects which would interfere with alertness or concentration. Driving may be permitted also if the mental illness is longstanding but maintained symptom-free on small doses of psychotropic medication with no side-effects likely to impair driving performance. Psychiatric reports may be required.
Psychosis Schizo-affective Acute psychosis Schizophrenia	6 months off the road after an acute episode requiring hospital admission. Licence restored after freedom from symptoms during this period, and the person demonstrates that he/she complies safely with recommended medication and shows insight into the condition. 1-, 2- or 3-year licence with medical review on renewal. Loss of insight or judgement will lead to recommendation to refuse/revoke.	Recommended refusal or revocation. At least 3 years off driving, during which must be stable and symptom-free, and not on major psychotropic or neuroleptic medication, except lithium. Consultant Psychiatric examination required before restoration of licence, to confirm that there is no residual impairment, the applicant has insight and would be able to recognise if he/she became unwell. There should be no significant likelihood of recurrence. Any psychotropic medication necessary must be of low dosage and not interfere with alertness or concentration or in any way impair driving performance.
Manic–depressive psychosis	6–12 months off the road after an acute episode of hypomania requiring hospital admission, depending upon the severity and frequency of relapses. Licence restored after freedom from symptoms during this period and safe compliance with medication. 1-, 2- or 3-year licence with medical review on renewal. Loss of insight or judgement will lead to recommendation to refuse/revoke.	As above for psychosis.

Table 21.1   (Continued)

Psychiatric disorder	Group 1 entitlement	Group 2 entitlement
Dementia Organic brain disorders; e.g. Alzheimer's disease NB: There is no single marker to determine fitness to drive but it is likely that driving may be permitted if there is retention of ability to cope with the general day to day needs of living, together with adequate levels of insight and judgement.	If early dementia, driving may be permitted if there is no significant disorientation in time and space, and there is adequate retention of insight and judgement. Annual medical review required. Likely to be recommended to be refused or revoked if disorientated in time and space, and especially if insight has been lost or judgement is impaired.	Recommended permanent refusal or revocation if the condition is likely to impair driving performance.
Severe mental handicap A state of arrested or incomplete development of mind which includes severe impairment of intelligence and social functioning	Severe mental handicap is a prescribed disability; licence must be refused or revoked. If stable, mild to moderate mental handicap it may be possible to hold a licence, but he/she will need to demonstrate adequate functional ability at the wheel, and be otherwise stable.	Recommended permanent refusal or revocation if severe. Minor degrees of mental handicap when the condition is stable with no medical or psychiatric complications may be able to have a licence. Will need to demonstrate functional ability at the wheel.
Personality disorder Including post head injury syndrome and psychopathic disorders	If seriously disturbed such as evidence of violent outbreaks or alcohol abuse and likely to be a source of danger at the wheel, licence would be refused or revoked. Licence restricted after medical reports that behaviour disturbances have been satisfactorily controlled.	Recommended refusal or revocation if associated with serious behaviour disturbance likely to be a source of danger at the wheel. If the person matures and psychiatric reports confirm stability supportive, licence may be permitted/restored. Consultant Psychiatrist report required.

N.B. A person holding entitlement to Group I (i.e. motor car/motor bike) or Group II (i.e. LGV/PCV), who has been relicensed following an acute psychotic episode, of whatever type, should be advised as part of follow-up that if the condition recurs, driving should cease and DVLA be notified. General guidance with respect to psychotropic/neuroleptic medication is contained under the appropriate section in the text. Alcohol and illicit drug misuse/dependency are dealt with under his or her specific sections. Reference is made in the introductory page to the current GMC guidance to doctors concerning disclosure in the public interest without the consent of the patient.

Table 21.2   *Advice of the DVLA to doctors with respect to fitness to drive in patients with alcohol problems*

Alcohol problem	Group 1 entitlement	Group 2 entitlement
Alcohol misuse/alcohol dependency See footnote	**Alcohol misuse** Alcohol misuse, confirmed by medical enquiry and by evidence of otherwise unexplained abnormal blood markers, requires licence revocation or refusal for a minimum 6-month period, during which time controlled drinking should be attained with normalization of blood parameters.	**Alcohol misuse** Alcohol misuse, confirmed by medical enquiry and by evidence of otherwise unexplained abnormal blood markers, will lead to revocation or refusal of a vocational licence for at least 1 year, during which time controlled drinking should be attained with normalization of blood parameters.

Alcohol problem	Group 1 entitlement	Group 2 entitlement
	Alcohol dependency Including detoxification and/or alcohol related fits. Alcohol dependency, confirmed by medical enquiry, requires a recommended 1-year period of licence revocation or refusal, to attain abstinence or controlled drinking and with normalization of blood parameters if relevant.	**Alcohol dependency** Vocational licensing will not be granted where there is a history of alcohol dependency within the past 3 years.
	Licence restoration Will require satisfactory independent medical examination, arranged by DVLA, with satisfactory blood results and medical reports from own doctors. Patient recommended to seek advice from medical or other sources during the period off the road.	**Licence restoration** On reapplication, independent medical examination arranged by DVLA, with satisfactory blood results and medical reports from own doctors. Consultant support/referral may be necessary. If an alcohol-related seizure or seizures have occurred, the vocational Epilepsy Regulations apply.
Alcohol-related seizure(s)	A licence will be revoked or refused for a minimum 1-year period from the date of the event. Where more than one seizure occurs, consideration under the Epilepsy Regulations may be necessary. Before licence restoration, medical enquiry will be required to confirm appropriate period free from alcohol misuse and/or dependency.	Vocational Epilepsy Regulations apply (see DVLA Guidelines).
Alcohol-related disorders e.g. severe hepatic cirrhosis, Wernicke's encephalopathy, Korsakoffs Psychosis, *et al.*	Licence recommended to be refused/revoked.	Recommended to be refused/revoked.

There is no single definition which embraces all the variables in these conditions. But as a guideline the following is offered: 'a state which because of consumption of alcohol, causes disturbance of behaviour, related disease or other consequences, likely to cause the patient, his family or society harm now or in the future and which may or may not be associated with dependency. In addition, assessment of the alcohol consumption with respect to current national advised guidelines is necessary.'
NB: A person who has been relicensed following alcohol misuse or dependancy must be advised as part of his/her follow-up that if his/her condition recurs he/she should cease driving and notify DVLA Medical Branch.
HIGH RISK OFFENDER SCHEME for drivers convicted of certain drink/driving offences:
1   One disqualification for drink/driving when the level of alcohol is 2.5 or more times the legal limit.
2   One disqualification that he/she failed, without reasonable excuse, to provide a specimen for analysis.
3   Two disqualifications within 10 years for being unfit through drink.
4   Two disqualifications within 10 years when the level of alcohol exceeds the legal limit. DVLA will be notified by courts. On application for licence, satisfactory independent medical examination with completion of structured questionnaire with satisfactory liver enzyme tests and MCV required. If favourable, Till 70 restored for Group I and can recommend issue Group II. If High Risk Offender associated with previous history of alcohol dependancy or misuse, after above satisfactory examination and blood tests, short-period licence only for ordinary and vocational use issued, depending on time interval between previous history and reapplication. High Risk Offender found to have current unfavourable alcohol misuse history and/or abnormal blood test analysis would have application refused.

Table 21.3 *Advice of the DVLA to doctors with respect to fitness to drive in patients with drug misuse and dependency*

Drug misuse and dependency	Group 1 entitlement	Group 2 entitlement
Cannabis Ecstasy and other 'recreational' psychoactive substances, including LSD and hallucinogens	The regular use of these substances, confirmed by medical enquiry, will lead to licence revocation or refusal for a 6-month period. Independent medical assessment and urine screen, arranged by DVLA, may be required.	Regular use of these substances will lead to refusal or revocation of a vocational licence for at least a 1-year period. Independent medical assessment and urine screen, arranged by DVLA, may be required.
Amphetamines Heroin Morphine Methadone* Cocaine Benzodiazepines	Regular use of, or dependency on, these substances, confirmed by medical enquiry, will lead to licence refusal or revocation for a minimum 1-year period. Independent medical assessment and urine screen, arranged by DVLA, may be required. In addition, favourable consultant or specialist report will be required on reapplication. * Applicants or drivers on consultant-supervised oral methadone withdrawal programme may be licensed, subject to annual medical review and favourable assessment.	Regular use of, or dependency on, these substances, will require revocation or refusal of a vocational licence for a minimum 3-year period. Independent medical assessment and urine screen, arranged by DVLA, may be required. In addition, favourable consultant or specialist report will be required before relicensing.
Seizure(s) associated with illicit drug usage	A seizure or seizures associated with illicit drug usage may require a licence to be refused or revoked for a 1-year period. Thereafter, licence restoration will require independent medical assessment, with urine analysis, together with favourable report from own doctor, to confirm no ongoing drug misuse. In addition, patients may be assessed against the Epilepsy Regulations.	Vocational Epilepsy Regulations apply.

NB: A person who has been relicensed following illicit drug misuse or dependency must be advised as part of his/her follow-up that if his/her condition recurs he/she should cease driving and notify DVLA Medical Branch.

22

Legal aspects of psychiatric care

NOTE

The Mental Health Act 1983 for England and Wales is detailed in this chapter; the equivalent Scottish treatment orders are also given. The mental health legislation relevant to your country of practice should be obtained and you should be familiar with its contents and use. The Misuse of Drugs legislation for England and Wales is considered in Chapter 26.

ENGLAND AND WALES: MENTAL HEALTH ACT 1983

DEFINITIONS

Section 1 of the Act contains the following definitions:

- *Mental disorder* – Mental illness, arrested or incomplete development of mind, psychopathic disorder and any other disorder or disability of mind.
- *Patient* – A person suffering from or appearing to suffer from mental disorder.
- *Severe mental impairment* – A state of arrested or incomplete development of mind which includes the severe impairment of intelligence and social functioning and is associated with abnormally aggressive or seriously irresponsible conduct on the part of the person concerned.
- *Mental impairment* – A state of arrested or incomplete development of mind (not amounting to severe mental impairment) which includes significant impairment of intelligence and social functioning and is associated with abnormally aggressive or seriously irresponsible conduct on the part of the person concerned.
- *Psychopathic disorder* – A persistent disorder or disability of mind (whether or not including significant impairment of intelligence) which results in abnormally aggressive or seriously irresponsible conduct on the part of the person concerned.
- *Medical treatment* – Includes nursing, and care and rehabilitation under medical supervision.
- *Responsible Medical Officer* (RMO) – The registered medical practitioner in charge of the treatment of the patient (i.e. the consultant psychiatrist); if that person is not available, the doctor who for the time being is in charge of the patient's treatment may deputize.

- *Approved doctor* – A registered medical practitioner approved under Section 12 of the Act by the Secretary of State (with authority being delegated to the Regional Health Authority) as having special experience in the diagnosis or treatment of mental disorder.
- *Approved social worker* (ASW) – An officer of a local social services authority with appropriate training who may make applications for compulsory admission; hospital senior social workers usually hold lists of approved social workers.
- *Nearest relative* – The first surviving person in the following list, with a full blood relative taking preference over half blood relatives, and the elder of two relatives of the same description or level of kinship taking preference also:
  - husband or wife
  - son or daughter
  - father or mother
  - brother or sister
  - grandparent
  - grandchild
  - uncle or aunt
  - nephew or niece.

  Preference is also given to a relative with whom the patient ordinarily lives or by whom he or she is cared for.

Note that the term *mental illness* is not formally defined; its operational definition is a matter of clinical judgement in each case. The Act states that a person may *not* be dealt with under the Mental Health Act as suffering from mental disorder 'by reason only of promiscuity or other immoral conduct, sexual deviancy or dependence on alcohol or drugs'.

CIVIL TREATMENT ORDERS

See Table 22.1.

Table 22.1   *Civil treatment orders under Mental Health Act 1983*

Section	Grounds	Application by	Medical recommendations	Maximum duration	Eligibility for appeal to Mental Health Review Tribunal
Section 2 Admission for assessment	Mental disorder	Nearest relative or approved social worker	Two doctors (one approved under Section 12)	28 days	Within 14 days
Section 3 Admission for treatment	Mental illness, psychopathic disorder, mental impairment, severe mental impairment (If psychopathic disorder or mental impairment, treatment must be likely to alleviate or prevent deterioration)	Nearest relative or approved social worker	Two doctors (one approved under Section 12)	6 months	Within first 6 months. If renewed, within second 6 months, then every year. Mandatory every 3 years.

Section	Grounds	Application by	Medical recommendations	Maximum duration	Eligibility for appeal to Mental Health Review Tribunal
Section 25 Supervised discharge	Same as section 3	CRMO	Social worker, one doctor	If renewed, 6 months	Within first 6 months. Renewable for 6 months, then every year. Hospital managers cannot discharge.
Section 4 Emergency admission for assessment	Mental disorder (urgent necessity)	Nearest relative or approved social worker	Any doctor	72 hours	
Section 5 (2) Urgent detention of voluntary in-patient	Danger to self or to others		Doctor in charge of patient's care	72 hours	
Section 5 (4) Nurses holding power of voluntary in-patient	Mental disorder (danger to self, health or others)	Registered mental nurse or registered nurse for mental handicap	None	6 hours	
Section 136 Admission by police	Mental disorder	Police officer	Allows patient in public place to be removed to 'place of safety'	72 hours	
Section 135	Mental disorder	Magistrates	Allows power of entry to home and removal of patient to place of safety	72 hours	

Reproduced with permission from Puri, B.K., Laking, P.J. & Treasaden, I.H. 2002: *Textbook of Psychiatry*, 2nd edn. Edinburgh: Churchill Livingstone.

CONSENT TO TREATMENT

See Table 22.2.

Table 22.2 *Consent to treatment under Mental Health Act 1983 – consent to treatment should be informed and voluntary (implies mental illness, e.g. dementia, does not affect judgement)*

Type of treatment	Informal	Detained
Urgent treatment	No consent	No consent
Section 57 Irreversible, hazardous or non-established treatments (e.g. psychosurgery such as leucotomy), hormone implants (for sex offenders), surgical operations (e.g. castration)	Consent and second opinion	Consent and second opinion
Section 58 Psychiatric drugs, ECT	Consent	Consent or second opinion

1 For first 3 months of treatment a detained patient's consent is not required for Section 58 medicines, but is for ECT.
2 Patients can withdraw voluntary consent at any time.
Reproduced with permission from Puri, B.K., Laking, P.J. & Treasaden, I.H. 2002: *Textbook of Psychiatry*, 2nd edn. Edinburgh: Churchill Livingstone.

FORENSIC TREATMENT ORDERS

See Table 22.3.

Table 22.3 *Forensic treatment orders for mentally abnormal offenders*

Section	Grounds	Made by	Medical recommendations	Maximum duration	Eligibility for appeal to Mental Health Review Tribunal
Section 35 Remand to hospital for report	Mental disorder	Magistrates or Crown Court	Any doctor	28 days Renewable at 28-day intervals Maximum 12 weeks	
Section 36 Remand to hospital for treatment	Mental illness, severe mental impairment (not if charged with murder)	Crown Court	Two doctors: one approved under Section 12	28 days Renewable at 28-day intervals Maximum 12 weeks	
Section 37 Hospital and guardianship orders	Mental disorder. (If psychopathic disorder or mental impairment must be likely to alleviate or prevent deterioration.) Accused of, or convicted for, an imprisonable offence	Magistrates or Crown Court	Two doctors, one approved under Section 12	6 months Renewable for further 6 months and then annually	During second 6 months, then every year Mandatory every 3 years.
Section 41 Restriction order	Added to Section 37 To protect public from serious harm	Crown Court	Oral evidence from one doctor	Usually without limit of time Effect: leave, transfer, or discharge only with consent of Home Secretary	As Section 37
Section 38 Interim hospital order	Mental disorder For trial of treatment	Magistrates or Crown Court	Two doctors: one approved under Section 12	12 weeks Renewable at 28-day intervals Maximum 6 months	None

Table 22.3 (*Continued*)

Section	Grounds	Made by	Medical recommendations	Maximum duration	Eligibility for appeal to Mental Health Review Tribunal
Section 47 Transfer of a sentenced prisoner to hospital	Mental disorder	Home Secretary	Two doctors: one approved under Section 12	Until earliest date of release from sentence	Once in the first 6 months Then once in the next 6 months Thereafter, once a year.
Section 48 Urgent transfer to hospital of remand prisoner	Mental disorder	Home Secretary	Two doctors: one approved under Section 12	Until date of trial	Once in the first 6 months Then once in the next 6 months Thereafter, once a year.
Section 49 Restriction direction	Added to Section 47 or Section 48	Home Secretary	–	Until end of Section 47 or 48 Effect: leave, transfer or discharge only with consent of Home Secretary	As for Section 47 and 48 to which applied

Reproduced with permission from Puri, B.K., Laking, P.J. & Treasaden, I.H. 2002: *Textbook of Psychiatry*, 2nd edn. Edinburgh: Churchill Livingstone.

MENTAL HEALTH (SCOTLAND) ACT 1984

See Table 22.4.

Table 22.4 *Equivalent Scottish and English Mental Health Act treatment orders*

Treatment order	Mental Health (England & Wales) Act 1983	Mental Health (Scotland) 1984
Emergency admission	Section 4	Section 24
Short-term detention	Section 2	Section 26
Admission for treatment	Section 3	Section 22
Nurses holding power of a voluntary inpatient	Section 5(4) (for 6 hours)	Section 25(2) for 2 hrs
Guardianship	Section 37	Section 37
Committal to hospital pending trial	Section 36	Sections 25 & 330 of the 1975 Act
Remand for enquiry into mental condition	Section 35	Sections 180 & 381 of the 1975 Act
Removal to hospital of persons in prison awaiting trial or sentence	Section 48	Section 70
Interim hospital order	Section 38	Sections 174a & 375a of the 1975 Act amended by the Mental Health (Amendment) (Scotland) Act 1983
Hospital order	Section 37	Sections 175 & 376 of the 1975 Act
Restriction order	Section 41	Sections 178 & 379 by the 1975 Act
Transfer of prisoner under sentence to hospital	Section 47	Section 71

Reproduced with permission from Puri, B.K., Laking, P.J. & Treasaden, I.H. 2002: *Textbook of Psychiatry*, 2nd edn. Edinburgh: Churchill Livingstone.

BIBLIOGRAPHY

Puri, B.K., Brown, R., McKee, H & Treasaden, I.H. 2004: *Mental Health Law Handbook*. London: Arnold.

Puri, B.K., Laking, P.J. & Treasaden, I.H. 2002: *Textbook of Psychiatry*, 2nd edn. Edinburgh: Churchill Livingstone.

23

Classification

ICD-10

ORGANIC, INCLUDING SYMPTOMATIC, MENTAL DISORDERS

F00 Dementia in Alzheimer's disease
F01 Vascular dementia
F02 Dementia in other diseases classified elsewhere
F03 Unspecified dementia
F04 Organic amnesic syndrome, not induced by alcohol and other psychoactive substances
F05 Delirum, not induced by alcohol and other psychoactive substances
F06 Other mental disorders caused by brain damage and dysfunction and by physical disease
F07 Personality and behavioural disorders caused by brain disease, damage and dysfunction
F09 Unspecified organic or symptomatic mental disorder.

MENTAL AND BEHAVIOURAL DISORDERS CAUSED BY PSYCHOACTIVE SUBSTANCE USE

F10 *Mental and behavioural disorders caused by the use of* alcohol
F11 ... ... opioids
F12 ... ... cannabinoids
F13 ... ... sedatives or hypnotics
F14 ... ... cocaine
F15 ... ... other stimulants, including caffeine
F16 ... ... hallucinogens
F17 ... ... tobacco
F18 ... ... volatile solvents
F19 ... ... multiple drug use and the use of other psychoactive substances.

SCHIZOPHRENIA, SCHIZOTYPAL AND DELUSIONAL DISORDERS

F20 Schizophrenia
F21 Schizotypal disorder

F22 Persistent delusional disorders
F23 Acute and transient psychotic disorders
F24 Induced delusional disorder
F25 Schizoaffective disorders
F28 Other nonorganic psychotic disorders
F29 Unspecified nonorganic psychosis.

MOOD (AFFECTIVE) DISORDERS

F30 Manic episode
F31 Bipolar affective disorder
F32 Depressive episode
F33 Recurrent depressive disorder
F34 Persistent mood (affective) disorders
F35 Other mood (affective) disorders
F39 Unspecified mood (affective) disorder.

NEUROTIC, STRESS-RELATED AND SOMATOFORM DISORDERS

F40 Phobic anxiety disorders
F41 Other anxiety disorders
F42 Obsessive–compulsive disorder
F43 Reaction to severe stress, and adjustment disorders
F44 Dissociative (conversion) disorders
F45 Somatoform disorders
F48 Other neurotic disorders.

BEHAVIOURAL SYNDROMES ASSOCIATED WITH PHYSIOLOGICAL DISTURBANCES AND PHYSICAL FACTORS

F50 Eating disorders
F51 Nonorganic sleep disorders
F52 Sexual dysfunction, not caused by organic disorder or disease
F53 Mental and behavioural disorders associated with the puerperium, not elsewhere classified
F54 Psychological and behavioural factors associated with disorders or diseases classified elsewhere
F55 Abuse of non-dependence-producing substances
F59 Unspecified behavioural syndromes associated with physiological disturbances and physical factors.

DISORDERS OF ADULT PERSONALITY AND BEHAVIOUR

F60 Specific personality disorders
F61 Mixed and other personality disorders
F62 Enduring personality changes, not attributable to brain damage and disease
F63 Habit and impulse disorders
F64 Gender identity disorders
F65 Disorders of sexual preference
F66 Psychological and behavioural disorders associated with sexual development and orientation
F68 Other disorders of adult personality and behaviour
F69 Unspecified disorder of adult personality and behaviour.

MENTAL RETARDATION

F70 Mild mental retardation
F71 Moderate mental retardation
F72 Severe mental retardation
F73 Profound mental retardation
F78 Other mental retardation
F79 Unspecified mental retardation.

DISORDERS OF PSYCHOLOGICAL DEVELOPMENT

F80 Specific developmental disorders of speech and language
F81 Specific developmental disorders of scholastic skills
F82 Specific developmental disorder of motor function
F83 Mixed specific developmental disorders
F84 Pervasive developmental disorders
F88 Other disorders of psychological development
F89 Unspecified disorder of psychological development.

BEHAVIOURAL AND EMOTIONAL DISORDERS WITH ONSET USUALLY OCCURRING IN CHILDHOOD AND ADOLESCENCE

F90 Hyperkinetic disorders
F91 Conduct disorders
F92 Mixed disorders of conduct and emotions
F93 Emotional disorders with onset specific to childhood
F94 Disorders of social functioning with onset specific to childhood and adolescence
F95 Tic disorders
F98 Other behavioural and emotional disorders with onset usually occurring in childhood and adolescence.

UNSPECIFIED MENTAL DISORDER

F99 Mental disorder, not otherwise specified.

DSM–IV–TR

The fourth edition of the *Diagnostic and Statistical Manual of Mental Disorders, text revision* (DSM-IV-TR), published by the American Psychiatric Association in 2000, is a multiaxial classification with the following five axes:

Axis I: Clinical disorders, and other conditions that may be a focus of clinical attention
Axis II: Personality disorders, and mental retardation
Axis III: General medical conditions
Axis IV: Psychosocial and environmental problems
Axis V: Global assessment of functioning.

In the following summary, NOS stands for 'not otherwise specified'.

AXIS I: Clinical disorders, and other conditions that may be a focus of clinical attention

DISORDERS USUALLY FIRST DIAGNOSED IN INFANCY, CHILDHOOD OR ADOLESCENCE (EXCLUDING MENTAL RATARDATION, WHICH IS DIAGNOSED ON AXIS II)

- Learning disorder
- Motor skills disorder
- Communication disorders
- Pervasive developmental disorders:
  - Autistic disorder
  - Rett's disorder
  - Childhood disintegrative disorder
  - Asperger's disorder
  - NOS
- Attention-deficit and disruptive behaviour disorders
- Feeding and eating disorders of infancy and early childhood
- Tic disorders
- Elimination disorders:
  - Encopresis
  - Enuresis
- Other disorders of infancy, childhood or adolescence.

DELIRIUM, DEMENTIA, AND AMNESTIC AND OTHER COGNITIVE DISORDERS

- Delirium
- Dementia
- Amnestic disorders
- Other cognitive disorders.

MENTAL DISORDERS CAUSED BY A GENERAL MEDICAL CONDITION

SUBSTANCE-RELATED DISORDERS

- Alcohol-related disorders
- Amphetamine (or amphetamine-like)-related disorders
- Caffeine-related disorders
- Cannabis-related disorders
- Cocaine-related disorders
- Hallucinogen-related disorders
- Inhalant-related disorders
- Nicotine-related disorders
- Opioid-related disorders
- Phencyclidine (or phencyclidine-like)-related disorders
- Sedative-, hypnotic- or anxiolytic-related disorders
- Polysubstance-related disorders
- Other (or unknown) substance-related disorders.

SCHIZOPHRENIA AND OTHER PSYCHOTIC DISORDERS

- Schizophrenia
- Schizophreniform disorder

- Schizoaffective disorder
- Delusional disorder
- Brief psychotic disorder
- Shared psychotic disorder
- Psychotic disorder caused by a general medical condition
- Substance-induced psychotic disorder
- Psychotic disorder NOS.

MOOD DISORDERS

- Depressive disorders
- Bipolar disorders.

ANXIETY DISORDERS

- Panic disorder without agoraphobia
- Panic disorder with agoraphobia
- Agoraphobia without history of panic disorder
- Specific phobia
- Social phobia
- Obsessive–compulsive disorder
- Post-traumatic stress disorder
- Acute stress disorder
- Generalized anxiety disorder
- Anxiety disorder caused by a general medical condition
- Substance-induced anxiety disorder
- NOS.

SOMATOFORM DISORDERS

- Somatization disorder
- Undifferentiated somatoform disorder
- Conversion disorder
- Pain disorder
- Hypochondriasis
- Body dysmorphic disorder
- NOS.

FACTITIOUS DISORDERS

DISSOCIATIVE DISORDERS

- Dissociative amnesia
- Dissociative fugue
- Dissociative identity disorder
- Depersonalization disorder
- NOS.

SEXUAL AND GENDER IDENTITY DISORDERS

- Sexual dysfunctions
  - Sexual desire disorders

- Sexual arousal disorders
- Orgasmic disorders
- Sexual pain disorders
- Sexual dysfunction caused by a general medical condition
- Paraphilias
  - Exhibitionism
  - Fetishism
  - Frotteurism
  - Pedophilia
  - Sexual masochism
  - Sexual sadism
  - Transvestic fetishism
  - Voyeurism
  - NOS
- Gender identity disorders.

EATING DISORDERS

- Anorexia nervosa
- Bulimia nervosa
- NOS.

SLEEP DISORDERS

- Primary sleep disorders
  - Dyssomnias
  - Parasomnias
- Sleep disorders related to another medical disorder
- Other sleep disorders.

IMPULSE–CONTROL DISORDERS NOT ELSEWHERE CLASSIFIED

ADJUSTMENT DISORDERS

OTHER CONDITIONS THAT MAY BE A FOCUS OF CLINICAL ATTENTION

AXIS II: Personality disorders, and mental retardation

PERSONALITY DISORDERS

- Paranoid personality disorder
- Schizoid personality disorder
- Schizotypal personality disorder
- Antisocial personality disorder
- Borderline personality disorder
- Histrionic personality disorder
- Narcissistic personality disorder
- Avoidant personality disorder

- Dependent personality disorder
- Obsessive–compulsive personality disorder
- NOS.

MENTAL RETARDATION

- Mild mental retardation
- Moderate mental retardation
- Severe mental retardation
- Profound mental retardation
- Mental retardation, severity unspecified.

AXIS III: General medical conditions

- Infectious and parasitic diseases
- Neoplasms
- Endocrine, nutritional, and metabolic diseases and immunity disorders
- Diseases of the blood and blood-forming organs
- Diseases of the nervous system and sense organs
- Diseases of the circulatory system
- Diseases of the respiratory system
- Diseases of the digestive system
- Diseases of the genitourinary system
- Complications of pregnancy, childbirth and the puerperium
- Diseases of the skin and subcutaneous tissue
- Diseases of the musculoskeletal system and connective tissue
- Congenital anomalies
- Certain conditions originating in the perinatal period
- Symptoms, signs and ill-defined conditions
- Injury and poisoning.

AXIS IV: Psychosocial and environmental problems

- Problems with the primary support group
- Problems related to the social environment
- Educational problems
- Occupational problems
- Housing problems
- Economic problems
- Problems with access to healthcare services
- Problems related to interaction with the legal system/crime
- Other psychosocial and environmental problems.

AXIS V: Global assessment of functioning

The final axis allows for a global assessment of functioning of the individual.

BIBLIOGRAPHY

American Psychiatric Association 2000: *Diagnostic and Statistical Manual of Mental Disorders, text revision.* Washington, DC: APA.

World Health Organization 1992: *The ICD-10 Classification of Mental and Behavioural Disorders.* Geneva: WHO.

24

Physical therapies

NOTE

Pharmacotherapy is considered in Chapters 15–18.

ELECTROCONVULSIVE THERAPY (ECT)

The following are key historical points in the development of electroconvulsive therapy:

- During the early twentieth century it was hypothesized that schizophrenia and epilepsy are more or less mutually exclusive disorders.
- In 1934, Meduna, on the basis of this hypothesis, attempted to treat schizophrenia by inducing seizures chemically.
- In 1938, Cerletti and Bini induced seizures electrically.

ECT indications, contraindications and side-effects

INDICATIONS FOR ECT

The main indications for ECT are:

- severe depressive illness
- puerperal depressive illness
- mania
- catatonic schizophrenia
- schizoaffective disorder.

CONTRAINDICATIONS AGAINST ECT

Raised intracranial pressure is an absolute contraindication to ECT. Relative contraindications include:

- cerebral aneurysm
- recent myocardial infarction
- cardiac arrhythmia
- intracerebral haemorrhage
- acute/impending retinal detachment
- pheochromocytoma
- raised anaesthetic risk
- unstable vascular aneurysm or malformation.

SIDE-EFFECTS OF ECT

The main early side-effects include:

- headache
- temporary confusion
- some loss of short-term memory.

ECT may cause depressed patients with bipolar mood disorder to become manic. In the long term, patients may complain of memory impairment.

Administration of ECT

- A patient receiving ECT in the morning should remain 'nil by mouth' from the previous midnight.
- A muscle relaxant is administered in order to prevent violent movements during the convulsion.
- Atropine is administered in order to reduce secretions and prevent the muscarinic actions of the muscle relaxant.
- If there is any possibility that the patient may have low or atypical plasma pseudocholinesterase enzymes, the anaesthetist must be informed as this could lead to prolonged muscle paralysis with the muscle relaxant.
- Bilateral or unilateral (to the non-dominant cerebral hemisphere) ECT is administered under a short-acting general anaesthetic.
- A bite is placed in the patient's mouth in order to prevent damage from biting during the convulsion.

NICE guidelines on ECT

NICE, the National Institute for Clinical Excellence, is part of the British National Health Service (NHS). It produces guidance for both the NHS and patients on the use of medicines, medical equipment, diagnostic tests and clinical and surgical procedures and under what circumstances they should be used. In 2003, NICE issued guidelines on ECT.

THE GUIDANCE

The NICE guidance contained the following ten main points.

Point 1
It is recommended that ECT be used only to achieve rapid and short-term improvement of severe symptoms after an adequate trial of other treatment options has proven ineffective

and/or when the condition is considered to be potentially life-threatening, in individuals with:

- severe depressive illness
- catatonia
- a prolonged or severe manic episode.

Point 2
The decision as to whether ECT is clinically indicated should be based on a documented assessment of the risks and potential benefits to the individual, including:

- the risks associated with the anaesthetic
- current co-morbidities
- anticipated adverse events, particularly cognitive impairment
- the risk of not having treatment.

Point 3
The risks associated with ECT may be enhanced in the following groups:

- pregnant women
- older people
- children and young people.

Therefore clinicians should exercise particular caution when considering ECT treatment in these groups.

Point 4
Valid consent should be obtained in all cases in which the individual has the ability to grant or refuse consent. The decision to use ECT should be made jointly by the individual and the clinician(s) responsible for treatment, on the basis of an informed discussion. This discussion should be enabled by the provision of full and appropriate information about the general risks associated with ECT (see guidance point 9 below) and about the risks and potential benefits specific to that individual. Consent should be obtained without pressure or coercion, which may occur as a result of the circumstances and clinical setting, and the individual should be reminded of his or her right to withdraw consent at any point. There should be strict adherence to recognized guidelines about consent, and the involvement of patient advocates and/or carers to facilitate informed discussion is strongly encouraged.

Point 5
In all situations in which informed discussion and consent is not possible, advance directives should be taken fully into account and the individual's advocate and/or carer should be consulted.

Point 6
Clinical status should be assessed following each ECT session and treatment should be stopped when a response has been achieved, or sooner if there is evidence of adverse effects. Cognitive function should be monitored on an ongoing basis, and at a minimum at the end of each course of treatment.

Point 7
It is recommended that a repeat course of ECT should be considered under the circumstances indicated in guidance point no. 1 (above) only for individuals who have severe depressive illness, catatonia or mania and who have previously responded well to ECT. In patients who are experiencing an acute episode but have not previously responded, a repeat trial of ECT should be

undertaken only after all other options have been considered and following discussion of the risks and benefits with the individual and/or where appropriate the carer/advocate.

Point 8

As the longer-term benefits and risks of ECT have not been clearly established, it is not recommended as a maintenance therapy in depressive illness.

Point 9

The current state of the evidence does not allow the general use of ECT in the management of schizophrenia to be recommended.

Point 10

National information leaflets should be developed through consultation with appropriate professional and user organizations to enable individuals and their carers/advocates to make informed decisions regarding the appropriateness of ECT for their circumstances. The leaflets should be evidence-based, include information about the risks of ECT and availability of alternative treatments, and be produced in formats and languages that make them accessible to a wide range of service users.

CRITICISMS OF GUIDANCE

A number of criticisms have been made of the above NICE guidelines on the use of ECT. For example, Cole and Tobiansky (2003) have made the following points:

- The potential benefits of maintenance ECT (also known as continuation ECT) seem to have been discounted.
- The recommendations have not acknowledged the different potential for memory disruption and cognitive side-effects arising from bilateral as opposed to unilateral ECT.
- In severely depressed patients who have previously shown a good response to ECT, it may be appropriate to consider it as a first-line treatment.
- While the NICE guidelines do not recommend ECT as a treatment for moderate depressive episodes, it should be noted that the randomized controlled trials that form the evidence base for ECT were carried out mainly on moderately or moderately severely depressed patients, excluding those with severe depressive episodes who were unable to give informed consent.

Certain of these points have in fact been addressed by NICE in statements relating to the clinical effectiveness of ECT (see below). In their editorial considering these NICE guidelines, Carney and Geddes (2003) concluded that:

> For too long electroconvulsive therapy has been a neglected service with widespread unexplained variations in practice and a low priority with managers: repeated audits by the Royal College of Psychiatrists have shown that many hospital trusts fail to adhere to the college's standards. The recommendations from NICE, together with the recently announced accreditation service from the Royal College of Psychiatrists, should provide the stimulus to ensure that services are brought up to acceptable standards throughout the United Kingdom.
>
> We predict that most parties will be reasonably satisfied with the NICE appraisal. Those concerned about potential overuse of the treatment can be reassured with the restrictions, increased safeguards, and improved consent procedures. Clinicians with the responsibility for helping the most severely ill patients will still have access to an effective treatment. So far, the process appears to have resulted in

an approach that is both evidence-based and broadly acceptable to most stakeholders. If this indeed is the result, it will be a substantial achievement in such a difficult area of clinical practice and a finely judged performance by NICE.

Clinical effectiveness of ECT

NICE published the following points in relation to the clinical effectiveness of ECT.

Point 1
The evidence presented in the Assessment Report was primarily drawn from a recent Cochrane Review of ECT in schizophrenia and a systematic review commissioned by the Department of Health on the use of ECT in schizophrenia, depressive illness and mania. Both reviews are of high quality and consider a total of 119 randomized controlled trials (RCTs) and a number of observational studies. Evidence submitted by patient and professional groups was also considered.

Point 2
There were problems with the design of many of the RCTs. A large proportion were conducted before the introduction of modern techniques of administering ECT, and therefore do not reflect current practice. There were large variations in the parameters of the ECT administered that included the machine used, the number of sessions, the dosage and waveform, electrode placement, and the type and dosage of concomitant therapy. A number of studies used fixed dosage rather than individual thresholds. There was little evidence to support the routine prescription of a set number of treatment sessions per course of ECT or of the value of continuation (maintenance) ECT. The validity of many of the measurement scales used in the studies to measure outcome has not been clearly established and no study adequately captured either users' views or quality of life.

Point 3
The Assessment Report reviews data from 90 RCTs in individuals with depressive illness, of different grades of clinical severity, who were referred for ECT. Overall, these RCTs provide evidence that real ECT (that is, where an electric current was applied) is more effective than sham ECT (where no electric current was applied) in the short term.

The data provide evidence that the stimulus parameters have an important influence on efficacy; at the end of a course of treatment, bilateral ECT was reported to be more effective than unilateral ECT. Raising the electrical stimulus above the individual's seizure threshold was found to increase the efficacy of unilateral ECT at the expense of increased cognitive impairment.

In trials comparing ECT with pharmacotherapy, ECT had greater benefit than the use of certain antidepressants but the trials were of variable quality and inadequate doses and durations of drug therapy were frequently used. The combination of ECT with pharmacotherapy was not shown to be superior to ECT alone, although the duration of the RCTs was insufficient to show whether pharmacotherapy was beneficial. Compared with placebo, continuation pharmacotherapy with tricyclic antidepressants and/or lithium reduced the rate of relapses in people who had responded to ECT.

Preliminary studies indicate that ECT is more effective than repetitive transcranial magnetic stimulation (rTMS).

Point 4
Evidence from 25 RCTs suggests that ECT may be effective in acute episodes of certain types of schizophrenia and reduce the occurrence of relapses, although the results are not conclusive and the

design of many of the studies did not reflect current practice. The data on differing efficacy related to electrode placement and stimulus parameters are equivocal and firm conclusions could not be drawn.

No RCT investigated the use of ECT in comparison with atypical antipsychotics, and the studies that included individuals with treatment-resistant schizophrenia did not consider the use of clozapine. The combined weight of evidence suggests that ECT is not more effective, and may be less effective, than antipsychotic medication. The combination of ECT and pharmacotherapy may be more effective than pharmacotherapy alone, but the evidence is not conclusive.

Point 5

The four RCTs reviewed in the Assessment Report suggest that ECT may be of benefit in the rapid control of mania and catatonia and this suggestion is supported by evidence from a number of observational studies and testimony from clinical experts. However, the evidence on which to base any general conclusions about the effectiveness of ECT or to determine the most appropriate therapeutic strategy is weak.

Point 6

There is clear evidence that cognitive impairment occurs both immediately after administration of ECT and following a course of therapy, and this may cause considerable distress to those affected. The impairment is greater in individuals who have had electrodes applied bilaterally than in those who have had them placed unilaterally, and unilateral placement to the dominant hemisphere causes more impairment than placement to the non-dominant hemisphere. A reduction in the risk of cognitive impairment is, however, mirrored by a reduction in efficacy.

There is some limited evidence from RCTs to suggest that the effects on cognitive function may not last beyond six months, but this has been inadequately researched.

There is also evidence to suggest that the impairment of cognitive function associated with ECT differs between individuals and that it is linked to the dose administered, although the relationship with the seizure threshold has not been adequately defined. There is no evidence to suggest that the effect of ECT on cognitive function differs between diagnoses.

Point 7

In addition to testimony from user groups, a systematic review of evidence from non-randomized studies relating to patients' accounts and experiences of ECT was also considered. This provided important evidence on the experiences of individuals receiving ECT, particularly cognitive impairment and its impact, and the validity of neuropsychological instruments used in clinical trials.

There was evidence that the measurement scales used in RCTs do not adequately capture the nature and extent of cognitive impairment, and qualitative studies have indicated that the impairment may be prolonged or permanent. Additionally, there was testimony that individuals are not provided with sufficient information on which to base a decision regarding consent. Also, some individuals are unaware of their rights to refuse treatment, or may feel unable to do so because of the perceived threat of detainment under the Mental Health Act.

Point 8

There was no evidence to suggest that the mortality associated with ECT is greater than that associated with minor procedures involving general anaesthetics, and there were limited data on mortality extending beyond the trial periods.

The six reviewed studies that used brain-scanning techniques did not provide any evidence that ECT causes brain damage.

While there is no evidence to suggest that benefits and safety are age-dependent, there are no studies on the impact of ECT on the developing brain. Furthermore, it is likely that co-morbidities could increase the risk of harm. The use of ECT during pregnancy is known to cause complications, but the risks associated with ECT need to be balanced against the risks of using alternative (drug) treatments.

REPETITIVE TRANSCRANIAL MAGNETIC STIMULATION

The use of repetitive transcranial magnetic stimulation (rTMS) is gaining support amongst psychiatrists as evidence emerges suggesting that it may provide an alternative to ECT in treating depression and other psychiatric disorders.

The following are key historical points in the development of transcranial magnetic stimulation (TMS) and repetitive transcranial magnetic stimulation:

- In 1896, d'Arsonval observed the occurrence of phosphenes and vertigo when a subject's head is put into a coil (driven at 42 Hz).
- In 1959, Kolin and colleagues stimulated the exposed frog sciatic nerve looped around the pole piece of an electromagnet and caused the gastrocnemius to contract (driven at 60 Hz and 1 kHz).
- In 1965, Bickford and Freeming successfully demonstrated non-invasive stimulation of human peripheral nerves.
- In 1985, Barker (in Sheffield, England) reported the first magnetic stimulation of the human motor cortex.

Indications for rTMS

At the time of writing there is evidence that the administration of repetitive transcranial magnetic stimulation to humans may be able to:

- lift mood in depression
- induce long-term potentiation.

In addition, rTMS with appropriate stimulation parameters may result in long-term effects on synaptic efficacy.

The development of magnetic seizure therapy (MST) holds out the promise of using transcranial magnetic stimulation to induce focal seizures limited to targeted cerebral regions, without causing side-effects related to the stimulation of other cerebral regions.

ECT versus rTMS/MST

ECT is compared with repetitive transcranial magnetic stimulation in Table 24.1.

Table 24.1   A comparison of ECT with rTMS

	ECT	rTMS
Anaesthesia	Required	Not required
Seizure	Required	Not required
Treatment frequency	2–3 per week	Every day
Occurrence of amnesia	Yes	No
Focality	Relatively non-focal	More focal
Tissue impedance	Shunting occurs	No shunting
Pulse width	0.5–2 ms	0.2 ms

PHOTOTHERAPY

This is treatment with high-intensity artificial light, and may be used to treat patients suffering from seasonal affective disorder (SAD).

The light boxes used typically emit light of a strength of around 10 000 lux. By comparison, on a sunny day the level of illumination may reach 100 000 lux, while the home environment may typically be illuminated at around 250 lux. The light spectrum used tends to be balanced, but usually with potentially harmful ultraviolet B (UVB) frequencies filtered out. Patients are usually instructed to sit at a specified distance from the light box for a specified length of time each day.

SLEEP DEPRIVATION

INDICATIONS

The clinical indications for sleep deprivation in mood disorders include:

* as an antidepressant in treatment-resistant patients
* to augment the response to antidepressants
* to hasten the onset of action of antidepressant medication or of lithium
* as a prophylaxis in recurrent mood cycles
* as an aid to diagnosis
* to predict the response to antidepressants or ECT.

ADMINISTRATION

In total sleep deprivation, the patient is kept awake for 36 hours. One variation is late partial sleep deprivation, in which the patient is kept awake from 2 a.m. until 10 p.m. Another variation entails depriving the patient only of rapid-eye-movement (REM) sleep.

PSYCHOSURGERY

The following are key points in the history of psychosurgery:

* From 3000 to 2000 BC there is evidence of trepanation.
* In the nineteenth century, Burckhardt removed postcentral, temporal and frontal cortices from patients.
* In 1910, Pusepp resected fibres between the frontal and parietal lobes in patients with bipolar mood disorder.
* In 1936, Ody resected the right prefrontal lobe of a patient with so-called childhood-onset schizophrenia.
* In 1935, after learning of the work of Fulton and Jacobsen involving bilateral ablation of the prefrontal cortex in chimpanzees, Moniz carried out human frontal leucotomy (work published in 1936).

Indications for psychosurgery

Psychosurgery is a last-resort treatment for:

- chronic severe intractable depression
- chronic severe intractable obsessive–compulsive disorder
- chronic severe intractable anxiety states.

Psychosurgery practice

Current methods for making sterotaxic lesions include:

- electrocautery
- radioactive yttrium implantation
- thermocoagulation
- gamma knife.

Some of the specific operations that may be used currently include:

- frontal-lobe lesioning
- cingulotomy
- capsulotomy
- subcaudate tractotomy
- limbic leucotomy.

VAGAL NERVE STIMULATION

Vagal nerve stimulation (VNS) is generally carried out by surgically implanting a vagus nerve stimulator (a pulse generator) into the subcutaneous tissues of the upper left chest, in order to deliver pulsed electrical stimulation to the cervical vagal trunk. VNS is of particular use in the treatment of epilepsy.

The first use of VNS in humans was by Penry and Dean (published in 1990) for the prevention of partial seizures. Later, a neurocybernetic prosthesis implant was used in a patient with depression at the Medical University of South Carolina (Charleston, USA).

Indications for VNS

There are two major indications for VNS:

- epilepsy
- treatment-resistant depression.

The rationale for using VNS in treatment-resistant depression is based partly on the following findings:

- VNS has been found to reduce depressive symptoms in epileptic patients.
- Limbic blood flow is altered by VNS.

- CSF monoamine concentrations are altered by VNS.
- Antiepileptic drugs may affect mood.

Preliminary results with VNS appear to support its efficacy in treatment-resistant depression (Rush *et al.*, 2000).

BIBLIOGRAPHY

Carney, S. & Geddes, J. 2003: Electroconvulsive therapy: recent recommendations are likely to improve standards and uniformity of use. *British Medical Journal* 326:1343–1344.

Cole, C. & Tobiansky, R. 2003: Electroconvulsive therapy: NICE guidance may deny many patients treatment that they might benefit from. *British Medical Journal* 327:621.

Lisanby, S.H. & Sackeim, H.A. 2002: Transcranial magnetic stimulation and electroconvulsive therapy: similarities and differences. In Pascual-Leone, A., Davey, N.J., Rothwell, J., Wassermann, E.M. & Puri, B.K. (eds) *Handbook of Transcranial Magnetic Stimulation*. London: Arnold.

Pascual-Leone, A., Davey, N.J., Rothwell, J., Wassermann, E.M. and Puri, B.K. (eds) 2002: *Handbook of Transcranial Magnetic Stimulation*. London: Arnold.

Puri, B.K., Laking, P.J. & Treasaden, I.H. 2002: *Textbook of Psychiatry*, 2nd edn. Edinburgh: Churchill Livingstone.

Rush, A.J., George, M.S., Sackeim, H.A. *et al.* 2000: Vagus nerve stimulation (VNS) for treatment-resistant depressions: a multicenter study. *Biological Psychiatry* 47:276–286.

Schachter, S. & Schmidt, D. (eds) 2001: *Vagus Nerve Stimulation*. London: Martin Dunitz.

Trimble, M.R. 1996: *Neuropsychiatry*, 2nd edn. Chichester: John Wiley.

25

Organic psychiatry

General issues

In ICD-10, organic mental disorders are grouped on the basis of a common demonstrable aetiology being present in the form of cerebral disorder, injury to the brain, or other insult leading to cerebral dysfunction, which may be:

- primary – disorders, injuries and insults affecting the brain directly or with predilection, such as Alzheimer's disease
- secondary – systemic disorders affecting the brain only in so far as it is one of the multiple organs or body systems involved (e.g. hypothyroidism).

By convention the following disorders are excluded from the category of organic mental disorders and considered separately:

- psychoactive substance use disorders (including brain disorder resulting from alcohol and other psychoactive drugs)
- certain sleep disorders
- the causes of learning disability (mental retardation).

The dementias and delirium are considered in Chapters 11 and 38, while Wernicke's encephalopathy and Korsakov's syndrome are considered in Chapter 26. The clinical features of focal cerebral disorders have been outlined in Chapter 10.

The causes of dementia are conveniently summarized here:

- degenerative diseases of the central nervous system:
  - Alzheimer's disease
  - Pick's disease
  - Huntington's disease
  - Creutzfeldt–Jakob disease
  - normal-pressure hydrocephalus
  - multiple sclerosis
  - Lewy body disease
- intoxication
  - alcohol

- heavy metals such as lead, arsenic, thallium and mercury
- carbon monoxide
- withdrawal from drugs
- withdrawal from alcohol
- intracranial
  - space-occupying lesions such as tumours, chronic subdural haematomas, aneurysms and chronic abscesses
  - infections
  - head injury
  - punch-drunk syndrome
- endocrine disorders
  - Addison's disease
  - Cushing's syndrome
  - hyperinsulinism
  - hypothyroidism
  - hypopituitarism
  - hypoparathyroidism
  - hyperparathyroidism
- metabolic disorders
  - hepatic failure
  - renal failure
  - respiratory failure
  - hypoxia
  - renal dialysis
  - chronic uraemia
  - chronic electrolyte imbalance ($\uparrow Ca^{2+}$, $\downarrow Ca^{2+}$, $\downarrow K^+$, $\uparrow Na^+$, $\downarrow Na^+$)
  - porphyria
  - Paget's disease
  - remote effects of carcinoma or lymphoma
  - hepatolenticular degeneration (Wilson's disease)
  - vitamin deficiency (thiamine, nicotinic acid, folate, B_{12})
  - vitamin intoxication (A, D)
- vascular
  - multi-infarct (vascular) dementia
  - cerebral artery occlusion
  - cranial arteritis
  - arteriovenous malformation
  - Binswanger's disease.

ORGANIC MENTAL DISORDERS

The treatment, course and prognosis for the following disorders are essentially those of the underlying pathology.

ORGANIC HALLUCINOSIS

In ICD-10, organic hallucinosis is defined as being a disorder of persistent or recurrent hallucinations, in any modality but usually visual or auditory, that occur in clear consciousness without any significant intellectual decline and that may or may not be recognized by the subject as such; delusional elaboration of the hallucinations may occur, but often insight is preserved. The causes of organic hallucinosis are shown in Table 25.1.

Table 25.1 *Causes of organic hallucinosis*

Psychoactive substance use	Alcohol abuse (alcoholic hallucinosis)
	Amphetamine and related sympathomimetics
	Cocaine
	Hallucinogens, e.g. LSD
	Flashback phenomena following the use of hallucinogens
Intoxication	Drugs – amantadine, bromocriptine, ephedrine, levodopa, lysuride
Intracranial causes	Brain tumour
	Head injury
	Migraine
	Infections, e.g. neurosyphilis
	Epilepsy, particularly temporal lobe epilepsy
Sensory deprivation	Deafness
	Poor vision, e.g. cataract
	Torture, e.g. in prisoners of war
Endocrine	Hypothyroidism – 'myxoedematous madness'
Huntington's disease	

Reproduced with permission from Puri, B.K., Laking, P.J. & Treasaden, I.H. 2002: *Textbook of Psychiatry*, 2nd edn. Edinburgh: Churchill Livingstone.

ORGANIC CATATONIC DISORDER

In ICD-10, organic catatonic disorder is defined as being a disorder of diminished (stupor) or increased (excitement) psychomotor activity associated with catatonic symptoms; the extremes of psychomotor disturbance may alternate. The stuporose symptoms may include complete mutism, negativism and rigid posturing, while excitement manifests as gross hypermotility. Other catatonic symptoms include sterotypies and waxy flexibility. Important causes of organic catatonic disorder include:

* encephalitis
* carbon monoxide poisoning.

ORGANIC DELUSIONAL OR SCHIZOPHRENIA-LIKE DISORDER

In ICD-10, organic delusional or schizophrenia-like disorder is defined as a disorder in which the clinical picture is dominated by persistent or recurrent delusions, with or without hallucinations. The delusions are most often persecutory, but grandiose delusions or delusions of bodily change, jealousy, disease or death may occur. Memory and consciousness are unaffected. Causes include:

* psychoactive substance use
    * amphetamine and related substances
    * cocaine
    * hallucinogens
* intracranial causes affecting the temporal lobe (e.g. tumours, epilepsy)
* Huntington's disease.

ORGANIC MOOD DISORDER

Organic mood disorder is a disorder characterized by a change in mood, usually accompanied by a change in the overall level of activity, caused by organic pathology. Table 25.2 gives the main causes of organic mood disorder.

Table 25.2   *Causes of organic mood disorder*

Psychoactive substance use	Amphetamine and related sympathomimetics Hallucinogens, e.g. LSD
Medication	Corticosteroids Levodopa Centrally acting antihypertensives – clonidine, methyldopa, reserpine and rauwolfia alkaloids Cycloserine Oestrogens – hormone replacement therapy, oral contraceptives Clomiphene
Endocrine disorders	Hypothyroidism, hyperthyroidism Addison's disease Cushing's syndrome Hypoglycaemia, diabetes mellitus Hyperparathyroidism Hypopituitarism
Other systemic disorders	Pernicious anaemia Hepatic failure Renal failure Rheumatoid arthritis Systemic lupus erythematosus Neoplasia, particularly carcinoma of the pancreas, carcinoid syndrome Viral infection, e.g. influenza, pneumonia, infections mononucleosis (glandular fever), hepatitis
Intracranial causes	Brain tumour Head injury Parkinson's disease Infections, e.g. neurosyphilis

Reproduced with permission from Puri, B.K., Laking, P.J. & Treasaden, I.H. 2002: *Textbook of Psychiatry*, 2nd edn. Edinburgh: Churchill Livingstone.

ORGANIC ANXIETY DISORDER

Organic anxiety disorder is characterized by the occurrence of the features of generalized anxiety disorder and/or panic disorder caused by organic pathology. Some of the symptoms of anxiety, which include tremor, paraesthesia, choking, palpitations, chest pain, dry mouth, nausea, abdominal pain, loose motions and increased frequency of micturition, are secondary to hyperventilation. Secondary cognitive impairment may occur. Table 25.3 shows the main causes of organic anxiety disorder; of these, it is particularly important to exclude hyperthyroidism, phaeochromocytoma and hypoglycaemia in clinical practice.

Table 25.3   *Causes of organic anxiety disorder*

Psychoactive substance use	Alcohol and drug withdrawal Amphetamine and related sympathomimetics Cannabis
Intoxication	Drugs – penicillin, sulphonamides Caffeine and caffeine withdrawal Poisons – aresenic, mercury, organophosphates, phosphorus, benzene Aspirin intolerance
Intracranial causes	Brain tumour Head injury Migraine Cerebrovascular disease Subarachnoid haemorrhage Infections – encephalitis, neurosyphilis Multiple sclerosis Hepatolenticular degeneration (Wilson's disease) Huntington's disease Epilepsy
Endocrine	Pituitary dysfunction Thyroid dysfunction Parathyroid dysfunction Adrenal dysfunction Phaeochromocytoma dysfunction Hypoglycaemia Virilization disorders of females
Inflammatory disorders	Systemic lupus erythematosus Rheumatoid arthritis Polyarteritis nodosa Temporal arteritis
Vitamin deficiency	Vitamin B_{12} deficiency Pellagra (nicotinic acid deficiency)
Other systemic disorders	Hypoxia Cardiovascular disease Cardiac arrhythmias Pulmonary insufficiency Anaemia Carcinoid syndrome Systemic neoplasia Febrile illnesses and chronic infections Porphyria Infectious mononucleosis (glandular fever) Posthepatic syndrome Uraemia Premenstrual syndrome

Based on Cummings, J. 1985: *Clinical Neuropsychiatry*. Orlando: Grune & Stratton.
Reproduced with permission from Puri, B.K., Laking, P.J. & Treasaden, I.H. 2002: *Textbook of Psychiatry*, 2nd edn. Edinburgh: Churchill Livingstone.

ORGANIC PERSONALITY DISORDER

In ICD-10, organic personality disorder is defined as being characterized by a significant alteration of the habitual patterns of behaviour displayed by the subject premorbidly. Such alteration always involves more profoundly the expression of emotions, needs and impulses. Cognition may be defective mostly or exclusively in the areas of planning one's own actions and anticipating their likely personal and social consequences. The causes of organic personality disorder include:

- intracranial (particularly affecting the frontal or temporal lobes)
  - head injury
  - tumours
  - abscesses
  - subarachnoid haemorrhage
  - neurosyphilis
  - epilepsy
- Huntington's disease
- hepatolenticular degeneration (Wilson's disease)
- medication (e.g. corticosteroids)
- psychoactive substance use
- endocrinopathies.

BIBLIOGRAPHY

Cummings, J. 1985: *Clinical Neuropsychiatry.* Orlando, FL: Grune & Stratton.

Lishman, W.A. 1997: *Organic Psychiatry: The Psychological Consequences of Cerebral Disorder,* 3rd edn. Oxford: Blackwell Scientific.

Marsden, C.D. & Fowler, T.J. 1989: *Clinical Neurology.* London: Edward Arnold.

Yudofsky, S.C. & Hales, R.E. (eds) 1992: *The American Psychiatric Press Textbook of Neuropsychiatry,* 2nd edn. Washington, DC: APP.

26

Psychoactive substance use disorders

CLASSIFICATION AND DEFINITIONS

ICD-10 classification of mental and behavioural disorders caused by psychoactive substance use

F10 *Mental and behavioural disorders caused by the use of* alcohol
F11 ... ... opioids
F12 ... ... cannabinoids
F13 ... ... sedatives or hypnotics
F14 ... ... cocaine
F15 ... ... stimulants, including caffeine
F16 ... ... hallucinogens
F17 ... ... tobacco
F18 ... ... volatile solvents
F19 ... ... multiple drug use and use of other psychoactive substances.

Specific clinical conditions are additionally coded as follows:

0   Acute intoxication
1   Harmful use
2   Dependence syndrome
3   Withdrawal state
4   Withdrawal state with delirium
5   Psychotic disorder
6   Amnesic syndrome
7   Residual and late-onset psychotic disorder
8   Other mental and behavioural disorders
9   Unspecified mental and behavioural disorder.

ACUTE INTOXICATION

This is a transient condition following the use of a psychoactive substance, resulting in disturbance of one or more of the following:

- consciousness level
- cognition
- perception
- affect
- behaviour.

Its intensity is closely related to dose, lessening with time, and the effects disappear when following cessation of the intake of the psychoactive substance. Recovery is usually complete.

Pathological intoxication applies only to alcohol, and refers to sudden aggressive behaviour, out of character, after drinking small amounts which would not produce intoxication in most people.

HARMFUL USE

This is use that is causing damage to physical or mental health. It does not refer to adverse social consequences.

DEPENDENCE SYNDROME

This is diagnosed if three or more of the following have been present together at some time in the previous year:

- compulsion to take the substance
- difficulties in controlling substance-taking behaviour: onset, termination or levels of use
- characteristic physiological withdrawal state when substance reduced or withdrawn; use of substance to avoid or relieve withdrawal symptoms
- increased tolerance, so larger doses are required to achieve effect originally produced by lower doses
- progressive neglect of other activities with increasing time spent in acquiring, taking or recovering from the effects of the substance
- persisting with substance use despite evidence of harmful consequences.

WITHDRAWAL STATE

Symptoms occur upon withdrawal or reduction of a substance after repeated, usually high dose, and prolonged use. Onset and course are time-limited, dose-related and differ according to the substance involved. Convulsions may complicate withdrawal.

WITHDRAWAL STATE WITH DELIRIUM

This is where the withdrawal state is complicated by delirium. Alcohol-induced *delirium tremens* is a short-lived, sometimes life-threatening toxic confusional state precipitated by relative or absolute alcohol withdrawal in severely dependent users. Classic symptoms include:

- clouding of consciousness
- hallucinations and illusions
- marked tremor.

It involves prodromal symptoms of:

- insomnia
- tremulousness
- fearful affect.

It is usually accompanied by

- delusions
- agitation
- insomnia
- autonomic over-activity.

In addition, convulsions may occur.

PSYCHOTIC DISORDER

Psychotic symptoms occur during or immediately after psychoactive substance use, in relatively clear sensorium (some clouding of consciousness but not severe confusion). It is not a manifestation of drug withdrawal or a functional psychosis. The characteristics of the psychosis vary according to the substance used, but the following are common:

- vivid hallucinations in more than one modality
- delusions
- psychomotor disturbances
- abnormal affect.

Stimulant-induced psychotic disorders are generally related to prolonged high-dose use. Typically it resolves at least partially within 1 month and fully within 6 months.

In ICD-10, further subdivisions may be specified:

- schizophrenia-like
- predominantly delusional
- predominantly hallucinatory (includes alcoholic hallucinosis)
- predominantly polymorphic
- predominantly depressive symptoms
- predominantly manic symptoms
- mixed.

AMNESIC SYNDROME

This is induced by alcohol or other psychoactive substances. Requirements for diagnosis include:

- chronic prominent impairment of recent memory; remote memory may be impaired; difficulty learning new material; disturbance of time sense
- immediate recall preserved; other cognitive functions are usually relatively preserved and consciousness is clear
- a history of chronic and usually high-dose use of alcohol or drugs.

Confabulation may be present, but not invariably so. Korsakov's psychosis is included here.

RESIDUAL AND LATE-ONSET PSYCHOTIC DISORDER

Alcohol- or psychoactive substance-induced changes of cognition, affect, personality or behaviour persist beyond the period during which the substance might reasonably be assumed to be operating. The onset is directly related to substance use.

Residual and late-onset psychotic disorder is further subdivided by ICD-10 into:

- flashbacks – episodic psychotic experiences which duplicate previous drug-related experiences and are usually very short-lived (seconds or minutes)
- personality or behaviour disorder
- organic mood disorder
- dementia – may be reversible after an extended period of abstinence
- other persisting cognitive impairment.

ALCOHOL

The concentration of alcohol in beverages is stated in terms of 'proof' scales. In the USA, one-degree (1°) proof is equal to a concentration of 0.5% by volume (v/v). In the UK, one-degree proof is equal to 0.5715% by volume (v/v).

One unit of alcohol is approximately 8–10 g of ethanol (C_2H_5OH), and is the amount contained in:

- a standard measure of spirits
- a standard glass of sherry or fortified wine
- a standard glass of table wine
- one half-pint of beer or lager of standard strength (3–3.5% by volume).

LEVELS OF CONSUMPTION

Up to 21 units of alcohol per week for men, and up to 14 units of alcohol per week for women, not consumed in one go and not consumed every day, are considered to be *low-risk levels* of intake. Women are more susceptible to the harmful effects of alcohol because their lower lean body mass results in higher blood alcohol levels per unit taken.

Consumption in greater amounts constitutes *excessive consumption*, carrying much greater risks of developing alcohol-related disability and alcohol dependence.

- *Increasing hazard* corresponds to an intake of alcohol of between 21 and 50 units per week for men, and between 14 and 35 units per week for women.
- *Dangerous levels* of alcohol consumption correspond to an alcohol intake of over 50 units per week for men, and over 35 units per week for women.

Abstinence or minimal alcohol intake is recommended in pregnancy, because of the risk of the development of fetal alcohol syndrome.

ALCOHOL-RELATED DISABILITIES

Excessive alcohol intake can lead to:

- physical morbidity
- psychiatric morbidity
- social morbidity.

Physical (medical) morbidity of alcohol consumption

Alcohol accounts for one-fifth to one-third of medical admissions to hospital.

Gastrointestinal disorders

These include:

- nausea and vomiting, particularly in the morning, prevented by drinking more alcohol
- gastritis
- peptic ulcers
- diarrhoea
- Mallory–Weiss tears
- oesophageal varices.

Malnutrition

This may result from:

- poor intake
- malabsorption
- impaired metabolism.

Results of malnutrition may include:

- thiamine deficiency presenting with Wernicke's encephalopathy acutely, leading in a high proportion of cases to Korsakov's psychosis (may also present with high output heart failure of beri-beri)
- niacin deficiency (vitamin B_3) presenting with pellagra, causing confusion, diarrhoea and light-sensitive rash
- vitamin C deficiency presenting with skin haemorrhages and gingivitis.

Liver

Hepatic damage is another important result of excessive alcohol intake. Fatty infiltration leading to an acute increase in the size of the liver occurs within a few days of excessive intake; it may cause pain in the right hypochondrium, nausea and vomiting, but is usually not detected. It is reversible with abstinence. Alcoholic hepatitis may occur secondary to long-term heavy daily drinking.

Liver cell necrosis and inflammation occurs, presenting with right hypochondrial pain and jaundice, sometimes accompanied by ascites and encephalopathy.

Cirrhosis with permanent fibrotic changes occurs. This may present with signs of liver failure, including:

- ascites
- encephalopathy
- bleeding oesophageal varices.

However, cirrhosis may be symptomless initially.

Pancreas

Acute and chronic pancreatitis lead to food malabsorption and diabetes in some cases.

Cardiovascular system

Cardiovascular system disorders include:

- hypertension, poorly responsive to conventional treatment but responsive to abstinence
- cardiac arrhythmias particularly after binge-drinking (holiday heart syndrome)
- cardiomyopathy, presenting with gradual onset of heart failure (the prognosis is poor with continued drinking)
- haemorrhagic and thrombotic CVA, even in the young.

Blood

Haematological changes may occur, since alcohol is a bone marrow toxin, resulting in the following:

- macrocytosis
- folate deficiency
- impaired clotting caused by vitamin K deficiency and/or reduced platelet functioning
- iron-deficiency anaemia, often as a result of gastrointestinal haemorrhage.

Endocrine and sexual disorders

Endocrine and sexual disorders can occur. There is gonadal atrophy which affects both sexes. Direct toxic effects upon the gonads result in reduced sex hormone synthesis. Liver disease results in oestrogenization in men resulting in gynaecomastia. Fertility may recover with abstinence. Autonomic nervous system dysfunction may result in erectile impotence and central effects cause anorgasmia. There is an increased risk of miscarriage and recurrent abortion in women.

Alcoholic pseudo-Cushing's syndrome may cause:

- obesity
- hirsuitism
- hypertension.

Neoplasms

There is an increased incidence of the following types of cancer:

- oropharygeal
- oesophageal
- colorectal
- pancreatic
- hepatic
- lung.

Pregnancy

Excessive alcohol consumption in pregnancy can lead to permanent fetal damage. Features of the resulting *fetal alcohol syndrome* include:

- low IQ (mean 70)
- cardiac abnormalities (e.g. atrial septal defect)
- low-set ears
- absent philtrum
- long upper lip with narrow vermilion border
- depressed bridge of the nose
- small nose
- ocular hypertelorism
- microcephaly
- strabismus
- pectus excavatum
- poor growth
- increased neonatal mortality.

Trauma

Accidents and trauma may result from alcohol consumption. These include:

- road accidents
- assaults (including head injuries)
- falls (including head injuries)
- drowning
- burns
- death by fire.

The most common traumatic injuries include:

- rib fractures
- head injuries
- subdural/extradural haematomata
- long-bone fractures.

Infections

There is an increased risk of infections such as tuberculosis and pneumonia, particularly in the homeless.

Metabolism

A variety of metabolic abnormalities may occur, including:

- alcohol-induced lactic acidosis
- alcoholic ketoacidosis
- hyperlipidemia in one-third of alcohol-dependent subjects (low levels of intake appear protective, however)
- hypoglycaemia
- hyperuricaemia
- haemochromatosis
- porphyria cutanea tarda.

Skin, muscle and skeleton

Dermatological disorders that may occur include acne and rhinophyma.
Musculoskeletal disorders that are associated with excessive drinking include:

- myopathy, presenting acutely with pain and tenderness of swollen muscles (usually symmetrical; if severe may cause renal failure due to myoglobinuria)
- proximal muscle weakness and wasting (common in alcoholics)
- osteoporosis
- avascular necrosis.

Nervous system

Neurological disorders that are associated with excessive drinking include:

- peripheral neuropathy resulting in numbness and paraesthesias in glove and stocking distribution
- cerebellar degeneration, affecting mainly the vermis, resulting in ataxia of gait
- convulsions occurring mainly secondary to alcohol withdrawal, within the first 48 hours (also secondary to brain damage or hypoglycaemia)
- optic atrophy
- central pontine myelinolysis.

Marchiafava–Bignami disease is a rare fatal demyelinating disease characterized neuropathologically by widespread demyelination affecting the central corpus callosum, and often also the middle cerebellar peduncles, the white matter of the cerebral hemispheres, and the optic tracts. It presents clinically with emotional disturbance and cognitive impairment followed by epilepsy, delirium, paralysis and coma.

Psychiatric morbidity of alcohol consumption

The major types of psychiatric morbidity that are associated with excessive alcohol intake are:

- mood disorders
- personality disorder
- alcoholic hallucinosis
- pathological jealousy
- neurotic disorders
- psychosexual disorders
- organic brain syndromes.

Each of these is now considered in turn.

Mood disorder

Chronic heavy drinking can itself produce severe, usually transient depressive symptoms, which generally improve with abstinence. If symptoms persist with abstinence, antidepressants should be considered. The suicide rate is at least 50 times greater in alcoholics than in the general population. Between one-quarter and one-third of completed suicides occur in alcoholics and up to four-fifths of those who kill themselves have been drinking.

Personality disorder

Those with sociopathic personality disorder engage in excessive drinking and those who drink heavily often engage in antisocial acts. If antisocial behaviour predates alcoholism by several years then the primary diagnosis is of personality disorder.

Cloninger (1987) described two types of alcoholic:

- *Type 1* (milieu-limited). This is the least severe, occurring in men and women, in dependent, anxious, rigid, less aggressive types, whose biological father or mother may have a mild adult-onset alcohol problem. It is thought that genetic predisposition and postnatal provocation are required to initiate this type of alcoholism.
- *Type 2*. This is severe and of early onset, occurring in men who are socially detached and confident, whose biological fathers (but not mothers) often have teenage-onset alcoholism and criminality. This type is thought by some to be alcoholism secondary to sociopathic personality disorder. Genetic predisposition has a powerful aetiological effect, with little contribution from the environment.

There does *not* appear to be a relationship between schizophrenia and alcoholism other than that occurring by chance. Genetic studies find that people suffering from alcoholism and schizophrenia have a predisposition to each condition separately.

Alcoholic hallucinosis

A rare disorder caused by chronic alcohol intake is alcoholic hallucinosis, characterized by auditory hallucinations in clear consciousness. It is distinguished from schizophrenia by the following features:

- association with alcohol abuse
- lack of family history
- onset at an older age (40 or 50 years)
- more acute presentation with resolution commonly within a month (if abstinent)
- absence of thought disorder
- more appropriate affect.

It may follow abstinence but can present or recur in those who are still drinking. If it persists for longer than 6 months the likely diagnosis is schizophrenia.

Pathological jealousy

Pathological jealousy is a well-recognized association with alcoholism, but may occur with other conditions such as schizophrenia and depression.

Neurotic disorders

Neurotic disorders may predispose to alcoholism in an attempt by the patient to self-medicate. Generalized anxiety, panic attacks and phobic disorders, particularly agoraphobia, may precede alcoholism. The patient should be reassessed once abstinent and any underlying condition should be appropriately managed.

Psychosexual disorders

Psychosexual disorders are a common association with excessive alcohol intake. In men, intoxication leads to erectile impotence and delayed ejaculation. Chronic heavy drinking in men can cause:

- loss of libido
- reduction in the size of the testes
- reduction in the size of the penis
- loss of body hair
- gynaecomastia.

In women, chronic heavy drinking can cause:

- menstrual cycle abnormalities
- loss of breast tissue
- vaginal dryness.

Organic brain syndromes

Organic brain syndromes that are associated with excessive alcohol intake may be considered under the headings of:

- acute/subacute syndromes:
  - alcoholic blackouts
  - delirium tremens
  - withdrawal fits
  - Wernicke's encephalopathy
- chronic syndromes:
  - Korsakov's syndrome
  - alcoholic dementia.

Each of these is now described.

ORGANIC BRAIN SYNDROMES

Alcoholic blackouts

Intoxication frequently leads to episodes of short-term amnesia or blackouts. These may occur after just one bout of heavy drinking, and are estimated to have been experienced by 15–20% of those who drink.

Three types of blackout are recognized, which, in order of increasing severity, are as follows:

1 *State-dependent memory loss.* Memory for events occurring while intoxicated are lost when sober, but return when next intoxicated.
2 *Fragmentary blackouts.* There is no clear demarcation of memory loss, and islets of memory exist within the gap. Some recovery occurs with time.
3 *En bloc blackouts.* There is a clearly demarcated total memory loss, with no recovery of this lost memory over time. If this memory loss extends for days the subject experiences a fugue-like state in which he or she may travel some distance before coming around, with no memory of the events occurring during this time.

Delirium tremens

In chronic heavy drinkers a fall in the blood alcohol concentration leads to withdrawal symptoms including delirium tremens. The peak onset is within two days of abstinence and it usually lasts for about five days. There is a prodromal period with:

- anxiety
- insomnia
- tachycardia
- tremor
- sweating.

The onset of delirium is marked by:

- disorientation
- fluctuating level of consciousness
- intensely fearful affect
- hallucinations
- misperceptions
- tremor
- restlessness
- autonomic over-activity.

The hallucinations are often visual and are commonly Lilliputian in nature. Auditory and tactile hallucinations, and secondary delusions, may also be present. There is a mortality rate of about 5%, associated with cardiovascular collapse or infection. The treatment of delirium tremens is supportive with sedation, fluid and electrolyte replacement, high-potency vitamins (especially thiamine to prevent an unrecognized Wernicke's encephalopathy progressing to Korsakov's psychosis – see below).

Withdrawal fits

Withdrawal fits may take place within 48 hours of stopping drinking.

Wernicke's encephalopathy

Wernicke's encephalopathy is caused by severe deficiency of thiamine (vitamin B_1), which is usually caused by alcohol abuse in Western countries. Other causes include:

- lesions of the stomach (e.g. carcinoma) causing malabsorption
- lesions of the duodenum causing malabsorption
- lesions of the jejunum causing malabsorption
- hyperemesis
- starvation.

Important clinical features of Wernicke's encephalopathy include:

- ophthalmoplegia
- nystagmus
- ataxia
- clouding of consciousness.

Peripheral neuropathy may also be present.

Wernicke's encephalopathy and Korsakov's psychosis (see below) have overlapping pathology and the former may culminate in the latter if untreated. Wernicke's encephalopathy is a medical emergency and should be treated with intravenous thiamine plus other B vitamins. Post-mortem examination of the brains of those dying of Wernicke's encephalopathy reveal petechial haemorrhages in the:

- mammillary bodies
- walls of the third ventricle (less commonly than in the mammillary bodies)
- periaqueductal grey matter (less commonly than in the mammillary bodies)
- floor of the fourth ventricle (less commonly than in the mammillary bodies)
- inferior colliculi (less commonly than in the mammillary bodies).

Nicotinic acid depletion can sometimes give rise to pellagra encephalopathy, a confusional state resembling Wernicke's encephalopathy.

Korsakov's syndrome

Korsakov's syndrome is an alcohol-induced amnesic syndrome that, as mentioned above, is frequently preceded by Wernicke's encephalopathy. It has been described as being 'an abnormal state in which memory and learning are affected out of all proportion to other cognitive functions in an otherwise alert and responsive patient' (Victor *et al.*, 1971). Clinical features include:

- retrograde amnesia
- anterograde amnesia
- sparing of immediate recall
- disorientation in time
- inability to recall the temporal sequence of events
- confabulation
- peripheral neuropathy.

Neuropathologically there is scarring and atrophy of the mammillary bodies and anterior thalamus, with substantial frontal lobe dysfunction on neuroimaging. Improvement may occur with abstinence and high-dose thiamine and replacement of other B vitamins, which should be continued for 6 months.

Alcoholic dementia

Those who have abused alcohol for some years commonly suffer mild to moderate cognitive impairment, which may improve over a number of years of abstinence. Women, who are known to suffer physical complications of alcohol abuse earlier than men, also develop cognitive impairment earlier in their drinking histories. A CT or structural MRI scan of the brain in alcoholics commonly shows ventricular enlargement and sulcal widening, which does not correlate with the degree of cognitive impairment and largely reverses with abstinence.

Chronic alcoholics show a coarsening of personality which appears to be related to frontal lobe atrophy.

Social morbidity of alcohol consumption

Heavy drinking is often associated with gambling and the use of other psychoactive substances. The social costs of excessive alcohol consumption are high. They include:

- family breakdown
- crime
- accidents and trauma
- economic harm.

One-third of problem drinkers cite marital discord as one of their problems; one-third of divorce petitions cite alcohol as a contributory factor; three-quarters of battered wives describe their husbands as frequently drunk or subject to heavy drinking. Children of alcoholics often suffer neglect, poverty or physical violence.

Alcohol misuse is strongly associated with crime, particularly against the person and against property. Half of those committing homicide have been drinking at the time of the offence, and half of victims are intoxicated. Half of rapists were drinking at the time of the offence. One- to two-thirds of burglaries are committed under the influence of alcohol.

In 1978, 31% of vehicle drivers and 29% of motorcyclists killed in accidents in the UK had blood alcohol levels above the legal limit of 80 mg per 100 mL, as did 30% of passengers and 21% of pedestrians. It is estimated that 1200 deaths each year, representing one-fifth of all deaths on the roads, result from drink-driving. Alcohol is implicated in one-third of accidents at home and deaths by drowning, and 40% of deaths by fire and falling.

Major costs to the country associated with the use of alcohol are incurred through:

- lost productivity and unemployment
- damage
- medical costs
- legal costs
- social costs.

Alcohol dependence

Edwards and Gross (1976) described the alcohol-dependence syndrome which was later also applied to other psychoactive substances:

1 *Increased tolerance.* Repeated doses of the drug produce less effect, resulting in escalating doses to achieve the original effect. The rate at which tolerance develops varies with the substance used: it is generally rapid with heroin, but much slower with alcohol.
2 *Repeated withdrawal symptoms.* A fall in blood alcohol concentration leads to unpleasant withdrawal symptoms within 12 hours of the last intake, relieved by drinking more alcohol.
3 *Subjective awareness of a compulsion to drink.* Attempted abstinence leads to tension and an increased craving for alcohol.

4   *Salience of drink-seeking behaviour.* Acquiring and drinking alcohol take primacy over other
     activities such as family, career and social position.
5   *Relief or avoidance of withdrawal symptoms.* This is achieved by further drinking.
6   *Narrowing of the drinking repertoire.* The pattern of drinking becomes increasingly stereotyped
     with increasing dependence. A daily routine develops and a certain drink will be favoured over
     others.
7   *Rapid reinstatement following abstinence.* After a period of abstinence the drinker may attempt to
     drink in moderation. The intake is likely to escalate rapidly as tolerance and dependence
     reappear within a few days.

Epidemiology of alcohol consumption

There is a close association between liver cirrhosis mortality and the national consumption of
alcohol. Mortality figures are a useful index of national alcohol consumption. Other indices
include the number of arrests for drunkenness, drunken driving, cases of assault and battery, and
deaths from alcohol poisoning. Ten per cent of the drinking population drinks half of all the alcohol drunk.

Price greatly affects levels of drinking. Countries with cheap alcohol consume more than
countries with more expensive alcohol. As the prices of alcoholic beverages rise, the quantity drunk
by even chronic dependent drinkers falls, and the amount of alcohol-related morbidity falls.

It is estimated that of the 55 million UK population, 36 million are regular drinkers; 2 million are
heavy drinkers (> 80 g alcohol daily for men, and > 40 g for women); 700 000 are problem drinkers
and 200 000 are dependent drinkers.

Men outnumber women, but the sex ratio of alcohol-related problems is falling. About fifteen
years ago, alcoholic cirrhosis was five times as common in men as in women, but the sex ratio has
fallen to about 2:1.

The age of first drinking has fallen to between 12 and 14 years in both sexes. The highest rates of
heavy drinking are seen between adolescence and the early twenties.

Certain occupational groups are at greater risk of drinking problems. Those with jobs in the
drink industry are at highest risk, including publicans, bartenders and brewers. Those whose jobs
take them away from home, such as fishermen, armed service personnel and executives, and those
with professional autonomy, such as doctors, are also at higher risk.

Aetiology of alcohol consumption

GENETIC FACTORS

There is good evidence that heavy drinking runs in families. The relatives of alcoholics have higher
rates of alcoholism than the relatives of controls.

Twin studies indicate that monozygotic twins have a higher concordance rate than dizygotic
twins. In normal twins, approximately one-third of the variance in drinking habits has been
estimated to be genetic in origin.

Adoption studies support the hypothesis of the genetic transmission of alcoholism. The sons of
alcoholic parents are three to four times more likely to become alcoholic than the sons of non-
alcoholics, irrespective of the home environment.

Strains of rats have been bred which voluntarily consume large quantities of alcohol. These rats
appear to have abnormalities in brain levels of serotonin, noradrenaline and dopamine.

PERSONALITY FACTORS

It has been suggested that some problem drinkers are predisposed to harmful drinking by their personality; however, studies in this area give contradictory results. It is known that those with sociopathic personality disorder have a high prevalence of heavy drinking and alcoholism. However, there is no typical pre-alcoholic personality.

BIOLOGICAL FACTORS

The EEG of sober, awake alcoholics shows an excess of fast activity and a deficiency of α, θ and δ activity. The sons of alcoholics also show an excess of fast activity when compared to controls, leading to speculation that this may be a specific marker for alcoholism.

Electrically evoked responses show reduced P3 voltage in both abstinent chronic alcoholics and in the young sons of alcoholics when compared to controls.

The metabolism of alcohol is genetically determined and varies between individuals. Over half of Orientals develop an unpleasant flushing response when alcohol is ingested, related to the accumulation of acetaldehyde, caused by the absence of the isoenzyme ALDH2: aldehyde dehydrogenase. It is thought that this intolerance of alcohol protects them from developing alcoholism, since it is much less prevalent in those of oriental heritage.

Ethanol at low concentrations (5–10 mmol/L) inhibits the action of NMDA-glutamate controlled ion channels, and potentiates the actions of GABA type A controlled ion channels. These are the main excitatory and inhibitory systems of the brain; the overall effect of ethanol is therefore as a central nervous depressant.

At slightly higher ethanol concentrations the actions of voltage-sensitive calcium channels and channels controlled by serotonin are affected.

Ethanol promotes the CNS release of dopamine particularly from the nucleus accumbens.

Chronic administration of ethanol produces alterations in the GABA, NMDA and voltage-sensitive calcium channel systems. Reduction in the production of subunits of the GABA receptors are seen particularly in mice prone to withdrawal convulsions. Chronic ethanol administration also causes an up-regulation of NMDA receptors in mouse hippocampus, more evident in mice prone to withdrawal convulsions. Both of these receptor changes promote CNS excitability and increase the likelihood of convulsions.

Excessive glutamate stimulation is toxic to the nerve cell and results in damage or cell death. Although ethanol exposure is the cause of increased numbers of NMDA receptors, its presence protects against the neurotoxicity of glutamate over-stimulation. The acute withdrawal of ethanol in the dependent subject results in convulsions and neurotoxicity.

PSYCHOLOGICAL FACTORS

There are three main components to psychological theories of dependence:

- *Withdrawal avoidance.* Prolonged drug use results in tolerance, with CNS adaptation to allow normal functioning despite the chronic presence of the psychoactive drug. If the drug is suddenly withdrawn, this adaptation results in drug-withdrawal symptoms, which are usually opposite to the effects of the drug. Thus in terms of this theory the dependent person continues drug use in order to avoid the adverse effects of drug withdrawal.
- *Positive effects of the drug.* According to this theory, the pleasant effects of the drug reinforce drug-taking behaviour, despite adverse social and physical consequences.
- *Motivational distortion.* According to this theory, the repetition of drug-taking behaviour, or the effects of the drugs themselves, change the motivational system supporting that behaviour.

Habit strength is a term describing the strength of the link between a stimulus that cues a behaviour. It is possible that it involves habituation at the neuronal level.

Each of these theories accounts for some but not all aspects of addiction.

CULTURAL FACTORS

There are high rates of alcoholism in countries where alcohol is drunk routinely with family meals, and in places where it is cheap.

PSYCHIATRIC ILLNESS

This can predispose patients to harmful drinking, particularly anxiety disorders, phobic disorders, depression and bereavement and mania.

Management of alcohol over-consumption

History taking
For screening purposes the CAGE questionnaire is widely used. Positive answers to two or more of the four questions is indicative of problem drinking. The CAGE questionnaire is:

- Have you ever felt you should **c**ut down on your drinking?
- Have people ever **a**nnoyed you by criticizing your drinking?
- Have you ever felt **g**uilty about your drinking?
- Have you ever had a drink first thing in the morning to steady your nerves or get over a hangover? (an **e**ye-opener)

The alcohol consumption history should include the average number of units of alcohol consumed weekly, and the drinking pattern. It should also include: information about the evolution of the problem (drinking career, drink-related problems, dependence); typical recent drinking day (initial, then hourly quantification of alcohol intake, waking nausea, tremor, nightmares and night sweats); and an interview with the spouse or partner.

When alcohol dependence is suspected or diagnosed, it is essential to carry out a full physical examination bearing in mind the multiple organ systems damaged by this substance.

Investigations
Blood investigations include alcohol levels in the intoxicated (breathalyzers can be useful to give an indication of levels of recent drinking). Alcoholism is the most common cause of raised mean corpuscular volume (MCV), and it is raised in 60% of alcohol abusers. Since the life of a red blood cell is 120 days, the MCV should return to normal 4 months after continued abstinence. Raised γ-glutamyl transferase may occur; this is good for screening as an indication of recent alcohol use, but it can be raised after only one heavy drinking session. Liver function tests (e.g. aspartate transaminase) may be abnormal, particularly during acute alcoholic hepatitis, less so in fatty liver, and may be normal in cirrhosis.

Treatment
Detoxification can usually be conducted as an outpatient unless severe withdrawal effects such as delirium tremens or convulsions are likely to occur; the patient's mental state causes concern; or there are severe social problems, in which case inpatient care should be organized. The aim should be for abstinence; education, support and counselling will be required.

After the assessment of the severity of withdrawal symptoms, a substitute sedative is started. Benzodiazepines such as diazepam or chlordiazepoxide are commonly used in a reducing regimen. Ethanol withdrawal increases glutamate in the brain which damages neurones. Repeated withdrawal causes increased neuronal death. Valium withdrawal is not neuroprotective. However, acamprosate blocks increased glutamate in withdrawal and is neuroprotective. Acamprosate should be started with detoxification if it is intended for use afterwards. Attention should be paid to the state of hydration and nutrition of the patient. Thiamine should always be given. If malabsorption is likely, intravenous thiamine and other B vitamins should be given in the first instance. A glucose load should be avoided as this can precipitate or exacerbate thiamine deficiency; ascorbic acid may also be required. The suicide risk should be assessed.

Alcoholics Anonymous is a self-help group which some alcoholics find helpful. Al-Anon supports the families of alcoholics, and Al-Ateen the teenage children of alcoholics.

Supportive therapy is helpful. Other forms of psychotherapy are also useful. Cognitive–behavioural models appear to be particularly effective in relapse prevention. Such therapies include cue exposure, relapse prevention strategies, contingency management, social skills and assertiveness training.

Medication can be used in the detoxified alcoholic to help maintain abstinence.

Aversive agents, disulfiram (Antabuse) and citrated calcium carbimide, both inhibit aldehyde dehydrogenase leading to the accumulation of aldehyde if alcohol is ingested. The patient experiences very unpleasant symptoms of flushing, headache, palpitations, tachycardia, nausea and vomiting with ingestion of small amounts of alcohol, and air hunger, arrhythmias and severe hypotension with large amounts of alcohol. These agents are contraindicated in ischaemic heart disease, in pregnancy or if there is a history of convulsions. Patients must be well motivated and aware of the risks of taking alcohol with these agents. Efficacy requires compliance with taking the aversive agent; involving the spouse or partner in administration can improve the success rate.

Acamprosate, in combination with counselling, may also be helpful in maintaining abstinence. It should be initiated as soon as is possible after the achievement of abstinence. It should be maintained if a relapse occurs. Acamprosate is contraindicated in cases in which there is renal or hepatic impairment, noradrenaline and also during pregnancy and lactation. Side-effects of this drug include diarrhoea, nausea, vomiting, abdominal pain and pruritus.

Prognosis

Good prognostic factors include:

- good insight
- strong motivation
- good social and family support.

Relapse can be precipitated by:

- emotional stress
- interpersonal conflict
- social pressures.

Long-term follow-up of alcoholics over a period of 10 years finds that:

- 25% continue troubled drinking
- 12% are abstinent.

The remainder follow a pattern of intermittent troubled drinking and abstinence.

NON-ALCOHOLIC PSYCHOACTIVE SUBSTANCES: LEGAL ASPECTS IN THE UNITED KINGDOM

NOTE

Colloquial names for some abused drugs are given in Table 26.1.

Table 26.1   *Colloquial names for some abused drugs*

Drug	Colloquial name
Heroin	Smack
Cannabinoids	Grass, hash, ganja, pot
Temazepam capsules	Jellies
Barbiturates	Downers
Cocaine	Snow, coke, girl, lady
Amphetamines	Speed, whizz
LSD	Acid
PCP	Angel dust, peace pill
MDMA	Ecstacy, XTC, Adam, E

MISUSE OF DRUGS ACT 1971

This Act specifies the classes of controlled drugs according to perceived dangerousness:

- *Class A.* This includes most opiates (heroin, morphine, opium, pethidine, methadone), cocaine, and hallucinogens and psychotomimetics (LSD, mescaline, PCP).
- *Class B.* This includes cannabis, codeine, amphetamines and barbiturates. Injectable preparations of class B drugs are designated as class A.
- *Class C.* This includes certain drugs related to the amphetamines such as benzfetamine and chlorphentermine, buprenorphine, diethylpropion, mazindol, meprobamate, pemoline, pipradrol, most benzodiazepines, zolpidem, androgenic and anabolic steroids, clenbuterol, chorionic gonadotrophin (HCG), non-human chorionic gonadotrophin, somatotropin, somatrem and somatropin.

The penalties for drug use and supply are related to these classes.

HOME OFFICE NOTIFICATION

The Misuse of Drugs (Notification of and Supply to Addicts) Regulations 1973 required any doctor to notify the Chief Medical Officer at the Home Office in writing within 7 days of attending to a patient who is considered or suspected (on reasonable grounds) to be addicted to any of the following controlled drugs:

cocaine
dextromoramide (Palfium)
diamorphine (heroin)
dipipanone (Diconal)
hydrocodone
hydromorphone
levorphanol

methadone
morphine
opium
oxycodone
pethidine
phenazocine
piritramide.

Notifications were compiled in the Addicts Index, which provided epidemiological information for use in the planning of services. A doctor could also contact the Index by telephone to check whether a presenting patient was currently known to another service. It thus acted as a safeguard against multiple scripting.

From 1 May 1997, the Addicts Index was closed and the statutory duty for doctors to notify details of addicts to the Addicts Index was removed.

MISUSE OF DRUGS REGULATIONS 2001

These regulations divide drugs into the following five schedules which specify the requirements that govern such issues as their supply, possession, prescription and record-keeping:

- *Schedule 1* includes drugs such as cannabis and lysergide which are not used medicinally. Possession and supply are prohibited except in accordance with the authority of the Home Office.
- *Schedule 2* includes drugs such as diamorphine (heroin), morphine, remifentanil, pethidine, secobarbital, glutethimide, amfetamine and cocaine, and are subject to the full controlled drug requirements relating to prescriptions, safe custody (except for secobarbital), the need to keep registers, etc. (unless exempted in schedule 5).
- *Schedule 3* includes the barbiturates (except secobarbital, which is in schedule 2), buprenorphine, diethylpropion, flunitrazepam, mazindol, meprobamate, pentazocine, phentermine and temazepam. They are subject to the special prescription requirements (except for phenobarbital and temazepam) but not to the safe custody requirements (except for buprenorphine, diethylpropion, flunitrazepam and temazepam) nor to the need to keep registers (although there are requirements for the retention of invoices for two years).
- *Schedule 4* includes, in Part I, benzodiazepines (except flunitrazepam and temazepam which are in schedule 3) and zolpidem, which are subject to minimal control. Part II includes androgenic and anabolic steroids, clenbuterol, chorionic gonadotrophin (HCG), non-human chorionic gonadotrophin, somatotropin, somatrem and somatropin. Controlled drug prescription requirements do not apply, and schedule 4 controlled drugs are not subject to safe custody requirements.
- *Schedule 5* includes those preparations which, because of their strength, are exempt from virtually all controlled drug requirements other than retention of invoices for two years.

MISUSE OF DRUGS ACT 1971 (MODIFICATION) ORDER 2003 AND MISUSE OF DRUGS REGULATIONS 2003

Changes were made to the legislation on the misuse of drugs by these regulations, which came into force on 1 July 2003. The following eight substances were brought under the control of the Misuse of Drugs Act 1971 and its associated subordinate legislation for the first time:

remifentanil	4-androstene-3, 17-dione
dihydroetorphine	19-nor-4-androstene-3, 17-dione
gamma-hydroxy-butyrate	5-androstene-3, 17-diol
zolpidem	19-nor-5-androstene-3, 17- diol.

Remifentanil and dihydroetorphine are controlled as class A drugs. Both are powerful opiates and have similar pharmacological properties to existing class A drugs. Both are listed under Schedule 2 of the Misuse of Drugs Regulations 2001.

4-hydroxy-*n*-butyric acid or gamma-hydroxy-butyrate (GHB) and zolpidem are controlled as class C drugs. Both are listed under Schedule 4 (Part I) of the 2001 Regulations. GHB has been used as an anaesthetic and to treat alcohol and drug dependence but has also been misused by clubbers. Zolpidem is a prescription medicine (a non-benzodiazepine hypnotic with a short duration of action) and acts in a similar same way as some sedatives such as benzodiazepines.

The following four anabolic substances are listed in Schedule 4 (Part II) of the 2001 Regulations:

4-androstene-3, 17-dione

5-androstene-3, 17-diol

19-nor-4-androstene-3, 17-dione

19-nor-5-androstene-3, 17- diol.

They are now controlled as class C drugs.

According to the Home Office, there is some evidence to suggest that some of the above eight substances have been produced in clandestine laboratories for the illicit drugs market in the last few years, and there have been a few police seizures of some of these substances in the UK.

Note that Schedule 2 drugs are subject to the additional prescription requirements of Regulation 15 (see below; amongst other things, prescriptions must be handwritten by doctors). Regulations 14 (documentation), 16 (supply on prescription), 18 (marking of containers), 19, 20, 21, 23 (keeping and preservation of registers), 26 (furnishing of information) and 27 (destruction) also apply to Schedule 2 drugs. Most Schedule 2 drugs are also subject to the statutory safe custody requirements.

Schedule 4 (*Part I*) includes benzodiazepines (e.g. diazepam, lorazepam and nitrazepam). Gamma-hydroxy-butyrate (GHB) and zolpidem have been added to the list of drugs in Schedule 4 (Part I). Persons already authorized by the Regulations (e.g. doctors and pharmacists), or by a written Home Office authority to produce, supply or possess Schedule 4 (Part I) drugs, are automatically so authorized in respect of GHB and zolpidem. In other cases an appropriate written Home Office authority is required. The Regulation 15 prescription requirements (including handwriting) do not apply to Schedule 4 (Part I) drugs. Regulations 22, 23 (keeping and preservation of records), 26 (furnishing of information) and 27 (destruction – holders of written authorities to produce only) also apply to Schedule 4 (Part I) drugs. Schedule 4 (Part I) drugs are not subject to the safe custody requirements.

Schedule 4 (*Part II*) now comprises 54 anabolic substances; examples are nandrolone and testosterone (and the four newly added anabolic substances: 4-androstene-3, 17-dione; 19-nor-4-androstene-3, 17-dione; 5-androstene-3, 17-diol; and 19-nor-5-androstene-3, 17-diol). Persons already authorized by the 2001 Regulations (e.g. doctors and pharmacists) or by a written Home Office authority to produce, supply or possess Schedule 4 (Part II) drugs are authorized in respect of the four newly added drugs; in other cases an appropriate written Home Office authority is required. (Note that *possession* licences are not required if the substances are in medicinal product form.) The Regulation 15 prescription requirements (including handwriting) do not apply to Schedule 4 (Part II drugs). Regulations 22, 23 (keeping and preservation of records), 26 (furnishing of information) and 27 (destruction – holders of written authorities to produce only) also apply to Schedule 4 Part II drugs. Schedule 4 Part II drugs are not subject to the statutory safe custody requirements.

PRESCRIBING CONTROLLED DRUGS

The main regulations relating to prescriptions for controlled drugs specified in Schedules 2 and 3, under the Misuse of Drugs Regulations 2001, are as follows.

Prescriptions ordering controlled drugs subject to prescription requirements must be *signed* and *dated* by the prescriber and specify the *prescriber's address*. The prescription must always state *in the prescriber's own handwriting* in ink or otherwise so as to be indelible:

- the name and address of the patient
- in the case of a preparation, the form and where appropriate the strength of the preparation
- the total quantity of the preparation, or the number of dose units, *in both words and figures*

- the dose
- the words 'for dental treatment only' if issued by a dentist.

A prescription may order a controlled drug to be dispensed by instalments. If so, the amount of the instalments and the intervals to be observed must be specified. Prescriptions ordering 'repeats' on the same form are not permitted. A prescription is valid for 13 weeks from the date stated thereon.

It is an offence for a prescriber to issue an incomplete prescription, and a pharmacist is not allowed to dispense a controlled drug unless all the information required by law is given on the prescription.

OPIOIDS

Note: Drugs derived from opium poppies are known as *opiates*. Synthetically derived opiates are known as *opioids*.

Heroin (gear, smack, scag ...)

Heroin (3,6-diacetylmorphine) is produced from morphine which is derived from the sap of the opium poppy. It may be smoked or chased by heating on tin foil and inhaling the sublimate. It is also injected intravenously, and much less commonly subcutaneously (skin-popping). Street heroin is usually 30–60% pure, and 0.25–0.75 g is a common daily consumption for addicts.

EPIDEMIOLOGY

The number of addicts notified to the Home Office has increased dramatically over the last 30 years. This is thought to be related to the wider availability of cheap opiates imported from the Middle East. Youth culture has become much more accepting of drug use, and poly-drug use is much more common than it used to be. The approximate numbers of notifications have been:

1960   500
1980   5000
1990   15 000

Most heroin users are aged between 20 and 30 years. The steepest increase has occurred in those aged 16–24 years. The male:female ratio is 2:1.

DRUG ACTION

The stimulation of opiate receptors produces analgesia, euphoria, miosis, hypotension, bradycardia and respiratory depression.

Opioid receptors fall into different types, each of which has subtypes. The main types are μ, κ and δ receptors. The effects of a particular opiate drug depend upon the combination of receptors stimulated. Most of the effects of morphine are mediated through μ receptors.

Euphoria is initially intense and is related in part to the method of administration. Thus methods delivering a large bolus quickly to the CNS are associated with a greater initial rush. Intravenous and inhalational techniques fulfil these conditions, oral and subcutaneous methods do not.

Dependence may arise within weeks of regular use.

EFFECTS OF DRUG WITHDRAWAL

These begin within 4–12 hours of last heroin use. Peak intensity is at about 48 hours, and the main symptoms disappear within a week of abstinence. Physical symptoms include intense dysphoria, aching limbs, nausea, diarrhoea, dilated pupils, shivering, sweating, yawning, sneezing, rhinorrhoea, lacrimation, fatigue, insomnia, and craving for the drug which may continue for weeks. Although it is unpleasant, opiate withdrawal is not generally dangerous (exceptions include pregnancy, when abortion may result from precipitous withdrawal).

HARMFUL EFFECTS

Effects of the drug itself

Overdose can be caused by the uncertain concentration of street drugs, or to reduced tolerance following a period of abstinence (e.g. upon release from prison). The clinical features of opiate overdose include stupor or coma, pinpoint pupils, pallor, severe respiratory depression, and pulmonary oedema. Supportive treatment and administration of an opioid antagonist such as nalaxone is indicated. The half-life of opioid antagonists is less than that of most opiate drugs, so the patient must be observed for several hours to ensure that the underlying opiate overdose has passed.

Intoxication

These include accidents.

Inhalation

The inhalation of heroin commonly exacerbates or causes lung conditions such as asthma. There are increased rates of pneumonia and tuberculosis in those who are HIV-positive.

Intravenous use

The hazards of intravenous use are many, and include the transmission of infection through the use of shared needles. HIV and hepatitis B, C and D are commonly transmitted through this route. Those who are HIV-positive have a poorer outcome if they continue to inject.

Bacterial infection

Bacterial infection results from the lack of aseptic technique; the risk is not eliminated by using clean needles since the drug itself is not of pharmaceutical quality, has often been adulterated with other substances, and is often not suitable for intravenous administration because of the presence of non-soluble components.

Skin infection

Skin infection at injection sites leads to abscess formation, and thrombophlebitis. *Staphylococcus aureus* and *Streptococcus pyogenes* are often responsible.

Blood infection

Most injecting results in transient bacteraemia. This can result in septicaemia and/or bacterial endocarditis, even in those with previously normal heart valves. Septic emboli may be carried to distant sites. Septic embolism can result in osteomyelitis.

Fungal infection

Systemic fungal infections have been reported which are difficult to treat and result in death or blindness because of ophthalmic involvement.

Vascular complications

Vascular complications include the obliteration of the lung vascular bed with continued prolonged injection of particulate matter. The same effect is seen in the lymphatic system, resulting in puffy hands. Deep vein thrombosis may develop at the site of femoral administration. Arterial administration can result in occlusion caused by spasm or embolism. The loss of a limb may result.

Long-term physical effects

Long-term users may develop membranous glomerulonephritis or amyloid disease.

Social effects

Because of the effects of tolerance and dependence, heroin users usually escalate the dose of drug taken in an attempt to continue to achieve the euphoriant effects and to keep the unpleasant withdrawal effects of the drug at bay. The result is often that the addict turns to acquisitive crime in order to fund the growing drug habit. It is estimated that the stabilization of heroin addicts on to methadone costs the NHS over £1000 per year per addict, but that this saves society over £30 000 per addict in drug-related crime. Relationships and family commitments usually come second to drug-related activities, and family breakdown often results. It is difficult to continue in employment when seriously addicted to heroin.

Methadone (Physeptone)

Methadone is a synthetic opiate (opioid) which can be taken orally or intravenously. Its half-life is longer than that of heroin (16–24 hours), allowing once-daily oral prescribing. It has little euphoric effect when administered orally, but has some street value, particularly in injectable form. It is frequently prescribed in the management of opiate dependence. In this case the elixir is the preferred preparation as it is less likely to be abused. Tablet form and sugar-free elixir should not be used routinely as both are more likely to be injected.

Dipipanone (Diconal)

Diconal consists of a combination of the opiate analgesic dipipanone and cyclizine. Intravenous use produces intense euphoria, but there is a danger of CVA, arterial spasm and gangrene if injected into an artery.

Codeine

Misuse of codeine preparations is common. Preparations include DF118 (dihydrocodeine 30 mg) and codeine linctus (codeine phosphate 15 mg/5 mL).

Management of opiate/opioid dependence

AIMS

The aims of management are to:

- help the person to deal with drug-related problems
- reduce damage occurring during drug use

- reduce duration of episodes of drug use
- reduce the chance of relapse
- help the person to remain healthy until he or she manages to attain a drug-free state.

HISTORY AND EXAMINATION

Before any treatment is initiated it is essential to establish that the person is in fact drug-dependent. A history of drug use, past and current, an account of withdrawal symptoms experienced upon cessation of the drug, a social history including sources of support, accommodation and employment, the funding of the drug habit, and a medical and psychiatric history are all considered necessary.

Physical examination should seek signs of current drug use and of complications related to the route of administration. It is essential to test urine for a drug screen, to establish that on two separate occasions the person was taking the drugs claimed. Most drugs will show up on urine screens for at least 24 hours after ingestion.

Once it is established that the person is opiate-dependent, it is necessary to assess his or her motivation for treatment, and to reach an agreement about the aims of treatment.

The Home Office should be notified. The person should be informed that there is a legal obligation upon the doctor to do this, but that the information will not be made available to the police.

Patients should receive information about harm minimization, and HIV and hepatitis testing should be arranged after counselling and with the person's consent.

The ultimate aim of treatment is to achieve opiate abstinence. However, this is unacceptable to some patients, in which case the aim is to minimize the harm associated with opiate abuse (harm minimization).

HARM MINIMIZATION

The aims are to stop or reduce the use of contaminated injecting equipment, to prevent the sharing of injecting equipment, to stop or reduce drug use, to stop or reduce unsafe sexual practices, to encourage health consciousness and a more stable lifestyle, and to establish and retain contact with the drug services.

To achieve these aims, education about the potential hazards is important. Sterile injecting equipment and condoms should be provided, non-immune individuals should be offered hepatitis B vaccination, and substitute oral opiates such as methadone should be prescribed.

SUBSTITUTE PRESCRIBING

Non-opiate substitutes

If dependence is not severe, reassurance, support and symptomatic treatment with non-opiate drugs may suffice. The following may be used:

- *clonidine* – an α-adrenergic antagonist that can give some symptomatic relief in opiate withdrawal (hypotension can be a problem)
- *lofexidine* – which acts centrally to reduce sympathetic tone (reduction in blood pressure is less marked than that produced by clonidine)
- *propranolol* – for somatic anxiety
- *thioridazine* – relieves anxiety in low doses
- *promethazine* – a sedative antihistamine effective for mild withdrawal
- *benzodiazepines* – for anxiety (do not give for longer than 2 weeks).

Substitute opioids

Oral methadone mixture 1 mg/mL is the usual choice. Any doctor can prescribe methadone to a drug misuser. Daily dispensing reduces the risk of overdose and abuse.

- For maintenance, a substitute opiate is prescribed indefinitely in an effort to stabilize the addict's life, and reduce risks of intravenous use.
- For long-term withdrawal, substitute prescribing takes place over a period of months to years with the long-term aim of opiate abstinence.
- For rapid withdrawal, withdrawal takes place over a period of weeks by the use of a substitute drug in decreasing doses.
- For gradual withdrawal, withdrawal takes place over a period of months by the use of a substitute drug in decreasing doses.

Treatment should be undertaken initially by the general practitioner, possibly with help from the local community drugs team. If these approaches fail, referral to the more specialized drug dependency unit may be required.

People who are dependent on more than one drug, those with a history of several failed attempts, those with coexisting mental or physical disease, those who are violent or highly manipulative, and those requiring injectable or high doses of substitute drugs should be considered for specialist referral.

PSYCHOLOGICAL METHODS

Therapeutic outcome is improved if substitute prescribing is combined with various forms of behaviour therapy.

Motivational interviewing

Confrontational approaches have traditionally been used to deal with issues of denial. However, it seems that confrontational techniques increase rather than reduce resistance to treatment. Motivational interviewing is a cognitive–behavioural approach that takes into account the patient's stage of preparedness for change, and prompts the patient to consider the favourable reasons to change.

Relapse prevention

Described by Marlatt, this is a short-term intervention with extensive follow-up and preparation of the patient to anticipate urges to return to the drug-taking behaviour for a considerable period after abstinence has been achieved.

People undergoing relapse prevention therapy are more likely to internally attribute change, and are more likely to remain opiate-free during follow-up, or to contain a temporary relapse. The internal attribution of control over drug use maximizes treatment effects.

Naltrexone is a long-acting opioid antagonist which precipitates a withdrawal syndrome in the opiate-dependent person. It is used in the detoxified addict who requires additional help to remain drug-free. The euphoriant effects of opiates are abolished, thus aiding abstinence. It is particularly helpful if a partner administers it, and if used in conjunction with cognitive–behavioural therapy.

PROGNOSIS

The mortality rate for intravenous drug abusers is twenty times that of their non-drug-using peers. Since the 1980s the prevalence of HIV infection among intravenous drug users has increased to approximately 50–60% in some groups (e.g. New York, Edinburgh), and mortality among this group has increased further.

STIMULANTS

Stimulants considered here are cocaine, amphetamines and caffeine.

Cocaine (coke, snow, crack ...)

Cocaine is derived from the leaves of the coca shrub. Coca leaves are chewed, and the paste derived from the leaves is smoked.

Cocaine hydrochloride, a white powder usually snorted, may be injected. Crack cocaine (rock) and freebase, alkaloid forms may also be smoked. This provides a powerful hit which produces strong psychological dependence.

It is a class A drug, requiring notification.

EPIDEMIOLOGY

There has been an epidemic of cocaine use in the USA. It remains relatively expensive in the UK, although its use is increasing. Amphetamines tend to be the preferred stimulant of abuse in the UK.

Fewer than 10% of cocaine addicts are notified to the Home Office.

DRUG ACTION

Cocaine blocks dopamine uptake at the dopamine re-uptake site. Extracellular levels of dopamine are markedly increased. Dopaminergic activity, particularly at the nucleus accumbens, has been found to have a major role in the pleasurable and reinforcing effects of cocaine, amphetamine, phencyclidine, nicotine and alcohol. Genetic polymorphisms at the dopamine re-uptake site may contribute to an individual's liability to become dependent.

Acute effects last about 20 minutes and include euphoria, reduced hunger, tirelessness, agitation, tachycardia, raised blood pressure, sweating, nausea, vomiting, dilated pupils, and impairment of judgement and social functioning. High doses may lead to an acute toxic psychosis with marked agitation, paranoia and auditory, visual and tactile hallucinations (cocaine bug).

Chronic use leads to tolerance, withdrawal symptoms and a chronically anxious state, possibly caused by dopamine depletion.

DRUG WITHDRAWAL

Following the initial rush of wellbeing and confidence, when the effects of the drug wear off there follows a rebound crash. This consists of dysphoria, anxiety, irritability, depression, fatigue and intense craving for the drug. The crash phase lasts nine hours to four days. The withdrawal phase of 1–10 weeks is the period of the greatest risk of relapse. The final phase is of unlimited duration, when stimuli can trigger craving.

HARMFUL EFFECTS

At high doses, convulsions, hyperthermia, coma and death may occur. Excessive use can also lead to hypertension with cardiac failure, myocardial infarction, subarachnoid haemorrhage and cerebrovascular accidents.

Perforation of the nasal septum can follow long-term administration by the nasal route because of the vasoconstriction caused by cocaine. Intravenous use carries with it the risks described above.

Cocaine abusers often take sedatives, including heroin, alcohol and benzodiazepines. As well as taking the edge off the high produced by cocaine, some of the metabolites of the cocaine–alcohol interaction have been found to have a much longer half-life than cocaine alone. It is possible that this prolongation of the effects of cocaine contributes to its use with alcohol.

Long-term stimulant abuse results in a stereotyped compulsive repetitive pattern of behaviour and paranoid psychosis resembling schizophrenia.

Amphetamines (speed, whizz, sulphate ...)

These stimulants are cheap and widely available in the UK and the USA. They are used clinically in the treatment of narcolepsy, as appetite suppressants and selectively in the hyperkinesis of childhood. They are administered orally and intravenously. Methamphetamine may be inhaled.

Drug action, clinical effects and withdrawal effects are similar to those of cocaine (see above).

The toxic psychosis produced by amphetamine abuse can be indistinguishable from schizophrenia. It usually resolves with abstinence, but may continue for some months. Marked tolerance can develop. Following chronic use profound depression and fatigue occur. Long-term use leads to central nervous system serotonergic neuronal destruction.

Caffeine

Caffeine is widely available in coffee, tea and chocolate, and is added to soft drinks and proprietary cold preparations.

Coffee contains about 80–150 mg of caffeine per cup depending upon the brewing method. Peak blood levels occur 15–45 minutes following oral administration; the half-life is 6 hours. Metabolism is increased by smoking, and reduced by oral contraceptives and pregnancy. Neonates cannot metabolize caffeine, therefore there is a very long half-life.

DRUG EFFECTS

A dose of 80–200 mg produces mood elevation, increased alertness and clarity of thought, increased gastric secretion, tachycardia, raised blood pressure, diuresis, and increased productivity.

In overdose (greater than 250 mg per day) caffeinism occurs. This results in anxiety, restlessness and nausea, and facial flushing.

At levels of intake in excess of 600 mg per day, dysphoria replaces euphoria, anxiety and mood disturbances become prominent, and insomnia, muscle-twitching, tachycardia and sometimes cardiac arrhythmias occur.

DRUG WITHDRAWAL

At high daily doses a withdrawal syndrome occurs with abstinence. This comprises restlessness, irritability, dizziness, severe headache, rhinorrhoea, depression and poor work performance.

Management of stimulant dependence

There is no case for substitute prescribing since these drugs do not produce a major withdrawal syndrome. Drugs should be withdrawn abruptly. Following stimulant withdrawal, insomnia, depression and intense craving for the drug may occur. Antidepressants may be helpful.

Desipramine has been found to reduce the intensity of cocaine craving irrespective of other psychopathology. Most patients can be managed as outpatients, but some become acutely suicidal and need observation.

Psychological support is helpful, and relapse prevention techniques incorporated into treatment packages increase the chances of success.

SEDATIVES

Central nervous system sedatives depress CNS activity with little analgesic effect. They include alcohol (see above), barbiturates, benzodiazepines and carbamates. All the CNS depressants have abuse potential and cause both psychological and physical dependence. Cross-tolerance between groups occurs, and the withdrawal syndromes are similar. When taken repeatedly in high doses all these drugs produce sadness/depression, a worsening of confusional states, and withdrawal syndromes in which anxiety is prominent.

Benzodiazepines

Widely prescribed, these have widespread physical dependence among licit users, and are very popular with illicit substance abusers.

The most common route of administration is oral, but some abusers attempt to inject the contents of capsules or ground tablets intravenously.

EPIDEMIOLOGY

Over one million of the UK population use benzodiazepines continuously for more than one year.

DRUG ACTION

This group of sedatives potentiates the inhibitory actions of the GABA-A receptor in the limbic areas of the brain. They have anxiolytic, hypnotic and anticonvulsant properties at normal doses.

The clinical signs of intoxication include slurred speech, uncoordination, unsteady gait, impaired attention or memory, psychological effects such as paradoxical aggression and disinhibition, lability of mood, impaired judgement and impaired social or occupational functioning.

DRUG WITHDRAWAL

Tolerance occurs rapidly. There is rebound anxiety after 4 weeks of use; dependence is seen in 45% of users after 3 months.

The onset and intensity of withdrawal symptoms are related in part to the half-life of the drug used (shorter half-lives lead to a more abrupt and intense withdrawal syndrome). The withdrawal syndrome is also related to the dose used. Onset is usually within 1–14 days after drug reduction/cessation, and may last for months.

Withdrawal symptoms include somatic effects such as autonomic hyperactivity (tachycardia, sweating, anorexia, weight loss, pyrexia, tremor of hands, tongue and eyelids, GI disturbance, sleep disturbance with vivid dreams due to REM rebound), malaise and weakness, tinnitus and grand mal convulsions.

There are cognitive effects with impaired memory and concentration. There are also perceptual effects with hypersensitivity to sound, light and touch, depersonalization and derealization. Delirium may develop within a week of cessation, associated with visual, auditory and tactile hallucinations, and delusions.

Affective effects such as irritability, anxiety and phobic symptoms may also occur.

HARMFUL EFFECTS

In a high-dose abuser, severe withdrawal symptoms occur if the person is unable to acquire the usual dose of drug. As in these doses the drugs have usually been acquired illicitly, supply cannot be guaranteed.

Benzodiazepines are relatively safe in overdose, but are liable to produce respiratory depression, and in combination with other drugs they can be lethal.

The injection of street benzodiazepines incurs all the dangers of injecting described above, but is particularly liable to cause limb ischaemia and gangrene, with resulting amputation.

MANAGEMENT

Withdrawal from sedative drugs is potentially lethal and should usually be managed on a medical ward.

Barbiturates

Although the prescribing of barbiturates has largely been superseded by the safer benzodiazepines, they still appear in the form of phenobarbitone, amylobarbitone and quinalbarbitone (Tuinal) and are widely available.

DRUG ACTION

Barbiturates potentiate action at the GABA-A receptor thus increasing CNS depression. This is particularly marked in the reticular activating system and cerebral cortex.

Clinical effects include impaired concentration, reduced anxiety and dysphoria. In increasing doses dysarthria, ataxia, drowsiness, coma, respiratory depression and death occur.

Chronic use results in tolerance caused by hepatic enzyme induction, cross-tolerance with alcohol, personality change, persistent intoxication, labile affect, poor concentration, impaired judgement and incoordination.

DRUG WITHDRAWAL

This causes anxiety, tremor, sweating, insomnia with marked REM rebound, irritability, agitation, twitching, vomiting, nausea, tachycardia, orthostatic hypotension, delirium and convulsions.

HARMFUL EFFECTS

Barbiturates are dangerous in overdose. Their therapeutic index is low. Tolerance to psychotropic effects exceeds tolerance to respiratory depression.

Parenteral administration of oral preparations is attempted by some addicts, incurring all the risks described.

MANAGEMENT

A gradual tapering of the dose is considered to be the most appropriate way to manage barbiturate dependence. Short-acting compounds should first be substituted by long-acting compounds, diazepam being the most commonly used form for the purposes of withdrawal. After stabilizing on diazepam, dose reduction is commenced. At high doses this can occur quite rapidly (e.g. at 5 mg per week) until the patient starts to complain of unpleasant effects, when the rate of reduction can be reduced. If symptoms of depression are present an antidepressant is indicated. Propranolol may help with some of the somatic symptoms of anxiety.

Psychological support is very important, with weekly contact initially. The family should be involved in the process.

The withdrawal of barbiturates similarly needs phased withdrawal; inpatient admission is often necessary.

HALLUCINOGENS

Hallucinogens are substances that give rise to marked perceptual disturbances when taken in relatively small quantities.

Lysergic acid diethylamine (LSD, acid, microdots, supermans ...)

LSD is chemically related to 5-HT. It is available in tablets or absorbed on to paper. Minute amounts (≤100 micrograms) produce marked psychoactive effects. These peak at 2–4 hours and subside after about 12 hours. It is taken orally; intravenous use is not common because the onset of the trip is very rapid with oral ingestion (15 minutes). Tolerance develops rapidly; sensitivity to its effects returns rapidly with abstinence.

DRUG ACTION

The substance acts at multiple sites in the central nervous system, the effects being thought to be related to 5-HT antagonism. The effects are dose-related.

Psychic effects include the heightening of perceptions, with perceptual distortion of shape, intensification of colour and sound, apparent movement of stationary objects, and changes in sense of time and place. Hallucinations may occur, but are relatively rare. The user usually retains insight into the nature of the experiences. Delusions (e.g. belief in the ability to fly) may occur. Emotional lability, heightened self-awareness and ecstatic experiences can occur. Synaesthesias in which a stimulus in one sensory modality is experienced in another modality (e.g. hearing colours) are common.

The physical effects are sympathomimetic, with tachycardia, hypertension and dilated pupils.

Unpleasant experiences may occur (bad trips), and these are more likely in the inexperienced, or if the ambient mood is disturbed. Users generally avoid being alone, in case of bad trips or dangerous behaviour while under the influence. The features of adverse experiences include anxiety, depression, dizziness and disorientation, and a short-lived psychotic episode characterized by hallucinations and paranoid delusions. With heavy use, an acute schizophreniform psychosis may persist.

Flashback phenomena (post-hallucinogen perception disorder) occur, in which aspects of the LSD experience occur spontaneously some time after LSD use. These are usually fleeting.

DRUG WITHDRAWAL

Physical withdrawal symptoms do not occur following the abrupt discontinuation of LSD or other hallucinogens.

HARMFUL EFFECTS

Accidents may occur while under the influence of hallucinogens, such as jumping from a height because of the delusional belief that the user can fly.

Flashback phenomena occur many months after drug elimination, giving rise to the possibility that these substances may cause permanent neurological changes.

Hallucinogenic mushrooms (magic mushrooms)

There are a number of fungi growing in the UK that contain psychoactive substances such as psilocybin and psilocin. Liberty cap and fly agaric mushrooms are the ones most commonly used for their psychoactive effects. Ingestion of these in the raw state is legal, but any attempt to process them, such as by cooking, drying or freezing, is illegal.

Ingestion causes mild LSD-like effects, with marked euphoria. At high doses, hallucinations, bad trips and acute psychoses can occur.

Mescaline

Mescaline is the active component of the Mexican peyote cactus. Mescaline is similar to noradrenaline. It is hallucinogenic, and is orally administered.

LSD is 200 times as potent as psilocybin, which is 30 times as potent as mescaline.

Phencyclidine (PCP, angel dust)

Phencyclidine is an arylcyclohexylamine related to ketamine. It is taken by smoking, snorting and injecting.

It produces stimulant, anaesthetic, analgesic and hallucinogenic effects. At low doses it induces euphoria, and a feeling of weightlessness. At high doses visual hallucinations and synaesthesias occur.

Psychosis, violence, paranoia and depression can occur following a single dose.

Physical effects include uncoordination, slurred speech, blurred vision, convulsions, coma and respiratory arrest.

Prolonged use can result in a withdrawal syndrome upon cessation.

3,4–methylenedioxymethamphetamine (MDMA, ecstasy, XTC, E, adam ...)

MDMA is a hallucinogenic amphetamine. It possesses both stimulant and mild hallucinogenic properties. It is widely used at parties or raves by young people, particularly in the last decade. Taken orally in tablet or capsule form, it is often impure. Its effects last 4–6 hours; multiple dosing is tried, but tolerance develops rapidly, and subsequent doses have less potency. Physical dependence does not occur.

DRUG ACTION

MDMA produces a positive mood, with feelings of euphoria, intimacy and closeness to others. The stimulant effects resemble those of amphetamine, and hallucinogenic effects resemble those of LSD. The physical effects include anorexia, tachycardia, jaw-tightening and bruxism, and sweating.

HARMFUL EFFECTS

Deaths have occurred in those with pre-existing cardiac disease caused by cardiac arrhythmias. In the fit user at normal doses deaths have occurred as a result of hyperpyrexia, resulting in disseminated intravascular coagulation, rhabdomyolysis, and renal failure.

Convulsions can also occur. Most deaths of this nature occur when the user has been dancing vigorously for a considerable period, in high ambient temperatures, with inadequate fluid replacement. MDMA has a direct effect upon the thermoregulatory mechanisms which compound these conditions.

Hypertensive crises may occur leading to CVA in some.

Toxic hepatitis has been reported in MDMA users possibly related to impurities in the preparation.

Psychiatric conditions (psychosis, depression, anxiety) in previously vulnerable individuals can occur following MDMA use.

Neurotoxicity is an established fact. Serotonergic nerve terminals are damaged by this drug, and although rat studies indicate that this is reversible, primate studies indicate the opposite. The long-term consequences of MDMA-induced serotonergic neurotoxicity in humans are not known.

MANAGEMENT

Abrupt discontinuation is recommended, there being no advantage to gradual withdrawal. Psychiatric disturbance should be treated accordingly.

CANNABIS (GRASS, HASH, GANJA, POT ...)

The major active constituent in cannabis is 9-tetrahydrocannabinol. It is derived from cannabis salva, the Indian hemp plant; the dried leaves contain 1–10% (marijuana); the resin contains 8–15% (hashish). It is usually smoked, but it can be eaten, and it is widely used. It is highly lipophilic, so it can be detected in the blood 20 hours following a single dose.

DRUG ACTION

Tetrahydrocannabinol has anticholinergic effects, and its action is particularly marked in the hippocampus. It thus has adverse effects on memory, cognition and other higher mental functions. The psychological effects include euphoria, relaxation, suspiciousness, a feeling that time has slowed down, impaired judgement, heightened sensory awareness and social withdrawal. Hunger and anxiety may occur. Physical effects include tachycardia, raised blood pressure, dry mouth, thirst, constipation, reduced intraocular pressure, ataxia and, rarely, photophobia and nystagmus. In high-dosage perceptual distortions, confusion, drowsiness, bradycardia, hypotension, hypothermia, bronchodilatation and peripheral vasoconstriction can occur. An acute toxic psychosis which resolves with abstinence may occur.

DRUG WITHDRAWAL

In chronic users, cessation of cannabis is often followed by a withdrawal syndrome consisting of irritability, restlessness, anorexia, nausea and insomnia. Craving and psychological dependence do not occur.

HARMFUL EFFECTS

Chronic cannabis use can lead to a deterioration in personality. An increase in aggressiveness may also occur. Flashbacks, and prolonged depersonalization and derealization, may occur.

Cognitive and psychomotor impairment resulting from even small amounts of cannabis make the performance of skilled tasks (such as driving) hazardous.

VOLATILE SOLVENTS

Volatile substances are inhaled (glue-sniffing) in order to experience their psychoactive effects. Solvents from glue (such as toluene), correction fluids (for example, trichloroethane), butane gas and other aerosol propellants are popular.

Solvents have been tried by 3–5% of 15-year-olds. Often fumes are rebreathed from a plastic bag, but sometimes an aerosol is sprayed directly into the oropharynx (this is particularly dangerous). Rapidly absorbed, its effects last about 30 minutes.

DRUG ACTION

The clinical effects include euphoria, disinhibition, dizziness, perceptual distortions and frank hallucinations, tinnitus, ataxia, confusion, slurred speech, nystagmus, decreased reflexes, tremor and muscle weakness. High doses cause stupor and death. Aspiration of vomit can occur at any time.

DRUG WITHDRAWAL

There is no physical withdrawal syndrome.

HARMFUL EFFECTS

Acute intoxication can lead to fatal accidents, particularly through falling or drowning. However, the greatest risk of death is during an episode of sniffing. Butane squirted directly into the mouth can cause cardiac arrest. Propellants squirted directly into the mouth are cooled to −20°C, which can cause burns to the throat and lungs, and may freeze the larynx, causing cardiac arrest through vagal nerve stimulation. Rebreathing from plastic bags can result in asphyxiation.

There are approximately 100 deaths per annum in the UK, with 20% of these occurring in first-time users, and the majority in those aged under 20 years.

There are reports of long-term damage to the CNS, heart, liver and kidneys. Chronic use may cause a persistent cerebellar syndrome, and peripheral neuropathy.

MANAGEMENT

Abrupt discontinuation is recommended. Advice from social services and/or a child psychiatrist may be needed.

DRUG ABUSE IN PREGNANCY

Drug abuse in pregnancy often results in poor antenatal care and the risk of infection. Women at this time may have an increased motivation to change their behaviour, and it is important to take this opportunity to engage them in services. Education and harm minimization should be attempted.

ANTENATAL CARE

Drug misusers are at a high risk of obstetric complications. There is a high incidence of intrauterine growth retardation and premature labour. HIV-positive women need counselling about risks to themselves and their fetus.

Drug withdrawal is best attempted gradually during the second trimester of pregnancy. If this is not possible then attempts should be made to ensure that the practice is as safe as possible (e.g. changing to non-injecting modes of administration). Sudden withdrawal should be avoided because of the risk of intrauterine death. Abstinence 4–6 weeks before birth minimizes the risks of neonatal withdrawal symptoms.

If the mother is HIV-positive or receiving high doses of opioids, breast-feeding should be avoided.

POSTNATAL CARE

Following the birth, an assessment should be made of the amount of social support the mother is likely to need. Continuing support after delivery is essential.

BIBLIOGRAPHY

Cloninger, C.R. 1987: Neurogenetic adaptive mechanisms in alcoholism. *Science* 23:410–415.

Department of Health, Scottish Office Home and Health Department, Welsh Office 1991: *Drug Misuse and Dependence: Guidelines on Clinical Management.* London: HMSO.

Edwards, G. & Gross, M. 1976: Alcohol dependence: provisional description of a clinical syndrome. *British Medical Journal* i:1058.

Glass, I.B. 1991: *The International Handbook of Addiction Behaviour.* London: Routledge.

Jarman, C.M.B. & Kellett, J.M. 1979: Alcoholism in the general hospital. *British Medical Journal* i:469–471.

Jaswrilla, A.G., Adams, P.H. & Hore, B.D. 1979: Alcohol and acute general medical admissions. *Health Trends* 11:95–97.

Kendler, K.S. 1985: A twin study of individuals with both schizophrenia and alcoholism. *British Journal of Psychiatry* 147:48–53.

Mattick, R.P. & Heather, N. 1993: Developments in cognitive and behavioural approaches to substance misuse. *Current Opinion in Psychiatry* 6:424–429.

Paton, A. 1988: *ABC of Alcohol*, 2nd edn. London: British Medical Journal.

Raistrick, D.S. & Davidson, R. 1986: *Alcoholism and Drug Addiction.* Edinburgh: Churchill Livingstone.

Royal College of Psychiatrists 1986: *Alcohol: Our Favourite Drug.* London: Tavistock.

Solowij, N. 1993: Ecstasy (3,4-methylenedioxymethamphetamine). *Current Opinion in Psychiatry* 6:411–415.

Tabakoff, B. & Hoffman, P.L. 1993: The neurochemist. *Psychiatry* 6:388–394.

Taylor, C., Brown, D., Duckitt, A. *et al.* 1985: Patterns of outcome: drinking histories over ten years among a group of alcoholics. *British Journal of Addiction* 80:45–50.

Victor, M., Adams, R.D. & Collins, G.H. 1971: *The Wernicke-Korsakoff Syndrome.* Oxford: Blackwell.

27

Schizophrenia and delusional (paranoid) disorders

SCHIZOPHRENIA

HISTORY

- In 1860, Morel used the term *démence précoce* for a disorder of deteriorating adolescent psychosis.
- In 1863, Kahlbaum described katatonie.
- In 1871, Hecker described hebephrenie.
- In 1894, Sommer included deteriorating paranoid syndromes in the concept of primary dementia.
- In 1868, Griesinger believed that insanity could develop in the absence of mood disturbance, primary insanity (primäre Verücktheit), and that all functional psychoses were expressions of single disease entity (Einheitspsychoses).
- In 1896, Emil Kraepelin grouped together catatonia, hebephrenia and the deteriorating paranoid psychoses under the name *dementia praecox*. He differentiated dementia praecox with its poor prognosis from the manic depressive psychoses with their relatively better prognoses. He considered dementia praecox to be a disease of the brain.
- In 1911, Bleuler introduced the term *schizophrenia*, applied it to Kraepelin's cases of dementia praecox, and expanded the concept to include what today may be considered schizophrenic spectrum disorders. He considered symptoms of ambivalence, autism, affective incongruity and disturbance of association of thought to be fundamental (the 'four As'), with delusions and hallucinations assuming secondary status. Bleuler was influenced by the writings of Sigmund Freud. He added *schizophrenia simplex* to Kraepelin's list.
- In 1931, Hughlings-Jackson considered positive symptoms as 'release phenomena' occurring in healthy tissue; negative symptoms were attributed to neuronal loss.
- In 1959, Kurt Schneider emphasized the importance of delusions and hallucinations in defining his first-rank symptoms.
- In 1960, Langfeldt sought to distinguish between schizophrenia and the better-prognosis *schizophreniform psychoses*; process versus non-process schizophrenia.
- In 1972, Cooper compared patients admitted to psychiatric hospitals in New York and London. He found identical symptomatology, but schizophrenia diagnosed nearly twice as often in New York compared to London.

- In 1973, the WHO conducted the International Pilot Study of Schizophrenia. This study found, using narrow criteria, a one-year incidence of schizophrenia of 0.7–1.4 per 10 000 population aged 15–54, across all countries. It was confirmed that psychiatrists in the USA and the former USSR diagnosed schizophrenia twice as often as those in seven other countries (Columbia, Czechoslovakia, Denmark, Nigeria, India, Taiwan and the UK). This led to a realization that psychiatric diagnoses had to be defined operationally.

CLASSIFICATION OF SCHIZOPHRENIA

SCHNEIDERIAN FIRST-RANK SYMPTOMS

In defining his first-rank symptoms, Schneider stated that in the absence of organic brain disease the following are highly suggestive of schizophrenia:

- auditory hallucinations
  - repeat the thoughts out loud (e.g. Gedankenlautwerden, écho de la pensée)
  - in the third person
  - in the form of a running commentary
- delusions of passivity
  - thought insertion, withdrawal and broadcasting
  - made feelings, impulses and actions
- somatic passivity
- delusional perception.

Second-rank symptoms include perplexity, emotional blunting, hallucinations and other delusions.

First-rank symptoms can occur in other psychoses and, although highly suggestive of schizophrenia, are not pathognomonic.

ST LOUIS CRITERIA (FEIGHNER ET AL., 1972)

The sufferer is continuously ill for at least 6 months, with no prominent affective symptoms, presence of delusions, hallucinations or thought disorder. Personal and family history are taken into account (e.g. marital status, age under 40, premorbid social adjustment).

CATEGO (WING ET AL., 1974)

This uses the Present State examination to generate diagnoses by means of a computer program. It is based on the Schneiderian concept of schizophrenia. No account is taken of symptom duration.

RESEARCH DIAGNOSTIC CRITERIA (SPITZER ET AL., 1975)

There is a two-week duration, lack of affective symptoms, presence of thought disorder, hallucinations or delusions similar to Schneider's first-rank symptoms.

INTERNATIONAL CLASSIFICATION OF DISEASES, TENTH REVISION: ICD-10 (WHO, 1992)

There are fundamental, characteristic distortions of thinking and perception, and inappropriate or blunted affect. There is clear consciousness. Intellectual capacity is usually maintained, but some cognitive deficits can evolve over time (see Table 27.1).

Table 27.1 *ICD-10 classification of schizophrenia and delusional disorders*

F20 Schizophrenia	F20.0 Paranoid schizophrenia F20.1 Hebephrenic schizophrenia F20.2 Catatonic schizophrenia F20.3 Undifferentiated schizophrenia F20.4 Post-schizophrenic depression F20.5 Residual schizophrenia F20.6 Simple schizophrenia F20.8 Other schizophrenia F20.9 Schizophrenia, unspecified
F22 Persistent delusional disorders	F22.0 Delusional disorder F22.8 Other persistent delusional disorders F22.9 Persistent delusional disorder, unspecified
F23 Acute and transient psychotic disorders	F23.0 Acute polymorphic psychotic disorder without symptoms of schizophrenia F23.1 Acute polymorphic psychotic disorder with symptoms of schizophrenia F23.2 Acute schizophrenia-like psychotic disorder F23.3 Other acute predominantly delusional psychotic disorder F23.8 Other acute and transient psychotic disorders F23.9 Acute and transient psychotic disorder, unspecified
F24 Induced delusional disorder	
F25 Schizoaffective disorders	F25.0 Schizoaffective disorder, manic type F25.1 Schizoaffective disorder, depressive type F25.2 Schizoaffective disorder, mixed type F25.8 Other schizoaffective disorders F25.9 Schizoaffective disorder, unspecified
F28 Other nonorganic psychotic disorders	
F29 Unspecified nonorganic psychosis	

Symptoms are divided into groups:

(a) thought echo and thought alienation
(b) delusions of passivity; delusional perception
(c) auditory hallucinations in the form of a running commentary, or discussing the patient, or hallucinatory voices coming from some part of the body
(d) persistent delusions, culturally inappropriate and impossible
(e) persistent hallucinations in any modality, accompanied by fleeting delusions without affective content, or by persistent over-valued ideas, or occurring every day for weeks
(f) formal thought disorder comprising interruptions in the train of thought, incoherence, irrelevant speech, or neologisms
(g) catatonic behaviour (e.g. excitement, stupor, posturing, waxy flexibility, negativism and mutism)
(h) negative symptoms (e.g. apathy, paucity of speech, blunted or incongruous affect)

(i) a significant and consistent change in the overall quality of some aspects of personal behaviour (e.g. loss of interest, aimlessness, idleness, self-absorbed attitude, social withdrawal).

Diagnostic guidelines require a minimum of one clear symptom (two if less clear-cut) belonging to groups (a) to (d), or symptoms from at least two of the groups (e) to (h) should have been present for most of the time during a period of one month or more.

Symptom (i) applies only to a diagnosis of simple schizophrenia, and a duration of at least one year is required.

Schizophrenia is not diagnosed if extensive affective symptoms are present, unless they postdate the schizophrenic syndrome. If both schizophrenic and affective symptoms develop together and are evenly balanced, the diagnosis of schizoaffective disorder is made.

Schizophrenia is not diagnosed in the presence of overt brain disease, or during drug intoxication or withdrawal.

The pattern of course is classified as: (i) continuous; (ii) episodic, progressive deficit; (iii) episodic, stable deficit; (iv) episodic, remittent; (v) incomplete remission; (vi) complete remission.

Subtypes

In ICD-10 the following subtypes of schizophrenia are distinguished:

- *Paranoid schizophrenia*. This is the commonest subtype. Hallucinations and/or delusions are prominent. Disturbances of affect, volition, speech and catatonic symptoms are relatively inconspicuous. Auditory, olfactory, gustatory and somatic hallucinations, and visual hallucinations may occur. Commonly there are delusions of control, influence, passivity and persecution.
- *Hebephrenic schizophrenia*. The age of onset is usually between 15 and 25 years. There is a poor prognosis. Affective changes are prominent. Fleeting and fragmentary delusions and hallucinations, irresponsible behaviour, fatuous, disorganized thought, rambling speech, and mannerisms are common. Negative symptoms, particularly flattening of affect and loss of volition, are prominent. Drive and determination are lost, goals abandoned, behaviour becomes aimless and empty. The premorbid personality is characteristically shy and solitary.
- *Catatonic schizophrenia*. One or more of the following behaviours dominate: stupor, excitement, posturing, negativism, rigidity, waxy flexibility, command automatism and perseveration of words or phrases. Catatonic symptoms alone are not diagnostic of schizophrenia; they may be provoked by brain disease, metabolic disturbance, alcohol and drugs and mood disorders. Psychomotor disturbances may alternate between extremes; violent excitement may occur. It may be combined with a dream-like state with vivid scenic hallucinations.
- *Simple schizophrenia*. There is an insidious onset of decline in functioning. Negative symptoms develop without preceding positive symptoms. Diagnosis requires changes in behaviour over at least a year, with marked loss of interest, idleness and social withdrawal.
- *Residual or chronic schizophrenia*. This is characterized by negative symptoms. There is past evidence of at least one schizophrenic episode, and a period of at least one year in which frequency of positive symptoms has been minimal and negative schizophrenic syndrome has been present. There is absence of depression, institutionalization, or dementia or other brain disorder.
- *Undifferentiated schizophrenia*. General criteria for schizophrenia are satisfied, but not conforming to the above syndromes.
- *Post-schizophrenic depression*. This is a depressive episode arising after a schizophrenic illness. Schizophrenic illness must have occurred within the last 12 months, some symptoms still being present. Depressive symptoms fulfil at least the criteria for a depressive episode, and are present for at least 2 weeks. There is an increased risk of suicide.

TYPE 1 AND TYPE 2 SCHIZOPHRENIA (Crow, 1980)

Crow described a two-syndrome hypothesis of schizophrenia – a categorical approach.

- *Type 1 schizophrenia.* This type is characterized by prominent positive symptoms, acute onset, good premorbid adjustment, good treatment response, intact cognition, intact brain structure and a reversible neurochemical disturbance.
- *Type 2 schizophrenia.* This type is characterized by prominent negative symptoms, insidious onset, poor premorbid adjustment, poor treatment response, impaired cognition, structural brain abnormalities (ventricular enlargement) and an underlying pathology based on neuronal loss, therefore irreversible.

SAPS AND SANS

In 1984, Andreasen developed structured scales for the assessment of positive and negative symptoms: the Scale for the Assessment of Positive Symptoms (SAPS) and the Scale for the Assessment of Negative Symptoms (SANS).

LIDDLE'S SYNDROMES (Liddle, 1987)

Liddle found that the pattern of symptoms in schizophrenia segregated into three distinguishable syndromes – a dimensional approach:

- *Psychomotor poverty syndrome.* There is poverty of speech, flatness of affect and decreased spontaneous movement.
- *Disorganization syndrome.* There are disorders of the form of thought and inappropriate affect.
- *Reality distortion syndrome.* There are delusions and hallucinations.

A subsequent PET study of regional cerebral blood flow (Liddle *et al.*, 1992) showed that each of these three syndromes is associated with a specific pattern of perfusion:

Psychomotor poverty syndrome
Hypoperfusion of the left dorsal prefrontal cortex extends to medial prefrontal cortex and anterior cingulate cortex. There is hyperperfusion in the head of the caudate nucleus which receives substantial projections from the dorsolateral prefrontal cortex. Some changes are also found on the right (laterality only a matter of degree). Hypofrontality in schizophrenia is more often seen in chronic patients and is associated with inactivity and catatonic symptoms. In normal subjects, prefrontal activity increases when involved in internal generation of action.

Disorganization syndrome
There is hypoperfusion of the right ventral prefrontal cortex, and increased activity in anterior cingulate and dorsomedial thalamic nuclei which project to the prefrontal cortex. There is relative hypoperfusion of Broca's area and bilateral hypoperfusion of parietal association cortex. Evidence suggests that in primates the ventral prefrontal cortex plays a role in suppression of interference from irrelevant mental activity. The anterior cingulate plays a role in attentional mechanisms. The suggestion is that these patients are engaged in an ineffective struggle to suppress inappropriate mental activity.

Reality distortion syndrome
There is increased activity in the left parahippocampal region and left striatum. This is consistent with the proposal that delusions and hallucinations arise from a disorder of internal monitoring

resulting in failure to recognize internally generated mental acts. Abnormalities of function underlying schizophrenic symptoms are not confined to single loci, but involve distributed neuronal networks.

NEURODEVELOPMENTAL CLASSIFICATION (MURRAY ET AL., 1992)

On the basis of genetic, epidemiological, neuropathological, neuroimaging and gender difference studies, schizophrenia has been subdivided into the following three groups:

- *Congenital schizophrenia.* The abnormality is present at birth and may be caused by genetic predisposition and/or environmental insult (e.g. maternal influenza, obstetric complication, early brain injury or infection). The person is more likely to have minor physical abnormalities, abnormal personality or social impairment in childhood; to present early; to exhibit negative symptoms; and to show morphological brain changes and cognitive impairment. The person is more likely to be male and to have a poor outcome.
- *Adult-onset schizophrenia.* The person is more likely to exhibit positive and affective symptoms. The person may have a genetic predisposition to manifest symptomatology anywhere along a continuum from bipolar mood disorder, schizoaffective disorder, to schizophrenia.
- *Late-onset schizophrenia.* This presents after age 60 years, with good premorbid functioning. It is most common in females. It is often associated with auditory and visual sensory deprivation. It is sometimes related to paranoid personality or to mood disorder. Organic brain dysfunction is often present.

EPIDEMIOLOGY OF SCHIZOPHRENIA

STATISTICS

- The incidence of schizophrenia is between 15 and 30 new cases per 100 000 of the population per year.
- The point prevalence is approximately 1%.
- The lifetime risk is approximately 1%.
- The age of onset is usually between 15 and 45 years, earlier in men than in women.
- It is equally common in males and females. There is a higher incidence in those not married.
- It is most common in social classes IV and V.
- Prevalence varies geographically. Rates from urban areas are generally higher than in rural areas, with marked exceptions – the highest prevalence measured (17.4 per 1000 population) was from a sparsely populated rural area in the west of Ireland.

THEORIES

The following are theories accounting for geographical variance in the prevalence of schizophrenia:

- *Social drift.* Goldberg and Morrison (1963) studied fathers' birth certificates, and found schizophrenic males had lower social class distribution than their fathers. They attributed these findings to social drift; i.e. migration of those affected to areas where social demands may be less. Men were more likely to drift into inner city areas.
- *Social residue.* Healthy people migrate away from undesirable areas, leaving schizophrenics behind.

- *'Breeder' or social causation.* This theory assumes that environmental factors are either causative or have to be present for the predisposed individual to develop schizophrenia. Castle *et al.* (1993) found that schizophrenic patients in Camberwell were more likely to have been born in a socially deprived area and to have fathers with manual jobs. Those developing schizophrenia were more likely than controls to have been born into socially deprived households. This suggested that some environmental factor of aetiological importance in schizophrenia is more likely to affect those born into households of lower socioeconomic status and in the inner city.

Theories emphasizing environmental influences need not exclude the importance of biological factors, such as exposure to toxins, increased incidence of obstetric complications and a higher rate of infectious disease in cities. Social factors more common in cities include stressful life-events, social isolation and social over-stimulation.

AETIOLOGY OF SCHIZOPHRENIA

Genetics in schizophrenia

Twin, family and adoption studies have consistently demonstrated familial aggregation of schizophrenia, largely attributable to genetic factors.

Family studies
Table 27.2 shows the approximate lifetime risks for the development of schizophrenia in the relatives of patients with schizophrenia.

Table 27.2   *Approximate lifetime risks for the development of schizophrenia in the relatives of patients with schizophrenia*

Relationship	Lifetime expectancy rate to the nearest percentage point
Parents	6
All siblings	10
Siblings (when one parent has schizophrenia)	17
Children	13
Children (when both parents have schizophrenia)	46
Grandchildren	4
Uncles, aunts, nephews and nieces	3

Twin studies
The concordance rate for monozygotic (MZ) twins is approximately 45%, that for dizygotic (DZ) twins approximately 10% (Gottesman & Shields, 1972).

Studying adult offspring of 21 MZ and 41 DZ twin pairs discordant for schizophrenia, Gottesman and Bertelsen found the risk of developing schizophrenia was 17% among the adult children of the MZ and DZ probands, 17% among the offspring of phenotypically normal MZ co-twins, and only 2% among the offspring of phenotypically normal DZ co-twins. This suggests that the normal MZ co-twins carried and transmitted the relevant genotype without expressing it themselves.

Adoption studies

When children of schizophrenic mothers have been adopted soon after birth by non-schizophrenic families, they have a similar likelihood of developing schizophrenia (approximately 13%) as the rates suggested by family studies. There appears to be no such increased risk of developing schizophrenia in the children of non-schizophrenic parents who are similarly adopted (Kety *et al.*, 1971).

The following are possible modes of inheritance:

- *Single major locus.* Some forms possibly exist but would account for a very small proportion of observed cases. To date no single genetic focus responsible for the development of schizophrenia has been reliably demonstrated.
- *Polygenic.* There might be a threshold of gene numbers required for expression of schizophrenia.
- *Multifactorial.* There may be aetiological heterogeneity with various genetic and environmental subtypes. There is probably a spectrum of causes ranging from wholly genetic, through those with mixed aetiology, to the totally environmental.

Linkage studies

Bassett and associates reported a man who presented with schizophrenia plus minor physical abnormalities both shared by his maternal uncle. Cytogenetic analysis revealed translocation of part of chromosome 5; this led the writers to postulate that this segment of chromosome 5 may be site of a putative schizophrenia gene.

Sherrington and associates collected seven extended schizophrenic families from Iceland and England, probed chromosome 5 and found evidence highly suggestive of linkage between markers on chromosome 5 and schizophrenia. However, this finding has never been replicated and the study has subsequently been criticized on methodological grounds.

There are problems in applying linkage methodology to schizophrenia:

- Schizophrenia is probably genetically heterogeneous.
- Linkage analysis is usually applied to conditions transmitted by simpler Mendelian inheritance.
- Diagnostic and penetrance problems probably require a much higher lod score than the usual +3 before linkage for psychiatric diagnoses can be regarded as proved.

Prenatal factors in schizophrenia

People developing schizophrenia as adults are born disproportionately more often during late winter and early spring. A similar but less marked seasonal effect is reported for bipolar affective disorders, but not for neurotic or personality disorders. Seasonally varying environmental causes have been sought, and prenatal infection is currently the most favoured explanation.

An excess of minor physical abnormalities is reported in schizophrenics; examples are low-set ears, greater distance between the eyes, and a single transverse palmar crease. Dermatoglyphics are determined by genes, and deleterious events in the second trimester of pregnancy can alter their form. Schizophrenics have deviations from normal in ridge patterns of fingers, palms and soles. Schizophrenic probands of monozygotic twin pairs discordant for schizophrenia have significantly more finger and palm epidermal ridge anomalies than their healthy co-twins (Bracha *et al.*, 1991).

Structural abnormalities in the brains of many schizophrenics suggest a neurodevelopmental rather than degenerative process. Most studies investigating brain morphology in schizophrenia report non-progressive ventricular and cortical sulcal enlargement, and structural abnormalities in the limbic areas. Structural changes reflect an early acquired hypoplasia, not degeneration. Cytoarchitectural changes in limbic and prefrontal areas are strong indicators of early disordered brain development. Altered distribution of cortical layers of NADPH-d neurones is consistent with a disturbance of development, in which the normal pattern of programmed cell death is compromised, resulting in defective migration of neurones.

Murray suggests that neural dysplasia results in premorbid cognitive deficits, abnormal personality, negative symptoms and abnormal CT scans in schizophrenia. Maturational brain changes in adolescence, possibly myelination or synaptic pruning, reveal immature neuronal circuitry with consequent onset of hallucinations and delusions.

The neurodevelopmental model of schizophrenia accounts for the following findings:

- Individuals who were in their second trimester of fetal life during the influenza epidemic in Finland in 1957 had an increased risk of later schizophrenia (Mednick *et al.*, 1988).
- The winter excess of births in schizophrenics is due to a seasonal prevalence of a viral infection or other perinatal hazard.
- Males have an earlier onset of schizophrenia than females, possibly due to increased vulnerability to neurodevelopmental damage (generally commoner in males).
- The smaller proportion of male schizophrenics is genetically determined; there is evidence that concordance rates for schizophrenia are lower in male than in female identical twins.

Obstetric complications are more frequent in schizophrenics than in normal controls. This is noted particularly in schizophrenics without a positive family history for psychosis, implying that obstetric factors may augment or substitute for a genetic cause.

Personality in schizophrenia

Only *schizotypal personality disorder* is aetiologically related to schizophrenia. Among the schizotypal criteria, eccentricity, affect constriction and excessive social anxiety are linked to schizophrenia. There may be a milder phenotype along the schizophrenia spectrum.

Social factors in schizophrenia

In 1968, Brown and Birley found that schizophrenics had experienced significantly more independent life events in the three weeks prior to onset of relapse than had controls. In 1976, Vaughn and Leff found an increased relapse rate of schizophrenia in those who lived with families in which the relatives displayed *high expressed emotion* (critical comments; over-involvement) (see Table 27.3). Changes in physiological arousal may account for this effect.

Table 27.3 *Relapse rates of 128 schizophrenics over a 9-month period (Vaughn & Leff, 1976)*

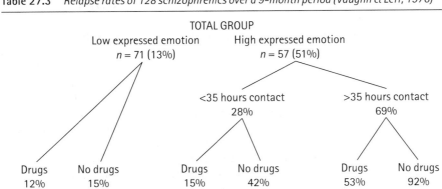

There was a *poverty of the social milieu* of patients with chronic schizophrenia, associated with increased negative symptoms, particularly social withdrawal, affective blunting and poverty of speech (Wing & Brown, 1961).

Neurotransmitters in schizophrenia

DOPAMINE

The *mesolimbic–mesocortical system* is a *dopaminergic* system originating in the ventral tegmental area of the brain. The mesolimbic system projects to the limbic system, while the mesocortical system innervates the cingulate, entorhinal and medial prefrontal cortices.

The *dopamine hypothesis of schizophrenia* asserts that the clinical features are the result of central dopaminergic hyperactivity in the mesolimbic–mesocortical system. The following is put as evidence in favour of the dopamine hypothesis:

- All clinically effective antipsychotic drugs occupy a substantial proportion of D_2 receptors in the brain (70–80% D_2 receptor occupancy in the striatum at normal doses).
- Amphetamine, a dopamine agonist, can cause a state similar to that of acute schizophrenia.
- Dopamine agonists exacerbate psychotic symptoms.
- Comparing actions of α and β isomers of flupenthixol in patients with acute schizophrenia, only those receiving the dopamine antagonist improved (Johnstone *et al.*, 1978).
- Postmortem studies have found increased D_2 receptors in the basal ganglia and limbic regions of schizophrenic brains.
- In animals, administration of dopamine agonists produces a behavioural picture said to be similar to human psychosis. This is reversed by giving dopamine antagonists.
- In drug-naive schizophrenics, the number of D_2 receptors in the striatum was 2–3 times that of controls as measured by PET (Wong *et al.*, 1986).

Evidence against the dopamine hypothesis includes:

- The concentration of dopamine metabolite HVA (homovanillic acid) in the cerebrospinal fluid in schizophrenics has generally not been found to be higher than in control subjects.
- D_2 receptor blockade caused by antipsychotics is an acute effect, but the therapeutic effect is observed 3–4 weeks later.
- 15–30% of schizophrenics fail to respond to dopamine antagonists.
- Antipsychotics have a better effect on positive than on negative symptoms.
- Clozapine, an effective antipsychotic, has less D_2 blocking activity than conventional antipsychotics.
- Some studies have failed to replicate Wongs' findings of increased D_2 receptors in striatum of brains of living schizophrenics.

Explanations which may account for contradictory results

- Schizophrenia is clinically complex, and the aetiology is heterogeneous.
- Schizophrenia may involve reduced dopaminergic activity in the prefrontal cortical area, and compensatory overactivity in subcortical or limbic areas.
- There are potential problems in patient selection and study methodology.
- Identification of D_1, D_3, D_4 and D_5 receptors has suggested that they alone or in addition to D2 receptors may be the appropriate target for antipsychotic drug therapy.

- Clozapine acts in part by antagonism of D_1, D_2, and particularly D_4 receptors; it is effective during long-term use in up to 60% of neuroleptic-resistant patients.
- D1 antagonist alone failed to show antipsychotic efficacy. Specific D_3 and D_4 antagonists have not yet been studied.
- During treatment with haloperidol, the ratio of dopamine metabolite (HVA) to serotonin and noradrenaline metabolites in CSF of schizophrenics increased significantly and correlated with reduction of symptoms. This supports the hypothesis that interactions between different monoamine neurotransmitters are involved in expression of schizophrenic symptoms.

SEROTONIN (5–HT)

There is some evidence that serotonergic dysfunction may be associated with schizophrenia:

- The hallucinogen LSD (see Chapter 26) acts at serotonin receptors.
- Antipsychotic risperidone is a potent $5-HT_2$ receptor antagonist (it also blocks D_2 receptors, however).
- Ritanserin, a selective $5-HT_2$ antagonist, reduced negative symptoms when given as adjunctive therapy in neuroleptic-treated schizophrenics.

GLUTAMATE

Glutamate stimulates the NMDA receptor. Phencyclidine ('angel dust' – see Chapter 26) causes schizophrenic-like effects by blocking NMDA receptors. A balance exists between excitatory glutamatergic and inhibitory dopaminergic terminals in the corpus striatum, regulating GABAergic neurones. These function in the 'thalamic filter' which seems to be hypoactive in schizophrenia. According to this theory, hypoactivity of GABA neurones is corrected by either reducing dopaminergic activity, or increasing glutamatergic activity.

Structural cerebral abnormalities in schizophrenia

Johnstone *et al.* (1976) conducted a CT scan study, finding that chronically hospitalized schizophrenic patients had larger lateral ventricles than controls. This has been confirmed by numerous neuroimaging studies.

In 1990, Andreasen conducted a large study in people matched for age, sex, height, weight and level of education. The ventricle/brain ratio was greater in schizophrenics than in controls. The differences were small, and there was overlap with the normal population; it was more marked in males.

MRI has shown a diffuse reduction in the volume of cortical grey matter in schizophrenic patients, this being associated with poor premorbid function. These findings are consistent with neurodevelopmental changes having taken place in such patients.

The following are further structural changes in schizophrenia found in some studies:

- reduced size of frontal lobes, or some division thereof
- reduced size of temporal lobe, particularly on the left
- reduced size of hippocampus and amygdala, particularly on the left
- reduced size of parahippocampal gyrus.

Neuropathological abnormalities in schizophrenia

Postmortem studies
Compared with control subjects, the brains of schizophrenic patients have shown in some studies:

- lower fixed brain weight
- reduced brain length
- reduced size of the parahippocampal gyrus.

Histological studies
Compared to controls, the brains of schizophrenics have shown in some studies:

- hippocampal pyramidal cell disarray
- reduced hippocampal cell numbers
- reduced cell numbers in the entorhinal cortex
- reduced hippocampal cell size
- disturbed cytoarchitecture in the entorhinal cortex.

Functional brain abnormalities in schizophrenia

Hypofrontality is associated with the presence of negative symptoms and autism.

Combining functional imaging with task activation, Weinberger *et al.* (1986) measured regional cerebral blood flow at rest and during the Wisconsin Card Sorting Test (activates frontal lobes normally). Impaired performance by schizophrenics was mirrored by a smaller increase in blood flow to prefrontal cortex.

MANAGEMENT OF SCHIZOPHRENIA

Hospitalization

Those with acute schizophrenia often require admission to hospital, if necessarily compulsorily, for assessment, investigations and treatment. Before discharge, Section 117 of the Mental Health Act 1983 for detained patients, and the care-programme approach for all patients, requires that an 'assessment of needs' be made. A key worker should be assigned to monitor a patient's progress and to administer depot medication.

Attendance at a day hospital or centre may be considered, and there should be appropriate communication with the patient's general practitioner.

Electroconvulsive therapy is used in the treatment of catatonic stupor.

See Appendix 1 for a summary of the National Institute of Clinical Excellence (NICE) guidelines on core interventions in the treatment and management of schizophrenia in primary and secondary care.

Drug treatments for schizophrenia

The efficacy of neuroleptics for acute symptoms has been demonstrated beyond doubt. 'Positive' symptoms respond better than 'negative' symptoms. Bear in mind the following:

- 5–25% of schizophrenics are unresponsive to conventional neuroleptics.
- 5–10% are intolerant owing to adverse neurological effects (parkinsonism, akathisia, dyskinesia).
- 40–60% of schizophrenics are non-compliant with oral medication. Possible reasons are:
  - limited insight into the disease
  - limited beneficial effect
  - unpleasant side effects
  - pressure from family and friends
  - poor communication with the medical team.
  Depot neuroleptics increase compliance, and reduce relapse rates.
- Continuous therapy is superior to intermittent treatment. It results in fewer relapses and a lower overall dose of neuroleptics.
- Of patients who stop medication, 60–70% relapse within a year, and 85% within 2 years, compared to 10–30% of those who continue on active medication.

USE OF ATYPICAL NEUROLEPTICS

If a patient has failed to respond to a trial of three neuroleptics of different classes, using an adequate dose for an adequate duration, an atypical agent such as clozapine can be tried. Clozapine can cause agranulocytosis, so regular blood counts are necessary. The incidence of agranulocytosis is 0.8% at 12 months and 0.9% at 18 months, with a peak risk in the third month; it is higher in women and older patients.

Atypical neuroleptics are distinguished from conventional neuroleptics by not producing catalepsy in animals, and not elevating prolactin levels in humans. There is a considerably lower potential for extrapyramidal side-effects and tardive dyskinesia. Extrapyramidal side-effects occur in up to 90% of patients taking neuroleptic medication.

Kane *et al.* (1988) showed that clozapine was significantly better than chlorpromazine in the treatment of schizophrenics previously resistant to haloperidol. Improvement was observed in both positive and negative symptoms.

NICE guidelines on atypical antipsychotics

In the UK, the NICE issued guidelines in June 2002 with respect to the prescription of atypical antipsychotics for patients with schizophrenia. They are as follows:

- The atypical antipsychotics (amisulpride, olanzapine, quetiapine, risperidone and zotepine) should be considered when deciding on the first-line treatment of newly diagnosed schizophrenia.
- An atypical antipsychotic is considered the treatment of choice for managing an acute schizophrenic episode when discussion with the individual is not possible.
- An atypical antipsychotic should be considered for an individual who is suffering from unacceptable side-effects with a conventional antipsychotic.
- An atypical antipsychotic should be considered for an individual in relapse whose symptoms were previously inadequately controlled.
- Changing to an atypical antipsychotic is not necessary if a conventional antipsychotic controls symptoms adequately and the individual does not suffer unacceptable side-effects.
- Clozapine should be introduced if schizophrenia is inadequately controlled despite the sequential use of two or more antipsychotics (one of which should be an atypical antipsychotic) each for at least 6–8 weeks.

Psychosocial treatments for schizophrenia

Social milieu
Wing and Brown (1970) found that negative symptoms varied in intensity with social stimulation within psychiatric institutions.

The TAPS study (Leff *et al.*, 1994) reported on long-stay patients discharged into the community. It found that, provided reprovision was well resourced with staffed homes for the more disabled, there was no increase in death rate, suicides, crime or vagrancy at 1- and 5-year follow-up, compared to matched controls. Between discharge and 5 years, negative symptoms reduced significantly in response to a more stimulating environment. Positive symptomatology remained stable.

Expressed emotion
Psychoeducational family programmes to increase medication compliance and coping with stressors are successful in reducing the risk of relapse. Families with high expressed emotion (EE) were identified using the Camberwell Family Interview. Education and family sessions in the home run in parallel with a relatives group. The programme is aimed at teaching problem-solving skills, lowering criticism and over-involvement, and reducing contact between patients and relatives whilst expanding social networks.

Prognosis for schizophrenia

Schizophrenia is a heterogeneous disorder, and there are no reliable predictors of outcome. Approximately 25% of cases of schizophrenia show good clinical and social recovery, while most studies show that fewer than a half of patients have a poor long-term outcome. Factors associated with a good prognosis include:

- being female
- being married
- an abrupt onset of the illness
- later onset of the illness
- an affective component to the illness
- paranoid, compared with non-paranoid
- good premorbid social adjustment
- family history of affective disorder
- short duration of illness prior to treatment
- good initial response to treatment
- lack of negative symptoms
- lack of cognitive impairment
- no ventricular enlargement.

Suicide
Ten per cent of schizophrenics commit suicide, and for most sufferers it happens early in their illness. Roy (1982) reported that suicide was more likely in the following cases:

- being male
- being young
- being unemployed
- having chronic illness, relapses and remissions

- having a high educational attainment prior to onset
- akathisia
- abrupt stoppage of drugs
- recent discharge from inpatient care.

Finally, paranoid schizophrenics are three times more likely than non-paranoid patients to commit suicide.

DELUSIONAL (PARANOID) DISORDERS

ICD-10 issues

According to ICD-10, a delusional disorder is an ill-defined condition, manifesting as a single delusion or a set of related delusions, being persistent, sometimes lifelong, and not having an identifiable organic basis. There are occasional or transitory auditory hallucinations, particularly in the elderly.

Delusions are the most conspicuous or only symptom and are present for at least 3 months. For the diagnosis there must be no evidence of schizophrenic symptoms or brain disease.

ICD-10 includes the previously used term *late paraphrenia*, although there is some evidence that there are differences between persistent delusional disorder and late paraphrenia. Howard *et al.* (1994) showed, using MRI scans in a group of late-onset schizophrenics and late-onset delusional disorders, that lateral ventricle volumes in the delusional disorder patients were much greater than those of schizophrenics, and almost twice those of controls.

Monodelusional disorders feature a stable, encapsulated delusional system, which takes over much of a person's life. The personality is preserved.

Epidemiology of delusional disorders

There is a point prevalence of 0.03% and a lifetime risk of 0.05–0.1%.

Munro (1991) reports from his series of patients with monodelusional disorder:

- a mean age of onset of 35 years for males and 45 years for females
- onset gradual and unremitting in 62%
- equal sex ratio of sufferers
- sufferers often unmarried, with high marital breakdown, low fecundity
- introverted, longstanding interpersonal difficulties
- family history of psychiatric disorder, but not of delusional disorder or schizophrenia
- evidence of minimal brain disorder in 16%.

Specific delusional (paranoid) disorders

PATHOLOGICAL (DELUSIONAL) JEALOUSY

This is also called the Othello syndrome, morbid jealousy, erotic jealousy, sexual jealousy, psychotic jealousy or conjugal paranoia. The person holds the delusional belief that his or her sexual partner is being unfaithful, and will go to great lengths to find evidence of infidelity. Underclothing may be examined for semen stains, belongings may be searched and the partner may be interrogated and followed. It is more common in men.

Pathological jealousy may be associated with the following conditions:

- organic disorders and psychoactive substance use disorders (e.g. alcohol dependence, cerebral tumour, endocrinopathy, dementia, cerebral infection, use of amphetamines or cocaine)
- paranoid schizophrenia
- depression
- neurosis or personality disorder.

Treatment should be directed at the underlying disorder. If no primary cause is identified, pharmacotherapy with a neuroleptic and/or psychotherapy may be helpful. There may be a risk of violence to the partner and it may be best to recommend that the couple separate.

EROTOMANIA (DE CLÉRAMBAULT'S SYNDROME)

The person holds the delusional belief that someone, usually of a higher social or professional status or a famous personality or in some other way 'unattainable', is in love with him or her. The patient may make repeated attempts to contact that other person. Eventually, rejections may lead to animosity and bitterness on the part of the patient towards the object of attention.

In hospital and outpatient clinical psychiatry, patients are more likely to be female than male, whereas in forensic psychiatry male patients are commoner. Overall, females outnumber males.

COTARD'S SYNDROME

This condition, also called *délire de négation*, is a nihilistic delusional disorder in which the patient believes that, for example, all his or her wealth has gone or that relatives or friends do not exist. It may take a somatic form with the patient believing that parts of his or her body do not exist. It can be secondary to very severe depression or to an organic disorder.

CAPGRAS SYNDROME

Although Capgras syndrome is also called *illusion des sosies*, or illusion of doubles, it is not an illusion but a delusional disorder. The essential feature of this rare condition is that a person who is familiar to the patient is believed to have been replaced by a double. It is more common in females. Common primary causes are schizophrenia, mood disorder and organic disorder. Derealization often occurs.

FREGOLI SYNDROME

In this very rare delusional disorder the patient believes that a familiar person, who is often believed to be the patient's persecutor, has taken on different appearances. Primary causes include schizophrenia and organic disorder.

INDUCED PSYCHOSIS (FOLIE À DEUX)

This rare delusional disorder is shared by two, or rarely more than two, people who are closely linked emotionally. One of the people has a genuine psychotic disorder; his or her delusional system is induced in the other person, who may be dependent or less intelligent than the first person. Geographical separation leads to recovery of the well person.

SCHIZOAFFECTIVE DISORDERS

Types of disorder

The term 'schizoaffective psychosis' was introduced by Kasanin in 1933 to describe a condition with both affective and schizophrenic symptoms, with sudden acute onset after good premorbid functioning, and usually with complete recovery.

ICD-10 describes these as disorders in which both affective and schizophrenic symptoms are prominent within the same episode of illness, either simultaneously or within a few days of each other. It distinguishes various types:

- *manic type* – the person usually makes a full recovery
- *depressive type* – prognosis not as good as that of the manic subtype, with a greater chance of developing 'negative' symptoms
- *mixed type*.

Relationship between affective and schizophrenic components

There is no consensus concerning the nosological status of schizoaffective disorder. Opposing views include the Kraepelinian binary system and continuum theories.

- *Binary theorists* (e.g. Winokur, Kendler) hold the traditional notion that there are two separate illnesses, schizophrenia and manic–depressive psychosis, having different aetiologies and requiring different treatments.
- *Continuum theorists* (e.g. Crow, Kendall) doubt that there are distinct illnesses, rather that features of psychosis vary quantitatively along a continuum, with schizophrenia and manic depression at opposing poles and schizoaffective disorder somewhere in between.

In 1991, Tsuang studied a subgroup of patients with strictly defined schizoaffective disorder. It was found that the morbid risk of schizophrenia in relatives of schizoaffectives was similar to that of a schizophrenic group, and fell between schizophrenia and affective disorder for the risk of affective disorder in relatives. It was concluded that this condition was different from schizophrenia or manic depression.

In 1993, Goldstein *et al.* found that, among probands with schizoaffective disorder, relatives had higher rates of schizophrenia and unipolar depression than relatives of males. Among relatives, males were at higher risk for schizophrenia spectrum disorders than females. This points to a stronger relationship between schizoaffective disorder to schizophrenia.

In 1994, DeLisi *et al.* reported the following in relationship to schizophrenia and affective disorder:

- At least one-third of schizophrenics have depressive symptoms.
- Affective disorder is more frequent in the families of schizophrenics than in controls.
- Unipolar depression is more common in families of schizoaffectives than schizophrenia-only probands. Bipolar disorder is as frequent in families of both.
- Affective disorder is frequently inherited from the same parental line as schizophrenia.
- Bipolar disorder is more frequent in male relatives and unipolar disorder more frequent in female relatives.

It was concluded that the same genes contribute to schizophrenia and affective disorder, and sex and phenotypic expression are related.

Prognosis for schizoaffective disorders

The prognosis of schizoaffective disorders lies between that of mood disorders and schizophrenia.

BIBLIOGRAPHY

Andreasen, N.C. 1983: *Scale for the Assessment of Negative Symptoms (SANS)*. Iowa City: University of Iowa.

Andreasen, N.C. 1984: *Scale for the Assessment of Positive Symptoms (SAPS)*. Iowa City: University of Iowa.

Andreasen, N.C., Swayze, V.W., Flaum, M. *et al.* 1990: Ventricular enlargement in schizophrenia evaluated with computed tomographic scanning. *Archives of General Psychiatry* 47:1008–1015.

Bassett, A., McGillivray, B., Jones, B. & Pantzar, J. 1985: Partial trisomy chromosome 5 cosegregating with schizophrenia. *Lancet* i:1023–1026.

Bracha, H.S., Torrey, E.F., Bigelow, L.B. *et al.* 1991: Subtle signs of prenatal maldevelopment of the hand ectoderm in schizophrenia: a preliminary monozygotic twin study. *Biological Psychiatry* 30:719–725.

Brown, G.W. & Birley, J.L.T. 1968: Crises and life changes and the onset of schizophrenia. *Journal of Health and Social Behaviour* 9:203.

Castle, D.J., Scott, K., Wessely, S. & Murray, R.M. 1993: Does social deprivation during gestation and early life predispose to later schizophrenia? *Social Psychiatry and Psychiatric Epidemiology* 28:1–4.

Chua, S.E. & McKenna, P.J. 1995: Schizophrenia – a brain disease? A critical review of structural and functional cerebral abnormality in the disorder. *British Journal of Psychiatry* 166:563–582.

DeLisi, L.E., Henn, S., Bass, N. *et al.* 1994: Depression in schizophrenia: is the Kraepelinian binary system dead? *Proceedings of the 9th World Congress of Psychiatry 1993*. Macclesfield: Gardiner–Caldwell Communications.

Duinkerke, S.J., Botter, P.A., Jansen, A.I.I. *et al.* 1993: Ritanserin, a selective 5-HT2/1c antagonist, and negative symptoms in schizophrenia: a placebo-controlled double-blind trial. *British Journal of Psychiatry* 163:451–455.

Feighner, J.P., Robins, E., Guze, S.B., Woodruff, R.A. Jr, Winokeer, G. & Munoz, R. 1972: Diagnostic criteria for use in psychiatric research. *Archives of General Psychiatry* 26:57–63.

Goldberg, E.M. & Morrison, S.L. 1963: Schizophrenia and social class. *British Journal of Psychiatry* 109: 785–802.

Goldstein, J.M., Faraone, S.V., Chen, W.J. & Tsuang, M.T. 1993: The role of gender in understanding the familial transmission of schizoaffective disorder. *British Journal of Psychiatry* 163:763–768.

Gottesman, I.I. & Shields, J. 1972: *Schizophrenia and Genetics: A Twin Study Vantage Point.* New York: Academic Press.

Howard, R.J., Almeida, O., Levy R. *et al.* 1994: Quantitative magnetic resonance imaging volumetry distinguishes delusional disorder from late onset schizophrenia. *British Journal of Psychiatry* 165:474–480.

Johnstone, E.C., Crow, T.J., Frith, C.D., Husband, J. & Kreel, L. 1976: Cerebral ventricular size and cognitive impairment in chronic schizophrenia. *Lancet* ii:924–926.

Johnstone, E.C., Crow, T.J., Frith, C.D. *et al.* 1978: Mechanism of the antipsychotic effect in the treatment of acute schizophrenia. *Lancet* ii:848–851.

Kahn, R.S., Davidson, M., Knott, P. *et al.* 1993: Effect of neuroleptic medication on cerebrospinal fluid monoamine metabolite concentrations in schizophrenia. *Archives of General Psychiatry* 50:599–605.

Kane, J.M. & Freeman, H.L. 1994: Towards more effective antipsychotic treatment. *British Journal of Psychiatry* 165 (Suppl. 25):22–31.

Kane, J.M., Honigfield, G., Singer, J. *et al.* 1988: Clozapine for the treatment-resistant schizophrenic: a double-blind comparison with chlorpromazine. *Archives of General Psychiatry* 45:789–796.

Kety, S.S., Rosenthal, D., Wender, P.H. *et al.* 1971: Mental illness in the biological and adoptive families of adopted schizophrenics. *American Journal of Psychiatry* 128:302.

Leff, J., Thornicroft, G., Coxhead, N. *et al.* 1994: The TAPS project: 22. A five-year follow-up of long-stay psychiatric patients discharged to the community. *British Journal of Psychiatry* 165 (Suppl. 25):13–17.

Lewis, S.W. & Murray, R.M. 1988: Obstetric complications, neurodevelopmental deviance and risk of schizophrenia. *Journal of Psychiatric Research* 21:473.

Liddle, P.F., Friston , K.J., Frith, C.D. *et al.* 1992: Patterns of cerebral blood flow in schizophrenia. *British Journal of Psychiatry* 160:179–186.

Lieberman, J.A. & Sobel, S.N. 1993: Predictors of treatment response and course of schizophrenia. *Current Opinion in Psychiatry* 6:63–69.

Mednick, S.A., Machon, R.A., Huttunen, M.O. & Bonnet, D. 1988: Adult schizophrenia following prenatal exposure to an influenza epidemic. *Archives of General Psychiatry* 45:189–192.

Meltzer, H.Y., Myung, A.L. & Ranjan, R. 1994: Recent advances in the pharmacotherapy of schizophrenia. *Acta Psychiatrica Scandinavica* 90 (Suppl. 384):95–101.

Murray, R.M., Lewis, S.W., Owen, M.J. & Foester, A. 1988: Neurodevelopmental origins of dementia praecox. In Bebbington, P. & McGuffin, P. (eds) *Schizophrenia: The Major Issue*. London: Heinemann.

Murray, R.M., O'Callaghan, E., Castle, D.J. & Lewis, S.W. 1992: A neurodevelopmental approach to the classification of schizophrenia. *Schizophrenia Bulletin* 18:319–332.

Roy, A. 1982: Suicide in chronic schizophrenia. *British Journal of Psychiatry* 141:171–177.

Sherrington, R., Brynjjolfsson, J., Petursson H. *et al.* 1988: Localisation of a susceptibility locus for schizophrenia on chromosome 5. *Nature* 336:164–167.

Spitzer, R.L., Endicott, J. & Robins, E. 1975: *Research Diagnostic Criteria (RDC) for a Selected Group of Functional Disorders*. New York: New York State Psychiatric Institute.

Syvälahti, E.K.G. 1994: Biological factors in schizophrenia: structural and functional aspects. *British Journal of Psychiatry* 164 (Suppl. 23):9–14.

Torgersen, S. 1994: Personality deviations within the schizophrenia spectrum. *Acta Psychiatrica Scandinavica* (Suppl. 384):40–44.

Tsuang, M.T. 1991: Morbidity risks of schizophrenia and affective disorders among first-degree relatives of patients with schizoaffective disorders. *British Journal of Psychiatry* 158:165–170.

Vaughn, C.E. & Leff, J.P. 1976: Influence of family and social factors on the course of psychiatric illness. *British Journal of Psychiatry* 129:125–137.

Weinberger, D.R., Berman, K.F. & Zec, R.F. 1986: Physiological dysfunction of dorsolateral prefrontal cortex in schizophrenia: I. Regional cerebral blood flow evidence. *Archives of General Psychiatry* 43:114–124.

Wing, J., Cooper, J.E. & Sartorius, N. 1974: *The Description of Psychiatric Symptoms: An Introduction Manual for the PSE and CATEGO System*. Cambridge: Cambridge University Press.

Wing, J.K. & Brown, G.W. 1961: Social treatment of chronic schizophrenia: a comparative survey of three mental hospitals. *Journal of Mental Science* 107:847.

Wing, J.K. & Brown, G.W. 1970: *Institutionalism and Schizophrenia*. Cambridge: Cambridge University Press.

Wong, D.F., Wagner, H.N., Tune, L.E. *et al.* 1986: Positron emission tomography reveals elevated D2 dopamine receptors in drug naive schizophrenics. *Science* 234:1558–1563.

World Health Organization 1973: *Report of the International Pilot Study of Schizophrenia*. Geneva: WHO.

World Health Organization 1992: *The ICD-10 Classification of Mental and Behavioural Disorders*. Geneva: WHO.

28

Mood disorders, suicide and parasuicide

HISTORY

- In 1921, Kraepelin divided the functional psychoses into two broad categories, *dementia praecox* and *manic–depressive insanity*. He thought of the latter as a disorder in which discrete episodes of illness alternated with clearly defined well periods during which patients returned to their previous state of health.
- In 1949, Cade first initiated the use of lithium, but it was not widely used until the 1960s.
- In the 1950s, tricyclic and monoamine oxidase inhibitor (MAOI) antidepressants were introduced.
- In the 1970s, anticonvulsants were first used for bipolar disorders. Specific psychological treatments (e.g. cognitive therapy) were introduced.
- In the 1980s, selective serotonin re-uptake inhibitors (SSRIs) were introduced.

CLASSIFICATIONS OF MOOD DISORDERS

ICD-10 classifications

BIPOLAR AFFECTIVE DISORDER

There are repeated episodes of mood disturbance, sometimes elevated, sometimes depressed.

Repeated episodes of *mania* are classified as bipolar (sufferers resemble those who also have depressive episodes in their family history, premorbid personality, age of onset and prognosis). It includes:

- bipolar affective disorder with:
  - current episode hypomanic, or
  - current episode manic without psychotic symptoms, or
  - current episode manic with psychotic symptoms
- bipolar affective disorder with:
  - current episode having mild/moderate depression, or
  - current episode having severe depression without psychotic symptoms, or

- current episode having severe depression with psychotic symptoms
- bipolar affective disorder with:
  - current episode mixed.

MANIC EPISODE

The fundamental disturbance is an elevation of mood to elation, with concomitant increase in activity level. Three degrees of manic episode are specified by ICD-10, all used for a single manic episode only:

- *Hypomania.* There is persistent elevated mood, increased energy and activity, feelings of wellbeing, and reduced need for sleep. Irritability may replace elation. Work is considerably disrupted. There are no hallucinations or delusions.
- *Mania without psychotic symptoms.* Mood is elevated, with almost uncontrollable excitement. There is over-activity, pressured speech, reduced sleep, distractible, inflated self-esteem, and grandiose thoughts. Perceptual heightening may occur. The person may spend excessively, become aggressive, amorous, or facetious.
- *Mania with psychotic symptoms.* The symptoms are as above, but with delusions and hallucinations, usually grandiose. There may be sustained physical activity, aggression and self-neglect.

DEPRESSIVE EPISODE

There is depression of mood, reduced energy and fatiguability. Mood is pervasively depressed. Other features are reduced attention and concentration, lowered self-esteem, ideas of guilt and worthlessness, pessimistic thoughts, thoughts of self-harm or suicide, and disturbed sleep.

Somatic changes include reduced appetite leading to weight loss (at least 5% of bodyweight in a month), constipation, early morning wakening (more than 2 hours before usual), diurnal variation of mood, anhedonia, loss of normal reactivity of mood, reduced libido, amenorrhoea, and psychomotor retardation or agitation.

A duration of 2 weeks is required for the diagnosis. This applies to the first episode only. Severity is graded:

- mild depressive episode
- moderate depressive episode
- severe depressive episode without psychotic symptoms
- severe depressive episode with psychotic symptoms.

RECURRENT DEPRESSIVE DISORDER

There are repeated episodes of depression, without episodes of mania. Recovery between episodes is usually complete, but a minority become chronic, especially in the elderly. It includes:

- recurrent depressive disorder with:
  - current episode mild, or
  - current episode moderate, or
  - current episode severe without psychotic symptoms, or
  - current episode severe with psychotic symptoms
- recurrent depressive disorder, currently in remission.

Other classifications of depression

Depression is variously classified, and the usefulness of differing categories is still under debate.

ENDOGENOUS VERSUS REACTIVE DEPRESSION

This is a distinction drawn by Roth and the Newcastle School in the 1950s.

- The *endogenous form* is thought to be of biological origin, with psychomotor retardation or agitation, loss of appetite and weight, anhedonia, early morning wakening and diurnal mood variation.
- The *reactive form* is thought to be of psychological origin. Depression is moderate; anxiety, irritability, initial insomnia and mood remains reactive.

However, triggering events are present in both types.

Kendall (1965) failed to find a point of rarity in symptomatology between neurotic/psychotic depression, so concluded that there are no essential differences between them.

UNIPOLAR VERSUS BIPOLAR DEPRESSION

This is a distinction due to Leonhard, Angst and Perris in the 1950s.

- *Unipolar depression* is more common in females. Episodes are longer, with somatic symptoms, anxiety, agitation, suicidal ideas, weight loss and initial insomnia.
- In *bipolar depression* a seasonal pattern and hypersomnia tend to be more commonly present. There are more male sufferers, more family history of mania, an earlier and more acute onset (15 years earlier than 'unipolars' on average), and more episodes.

No difference is observed in sleep EEGs of these two groups.

Bipolar I and bipolar II

- Bipolar I refers to major depression alternating with mania.
- Bipolar II refers to major depression alternating with hypomania.

Rapid–cycling bipolar disorder

This refers to those patients who experience four or more affective episodes in 12 months. It is more common in women, predicts poorer prognosis with more lifetime affective episodes and a poorer response to lithium and other treatments. Twenty per cent are induced by antidepressant drugs.

OTHER CLASSES

Dysthymia

This is a chronic, less severe depression, usually with an insidious onset. Symptoms include excessive guilt, difficulty in concentrating, loss of interest, pessimism, low self-esteem, low energy, irritability and reduced productivity. For the diagnosis it must be present for at least 2 years. ICD-10 and DSM-IV-TR criteria are similar.

Double depression

This is a major depression superimposed upon dysthymia.

Depressive stupor

The person is unresponsive, akinetic, mute and fully conscious. Following an episode, the patient can recall the events that took place at the time. Episodes of excitement may occur between episodes of stupor.

Recurrent brief depression

In 1990, Angst proposed diagnostic criteria for this condition: dysphoric mood or loss of interest for a duration of less than 2 weeks, with at least four of the following: poor appetite, sleep problems, agitation, loss of interest, fatigue, feelings of worthlessness, difficulty concentrating, and suicidality. One or two episodes per month for at least a year are characteristic.

Masked depression

In masked depression, depressed mood is not always complained of, rather somatic or other complaints. It is more common in the undeveloped world and in those unable to articulate their emotions (e.g. those with learning disability or dementia). The presence of biological symptoms is helpful in making the diagnosis. Diurnal variation in abnormal behaviour may mirror diurnal variation in mood.

Seasonal affective disorder (SAD)

In SAD there is a regular temporal relationship between the onset of depressive episodes and a particular time of year. Depressive episodes commence in autumn or winter months and end in the spring or summer months as the hours of daylight increase.

Note that the onset of bipolar disorders may be seasonal. Hyperphagia, hypersomnia and weight gain are more frequent than in matched non-seasonal patients.

Atypical depression

This is depression characterized by reversed neurovegetative symptoms such as psychomotor retardation, hypersomnia and hyperphagia with weight gain.

Mixed affective states

Kraepelin maintained that mood, cognition and behaviour may vary independently, producing mixed affective states which are usually transitional, but are sometimes persistent.

Bereavement reactions

Grief usually has three phases. The *stunned* phase lasts from a few hours to a few weeks. This gives way to the *mourning* phase, with intense yearning and autonomic symptoms. After several weeks the phase of *acceptance and adjustment* takes over. Grief typically lasts about six months.

Atypical grief is divided by Parkes (1985) into:

- unexpected grief syndrome
- ambivalent grief syndrome
- chronic grief.

EPIDEMIOLOGY OF MOOD DISORDERS

DEPRESSIVE EPISODES

Problems are encountered in epidemiological studies of mood disorders because of the differing use of diagnostic categories, screening instruments and definitions of caseness.

Broadly, depressive episodes are more common in females: the annual *incidence* in men in the population is between 80 and 200 per 100 000, the corresponding figure for women being between 250 and 7800 per 100 000. There is a raised incidence in those who are not married. The *point prevalence* in Western countries is 1.8–3.2% for men and 2.0–9.3% for women.

The point prevalence of depressive *symptoms* is 10–30% (women 18–34%, men 10–19%). In the general population of Western countries, the *lifetime risk* of suffering from depressive episodes is 5–12% for men and 9–26% for women.

The *average age of onset* of depressive episodes is around the late thirties; however, they can start at any age.

Brown and Harris (1978) found that 15% of urban women had severe depressive symptoms, and there was a higher prevalence in working-class than in middle-class women.

BIPOLAR MOOD DISORDER

The sex ratio is equal, and it is more common in the upper social classes. The *point prevalence* in Western countries is 0.4–1.2% in the adult population. In the general population of Western countries, the *lifetime risk* of suffering from a bipolar disorder is 0.6–1.1%. The *average age of onset* is around the mid-twenties.

AETIOLOGY OF MOOD DISORDERS

Genetic factors

Family studies
In unipolar probands there is an increased risk of unipolar depression in first-degree relatives, but the amount of bipolar illness is virtually the same as in the general population (combined risk = 7–8%). In bipolar probands there is an increased risk of both bipolar and unipolar disorder in first-degree relatives (combined risk = 18–20%).

Twin studies
In a large Danish twin study of affective disorder (Bertelson *et al.*, 1977), the concordance rate for monozygotic (MZ) twins was 67%, compared with 20% for dizygotic (DZ) twins. The MZ to DZ concordance ratio for bipolar disorder of 79:19 compared with 54:24 for unipolar disorder.

Adoption studies
In adoptees with bipolar disorder, 28% of biological parents suffer from a mood disorder compared with 12% of adoptive parents. By comparison, 26% of the biological parents of bipolar non-adoptees were found to suffer from a mood disorder.

Molecular genetics
In certain families, manic depressive illness has been cross-linked to colour blindness and glucose-6-phosphate deficiency.

Egeland *et al.* (1987) found linkage to chromosome 11 in an old-order Amish pedigree. This finding is now thought to have been a statistical artefact and has not been replicated. In linkage studies of complex diseases such as manic depressive disorder, spurious linkage may be produced because of phenotypic misclassification and misspecification of the disease model.

Personality factors in mood disorder

Cyclothymic personality disorder
This is characterized by persistent instability of mood with numerous periods of mild depression and mild elation. It may predispose to bipolar disorder.

Depressive personality disorder
This is related to the mood disorders, overlapping substantially with them, but not congruent with them. It often coexists with mood disorders. Core phenomena are excessive negative, pessimistic beliefs about oneself and others. Symptoms include unhappy, gloomy mood, low self-esteem, being self-critical, brooding, negativistic and judgemental towards others, pessimism and prone to feelings of guilt.

Psychosocial stressors in mood disorder

Vaughn and Leff (1976) showed that high expressed emotion (EE) increased the risks of relapse in depressed patients. Compared to schizophrenics, depressives were more sensitive to critical remarks. However, hostility and over-involvement did not add to the significant association. The effect of critical comments (criticism index) was not mitigated by reducing the number of hours depressed people spent in contact with their relatives (unlike schizophrenia, in which it was).

Excess life events occur in the six months before a depressive episode starts. Brown and Harris (1978), in a community survey in Camberwell, south London, identified *vulnerability factors* which increase the risk of depression if a *provoking agent* is present. Four vulnerability factors are:

- having three or more children at home under the age of 14 years
- not working outside the home
- lack of a confiding relationship
- loss of the mother before the age of 11 years.

Vulnerability factors may operate by reducing self-esteem.

Kendler *et al.* (1995) compared stressful life events in twins with and without depression. He found that, in those with the lowest risk (MZ co-twin unaffected), the probabilities of onset of major depression were 0.5% and 6.2% respectively for those unexposed and exposed to the life event. In those at highest genetic risk (MZ co-twin affected), these probabilities were 1.1% and 14.6% respectively. He concluded that genetic factors influence the risk of the onset of major depression in part by altering the sensitivity of individuals to the depression-inducing effect of stressful life events.

Physical illness in mood disorder

Viral infection, particularly influenza, hepatitis A and brucellosis, are sometimes accompanied or followed by depressed mood. More recently, a significant association has been found between the occurrence of anti-Borna Disease Virus (BDV) antibodies and mood disorder (unipolar and bipolar) (Terayama *et al.*, 2003).

Endocrine disorders commonly predispose to depression. Eighty-three per cent of people with Cushing's syndrome develop affective disorder during the course of their disorder. It is also seen in hypothyroidism and hypo- and hyperparathyroidism.

Psychological factors in mood disorder

Seligman gave naive dogs unavoidable electric shocks and found that, after learning that there was nothing that could be done to influence the outcome of events, the dogs finally developed a condition which he thought resembled depression in humans, with reduced appetite, reduced sex drive and disturbed sleep. He called this condition *learned helplessness.*

It has been suggested that in humans depression is more likely to occur if the helplessness is perceived to be attributable to a personal source, thus leading to lowered self-esteem. Global stable attributions are likely to be the longest lasting.

Beck *et al.* (1979) proposed a cognitive model of depression from which cognitive therapy has developed. Three concepts seek to explain the psychological substrate of depression:

- *Cognitive triad.* The depressed person has:
  - a negative personal view
  - a tendency to interpret his or her ongoing experiences in a negative way
  - a negative view of the future.
- *Schemas.* These are stable cognitive patterns forming the basis for the interpretation of situations.
- *Cognitive errors.* These are systematic errors in thinking that maintain depressed people's beliefs in negative concepts.

  Cognitive distortions include:

- arbitrary inference
- selective abstraction
- over-generalization
- personalization
- magnification and minimization
- dichotomous thinking.

Neurotransmitters in mood disorder

According to Schildkraut in 1965 the monoamine hypothesis of mood disorders stated that depression was associated with a depletion, and mania with an excess, of central monoamine. Evidence favouring this hypothesis includes the following findings:

- Tricyclic antidepressants inhibit the re-uptake of noradrenaline and serotonin by presynaptic neurones, leading to an increase in the availability of these monoamines in the synaptic cleft.
- Monoamine oxidase inhibitors increase the availability of monoamines, by inhibiting their metabolic degradation by monoamine oxidase.
- Selective serotonin re-uptake inhibitors (SSRIs) increase the availability of serotonin by inhibiting the re-uptake of serotonin.
- Use of antidepressants in bipolar disorder can precipitate mania.
- Amphetamine releases catecholamines from the neurones; it is a central nervous system stimulant that lifts mood.
- Reserpine, an antihypertensive drug derived from the Indian plant Rauwolfia, depletes central monoaminergic neuronal stores of catecholamines and serotonin. Its use can lead to severe depression and suicide.

- The cerebrospinal fluid level of the serotonin metabolite 5-hydroxyindole-acetic acid (5-HIAA) is often reported as being reduced in depressed patients.
- Impaired repression at a 5-hydroxytryptamine 1A receptor gene polymorphism is associated with major depression and suicide (Lemonde *et al.*, 2003).
- The antidepressant effects of light therapy combined with sleep deprivation are influenced by a functional polymorphism within the promoter of the serotonin transporter gene (Benedetti *et al.*, 2003).

Evidence against the monoamine hypothesis includes the following:

- Antidepressant pharmacotherapy takes at least a fortnight to effect a clinical improvement. This time interval is much greater than the relatively rapid onset of biochemical action.
- Not all drugs that act as monoamine re-uptake inhibitors have a therapeutic antidepressant action (e.g. cocaine).

Serotonin

Additional evidence for abnormal serotonergic function in mood disorders includes the following:

- In subgroups of depressed patients, low levels of 5-HIAA have been reported in cerebrospinal fluid.
- In depressed patients, a low density of brain and platelet serotonin transporter sites has been found, as well as a high density of brain and platelet serotonin binding sites.
- Dietary tryptophan depletion induced a prompt relapse in depressed patients who had responded to SSRIs.
- There is a low plasma tryptophan in depressed patients.
- All SSRIs are clinically effective antidepressants.
- Serotonin function is reduced in depression and may be normalized with active treatment.

Adaptive changes in receptors

During antidepressant treatment, changes take place in cerebral α- and β-adrenergic and serotonin receptors, showing only after 2 weeks of treatment, at the same time as the therapeutic effect. A decrease in the sensitivity (down-regulation) of β-adrenergic receptors is particularly evident.

Neuroendocrine factors in mood disorder

THE BRAIN–STEROID AXIS

Disturbances of the hypothalamic–pituitary–adrenal axis are reported in depression. In normal humans, cortisol secretion is episodic and follows a circadian rhythm. Peak cortisol secretion is in the morning; between noon and 4 a.m. secretion remains low, being lowest just after the onset of sleep.

In biological depression, there is disruption in the normal circadian rhythm of cortisol secretion, the morning peak being increased and longer lasting. A phase shift with the morning peak occurring earlier has been reported.

In depressed patients, increased secretion has been reported in corticotrophin (ACTH), cortisol, β-endorphin and prolactin.

In the dexamethasone suppression test (DST), plasma cortisol levels are measured following the administration of the long-acting potent synthetic steroid dexamethasone the previous evening. In normal subjects, dexamethasone leads to a suppression in the level of cortisol over the next 24 hours through negative feedback. In depressed patients with biological symptoms, non-suppression of cortisol has been reported in over 60%. The DST has not proved to be a useful laboratory test for depression because a relatively high level of cortisol non-suppression has been found in other psychiatric disorders. The DST can be affected by factors such as age, bodyweight, drugs, ECT and endocrinopathies. The DST is usually state-dependent and in most subjects normalizes as the patient recovers.

Corticotropin-releasing factor (CRH or CRF) is an important hypothalamic peptide in the regulation of appetite and eating. In the CRH stimulation test the administration of CRH to normal humans leads to the release of corticotropin. In depression there is a consistent reduction of corticotropin response.

The noradrenergic neurones of the locus coeruleus express glucocorticoid receptors, through which corticosteroids can regulate its functioning. It is hypothesized that steroids may be important in causing and perpetuating depression.

THE BRAIN–THYROID AXIS

Thyroid-releasing hormone (TRH) causes the release of thyroid-stimulating hormone (TSH) from the adenohypophysis. In normal subjects there is a circadian pattern of TSH secretion, with a nocturnal rise which is blunted in depression and returns with sleep deprivation. In the TRH stimulation test the TSH response to intravenous TRH is measured. About 25% of depressed patients show a blunted TSH response to TRH stimulation. This does not often normalize as the subject recovers from depression. Blunting is also found in panic disorder. TRH stimulation studies in depression have also shown that approximately 15% of patients have a raised TSH response; many of these patients have been found to have antimicrosomal thyroid and anti-thyroglobulin antibodies, indicating that depression can be associated with symptomless auto-immune thyroiditis.

MELATONIN

Patients with depression have disordered biological rhythms – short REM latency (time from falling asleep to onset of REM sleep), early morning wakening, and diurnal mood variation. The suprachiasmatic nucleus (SCN) of the hypothalamus plays a major role in regulating diurnal rhythms. Information about light conditions from the retina, via the retinohypothalamic pathway, controls the SCN. This influences the pineal which excretes melatonin. The biosynthesis of melatonin from its precursor, serotonin, occurs via *N*-acetylation followed by *O*-methylation. The step involving serotonin *N*-acetyltransferase is probably rate-limiting and is stimulated at night. Melatonin receptors are numerous in the SCN and parts of the hypothalamus where releasing and inhibiting hormones end. Darkness stimulates melatonin release and light blocks its synthesis. When compared with normal subjects, patients with seasonal affective disorder (SAD) have been found to have an increased sensitivity of melatonin biosynthesis to inhibition by phototherapy.

WATER AND ELECTROLYTE CHANGES

There are increases in the body's residual sodium (which is an index of intracellular sodium ion concentration) in both depression and mania. Erythrocyte sodium ion concentrations decrease following recovery from depression or mania as a result of increased Na^+–K^+-ATPase activity.

MANAGEMENT OF MOOD DISORDERS

Pharmacotherapy

UNIPOLAR DEPRESSION

Categories
Frank *et al.* (1991) have categorized outcomes of treatment according to the '5 Rs':

- *Response.*
- *Remission.* This is a return to the patient's premorbid self.
- *Relapse.* This is a return of depressive symptoms in the time between initial response and recovery. Risk is particularly high (40–60%) following the withdrawal of antidepressants within the first 4 months of achieving a response. The risk of relapse is reduced to 10–30% by continuation of pharmacotherapy.
- *Recovery.* A patient who has achieved a stable remission for at least 4–6 months is assumed to have recovered from the index episode.
- *Recurrence.* This is a return of depression after recovery from the index episode. Risk factors for recurrent depression include frequent and/or multiple prior episodes, seasonal pattern, and a family history of mood disorder.

Acute treatment
This is initial treatment which aims to achieve a response.

Continuation treatment
This begins when a patient has achieved a significant response to treatment. The aim is to prevent relapse and consolidate response into remission.

Maintenance treatment
This follows continuation treatment for those patients with a history of recurrent depression. A recurrence rate of 85% is seen in those patients with recurrent depression within 3 years following the discontinuation of pharmacotherapy. After 6 months, continuation becomes maintenance treatment by arbitrary definition.

In an MRC trial in 1965, 269 patients with operationally defined depression were randomly assigned to treatment groups, with the following results at 4 weeks:

- a tricyclic antidepressant (imipramine) response rate of 53%
- an MAOI (phenelzine) response rate of 30%
- a placebo response rate of 39%
- an ECT response rate of 71%.

Drugs
The first-line treatment of depression is with antidepressants. It is important that patients receive an adequate dose for an adequate duration, conventionally 6 weeks. Antidepressants should be continued for 4–6 months after the amelioration of symptoms of the acute episode. Maintenance therapy usually with the same agent is used to treat the acute and continuation phases.

Lithium is efficacious in preventing recurrent depressive episodes, but less so than tricyclic antidepressants.

Patients maintained on the full effective treatment dose of antidepressants have proportionately fewer relapses than those whose dose is cut down to a lower maintenance level.

ATYPICAL DEPRESSION

This responds better to monoamine oxidase inhibitors than to tricyclic antidepressants.

PSYCHOTIC DEPRESSION

Spiker *et al.* (1985) found a superior response when an antidepressant and an antipychotic were used in combination, in delusional depression:

- 41% responded to amitriptyline alone
- 19% responded to perphenazine alone
- 78% responded to a combination of amitriptyline and perphenazine.

RESISTANT MAJOR DEPRESSION

Up to 20% of patients may be resistant to first line treatment with antidepressant medication, and another 20–30% may have only a partial response. Patients with a partial response have a significantly higher rate of relapse during the first 6 months following response.

Those patients not showing a response to adequate first-line drug treatment may respond to augmentation with various agents including lithium, T_3 or tryptophan. ECT should be tried if these measures fail.

BIPOLAR AFFECTIVE DISORDER

The treatment of acute mania is with neuroleptic medication. Lithium carbonate and citrate are used in the prophylaxis of bipolar disorder. They can also be used in the treatment of acute mania, but neuroleptics are preferred in the first instance.

A maintenance strategy consisting of lithium carbonate monotherapy in bipolar disorder is likely to result in sustained remission in approximately 50% of cases.

The premature withdrawal of lithium in bipolar patients results in more than 80% of recurrences within 36 months, a 28-fold increase compared to those left on lithium. Low-dose maintenance strategies (less than the usual acute antimanic range of (0.8–1.2 mmol/L) lead to an increased risk of relapse.

In cases of bipolar disorder which are resistant to or intolerant of lithium, alternative prophylactic treatment with carbamazepine or sodium valproate are effective, both as acute antimanic treatment and as prophylaxis.

Electroconvulsive therapy (ECT) in mood disorder

Double-blind placebo-controlled trials have shown ECT to be superior to placebo, especially in delusional depression. It is considered the gold standard of antidepressant therapy and is often given to patients who have not responded to antidepressants. ECT is also used in the treatment of resistant mania or manic stupor.

Psychosocial treatments

PSYCHOTHERAPIES

This includes interpersonal therapy, cognitive therapy and behavioural therapy. Most progress has been made with psychotherapies for the acute treatment of major depression. Numerous trials have demonstrated the efficacy of psychotherapy in reducing the acute symptoms of depression, with greatest efficacy in more mildly ill patients. They are associated with a longer lag period for response than drug treatment. They may be a promising alternative to drugs during long-term maintenance treatment.

COMPUTERIZED CBT: NICE GUIDELINES (UK)

In 2002, the National Institute for Clinical Excellence issued guidance to the National Health Service on the use of computerized cognitive behavioural therapy (CCBT). The guidance states that current research shows that CCBT may be of value in the management of anxiety and depression, but that this evidence is not strong enough to recommend CCBT for general use in the NHS.

In particular, the committee concluded that it is still uncertain how CCBT works alongside other treatments such as therapist-led therapy. There were also uncertainties about the type, quantity and quality of support required from a facilitator to accompany CCBT, and about where and how CCBT should be delivered.

Prognosis for mood disorders

Depression is a chronic and recurrent condition. It has become increasingly clear that a significant proportion of patients followed in the long term after suffering from depression remain chronically ill, despite the previously held belief that patients tended to recover fully between depressive episodes. Factors predicting a prolonged time to recovery are the longer duration and the increased severity of the index episode, a history of non-affective psychiatric disorder, lower family income, and married status during the index episode.

It has been found that 15–20% of depressed patients develop a chronic course of illness and 75–80% suffer multiple episodes. The risk of relapse decreases the longer the patient remains well. For a first episode of depression, an older age and a history of previous non-affective psychiatric illness predicts a shorter time to relapse. Continuing high levels of medication in the first few months is associated with a higher chance of remaining well. Overall, there is a suicide rate of around 15%.

The time to recovery from the index episode of major depression in patients suffering from double depression is shorter than in patients suffering major depression alone, but they tend to relapse more frequently and rapidly.

PERSISTENT MOOD DISORDERS

ICD-10 describes persistent and usually fluctuating disorders of mood in which individual episodes are rarely sufficiently severe to warrant being described as hypomanic or mild depressive episodes. They may last for years at a time, sometimes for the greater part of adult life and involve considerable subjective distress and disability.

In ICD-10, the persistent mood disorders are classed with the mood disorders rather than with the personality disorders because of evidence from family studies which suggests that the persistent mood disorders are genetically related to other mood disorders.

The two most important persistent mood disorders are cyclothymia and dysthymia.

CYCLOTHYMIA

Cyclothymia is defined in ICD-10 as:

> A persistent instability of mood, involving numerous periods of mild depression and mild elation. This instability usually develops early in adult life and pursues a chronic course, although at times the mood may be normal and stable for months at a time. The lifetime risk of cyclothymia is between 0.4 and 3.5%, sex ratio equal. First-degree relatives of patients with cyclothymia are more likely than the general population to suffer from depressive episodes and bipolar disorder.

Some are treated successfully with lithium and/or with individual or group psychotherapy.

DYSTHYMIA

Dysthymia, also called *depressive neurosis*, is defined in ICD-10 as:

> A chronic depression of mood which does not fulfil the criteria for recurrent depressive disorder . . . . The balance between individual phases of mild depression and intervening periods of comparative normality is very variable. Sufferers usually have periods of days or weeks when they describe themselves as well, but most of the time . . . they feel tired and depressed; everything is an effort and nothing is enjoyed. They brood and complain, sleep badly and feel inadequate, but are usually able to cope with the basic demands of everyday life.

Dysthymia is probably more common in women than in men. It is more common in first-degree relatives of patients with a history of depressive episodes than in the general population.

Treatment with antidepressants, individual psychotherapy or cognitive therapy may be helpful.

SUICIDE AND PARASUICIDE (DELIBERATE SELF–HARM)

Suicide

EPIDEMIOLOGY

The annual incidence of suicide in England and Wales is approximately 1 in 10 000 of the population. It is more common in men than women and also more common in those aged over 45 years. The highest rates are in those who are divorced, single or widowed. The highest rates are in social classes I and V.

Suicide is associated with unemployment and retirement. Suicide rates fell in England and Wales during the First and Second World Wars.

There is a seasonal variation in suicide rates. In the northern hemisphere, suicide rates are highest during the months of spring and early summer. In the southern hemisphere, rates are highest in the months corresponding to spring and early summer.

There is evidence that the availability of method affects gross suicide rates as well as the choice of method. Suicide rates by hanging were constant until the 1960s when there was a rise after the abolition of capital punishment. A massive reduction in the number of deaths caused by gassing followed the switch from coal gas to the safer North Sea gas in the 1960s. A marked rise in poisoning in the early 1960s was because of the increased availability of medicines such as barbiturates.

AETIOLOGY OF SUICIDE

Statistics

Ninety per cent of people who commit suicide suffer from a psychiatric disorder. Of these, approximately 50% suffer depression, 25% alcoholism, 5% schizophrenia and 20% other (e.g. personality disorder, chronic neuroses, and psychoactive substance abuse disorders). The rate of suicide is increased by 50 times the population rate among psychiatric inpatients. There is also an association with physical illnesses, particularly chronic painful illnesses, epilepsy (especially temporal lobe epilepsy), cancer, peptic ulcer and gastric ulcer disease.

Following an act of deliberate self-harm the risk of completing suicide in the subsequent year is approximately 100 times that in the general population, and remains high in subsequent years.

Associations

Positive associations with suicide in the general population include:

- being male
- being elderly
- having suffered loss or bereavement
- being unemployed
- being retired
- childlessness
- living alone in a big, densely populated town
- a broken home in childhood
- mental or physical illness
- loss of role
- social disorganization, including overcrowding, criminality, drug and alcohol misuse.

Negative associations include:

- religious devoutness
- lots of children
- times of war.

Risk factors

Risk factors by psychiatric diagnosis are as follows:

- *Schizophrenia.* There is a 10% mortality from suicide. Roy (1982) characterized schizophrenics who commit suicide as young, male and unemployed, with chronic relapsing illness. Fewer schizophrenic patients give warning of their intention to commit suicide than patients in other diagnostic groups (23% versus 50%). The suicide is usually after recent discharge, with good insight.
- *Affective psychosis.* There is a 15% mortality from suicide. Men are older, separated, widowed or divorced, living alone and not working. Women are middle-aged, middle-class, with a history of parasuicide and threats made in the last month. Those with obsessive–compulsive symptoms are about six times less likely to commit suicide than those without.
- *Neuroses.* Nearly 90% have a history of parasuicide, and a high proportion have threatened suicide in the preceding month. There is a tendency after a failed attempt to resort to more violent means. There is a high risk in depressive neurosis and panic disorder, but a lower risk in obsessive–compulsive disorder.
- *Alcoholism.* There is a 15% mortality from suicide. It tends to occur later in the course of the illness, and those affected are often also depressed. Associated with completed suicide is poor physical health, a poor work record, previous parasuicide and a recent loss of a close relationship.

- *Personality disorder.* High risk factors are lability of mood, aggressiveness, impulsivity, alienation from peers and associated alcohol and substance misuse.

Life events and suicide
The risk of suicide increases, more among males than females, during the 5 years following the bereavement of a parent or a spouse.

Compared with psychiatric patient controls, suicides have experienced interpersonal losses more frequently, although schizophrenic suicides have experienced fewer losses than non-schizophrenic controls.

Age-related variations of stressors have been described, with conflict–separation–rejection more common in younger age groups, economic problems in middle-aged groups and medical illness among the older age groups.

Biochemical disturbances
Low 5-HIAA concentration in cerebral spinal fluid is associated with increased suicidal behaviour and aggression. Irrespective of the clinical diagnosis, the group in which CSF concentration of 5-HIAA is low often includes persons who have attempted a violent method of suicide. Serotonin may play an important role in the biology of aggression and the control of impulsive behaviour.

Postmortem ligand binding studies have found increased numbers of $5HT_2$ receptors in the prefrontal cortex of suicide victims, particularly those who used violent means. Low concentrations of serum cholesterol have been found to be prospectively associated with an increase in the risk of violent death or suicide. Biological mechanisms linking low serum cholesterol concentration and suicide have been hypothesized.

Sociological theory
Durkheim in 1897 used the phenomenon of suicide to describe society (see also Chapter 7). He described four types of suicide:

- *Altruistic.* The individual sets no value on life and renounces his or her personal being in order to be engulfed into something wider (e.g. religious or terrorist suicides).
- *Egoistic.* Suicide springs from excessive individuation of the individual from society.
- *Anomic.* This relates to how society regulates the individual. Suicide results from the fact that a human's activities lack regulation.
- *Fatalistic.* This is a rare type of suicide, the opposite of anomic, deriving from excessive regulation by oppressive regimes.

ASSESSMENT OF THE INDIVIDUAL FOR SUICIDE

Suicidal ideation should be explored in every patient and forms a part of the routine mental state examination. There is no evidence that asking patients about suicidal thoughts increases the risk of suicide.

The majority of people who commit suicide have told somebody beforehand of their thoughts. Two-thirds have seen their GP in the previous month. One-quarter have been psychiatric outpatients at the time of death; half of them will have seen a psychiatrist in the previous week.

MANAGEMENT OF SUICIDAL IDEATION

Once the need for treatment has been identified it should be provided quickly. The interval between GP referral to psychiatric services and consultation has been identified as a danger period and should be minimized.

If there is a serious risk of suicide the patient should be admitted to hospital. Any psychiatric disorder from which the patient suffers should be treated appropriately. If the patient is suffering from severe depression, electroconvulsive therapy may be required. Patients with manic depression have a mortality up to three times that of the general population, with suicide and cardiovascular disease being primarily responsible. In patients treated with lithium prophylaxis, cumulative mortality does not differ from that of the general population. A minimum of 2 years of lithium treatment is needed to reduce the high mortality resulting from manic depression. It is proposed that lithium exerts its anti-suicide effect as a result of improved serotonergic transmission.

Parasuicide

EPIDEMIOLOGY

There is an annual incidence of about three in 1000, but this is probably an under-estimate. It is most common in females and in those aged below 35 years. The highest rates are in those who are divorced or single, among the lower social classes, unemployed, and living in overcrowded urban areas in which there are high rates of juvenile delinquency.

Ninety per cent of cases involve deliberate self-poisoning with drugs. Forty per cent use minor tranquillizers and a further 30% use salicylates and paracetamol.

AETIOLOGY OF PARASUICIDE

Compared with the general population, life events are more common in the 6 months before an act of parasuicide. These include the break-up of a relationship, trouble with the law, physical illness and the illness of a loved one.

Predisposing factors include:

- marital difficulties
- unemployment
- physical illness, particularly epilepsy
- mental retardation
- parental neglect or abuse.

Motives include interruption, attention, communication, or a true wish to die.

ASSESSMENT OF THE INDIVIDUAL FOR SUICIDE

A high degree of suicidal intent is indicated by the following:

- The act was planned and prepared.
- Precautions were taken to avoid discovery.
- The person did not seek help after the act.
- The act involved a dangerous method.
- There were final acts such as making a will or leaving a suicide note.

In interviewing the parasuicidal:

- Establish rapport.
- Try to understand the attempt.
- Enquire about current problems.
- Elicit background information.
- Implement a mental state examination.

The presence of psychiatric disorders should be looked for, and any previous history of suicide attempts should be asked about. Social and financial support should also be detailed. Do not avoid asking about suicidal intent.

ASSESSMENT OF RISK FACTORS FOR SUBSEQUENT COMPLETION OF SUICIDE

Tuckman and Youngman (1968) devised the following checklist. One point is awarded for each of the following:

age > 45 years	recent medical treatment
male	psychiatric disorder
unemployed	violent attempt
not married	suicide note
living alone	previous attempt.
poor physical health	

Score– 2 to 5: subsequent suicide rate 7 per 1000
>10: subsequent suicide rate 60 per 1000

MANAGEMENT OF PARASUICIDE

The individual should be treated medically as appropriate. Assess fully. Identify the risk factors. Reduce the immediate risk and treat the causes. If the patient suffers from a psychiatric disorder this should be treated appropriately.

Management of suicidal feelings involves the following:

* Allow ventilation. Talking out avoids acting out.
* Strike a bargain on medication. Ask whether the person can cope with the responsibility of a bottle of tablets. If 'no', then admit to hospital.
* Agree a list of problem areas.
* Establish possible practical help.
* Allow for an under-estimate of the true risk.

Prevention involves:

* recognizing high-risk cases and taking them seriously
* asking patients about their suicidal ideas
* not removing hope
* prescribing the safest drugs
* treating underlying illness adequately.

BIBLIOGRAPHY

Ahrens, B., Måller-Oerlinghausen, B. & Grof, P. 1993: Length of lithium treatment needed to eliminate the high mortality of affective disorders. *British Journal of Psychiatry* 163 (Suppl. 21):27–29.

Beck, A.T., Rush, A.J., Shaw, B.F. & Emery, G. 1979: *Cognitive Therapy of Depression.* New York: Guilford Press.

Benedetti, F., Colombo, C., Serretti, A. *et al.* 2003: Antidepressant effects of light therapy combined with sleep deprivation are influenced by a functional polymorphism within the promoter of the serotonin transporter gene. *Biological Psychiatry* 54:687–692.

Bertelson, A., Harvald, B. & Hauge, M. 1977: A Danish twin study of manic–depressive disorders. *British Journal of Psychiatry* 130:330.

Brown, G.W. & Harris, T. 1978: Social origins of depression. London: Tavistock.

Cassano, G.B., Tundo, A. & Micheli, C. 1994: Bipolar and psychotic depressions. *Current Opinion in Psychiatry* 7:5–8.

Egeland, J.A., Gerhard, D.S., Paus, D.L. *et al.* 1987: Bipolar affective disorders linked to markers on chromosome 11. *Nature* 325:783–787.

Frank, E., Prien, R.F., Jarrett, D.B. *et al.* 1991: Conceptualization and rationale for consensus definitions of terms in major depressive disorder: response, remission, recovery, relapse, and recurrence. *Archives of General Psychiatry* 48:851–855.

Gallerani, M., Manfredini, R., Caracciolo, S. *et al.* 1995: Serum cholesterol concentrations in parasuicide. *British Medical Journal* 310:1632–1636.

Heikkinen, M., Aro, H. & Lînnqvist, J. 1994: Recent life events, social support and suicide. *Acta Psychiatrica Scandinavica* (Suppl. 377):65–72.

Hirschfield, R.M.A. 1994: Major depression, dysthymia and depressive personality disorder. *British Journal of Psychiatry* 165 (Suppl. 26):23–30.

Keller, M.B. 1994: Depression: a long-term illness. *British Journal of Psychiatry* 165 (Suppl. 26):9–15.

Kendler, K.S., Kessler, R., Walters, E.E. *et al.* 1995: Stressful life events, genetic liability and onset of an episode of major depression in women. *American Journal of Psychiatry* 152:833–842.

King, E. 1994: Suicide in the mentally ill: an epidemiological sample and implications for clinicians. *British Journal of Psychiatry* 165:658–663.

Kraepelin, E. 1921: Manic Depressive Insanity and Paranoia (ed. G.M. Robertson, trans. R.M. Barclay). Edinburgh: Churchill Livingstone.

Lemonde, S., Turecki, G., Bakish, D. *et al.* 2003: Impaired repression at a 5-hydroxytryptamine 1A receptor gene polymorphism associated with major depression and suicide. *Journal of Neuroscience* 23:8788–8799.

Medical Research Council 1965: Clinical trial of the treatment of depressive illness. *British Medical Journal* i:881.

Nemeroff, C.B., Knight, D.L., Franks, J. *et al.* 1994: Further studies on platelet binding in depression. *American Journal of Psychiatry* 151:1623–1625.

Parkes, C.M. 1985: Bereavement. *British Journal of Psychiatry* 146:11–17.

Roy, A. 1982: Suicide in chronic schizophrenia. *British Journal of Psychiatry* 141:171–177.

Spiker, D.G., Cofskyweiss, J., Dealy, R.S. *et al.* 1985: The pharmacological treatment of delusional depression. *American Journal of Psychiatry* 142:430–436.

Symonds, R.L. 1991: Books reconsidered. *Suicide: A Study in Sociology* by Emile Durkheim. *British Journal of Psychiatry* 159:739–741.

Syvälahti, E.K.G. 1994: Biological aspects of depression. *Acta Psychiatrica Scandinavica* (Suppl. 377):11–15.

Terayama, H., Nishino, Y., Kishi, M. *et al.* 2003: Detection of anti-Borna Disease Virus (BDV) antibodies from patients with schizophrenia and mood disorders in Japan. *Psychiatry Research* 120:201–206.

Thase, M.E. 1993: Maintenance treatments of recurrent affective disorder. *Current Opinion in Psychiatry* 6:16–21.

Tuckman, J. & Youngman, W.F. 1968: A scale for assessing risk of attempted suicides. *Journal of Clinical Psychology* 24:17–19.

Vaughn, C.E. & Leff, J.P. 1976: The influence of family and social factors on the course of psychiatric illness: a comparison of schizophrenic and depressed neurotic patients. *British Journal of Psychiatry* 129:125–137.

29

Neurotic, stress-related and somatoform disorders

HISTORY

- In 1869, Beard introduced neurasthenia, comprising almost all current anxiety disorders.
- In 1893, Hecker subdivided neurasthenia into different syndromes.
- In 1900, Sigmund Freud distinguished between:
    - *actual neuroses:* somatic causation, comprising neurasthenia, anxiety neurosis (generalized anxiety, panic disorder and agoraphobia) and hypochondriasis
    - *psychoneuroses:* psychological causation, comprising hysteria and obsessions (simple phobia, social phobia and obsessive–compulsive disorder).
- Libidinous impulses reaching the ego generate anxiety; repression and symptom formation follow.
- *Fright neurosis*, not related to repressed libido, was also described, similar to current post-traumatic stress disorder.

CLASSIFICATIONS OF NEUROSIS

NEUROTIC SYNDROME

Neurosis is increasingly split into categories, but there is debate as to the validity of this. Tyrer *et al.* (1993) favour a *general neurotic syndrome*, supported by the following facts:

- A lifetime experience of more than one neurosis is more common, while the frequency of a single neurotic diagnosis is less common than expected.
- Tyrer randomly assigned various neurotic groups to diazepam, dothiepin, cognitive–behavioural therapy, placebo and a self-help treatment programme. No difference in treatment response between diagnostic groups was found. Diazepam was less effective than dothiepin, cognitive–behavioural therapy or self-help, which were of similar efficacy in all groups.
- The effects of treatment were independent of neurotic subtype, so division of the neuroses into subtypes was not supported.

Major psychiatric classifications continue to divide the neuroses into subtypes.

ICD-10

The traditional division between neurosis and psychosis is not used in ICD-10. The following are delineated:

- *Phobic anxiety disorders:* agoraphobia, with and without panic disorder; social phobias and specific phobias
- *Other anxiety disorders:* panic disorder, generalized anxiety disorder and mixed anxiety and depressive disorder
- *Obsessive–compulsive disorder*
- *Reaction to severe stress, and adjustment disorders:* acute stress reaction, post-traumatic stress disorder, and adjustment disorders
- *Dissociative (conversion) disorders:* dissociative amnesia, fugue and stupor; trance and possession disorders; dissociative motor disorders, convulsions, anaesthesia and sensory loss; Ganser's syndrome, and multiple personality disorder
- *Somatoform disorders:* somatization disorder; hypochondriacal disorder; somatoform autonomic dysfunction and persistent pain disorder
- *Other neurotic disorders:* neurasthenia and depersonalization–derealization syndrome.

GENERAL ISSUES

The effect of childhood neurosis

Robins (1966) found that most children with neurotic disorders do not suffer neurosis in adulthood. Adult neurotics develop neurosis in adult life.

In childhood there is excess neurosis in males. After puberty there is excess in females.

Effect of personality disorder

The prevalence of personality disorder in neurosis is 12% in primary care and 40% in psychiatric outpatients. Psychological treatment, particularly self-help, is more effective in neurotic patients without personality disorder. Neurotic patients with personality disorder respond better to antidepressant drug treatment.

Mortality

There is increased mortality in severe neurotic disorder. The relative risk of death in the decade following treatment for neurosis is 1.7. The biggest cause of increased risk is accidental death, particularly suicide (relative risk = 6.1). There is also a major excess of deaths from nervous, circulatory and respiratory disease. Suicide is most likely in the first year after discharge.

PHOBIC ANXIETY DISORDERS

The Greek word *phobos* means panic or terror. In phobic anxiety disorders, anxiety is evoked predominantly by certain well-defined situations, characteristically avoided. Contemplation of a feared situation generates anticipatory anxiety.

In defining fear as phobic the following are considered:

- It is out of proportion to objective risks.
- It cannot be reasoned or explained away.
- It is beyond voluntary control.
- It leads to avoidance.

Marks *et al.* (1993) classify adult fears as normal or abnormal fears. The latter are grouped as follows:

- Phobias of *external stimuli*:
  - agoraphobia
  - social phobia
  - animal phobia
  - miscellaneous specific phobias
- Phobias of *internal stimuli*:
  - illness phobia
  - obsessive phobias.

Epidemiology of phobic anxiety disorder

The Epidemiological Catchment Areas study found:

- a lifetime prevalence for all phobias from 7.8% to 23.3% between sites
- a 6-month prevalence for agoraphobia of 2.8–5.8%
- a 6-month prevalence for simple phobia of 4.5–11.8%
- a 6-month prevalence for social phobia of 1.2–2.2%.

The Edmonton Study (Dick *et al.*, 1994) found:

- a lifetime prevalence for all phobias of 8.9% (females 11.7%, males 6.1%)
- age of first symptoms – 6 years in females, 12 years in males
- high rates of comorbidity with depression, alcohol abuse, drug abuse and obsessive–compulsive disorder in all types of phobia.

Phobic anxiety disorders affect females more than males (agoraphobia 75%, simple phobia 95%), except social phobia where the sex ratio is equal.

Aetiology of phobic anxiety disorder

GENETIC FACTORS

Phobic disorders or other psychiatric illnesses (neurosis, alcoholism, depressive illness) are more prevalent in families of phobic probands.

Kendler *et al.* (1993), using the twin registry, demonstrated that familial aggregation of phobia resulted from genetic liability, not from shared environmental factors.

The relatives of socially phobic probands have a three-fold elevated risk of social phobia.

PSYCHOLOGICAL FACTORS

- *Pavlovian classical conditioning.* Watson, in the 'Little Albert' experiment on an 18-month-old child, produced fear of a toy white rat by presenting it repeatedly with a loud noise. Fear is later generalized to all furry objects (see Chapter 1).

- *Operant conditioning.* Avoidance of a phobic situation is rewarded by a reduction in anxiety which reinforces avoidance.
- *Seligman's preparedness theory.* Anxiety is easily conditioned to certain stimuli (e.g. heights, snakes, spiders), and is resistant to extinction. Prepared stimuli were dangerous to primitive man and may have been acquired by natural selection.
- *Freudian psychoanalytic theory.* Phobias represent a conflict leading to avoidance of situations symbolic of that conflict. 'Little Hans' developed a phobia of horses after seeing a male horse urinate. Freud believed that fear of castration by his father was displaced on to horses after this viewing.

COMORBIDITY

There is overlap between anxiety disorders. For example, 55% of agoraphobics have social phobia and 30% of social phobics also have agoraphobia.

Persons with major depression have 15 times the risk of having agoraphobia and nine times the risk of simple phobia as controls.

Twenty-five per cent of phobics report alcohol abuse/dependence; there are higher rates in agoraphobics and social phobics than in simple phobias.

Management of phobic anxiety disorder

PSYCHOLOGICAL APPROACHES

Behaviour therapy is the treatment of choice. *Exposure techniques* are most widely used. Wolpe's systematic desensitization combines relaxation with graded exposure. *Reciprocal inhibition* prevents anxiety from being maintained when exposed to the phobic stimulus while relaxed.

Flooding entails maximal exposure to the feared stimulus until anxiety reduction occurs. This is not more effective than other exposure techniques.

Modelling requires the patient to observe the therapist engaging in non-avoidant behaviour when exposed to a feared stimulus.

Psychoanalytic psychotherapy has proved to be ineffective.

PHARMACOLOGICAL APPROACHES

Monoamine oxidase inhibitors are effective in agoraphobics and social phobics: 80–90% of pure social phobics are almost asymptomatic at week 16, but patients withdrawn from the active drug relapse (Versiani *et al.*, 1992).

Using fluoxetine, buspirone, phenelzine or moclobemide, two-thirds of socially phobic patients show significant improvement.

Benzodiazepines may help prevent the reinforcement of fear through avoidance.

Specific phobic disorders

AGORAPHOBIA

In 1871, Westphal first used the term to describe patients who experienced intense anxiety when walking across open spaces.

ICD-10

- Symptoms are manifestations of anxiety and are not secondary to other symptoms such as delusions or obsessional thoughts.
- Anxiety is restricted to at least two of the following: crowds, public places, travelling away from home and travelling alone.
- Avoidance of the phobic situation is prominent.

Course

Symptoms fluctuate, but the course is prolonged. Eighty per cent of agoraphobics are not free of symptoms after 5 years.

SOCIAL PHOBIAS

Social phobias are characterized by a fear of scrutiny by others in small groups. This may progress to panic attacks. Avoidance is often marked.

ICD-10

- Symptoms are manifestations of anxiety and not secondary to other symptoms.
- Anxiety is restricted to or predominates in particular social situations.
- The phobic situation is avoided whenever possible.

Course

The course is continuous but it may improve gradually. Alcohol and drug abuse are common.

ISOLATED PHOBIAS

Isolated phobias are restricted to highly specific situations. The seriousness of the handicap depends on how easily a feared situation can be avoided.

ICD-10

- Symptoms are manifestations of anxiety and not secondary to other symptoms.
- Anxiety is restricted to the particular phobic situation.
- The phobic situation is avoided whenever possible.

Course

Childhood phobias are always improved after 5 years. In adult phobias, 20% are unchanged, 40% are better, 40% are worse after 5 years.

PANIC DISORDER

This involves recurrent unpredictable attacks of severe anxiety lasting usually for a few minutes only. There can be a sudden onset of palpitations, chest pain, choking, dizziness, depersonalization and derealization, together with a secondary fear of dying, losing control or going mad. It often results in a hurried exit and a subsequent avoidance of similar situations; it may be followed by persistent fear of another attack.

ICD-10

- There is absence of phobias and depressive disorder.
- Several attacks occur within one month:
  - where there is no objective danger
  - not confined to predictable situations
  - with freedom from anxiety symptoms between attacks.

Epidemiology of panic disorder

The Epidemiological Catchment Areas study found that 3% of the population had experienced a panic attack in the previous 6 months. All socioeconomic groups were affected, and there was no relationship with race or education. Women aged 25–44 years, with a family history of panic disorder, divorced or separated were at highest risk. Other findings were:

- maximum period of onset from mid-teens to mid-thirties, rarely after the age of 40
- more common in females than males (2:1)
- a prevalence of strictly defined panic disorder of 0.1–0.4%
- a 1-year prevalence of 0.2–1.2%
- a lifetime prevalence of 1.4–1.5%.

Aetiology of panic disorder

GENETIC FACTORS

The morbid risk for panic disorder in relatives of probands is 15–30%, much higher than in the general population (2%). Female relatives are at higher risk than male relatives. There is an increased risk of alcoholism in the relatives of probands.

Kendler *et al.* (1993) estimated that the heritability for panic disorder with or without phobic avoidance is 35–40%.

COMORBIDITY

One-third develop secondary depression following the onset of panic disorder. If depression does occur, the course is poorer. Agoraphobia usually occurs with panic disorder, but can occur separately.

There is an increased lifetime prevalence of alcohol abuse/dependence (54%) and drug abuse/dependence (43%) in persons with panic disorder. Some use substances as a complication of panic disorder; others develop panic disorder as a result of withdrawal from substances.

Major controversy surrounds the relationship between anxiety disorders and depression. There is evidence supporting the unitary position, that anxiety and depression lie along the same continuum:

- high overlap of symptoms (65% of anxious patients have depressive symptoms) (Roth *et al.*, 1972)
- difficulty separating primary disorder in patients experiencing both panic attacks and depression
- no differences in family history for anxiety and mixed anxiety depression groups.

Evidence supporting separation

- Family studies show no excess of depression in the relatives of probands suffering from pure panic disorder (Leckman *et al.*, 1985).
- Children of probands with major depression show increased rates of major depression but not anxiety disorders.
- Children of probands with major depression and panic disorder have higher rates of major depression and anxiety disorders.
- There is an increased rate of panic disorder but not major depression or other anxiety disorders in the relatives of panic disorder probands.

LIFE EVENTS

There is an excess of stressful life events in the year prior to the onset of panic disorder, especially illness or death of a cohabitant or relative.

PHYSIOLOGICAL FACTORS

Pitts and McClure (1967) provoked panic attacks in patients with anxiety neurosis but not controls, by the intravenous infusion of sodium lactate. There were higher levels of autonomic arousal in preinfusion panickers compared to non-panickers.

No single biochemical or neuroendocrine finding explains lactate-induced panic. Yohimbine, a presynaptic α_2-adrenergic autoreceptor blocker, induced panic attacks in a subgroup of individuals. This group showed increased noradrenergic activity and blunted growth hormone response to clonidine, supporting the hypothesis of a dysregulation of the noradrenergic system and possibly the hypothalamus–pituitary–adrenal axis in a subgroup of panic-disorder patients. There were very low rates of non-suppression during a dexamethasone suppression test in panic disorder.

Panic attacks are associated with a reduced blood flow in the frontal lobes. Panic-disorder patients not having a panic attack have reduced perfusion of the hippocampus bilaterally and an increase in blood flow to the right inferior frontal cortex.

Mitral valve prolapse occurs in 40% of panic-disorder patients compared to 9% of controls. Patients suffering from mitral valve prolapse do not suffer more panic disorder than controls. An aetiological role for mitral valve prolapse in panic disorder is unlikely.

Panic-disorder patients have abnormal sleep breathing with increased irregularity in tidal volume during REM sleep and an increased rate of microapnoeas. One aetiological theory of panic disorder proposes that patients have a hypersensitive respiratory control system operating at the level of brainstem chemoreceptors. Their 'suffocation' alarm is thus at a pathologically low set point. Enhanced CO_2 sensitivity results in more frequent sighing to reduce CO_2 levels; this results in breathing pauses because the CO_2 stimulus for breathing is withdrawn.

Management of panic disorder

PHARMACOTHERAPY

The tricyclic antidepressants imipramine and clomipramine, MAOIs and SSRIs are efficacious in the treatment of panic disorder. The down-regulation of $5HT_2$ receptors may be responsible for therapeutic effects, which take up to 4 weeks to appear. Increased anxiety or panic may occur in the first week of treatment.

Maprotiline, a specific noradrenaline re-uptake inhibitor, is ineffective in the treatment of panic disorder.

Seventy-five per cent of patients with panic disorder and agoraphobia responsive to treatment with imipramine relapse within 6 months of drug discontinuation, compared to none maintained on treatment. There is superior resistance to relapse in patients treated for longer periods, suggesting that treatment may alter subsequent course in an enduring manner.

Benzodiazepines (e.g. alprazolam in high dosage) reduce the frequency of panic attacks in the short term. There is the need to maintain treatment in the long term, with the risk of dependency.

The re-emergence of symptoms following discontinuation of therapy is problematic.

PSYCHOLOGICAL TREATMENT

Cognitive–behavioural therapy involving the cognitive restructuring of catastrophic interpretations of bodily experience is efficacious in panic disorder, as are exposure techniques which generate bodily sensations of fear during therapy with the aim of habituating the subject to them. Agoraphobic avoidance is treated by situational exposure and relaxation techniques.

Marks *et al.* (1993), comparing alprazolam and exposure therapy in patients suffering from panic disorder and agoraphobia, found the effect size of exposure was twice that of alprazolam; during follow-up gains from alprazolam disappeared, but exposure gains were maintained. Treatment with a combination of exposure and alprazolam impaired improvement seen in the exposure-alone group.

Course

The course is highly variable. Sixty per cent suffer mild impairment. Ten per cent suffer severe disability. Poor outcome is predicted by lower social class and long duration of illness.

GENERALIZED ANXIETY DISORDER

The diagnostic reliability of generalized anxiety disorder (GAD) is lower than that of other anxiety disorders. Patients report uncontrollable worry. A negative response to the question 'Do you worry excessively over minor matters?' virtually rules out GAD as a diagnosis (negative predictive power 0.94). Symptoms of muscle and psychic tension are the most frequently reported by people with GAD.

GAD is associated with the highest rates of comorbidity of all anxiety disorders.

ICD-10

- There is generalized, persistent, free-floating anxiety. Continuous feelings of nervousness, trembling, muscular tension, sweating, light-headedness, palpitations, dizziness, and epigastric discomfort are common.
- Anxiety presents most days for several weeks. Symptoms include:
  - apprehension
  - motor tension
  - autonomic over-activity.

Epidemiology of generalized anxiety disorder

The Epidemiological Catchment Areas study found:

- a 6-month prevalence of GAD of 2.5–6.4%.
- an earlier age of onset (majority before age 20) and more gradual than other anxiety disorders.

Early-onset GAD is more likely to be in a female, in a person having a history of childhood fears and/or having marital or sexual disturbance. Later onset is more likely to develop after a stressful life event.

Aetiology of generalized anxiety disorder

GENETIC FACTORS

Some studies show familial aggregation of GAD, others do not. Kendler *et al.* (1993) concluded that GAD is a moderately familial disorder with a heritability of 30%.

ENVIRONMENTAL FACTORS

Torgersen (1983) reported that probands with GAD had lost their parents by death far more often than probands with panic disorder, suggesting that environmental factors contribute to a higher vulnerability for the development of GAD.

Management of generalized anxiety disorder

PHARMACOTHERAPY

Benzodiazepines were effective in 40%, although the effect was weak and short-lived.
Response to buspirone is slower than to benzodiazepines. There is an appreciable anxiolytic effect with no increase in psychopathology upon withdrawal.

PSYCHOLOGICAL THERAPIES

Patients respond less favourably to conventional cognitive–behavioural treatments than in other anxiety disorders. Treatments tend to be non-specific (e.g. relaxation training). Interventions specifically targeting the worry associated with GAD may be more effective.

Course
Follow-up after 6 years reveals stability of diagnosis; the most common change of diagnosis is to alcoholism. Sixty-eight per cent have mild or no residual impairment, 9% have severe impairment.

OBSESSIVE–COMPULSIVE DISORDER (OCD)

ICD-10
Obsessional symptoms or compulsive acts are present most days for at least two successive weeks causing distress or interfering with activities. Obsessional symptoms have the following characteristics:

- recognized as the individual's own
- at least one thought or act is resisted unsuccessfully

- the thought of carrying out the act must not in itself be pleasurable
- thoughts, images or impulses are unpleasantly repetitive.

Obsessional symptoms developing in the presence of schizophrenia, Tourette's syndrome or organic mental disorder are regarded as part of these conditions.

Epidemiology of OCD

The Epidemiological Catchment Areas study found that OCD is very rare in children. Rutter found no cases among 2000 10- and 11-year-olds on the Isle of Wight. Other findings were:

- a 6-month prevalence of OCD of 1.3–2.0%
- a lifetime prevalence of 1.9–3.0%.
- sex ratio equal
- bimodal age of onset with peaks occurring at 12–14 and 20–22 years of age (decline in onset after the age of 35)

The ECA study prevalance findings were consistently higher than earlier accepted estimates.

Aetiology of OCD

GENETIC FACTORS

First-degree relatives of OCD patients have a higher than normal incidence of psychiatric disorders, most commonly anxiety, phobias, depression and schizophrenia.

First-degree relatives of OCD patients have higher than normal obsessional traits; the risk of OCD among relatives is higher in early-onset OCD probands, suggesting aetiological heterogeneity.

Twin studies suggest that monozygotic twins are more likely to be concordant than dizygotic twins for OCD, but the literature conflicts.

Gilles de la Tourette's syndrome is a familial condition with a substantial genetic basis. Twin and family studies find high rates of OCD and obsessive–compulsive symptoms among Tourette's families. This suggests that some forms of OCD may be related to Tourette's syndrome.

OCD is equally frequent in families of Tourette's probands regardless of whether the proband has OCD. The rate of OCD alone is higher in female relatives and the rate of Tourette's and tics is higher in male relatives of a Tourette's proband. These findings suggest that some forms of OCD are familial.

Probands with no relatives affected by OCD may represent a sporadic form of OCD which is aetiologically distinct from the familial form.

NEUROLOGICAL FACTORS

The reported numbers of OCD cases increased following the 1915 and 1926 outbreaks of encephalitis lethargica.

OCD patients have more abnormal births than expected and more neurological disorders including Sydenham's chorea and encephalitis, suggestive of basal ganglia dysfunction. Flor-Henry observed neuropsychological deficits implicating left frontal lobe dysfunction.

Brain-imaging techniques show morphological changes of basal ganglia structures in OCD. Fronto-striatal abnormality is present. Functional neuroimaging studies show increased blood flow in the basal ganglia, orbital, prefrontal and anterior cingulate cortex. Caudate metabolic rate is reduced after treatment with drugs or behaviour therapy in those patients responsive to treatment, with the percentage change in symptom ratings correlating significantly with right caudate change.

PSYCHOLOGICAL FACTORS

In learning theory, obsessions are thoughts with which anxiety has become associated. Rituals or neutralizing thoughts terminate exposure to the stimulus; thus anxiety is reduced and the rituals are negatively reinforced. The use of rituals prevents the natural reduction in anxiety that would occur if exposure to the stimulus was not cut short by the ritual or neutralizing thought.

In a cognitive model, obsessional distortion concerns exaggerated the responsibility for thoughts, with a tendency to neutralize thoughts with rituals.

In psychoanalysis, OCD symptoms are seen as defensive responses to unconscious impulses. Obsessional symptoms arise from intrapsychic anxiety because of the conflicts being expressed by the defence mechanisms of displacement, undoing and reaction formation. The origin of obsessional personality is located at the anal-training stage of development; OCD is thought to represent regression to this stage.

Neuropsychological tests suggest the presence of amnestic deficits with respect to non-verbal memory and memory for actions. OCD patients also perform poorly on tests of frontal lobe function, particularly tests of shifting set.

Management of OCD

PHARMACOTHERAPY

Antidepressants are effective in the short-term treatment of OCD. Clomipramine and SSRIs have greater efficacy than antidepressants with no selective serotonergic properties. Concomitant depression is not necessary for serotonergic antidepressants to improve symptoms. There are success rates of 50–79%.

Relapse often follows discontinuation of treatment.

PSYCHOLOGICAL TREATMENTS

Behavioural methods (e.g. modelling, exposure and response prevention) are the most widely accepted psychological treatments; there are success rates of 60–85%.

The value of cognitive therapy in the treatment of OCD is not conclusive. Psychoanalytic therapy is not effective in the treatment of OCD.

PHYSICAL TREATMENTS

Psychosurgery may be indicated in the chronic unremitting OCD of at least 2 years' duration with severe life disruption, unresponsive to all recognized forms of therapy. Open, uncontrolled studies show that 65% of patients with OCD are improved or greatly improved with cingulotomy plus bifrontal operations.

Course

Favourable prognostic factors include:

- mild symptoms
- predominance of phobic ruminative ideas, absence of compulsions

- short duration of symptoms
- no childhood symptoms or abnormal personality traits.

Poor prognostic factors include:

- males with early onset
- symptoms involving the need for symmetry and exactness
- the presence of hopelessness, hallucinations or delusions
- a family history of OCD
- a continuous, episodic or deteriorating course.

ACUTE STRESS REACTION

This is a transient disorder developing in an individual without other mental disorder in response to exceptional stress. It usually subsides within hours or days. The risk is increased if physical exhaustion or organic factors are present.

ICD-10

- There is an immediate temporal connection between the impact of an exceptional stressor and onset of symptoms, which is within minutes.
- In addition, symptoms:
  - show a mixed and changing picture – initial state of daze, depression, anxiety, anger, despair, over-activity and withdrawal may all be seen, with no one symptom predominating for long
  - resolve rapidly, within a few hours if removal from the stressful environment is possible.

If stress continues, symptoms diminish after 24–48 hours.

POST-TRAUMATIC STRESS DISORDER (PTSD)

ICD-10

- PTSD arises within six months as a delayed and/or protracted response to a stressful event of an exceptionally threatening nature.
- Symptoms include repeated reliving of the trauma. Repetitive, intrusive memories (flashbacks), daytime imagery, or dreams of the event must be present.
- Emotional detachment, persisting background numbness, avoidance of stimuli reminiscent of original event are often present, but are not essential.
- Autonomic disturbances (hyperarousal with hypervigilance, enhanced startle reaction, and insomnia) and mood disorder contribute to the diagnosis but are not essential. Anxiety, depression and suicidal ideation are not uncommon. The excessive use of alcohol or drugs may complicate matters.

Aetiology of PTSD

GENERAL FACTORS

About 25% of people exposed to a potentially traumatic event develop PTSD. Low education and social class, pre-existing psychiatric problems and female gender are vulnerability factors. Viewing the dead body of a relative after a disaster is predictive of lower PTSD. Psychopathic traits are protective.

Sufferers of PTSD report childhood physical sexual abuse more often than expected.

BIOLOGICAL FACTORS

People with PTSD have exaggerated physiological responses (heart rate, skin conductance, electromyographic response) to traumatic imagery. They have a heightened physiological state specific to PTSD and which is difficult to simulate. This may be mediated by noradrenergic and dopaminergic neurotransmitter systems, and the HPA axis.

Initial mobilization and the subsequent depletion of noradrenaline following inescapable shock in animals indicates a possible catecholaminergic mediation of PTSD symptoms. Drugs effective in PTSD (MAOIs, tricyclics, benzodiazepines and clonidine) are also effective in preventing development of learned helplessness in animals when infused into the locus coeruleus.

There are similarities between PTSD symptoms and opioid withdrawal, leading to speculation that opioid function is disturbed in PTSD. Stress-induced analgesia is reversible by nalaxone in PTSD veterans exposed to traumatic stimulus.

Management of PTSD

A flexible, staged approach using several techniques is advocated.

PSYCHOLOGICAL THERAPY

Exposure to aversive memories is central, irrespective of the specific therapy used. Exposure to anxiety-producing stimuli *in a supportive setting* results in arousal, attenuation and symptom reduction or habituation. Another common element is some form of cognitive restructuring.

Behavioural techniques are most effective in relation to PTSD following simple trauma. For more complicated traumas, such as torture, these should be combined with cognitive methods.

PHARMACOTHERAPY

MAOIs and tricyclic antidepressants are beneficial in PTSD, particularly for intrusive symptoms. SSRIs are helpful with avoidant symptoms.

Carbamazepine, propranolol and clonidine reduce hyperarousal and intrusive symptoms; fluoxetine and lithium reduce explosiveness and improve mood. Buspirone may lessen fear-induced startle; it may play an adjunctive role.

Alprazolam is no more effective than placebo, but there have been some positive reports with clonazepam.

There is an almost total lack of response to placebo in chronic PTSD.

The drugs require at least 8 weeks' duration before the effects are evident. The magnitude of the drug effect is limited. Progressive and continued improvement has been noted over several months in chronic PTSD treated with tricyclics.

EYE MOVEMENT DESENSITIZATION

Involuntary multi-saccadic eye movements occur during disturbing thoughts. It is claimed that inducing these eye movements while experiencing intrusive thoughts stops symptoms of PTSD.

Course

Half of patients still have PTSD decades later. A dose–response relationship exists between the severity of the stressor and the degree of consequent psychological distress.

Most PTSD patients also have depression, anxiety disorders, substance abuse and/or sexual dysfunction.

ADJUSTMENT DISORDERS

States of distress and emotional disturbance arise in the period after a stressful life event. Individual predisposition plays a greater role than in other stress-induced conditions, but this condition would not have arisen without a stressor.

Manifestations vary. They include depressed mood, anxiety, worry, an inability to cope and some inability to manage the daily routine. Conduct disorders may be associated, especially in adolescents. Regressive phenomena in children are frequently seen.

Onset is within one month of the stressor. The duration is usually less than 6 months, except for prolonged depressive reaction.

Grief reactions considered abnormal because of their form or content are included in this category.

ICD-10

The following adjustment disorders are outlined in ICD-10:

- brief depressive reaction – less than 1 month
- prolonged depressive reaction – less than 2 years
- mixed anxiety and depressive reaction
- predominant disturbance of emotions and/or conduct.

DISSOCIATIVE (CONVERSION) DISORDERS

ICD-10

Dissociative (conversion) disorders are presumed to be psychogenic in origin. They are associated with traumatic events, insoluble problems or disturbed relationships. The unpleasant affect associated with these conflicts is transformed (converted) into symptoms.

Diagnostic guidelines are:

- no evidence of physical disorder that may explain symptoms
- evidence for psychological causation – a clear association in time with stressful events.

Specific dissociative conditions

DISSOCIATIVE AMNESIA

- Loss of memory of an important event is not due to organic disorder, fatigue or ordinary forgetfulness.

- Partial and selective amnesia is usually centred on traumatic events.
- The extent varies from day to day. A persistent core cannot be recalled while awake.
- Perplexity, distress or calm acceptance may accompany the amnesia.
- It begins and ends suddenly, following stress. It rarely lasts more than a couple of days, and recurrence is unusual.
- It is more common in young adults, but rare in the elderly.
- Recovery is complete.

DISSOCIATIVE FUGUE

- There are all the features of dissociative amnesia (see above), plus an apparently purposeful journey away from home. A new identity may be assumed.
- It s precipitated by severe stress.
- There is amnesia for the duration of the fugue, but self-care and social interaction are maintained.
- It lasts for hours to days, but recovery is abrupt and complete.

DISSOCIATIVE STUPOR

- The sufferer is stuporose, with no evidence of a physical or other psychiatric cause.
- Onset is sudden and stress-related.
- The person sits motionless for long periods, speech and movement absent. Muscle tone, posture, breathing and eye movements indicate that the individual is neither asleep nor unconscious.

TRANCE AND POSSESSION DISORDERS

- There is a temporary loss of personal identity and awareness of surroundings.
- Attention and awareness are limited to one or two aspects of the immediate environment.
- There are repeated movements, postures or utterances.

This includes only an involuntary or unwanted trance, occurring outside the culturally accepted situation.

DISSOCIATIVE DISORDERS OF MOVEMENT AND SENSATION

- There is loss of movement or sensations, usually cutaneous, with no physical cause.
- Symptoms often reflect the person's concept of disorder, which may be at variance with physiological or anatomical principles (e.g. glove and stocking anaesthesia).
- The resulting disability helps the person to escape conflict, or express dependency or resentment indirectly.
- There is calm acceptance (*la belle indifférence*), not common and not diagnostic. This is also seen in normal people facing serious illness.
- Premorbid personality and relationships are often abnormal.

DISSOCIATIVE CONVULSIONS

- Pseudoseizures mimic epileptic seizures, but tongue biting, serious bruising and incontinence of urine are uncommon.
- Loss of consciousness is absent or replaced by stupor or trance.

DISSOCIATIVE ANAESTHESIA AND SENSORY LOSS

- There are patches of sensory loss that do not correspond to anatomical dermatomes.
- Visual loss is rarely total.
- General mobility is well preserved.
- Dissociative deafness and anosmia are uncommon.

OTHER DISSOCIATIVE DISORDERS

Ganser's syndrome

This is a complex disorder described by Ganser, characterized by approximate answers and usually accompanied by several dissociative symptoms, often in circumstances that suggest psychogenic aetiology. The five main features of Ganser syndrome are:

- approximate answers (*Vorbeireden*)
- clouding of consciousness
- somatic conversion
- pseudohallucinations (often)
- subsequent amnesia.

Multiple personality disorder (MPD)

Controversy exists about whether MPD is iatrogenic or culture-specific. There is an apparent existence of two or more distinct personalities within an individual, of which only one is evident at any time. Each personality is complete, with its own memories, behaviour and preferences.

One personality is dominant. It does not have access to memories of the other, and is unaware of the existence of others. The change from one personality to another is sudden and associated with stress.

Psychoanalysis views MPD as a complex, chronic developmental dissociative disorder related to severe, repetitive childhood abuse or trauma, usually beginning before the age of 5 years. Dissociative defences are used to handle subsequent traumatic experiences.

Additionally, *mass hysteria* presents with abnormal illness behaviour transmitted in close communities spreading from individuals of high status down the hierarchy. Affected individuals are suggestible. *Couvade syndrome* presents in males whose partners are pregnant, with symptoms of morning sickness, abdominal pain and anxiety.

Epidemiology of dissociative disorder

Relatively high frequencies of dissociative experiences are reported in patients with PTSD, women with chronic pelvic pain, substance abusers (40%), patients with eating disorders and those with a history of childhood abuse. Intelligence quotient (IQ) is negatively correlated.

Aetiology of dissociative disorder

Sigmund Freud introduced the term *conversion* to describe the unconscious rendering of innocuous of threatening ideas by conversion into physical symptoms, which have symbolic significance. This results in the relief of emotional conflict (primary gain) and the direct advantages of assuming a sick role (secondary gain).

The spectrum of dissociation (multiple personality disorder is most extreme) with increasingly complex and symptomatic forms is related to increasingly severe childhood trauma.

Levels of psychological distress are highly correlated with dissociative experiences.

Of 100 substance-dependent subjects, 39 had dissociative disorder and 43 reported childhood abuse. Patients with dissociative disorder may use substances to block out more severe abuse memories and suppress dissociative symptoms.

Management of dissociative disorder

Do not confront the individual. Complete physical investigations and emphasize that serious illness is excluded. Minimize the advantages of a sick role, and praise healthy behaviour. Allow the patient to discard symptoms without losing face.

The main treatment of MPD is long-term psychoanalytic psychotherapy aimed at the unification of divided mental processes.

Course

Dissociative states tend to remit after a few weeks or months. Chronic states of more than one or two years are often resistant to therapy. Those with acute, recent onset, a good premorbid personality and resolvable conflict have a better prognosis.

In a classic paper, Slater (1965) reported on a 9-year follow-up of 85 patients who were diagnosed as hysterics by senior psychiatrists and neurologists. He found that 33% developed definite organic illness; 15% had a major mental illness; 12 patients died, four from suicide of whom two had demyelinating neurological conditions, and eight from natural causes which could have accounted for their original presentations. Of the original sample of 85, he was left with seven young patients who had experienced acute psychogenic reactions in the form of a conversion syndrome, and 14 who were suffering from lasting personality disorders. Slater concluded that the diagnosis of hysteria should not be made.

SOMATOFORM DISORDERS

ICD-10

- There is repeated presentation of physical symptoms with persistent requests for medical investigations.
- No physical basis is found.
- Attempts to discuss possible psychological causation are resisted.

Somatization disorder

There are multiple, recurrent, frequently changing physical symptoms. Most patients have multiple contacts with primary and specialist medical services; there are many negative investigations. Gastrointestinal and skin symptoms are most common. Sexual and menstrual complaints are also common. Onset after the age of 40 may indicate the onset of affective disorder.

ICD-10 requires the presence of all the following:

- 2 years of multiple and variable physical symptoms, with no physical explanation found
- persistent refusal to accept the advice of several doctors
- impairment of functioning attributable to symptoms and resulting behaviour.

The possibility of *developing* an independent physical disorder should be considered.

The emphasis on symptoms and their effects distinguishes this from hypochondriacal disorder (see below) where the emphasis of concern is on possible underlying disease.

Briquet's syndrome or St Louis hysteria is a multiple somatization disorder.

EPIDEMIOLOGY

- There is a 0.2–0.5% prevalence in the UK.
- Three per cent of repeated gut clinic attenders have somatization disorder.
- Using abridged criteria (four unexplained symptoms in males, six in females), the prevalence is :
  - community – 4.4%
  - patients with medically unexplained symptoms – 32%.
- It is far more common in women than men.
- It usually starts in early adult life.

AETIOLOGY

Genetic factors

Torgersen (1986) reported an MZ to DZ concordance in somatoform disorder of 29:10. This suggests that somatoform disorder has a familial transmission.

Environmental factors

The South London somatization study reported by Craig *et al.* in 1993 was a longitudinal study in primary care; it compared somatizers with those with pure emotional disorder and those with pure physical disorder. The physical symptoms of somatizers were less likely to improve; one-third went on to develop chronic somatoform disorders.

Changes in physical symptoms mirrored changes in emotional arousal. Somatizers were more likely to report parental physical illness and to have had more physical illness themselves in childhood. Emotionally disordered subjects reported more parental lack of care.

It was hypothesized that physical illness in childhood lessened the distress of lack of care, resulting in somatic rather than emotional responses as a means of attracting care or lessening hostility, which endures into adult life.

MANAGEMENT

Engage the patient and spouse. Conduct no more investigations, but listen empathically. Elicit childhood experience of illness and parental disability. Link physical symptoms to relevant life events (the reattribution model of Goldberg). Reduce all medication apart from antidepressants for the depressed. Limit the expectations of cure.

Alexithymia (limited ability to describe emotions verbally) is common in somatoform disorder. Traditional psychotherapy with alexithymic individuals is difficult. A more reality-based educational and supportive approach is better.

COURSE

The course is chronic and fluctuating. Treatments use disproportionate health resources. If engaged as above, this significantly reduces the use of resources. However, depression and anxiety are often present and may require treatment.

Hypochondriacal disorder

This is a persistent preoccupation with the possibility of having serious disease. Attention is usually focused on one or two organ systems only. It occurs in both men and women, with no familial characteristics.

ICD-10

- There is a persistent belief in the presence of at least one serious physical illness, despite repeated investigations revealing no physical explanation of presenting symptoms, or persistent preoccupation with presumed deformity.
- There is a persistent refusal to accept the advice of several different doctors that there is no physical illness underlying the symptoms.

If depressive symptoms are prominent and precede the onset of hypochondriacal ideas, then depressive disorder may be primary.

Somatoform autonomic dysfunction

Symptoms are presented as if caused by a disorder of a system or organ largely under autonomic control (e.g. cardiac neurosis, psychogenic hyperventilation, gastric neurosis, nervous diarrhoea).

ICD-10

- There are persistent and troublesome symptoms of autonomic arousal.
- Symptoms are referred to a specific organ system, with no evidence of organ pathology.
- There is distress about the possibility of disorder of the organ system, not responsive to repeated reassurance.

Persistent somatoform pain disorder

This presents with persistent, severe, distressing pain, not explained by physical disorder. Pain occurs in association with emotional conflict, and results in increased support and attention.

OTHER NEUROTIC DISORDERS

NEURASTHENIA

ICD-10

- There are persistent, distressing complaints of increased fatigue after mental effort, or persistent, distressing complaints of bodily weakness and exhaustion after minimal effort.
- At least two of the following are reported: muscular aches; dizziness; headaches; sleep disturbance; inability to relax; irritability or dyspepsia.

DEPERSONALIZATION–DEREALIZATION SYNDROME

It is uncommon to experience these in an isolated form.

ICD-10

- There are depersonalization symptoms and/or derealization symptoms.
- Insight is maintained.
- There is a clear sensorium and absence of toxic confusional state or epilepsy.

BIBLIOGRAPHY

Andrews, G., Stewart, G., Morris-Yates, A. *et al.* 1990: Evidence for a general neurotic syndrome. *British Journal of Psychiatry* 157:6–12.

Boer, J.A. den 1988: Serotonergic Mechanisms in Anxiety Disorders. An Enquiry into Serotonin Function in Panic Disorder. PhD thesis, University of Utrecht.

Brown, T.A., Barlow, D.H. & Liebowitz, M.R. 1994: The empirical basis of generalized anxiety disorder. *American Journal of Psychiatry* 151:1272–1280.

Craig, T.K.J., Boardman, A.P., Mills, K. *et al.* 1993: The South London somatisation study: I. Longitudinal course and the influence of early life experiences. *British Journal of Psychiatry* 163:579–588.

Davidson, J. 1992: Drug therapy of post-traumatic stress disorder. *British Journal of Psychiatry* 160:309–314.

Dick, C.L., Bland, R.C. & Newman, S.C. 1994: Panic disorder. *Acta Psychiatrica Scandinavica* (Suppl. 376):45–53.

Dick, C.L., Sowa, B., Bland, R.C. and Newman, S.C. 1994: Phobic disorders. *Acta Psychiatrica Scandinavica* (Suppl. 376):36–44.

James, I.A. & Blackburn, I.-M. 1995: Cognitive therapy with obsessive–compulsive disorder. *British Journal of Psychiatry* 166:444–450.

Kendler, K., Neale, M., Kessler, R. *et al.* 1993: Major depression and phobias: the genetic and environmental sources of comorbidity. *Psychological Medicine* 23:361–371.

Kendler, K., Neale, M., Kessler, R. *et al.* 1993: Panic disorder in women: a population based twin study. *Psychological Medicine* 23:397–406.

Klerman, G.L. 1986: The National Institute of Mental Health's Epidemiologic Catchment Areas (NIMH-ECA) program: background, preliminary findings and implications. *Social Psychiatry* 21:159–166.

Kolada, J.L., Bland, R.C. & Newman, S.C. 1994: Obsessive–compulsive disorder. *Acta Psychiatrica Scandinavica* (Suppl. 376):24–35.

Leckman, J.F., Weissman, M.M., Merikangas, K.R. *et al.* 1985: Major depression and panic disorder: a family study perspective. *Psychopharmacological Bulletin* 21:543–545.

Loewenstein, R.J. & Ross, D.R. 1992: Multiple personality and psychoanalysis: an introduction. *Psychoanalytic Inquiry* 12:3–48.

Marks, I.M. & Gelder, M.G. 1966: Different ages of onset in varieties of phobia. *American Journal of Psychiatry* 123:218–221.

Marks, I.M., Swinson, R.P., Basoglu, M. *et al.* 1993: Alprazolam and exposure alone and combined in panic disorder with agoraphobia. *British Journal of Psychiatry* 162:776–787.

McIvor, R.J. & Turner, S.W. 1995: Assessment and treatment approaches for survivors of torture. *British Journal of Psychiatry* 166:705–711.

Pauls, D.L., Alsobrook, J.P., Goodman, W. *et al.* 1995: A family study of obsessive–compulsive disorder. *American Journal of Psychiatry* 152:76–84.

Piccinelli, M., Pini, S., Bellantuono, C. *et al.* 1995: Efficacy of drug treatment in obsessive–compulsive disorder: a meta-analytic review. *British Journal of Psychiatry* 166:424–443.

Pitts, F.N. & McClure, J.N. 1967: Lactate metabolism in anxiety neurosis. *New England Journal of Medicine* 13:29–36.

Robins, L.N. 1966: *Deviant Children Grown Up.* Baltimore: Williams & Wilkins.

Roth, M., Gurney, C., Garside, R.F. *et al.* 1972: Studies in the classification of affective disorders: the relationship between anxiety states and depressive illnesses: I. *British Journal of Psychiatry* 121:147–161.

Sims, A. & Prior, P. 1978: The pattern of mortality in severe neuroses. *British Journal of Psychiatry* 133:299–305.

Slater, E. 1965: Diagnosis of hysteria. *British Medical Journal* i:1395–1399.

Spector, J. & Huthwaite, M. 1993: Eye-movement desensitisation to overcome post-traumatic stress disorder. *British Journal of Psychiatry* 163:106–108.

Stein, M.B., Millar, T.W., Larsen, D.K. *et al.* 1995: Irregular breathing during sleep in patients with panic disorder. *American Journal of Psychiatry* 152:1168–1173.

Tallis, F. 1995: Reading about obsessive–compulsive disorder. *British Journal of Psychiatry* 166:546–550.

Torgersen, S. 1983: Genetic factors in anxiety disorders. *Archives of General Psychiatry* 40:1085–1089.

Torgersen, S. 1985: Hereditary differentiation of anxiety and affective neuroses. *British Journal of Psychiatry* 146:530–534.

Torgersen, S. 1986: Genetics of somatoform disorders. *Archives of General Psychiatry* 43:502–505.

Tyrer, P., Seivewright, N., Murphy, S. *et al.* 1988: The Nottingham study of neurotic disorder: comparison of drug and psychological treatments. *Lancet* ii:235–240.

Tyrer, P., Seivewright, N., Ferguson, B. *et al.* 1993: The Nottingham study of neurotic disorder: effect of personality status on response to drug treatment, cognitive therapy and self-help over two years. *British Journal of Psychiatry* 162:219–226.

Versiani, M., Nardi, A.E., Mundim, F.D. *et al.* 1992: Pharmacotherapy of social phobia: a controlled study with moclobemide and phenelzine. *British Journal of Psychiatry* 161:353–360.

30

Disorders specific to women

PREMENSTRUAL SYNDROME (PMS)

Symptoms of PMS

Premenstrual syndrome includes emotional and/or physical symptoms occurring premenstrually (late luteal phase) but remitting usually during the week before menstruation (follicular phase).

More than 150 symptoms have been implicated in PMS. There are considerable differences in the patterns of symptoms, but there is strong support for cycle-related variability in most subjects. The existence of PMS as a discrete entity has often been questioned; there is a lack of consensus about its definition.

The common symptoms experienced by those women suffering PMS are listed in Table 30.1.

Table 30.1   *Common symptoms experienced by women suffering PMS*

Mood symptoms	Other symptoms
Irritability	Bloated abdomen
Easily angry or upset without good reason	Tender breasts
Tension	Carbohydrate craving
Emotional lability	Disturbed sleep
Depressed mood	Poor concentration
Violent feelings	Clumsiness
	Headaches
	Muscle and joint pain
	Spots

Epidemiology of PMS

Forty per cent of women experience some cyclical premenstrual symptoms; 2–10% report severe symptoms. There are associations with the following:

- There is a higher prevalence in those around 30 years of age.
- Prevalence increases with increasing parity.
- There is a higher prevalence in those women who have experienced natural menstrual cycles (unmodified by oral contraceptives and uninterrupted by pregnancy) for longer periods of time.
- Women using oral contraceptives, especially if nulliparous, have reduced rates of PMS.
- Prevalence is increased in those experiencing higher levels of psychosocial stress.

Aetiology of PMS

GENETIC FACTORS

Highly significant correlations between mother and daughter have been reported on a variety of menstrual variables including premenstrual tension.

Condon (1993) reported concordances for global PMS scores:

- 0.28 in DZ twin pairs
- 0.55 in MZ twin pairs.

Concordances for MZ twins exceeded those of DZ twins on every subscale. The findings support the hypothesis that the familial aggregation of PMS symptoms is determined largely by genetic factors.

NEUROENDOCRINE FACTORS

Beta-endorphin
Anxiety, food cravings and physical discomfort in PMS subjects are associated with a significant decline in β-endorphin (these symptoms are also found in opiate withdrawal).

Serotonin
Post-synaptic serotonergic responsivity is altered during the late luteal phase of the menstrual cycle. It is thought that gonadal hormones cause changes in the levels of activity of serotonergic systems. Carbohydrate craving and depression are linked to serotonergic brain changes which are marked in the late luteal phase.

Plasma taken from subjects suffering from PMS inhibits serotonin uptake in rat brain synaptosomes to a greater degree than serum taken from controls.

Noradrenaline
MHPG (3-methoxy-4-hydroxyphenylglycol, a metabolite of noradrenaline) in cerebrospinal fluid is elevated in PMS subjects premenstrually.

Androgens
Serum androgens are higher in women with premenstrual irritability and dysphoria than in controls. Serum-free testosterone levels are significantly higher in PMS subjects than in matched controls around ovulation, and 17-hydroxyprogesterone levels are higher in PMS women in the luteal phase.

Other
Various hypotheses have been explored, particularly in relation to the balance between oestrogen and progesterone with a relative lack of progesterone, excessive production of prolactin, aldosterone or antidiuretic hormone. None are conclusive.

NEUROPHYSIOLOGICAL FACTORS

The following have been reported:

- There are consistent cycle-dependent changes in electroencephalographic recordings, most prominent in the α range.
- There are alterations in response to dichotic auditory stimuli premenstrually in comparison with the follicular phase, most markedly in sufferers of PMS.
- There are alterations in skin conductance in response to auditory stimuli premenstrually in comparison with the follicular phase, most markedly in sufferers of PMS.

PERSONALITY FACTORS

Neuroticism may be an important determinant of women's experiences and reports of their menstrual cycle, and is higher in those reporting PMS.

Women with coronary-prone type-A behaviour experience 50% more PMS symptoms than women with non-coronary-prone type-B behaviour.

PSYCHOLOGICAL FACTORS

Psychological views of PMS attribute it to an impoverishment of the ego in relation to feminine self-acceptance and identification with the mother. It is suggested that popular beliefs that derogate femininity are internalized and form part of the socialization of women.

Self-report of PMS is strongly related to psychosocial stress, particularly unusual stress and unhappy relationships.

Management of PMS

Treatment should be supportive and directed towards symptom relief, psychosocial support, stress reduction and dietary change. No single medication has proven effective in the treatment of PMS.

Antidepressants

Favourable results are sometimes found particularly when a serotonergic antidepressant is used. Psychic, but not somatic, symptoms improve. A 70% reduction in premenstrual irritability and depressed mood is found using clomipramine, compared to a 45% reduction with placebo. Similar results have been obtained using fluoxetine, adding support to the hypothesis that a serotonergic imbalance is involved in premenstrual psychic symptoms.

Oral contraceptive pill

Somatic symptoms are improved but psychic symptoms are not. Oestrogenic effects are thought to exacerbate premenstrual irritability, and progestogenic effects exacerbate premenstrual depression.

Oral contraceptive users report significantly less menstrual pain and premenstrual breast tenderness than controls, but also show significantly less improvement in negative mood during the menstrual phase than non-users.

Gamma linolenic acid (GLA)

GLA, an n-6 essential fatty acid, has been reported to help with several PMS symptoms, such as mastalgia. It is found in products such as evening primrose oil.

Other treatments

Other treatments used for which there are conflicting reports of efficacy include:

- *alprazolam* – some reports of usefulness, but double-blind placebo-controlled trial showed absence of any therapeutic benefit
- *hysterectomy* – no change in cyclical mood changes following hysterectomy
- *vitamin B6* – produces a reduction in prolactin synthesis; use advocated, but little evidence of improvement in PMS symptoms
- *progesterones* – use advocated, but little evidence of improvement in PMS symptoms
- *diuretics* – produce some relief in symptoms of bloatedness, but no improvement in psychic symptoms
- *bromocriptine* – effective only in the relief of breast symptoms.

CYCLIC PSYCHOSIS

A few reports of cyclic psychoses related to menstruation exist in the literature. Psychotic symptoms appear suddenly a few days before menstruation, resolve with the onset of menstrual bleeding, and reappear with the next cycle. Between psychotic episodes the woman appears largely asymptomatic. Most cases do not show familial psychiatric morbidity. The first psychotic episode usually occurs at a young age.

The psychiatric picture is non-specific, and changes with every menstruation. Some common features include psychomotor retardation, anxiety, perplexity, disorientation and amnestic features. Transitory EEG abnormalities may occur, not amounting to epileptic activity.

It has been suggested that in some cases menstrual psychoses should be regarded as a specific variant of PMS.

Recommended treatments for menstrual cyclic psychosis include:

- bromocriptine which reduces prolactin
- progesterone which inhibits ovulation
- clomiphene citrate
- acetazolamide, a diuretic
- psychotropic medications (results inconclusive).

The prognosis is good, and spontaneous remission is usual.

PREGNANCY

Miscarriage

Miscarriage occurs in 12–15% of clinically recognized pregnancies. About one-half are associated with chromosomal abnormalities. Other recognized causes include uterine malformation, cervical incompetence, trauma, infection, endocrine disorder, toxins, irradiation and immune dysfunction.

Animal evidence shows that stress leads to abortion in a number of mammallian species including baboons.

O'Hare and Creed (1995) studied the relationship between life events and miscarriage in 48 case–control pairs matched for known predictors of miscarriage. They found that the miscarriage group were more likely to have experienced:

- a severe life event in the 3 months preceding miscarriage
- a major social difficulty
- life events of severe short-term threat in the fortnight immediately beforehand.

Fifty-four per cent of the miscarriage group had experienced some psychosocial stress, compared to only 15% of controls.

Other factors significantly associated with miscarriage include:

- childhood maternal separation
- poor relationships with partners
- few social contacts.

Stress-induced abortion may involve increased catecholamine levels and α-adrenergic stimulation of the myometrium. Serotonin, implicated in stress responses, promotes abortion. This may be mediated via reduced gonadotrophin output.

In the management of recurrent miscarriage, a psychosocial history should be taken in order to ascertain any sources of stress amenable to social intervention.

CONSEQUENCES OF MISCARRIAGE

A high percentage of women experience profound loss following miscarriage, reporting symptoms typical of the grief that follows bereavement. Friedman and Gath (1989) found that at 4 weeks after miscarriage 48% of women were psychiatric cases as measured on the PSE, all suffering depressive disorders. Many of the women were already recovering at this time.

Symptoms are increased in women who have experienced a previous miscarriage. Many women are fearful of experiencing loss in a future pregnancy.

Other factors increasing women's vulnerability to developing depressive symptoms are lack of a supportive partner, childlessness, neuroticism and previous psychiatric consultation.

Psychiatric morbidity can persist for several months. The duration of bereavement reaction is appreciably shortened by support and counselling.

Termination of pregnancy

Psychological disturbance occurring in association with therapeutic abortion are severe or persistent in only a minority, about 10% of women. Depression and anxiety are most common with psychosis reported very uncommonly, in 0.003% of cases. Of the latter, most have a previous psychiatric history.

Women at greater risk of adverse psychological sequelae include:

- those with a previous psychiatric history
- younger women
- those with poor social support
- those from cultural groups opposed to abortion.

About one-third of women experience feelings of loss, guilt and self-reproach at 6 months after abortion, particularly those ambivalent towards the termination of pregnancy. Those requiring therapeutic abortion because of fetal abnormalities or medical complications have poorer psychological outcomes.

Gilchrist *et al.* (1995) studied psychiatric morbidity following termination of pregnancy compared with other outcomes of unplanned pregnancy in a large prospective cohort study. They found:

- Rates of total psychiatric disorder were no higher after termination of pregnancy than after childbirth.
- Women with a previous psychiatric history were most at risk of disorder after the end of their pregnancy, whatever its outcome.
- Women without a past history of psychosis had a lower risk of psychosis after termination than after childbirth.
- In women without a past psychiatric history, deliberate self-harm was more common in those who were refused a termination (relative risk = 2.9), or who had a termination (relative risk = 1.7).
- There was no overall increase in psychiatric morbidity in those having a termination of pregnancy.

Mental disorders in pregnancy

MINOR MENTAL ILLNESS

There is an increased risk of minor mental illness in the first trimester. This usually resolves spontaneously by the second trimester, so reassurance and psychological interventions are usually most appropriate.

Benzodiazepines should be avoided particularly in the first and third trimesters.

MAJOR MENTAL ILLNESS

It was previously believed that pregnancy offered protection against mental illness. It is now known that this is not the case. The prevalence of depression in pregnancy is high.

It is always best to avoid drugs in pregnancy if possible. Stable patients may often be withdrawn from medication before conception. In those with great risks of relapse a judgement has to be made about the relative risk of relapse against the relative risk of taking medication.

Neuroleptics can be maintained at minimal doses during pregnancy if necessary. It is best to withdraw anticholinergics if possible since the risk of teratogenesis in humans is inconclusive.

Lithium is teratogenic and is contraindicated in pregnancy especially in the first and third trimesters. Women of child-bearing age started on lithium should be informed of its effects and the need to avoid pregnancy. Lithium should be withdrawn at least a month before conception and immediately if a woman is found to be pregnant.

The majority of studies report that the SSRI antidepressants are safe for use in pregnancy.

PUERPERAL DISORDERS

General issues

There are associations between the puerperal mental conditions. Severe *postnatal blues* can progress to *postnatal depression*; there may also be an association between postnatal blues and *puerperal psychosis*, since there is an excess of onset of the latter towards the end of the first week post-partum.

ICD-10 does not categorize puerperal mental disorders separately unless they do not meet criteria for disorders classified elsewhere. Thus under the chapter 'Behavioural syndromes associated with physiological disturbances and physical factors' is a section (F53) *Mental and behavioural disorders associated with the puerperium, not elsewhere classified* which includes mild, severe and other mental and behavioural disorders associated with the puerperium.

Postnatal blues

Postnatal blues is a brief psychological disturbance, characterized by tearfulness, emotional lability and confusion in mothers occurring in the first few days after childbirth.

EPIDEMIOLOGY

It occurs in about 50% of women, peaking at the third to fifth day post-partum.

AETIOLOGY

There is some evidence of links with biological factors, including:

- a history of premenstrual tension
- serum calcium levels
- monoamines, serum tryptophan, platelet α_2-adrenoceptors
- progesterone withdrawal post delivery – women experiencing severe blues have higher antenatal progesterone levels, a steeper rise in the last 2 weeks of pregnancy, a bigger decrement from antenatal levels to the day of peak blues score, and lower progesterone levels on the day of peak blues.

Postnatal blues have also been positively associated with:

- poor social adjustment
- poor marital relationship
- high scores on EPI neuroticism scale
- fear of labour
- anxious and depressed mood during pregnancy.

There is no association between the development of postnatal blues and life events, demographic and social factors or obstetric factors.

Postnatal women differ significantly from women undergoing elective gynaecological surgery in the frequencies of different symptoms at different times, suggesting that postnatal mood swings are characteristic of the puerperium and are not simply non-specific reactions to stress.

MANAGEMENT

The woman should receive reassurance.

Postnatal depression

Postnatal depression is a depressive illness not qualitatively different from non-psychotic depression in other settings. It is characterized by low mood, reduced self-esteem, tearfulness, anxiety, particularly about the baby's health, and an inability to cope. Mothers may experience reduced affection for their baby, and may have difficulty with breast-feeding.

EPIDEMIOLOGY

Postnatal depression occur in 10–15% of post-partum women usually within 3 months of childbirth. Those women who are emotionally unstable in the first week after childbirth are at an increased risk of developing postnatal depression.

Postnatal depression is not associated with social class or parity.

AETIOLOGY

Environmental factors

Of the puerperal psychiatric conditions, postnatal depression has the least biological cause. Onset after childbirth is spread over a few months, and studies have repeatedly indicated the importance of social stress in its causation.

Paykel *et al.* (1980) found the strongest associated factor in mild post-partum depressives was the occurrence of recent stressful life events. Younger age, poor marital relationships and absent social supports were also notable. Early post-partum blues was associated with postnatal depression in the absence of life events, suggesting a small subgroup of postnatal depression with a hormonal aetiology. A past psychiatric history was a strong risk factor with or without life events.

Murray *et al.* (1995) found that postnatal depression, but not control depression, was associated with a poor relationship with the woman's own mother.

Postnatal depression is more contingent upon the acute biopsychosocial stresses caused by the arrival of a child, whereas depression not associated with childbirth is more closely related to longer-term social adversity and deprivation.

Hormonal factors

Despite the modest association between progesterone levels and post-partum blues, no direct association has been demonstrated between progesterone levels and postnatal depression.

Oestrogens affect dopaminergic transmission in the CNS; their precipitate drop after delivery may be responsible for psychosis, and possibly also depression in predisposed women.

Puerperal women, whether depressed or not, are non-suppressers in terms of the dexamethasone-suppression test. However, no associations have been found between postnatal depression and cortisol.

Transient hypothyroidism, sometimes preceded by hyperthyroidism, occurs in up to 5% of women in the post-partum year, peaking at 4–5 months. Such post-partum thyroid dysfunction is associated with depression. It is estimated that 1% of post-partum women in the general population will experience a depressive episode associated with thyroid dysfunction.

MANAGEMENT

The education of health visitors and midwives is necessary to identify cases early. The Edinburgh Postnatal Depression Scale is a 10-item self-report questionnaire, used by health visitors to identify postnatal depression during the course of their normal contacts with new mothers.

Non-directive counselling by health visitors individually or in groups is effective in one-third of cases. Self-help groups and mother-and-baby groups are useful to combat isolation.

In those with more severe symptomatology, or those unresponsive to counselling, antidepressants are required. If depression is severe, admission, preferably with the baby to a mother-and-baby unit, may be required. Suicidal mothers may have thoughts of taking their babies with them, so questions about the safety of the child should form part of the normal assessment of mothers of young children. ECT may be required, particularly if worthlessness, hopelessness and despair are present.

Breast-feeding should not be routinely suspended. Tricyclic antidepressants are transmitted in reduced quantities in breast milk. They are, however, safe. Lithium is transmitted and should not be given to a breast-feeding mother because of the risk of toxicity to the child.

OUTCOME

If undetected, postnatal depression may last up to 2 years with serious consequences for the marital relationship and the development of the child. There is good evidence for a link between depressive disorders in mothers and emotional disturbance in their children.

The following are more frequent in the children of mothers suffering postnatal depression:

- insecure attachment
- behaviour problems
- difficulties in expressive language
- fewer positive, and more negative facial expressions
- mild cognitive abnormalities
- less affective sharing
- less initial sociability.

Social and marital difficulties are often associated with reduced quality of mother–child interactions.

Cooper and Murray (1995) distinguished between those whose postnatal depression was a recurrence of previous affective disturbance, and those for whom postnatal depression had arisen *de novo*. Those who were suffering from a recurrence of depression were at raised risk of further non-post-partum episodes but not post-partum episodes. Those for whom the depression had arisen *de novo* were at raised risk for further episodes of postnatal depression but not for non-post-partum episodes.

The relapse rate for subsequent non-psychotic depression is 1 in 6.

Puerperal psychosis

The risk of developing a psychotic illness is increased 20-fold in the first post-partum month. Certain symptoms that are distinctive are:

- abrupt onset, within the first 2 weeks after childbirth
- marked perplexity, but no detectable cognitive impairment
- rapid fluctuations in mental state, sometimes from hour to hour
- marked restlessness, fear and insomnia
- delusions, hallucinations and disturbed behaviour, which develop rapidly.

EPIDEMIOLOGY

Kendell *et al.* (1987) linked psychiatric and obstetric registers in Edinburgh and found the number of admissions for psychotic disorders to be substantially elevated in the puerperium. This is shown in Table 30.2.

Eighty per cent of puerperal psychoses are affective. Schizophreniform psychoses often have manic features. Those with a previous history of manic depressive illness have a substantially higher risk than those with a history of schizophrenia or depression.

The following factors are associated with women developing puerperal psychoses:

- increased rate of Caesarean section
- higher social class

Table 30.2 *Number of admissions to mental hospitals per month in the pre-
and post-partum periods*

	Non-psychotic	Psychotic
15 months pre-conception	8	2
During pregnancy	5	2
1st post-partum month	17	51
2nd post-partum month	14	25
3rd post-partum month	10	13
4th post-partum month	8	9
5th post-partum month	6	6
Mean for next 18 months	9	4

- older age at birth of first child
- primiparae.

Psychosis following childbirth is usually of an affective type with a particularly high proportion of manic episodes within the first 2 weeks.

Puerperal psychoses follow 20–30% of births in those with pre-existing bipolar mood disorders.

AETIOLOGY

Genetic factors

- Family studies of puerperal psychosis point to a familial aggregation of psychiatric disorder, particularly affective illness.
- Children of probands who have had puerperal psychosis have an increased psychiatric morbidity.
- Female relatives of puerperal probands have a higher rate of puerperal illness than the general population, but the majority of illness in the relatives of probands is non-puerperal.
- The weight of evidence from clinical and family studies suggests that most cases of puerperal psychosis of early onset are closely related to bipolar disorder.

Environmental factors

There is no evidence of any excess of life events in puerperal psychotics compared to matched normal puerperal controls. The absence of social stress in this group contrasts with the findings for post-partum depression and disorders with onset in pregnancy. These findings suggest that the aetiology of severe puerperal psychosis is predominantly biological and interactive with previous vulnerability.

Hormonal factors

The pathophysiology of puerperal psychosis is not well understood but it is likely that the precipitous fall in the levels of circulating sex steroid hormones such as oestrogen occurring at the time of parturition plays an important role.

In animals, the administration of oestrogen leads to increased striatal dopamine binding, and oestrogen withdrawal leads to dopamine receptor supersensitivity.

Wieck *et al.* (1991) have reported increased sensitivity of dopamine receptors in the hypothalamus associated with the onset of affective psychosis following childbirth. It is possible that these changes in sensitivity are mediated by changes in circulating oestrogen levels.

Supersensitivity of dopamine receptors is then thought to precipitate psychosis.

MANAGEMENT

The identification of high-risk patients during pregnancy is important in the planning of postnatal management. Admission to a psychiatric hospital is usually essential, and it is usually preferable to admit mothers with their babies.

The following are some advantages of joint admission:

- Most psychotic mothers are capable of looking after their babies with supervision and support.
- There is evidence suggesting that joint admission may reduce the duration of illness and relapse rates.

The following are some disadvantages of joint admission:

- There is a risk of non-accidental injury to the child from the mother or fellow patients. A nurse should be dedicated to the care and supervision of the child and a lockable nursery should be provided.
- Joint admission needs higher staffing levels.
- The long-term effects of admission upon the development of the child are not known.
- The woman's partner needs support and education.

Therapy

- Phenothiazines and lithium are effective in the treatment of manic episodes. Control of lithium levels in the immediate post-partum period can be difficult because of fluid and electrolyte changes.
- ECT is particularly effective in the treatment of puerperal psychoses, and accelerates recovery in all diagnostic categories. It is used generally if the drug treatment has failed.
- In breast-feeding mothers, lithium is contraindicated because it is excreted into breast milk and is toxic to the baby.
- Neuroleptics can be administered to breast-feeding mothers, but high doses should be avoided and the baby should be observed for signs of drowsiness, such as a failure to feed adequately.
- Neuroleptics should be maintained for at least 3 months following recovery. If there are further manic or depressive episodes, lithium should be considered.

COURSE

Following discharge from hospital the mother will require close support and follow-up. An assessment of the mother–baby interaction should be made prior to discharge.

The initial prognosis is quite good. Cases often settle within 6 weeks, and most are fully recovered by 6 months. A few, however, have a protracted course.

After one episode of puerperal psychosis the risk of a further episode in each subsequent pregnancy is between one in three and one in five. For those with a previous psychiatric history or a family history the risk is higher; for those whose puerperal episode was associated with life events or Caesarean section the subsequent risk is lower.

MENOPAUSE

General population surveys indicate no major effect of the menopause on a variety of common psychiatric symptoms. If anything, women in the post-menopausal years show less evidence of psychiatric disturbance than younger women.

Anxiety and depression in post-menopausal women do not respond to oestrogen therapy, but may respond to antidepressants. Where sexual symptoms are present, hormone replacement therapy may be effective. There is some evidence that hormone replacement therapy ameliorates psychological symptoms after surgical menopause.

BIBLIOGRAPHY

Ashby, C.R., Carr, L.A., Cook, C.L. *et al.* 1992: Inhibition of serotonin uptake in rat brain synaptosomes by plasma from patients with pre-menstrual syndrome. *Biological Psychiatry* 31:1169–1171.

Ballinger, C.B. 1990: Psychiatric aspects of the menopause. *British Journal of Psychiatry* 156:773–787.

Bancroft, J. & Rennie, D. 1993: The impact of oral contraceptives on the experience of premenstrual mood, clumsiness, food craving and other symptoms. *Journal of Psychosomatic Research* 37:195–202.

Condon, J.T. 1993: The pre-menstrual syndrome: a twin study. *British Journal of Psychiatry* 162:481–486.

Cooper, P.J. & Murray, L. 1995: Course and recurrence of postnatal depression: evidence for the specificity of the diagnostic concept. *British Journal of Psychiatry* 166:191–195.

Craddock, N., Brockington, I., Mant, R. *et al.* 1994: Bipolar affective puerperal psychosis associated with consanguinity. *British Journal of Psychiatry* 164:359–364.

Dowlatshahi, D. & Paykel, E.S. 1990: Life events and social stress in puerperal psychoses: absence of effect. *Psychological Medicine* 20:655–662.

Eriksson, E., Sundblad, C., Lisjo, P. *et al.* 1992: Serum levels of androgens are higher in women with pre-menstrual irritability and dysphoria than in controls. *Psychoneuroendocrinology* 17:195–204.

Friedman, T. & Gath, D. 1989: The psychiatric consequences of spontaneous abortion. *British Journal of Psychiatry* 155:810–813.

Giannini, A.J., Melemis, S.M., Martin, D.M. *et al.* 1994: Symptoms of pre-menstrual syndrome as a function of beta-endorphin: two subtypes. *Progress in Neuropsychopharmacology and Biological Psychiatry* 18:321–327.

Gilchrist, A.C., Hannaford, P.C., Frank, P. *et al.* 1995: Termination of pregnancy and psychiatric morbidity. *British Journal of Psychiatry* 167:243–248.

Hannah, P., Adams, D., Lee, A. *et al.* 1992: Links between early post-partum mood and post-natal depression. *British Journal of Psychiatry* 160:777–780.

Harris, B. 1994: Biological and hormonal aspects of postpartum depressed mood: working towards strategies for prophylaxis and treatment. *British Journal of Psychiatry* 164:288–292.

Hicks, R.A., Olsen, C. & Smith Robinson, D. 1986: Type A-B behaviour and the pre-menstrual syndrome. *Psychological Reports* 59:353–354.

Iles, S., Gath, D. & Kennerley, H. 1989: Maternity blues: II. A comparison between post-operative women and post-natal women. *British Journal of Psychiatry* 155:363–366.

Kantero, R. & Widholm, O. 1971: Correlations of menstrual traits between adolescent girls and their mothers. *Acta Obstetrica and Gynecologica Scandinavica* 14 (Suppl. 14):30–36.

Kendell, R.E., Chalmers, J.C. & Platz, C.L. 1987: Epidemiology of puerperal psychoses. *British Journal of Psychiatry* 150:662–673.

Kennerley, H. & Gath, D. 1989: Maternity blues: III. Associations with obstetric psychological and psychiatric factors. *British Journal of Psychiatry* 155:367–373.

Logue, C.M. & Moos, R.H. 1986: Pre-menstrual symptoms: prevalence and risk factors. *Psychosomatic Medicine* 48:388–414.

Murray, D., Cox, J.L. Chapman, G. *et al.* 1995: Childbirth: life event or start of a long term difficulty? Further data from the Stoke-on-Trent controlled study of postnatal depression. *British Journal of Psychiatry* 166:595–600.

O'Hare, T. & Creed, F. 1995: Life events and miscarriage. *British Journal of Psychiatry* 167:799–805.

Paykel, E.S., Emms, E.M., Fletcher, J. *et al.* 1980: Life events and social supports in puerperal depression. *British Journal of Psychiatry* 136:339–346.

Pearce, J., Hawton, K. & Blake, F. 1995: Psychological and sexual symptoms associated with the menopause and the effects of hormone replacement therapy. *British Journal of Psychiatry* 167:163–173.

Schmidt, P., Grover, G.N. & Rubinow, D.R. 1993: Alprazolam in the treatment of pre-menstrual syndrome: a double-blind placebo-controlled trial. *Archives of General Psychiatry* 50:467–473.

Stein, A., Gath, D.H., Bucher, J. *et al.* 1991: The relationship between post-natal depression and mother-child interaction. *British Journal of Psychiatry* 158:46–52.

Stein, D., Hanukoglu, S., Blank, S. *et al.* 1993: Cyclic psychosis associated with the menstrual cycle. *British Journal of Psychiatry* 163:824–828.

Sundblad, C., Hedberg, M.A. & Eriksson, E. 1993: Clomipramine administered during the luteal phase reduces the symptoms of pre-menstrual syndrome: a placebo controlled trial. *Neuropsychopharmacology* 9:133–145.

Warner, P. & Bancroft, J. 1990: Factors related to self-reporting of the pre-menstrual syndrome. *British Journal of Psychiatry* 157:249–260.

Wieck, A., Kumar, R., Hirst, A.D. *et al.* 1991: Increased sensitivity of dopamine receptors and recurrence of affective psychosis after childbirth. *British Medical Journal* 303:613–616.

Zolese, G. & Blacker, C.V.R. 1992: The psychological complications of therapeutic abortion. *British Journal of Psychiatry* 160:742–749.

31

Sexual disorders

HISTORY

- In 1910, Havelock Ellis, a British pioneer, was the first to subject normal as well as pathological sexuality to scientific investigation.
- Starting in 1948, Kinsey and associates conducted landmark research into human sexual experience in thousands of men and women. A wide range of human sexual expression was noted. Methodological problems included non-random sampling. Volunteers were recruited from a variety of sources, with a non-representative excess of college-educated people. Criminals and sex offenders were also over-represented. Despite these shortcomings, their findings have been generalized to the wider population and remained authoritative for decades in the absence of methodologically superior work.
- In 1981, acquired immune deficiency syndrome (AIDS) was first described in the USA. It was initially believed to be confined to a small group of promiscuous homosexual men. Subsequently a primarily heterosexual worldwide epidemic of major proportions has developed.

BRITISH SEXUAL BEHAVIOUR AND ATTITUDES

A major survey of British sexual attitudes and lifestyle (Johnson *et al.*, 1994) has provided the most comprehensive evaluation of sexual behaviour in the British public to date. It was motivated largely by the emergence in the 1980s of the lethal epidemic of sexually transmitted infection, HIV, and the lack of baseline measures of sexual behaviour. The survey involved 18 876 British men and women in a random population sample aged 16–59. The following statistics were among many that emerged.

FIRST HETEROSEXUAL INTERCOURSE

- Age at occurrence is decreasing over time. In the past four decades the median age of first heterosexual intercourse has fallen from 21 to 17 for women, and from 20 to 17 for men.

- The proportion occurring before age 16 has increased over time. Fewer than 1% of women aged 55 or over report heterosexual intercourse before the age of 16, compared to 20% of those in their teens.
- There has been a convergence in behaviour of men and women over time.
- People today are more likely to use contraception (usually condoms) than those of a previous generation. However, the earlier first intercourse occurs, the less likely it is that contraception is used.
- Early intercourse is associated with lower social class and lower educational level.
- Now there is more planning and less spontaneity than formerly.
- The majority of intercourse occurs within an established relationship.
- Young women tend to be initiated by an older male. Men's first partners tend to be age peers.
- It is very rare for men's first sexual intercourse to be with a prostitute.

HETEROSEXUAL PARTNERSHIPS

- Age and marital status are associated with multiple partnerships. The young and those previously married or single (including cohabitees) are most likely to report high partner numbers.
- There is increasing partner change with increasing social class.
- There are increasing numbers of partners over historical time.
- The proportion reporting multiple partnerships in the last five years declines with increasing age.
- Serial monogamy is more common in those aged 16–24. Concurrent partnerships are more common in those over the age of 35.
- Sex with a prostitute in the last five years is most common in the 25–34 year age group.
- Raised odds of ever using a prostitute are associated with age, previous marriage or current cohabitation, working away from home, and a history of having a homosexual partner.

HETEROSEXUAL PRACTICES

- Frequency of heterosexual sex (oral, vaginal or anal intercourse) shows wide variability, with a small proportion of the population reporting a very high frequency of sexual contact.
- Age is closely related to the number of acts, frequency peaking in mid-twenties, then gradually declining.
- Frequency is affected by partner availability, being highest in married and cohabiting groups of all ages.
- There is a strong association in all age groups between length of relationship and frequency of sex: a much lower frequency in longer relationships.
- Vaginal intercourse predominates. Seventy-five per cent have experience of non-penetrative sex and 70% have some experience of oral sex. Any experience of anal intercourse is reported by 14% of men and 13% of women.
- Practice of oral sex has increased, but not as a substitute to vaginal intercourse.
- Those not married have a wider repertoire of sexual practice. Prevalence of oral, anal and non-penetrative sex increases with increasing numbers of partners.
- Those outside married or cohabiting relationships have less frequent sex overall, but are more likely to have multiple partners, a wider range of practices and recent experience of high-risk practices.

SEXUAL DIVERSITY AND HOMOSEXUAL BEHAVIOUR

- No sexual attraction or experience of any kind is reported by 0.4% of men and 0.5% of women.
- Exclusively heterosexual attraction and experience is reported by 90% of men and 92% of women.
- Mostly or exclusively homosexual attraction and experience is reported by 1% of men and 0.25% of women.
- Some form of homosexual experience is reported by 6% of men and 3% of women.
- Lifetime experience of homosexual orientation is higher in higher social classes.
- Recent homosexual experience is strongly associated with region. Greater London has more than twice the proportion of men reporting homosexual experience and current practice than anywhere else in Britain.
- Those who had a boarding-school education are more likely to report any homosexual contact; this has little or no effect on homosexual practice in later life.
- Exclusively homosexual behaviour is rare. The majority of those with homosexual experience have had sex with both men and women. Ninety per cent of men and 95% of women reporting same-gender sexual partners in their lifetime have also had an opposite-gender partner.
- Men reporting anal sex do so usually (60%) as both the receptive and insertive partner.
- Highest levels of homosexual activity are reported by 25- to 34-year-olds, nearly a decade later than heterosexual partnerships, consistent with later age at first experience.

SEXUAL ATTITUDES

- Acceptance of premarital sex is now nearly universal, as is its practice.
- Disapproval of infidelity extends to all age groups, the young being marginally more tolerant than older people.
- The British public show widespread condemnation of homosexual relationships. Women are more tolerant than men.
- Sex is not considered the most important part of a relationship; a monogamous relationship is considered more likely to lead to greater sexual satisfaction.

PHYSICAL HEALTH

- Multiple sexual partnerships are significantly associated with smoking and increasing levels of alcohol consumption.
- Attendance at a clinic for sexually transmitted diseases (STDs) is strongly associated with the number of heterosexual partners and a history of homosexual partnerships.
- There is a strong relationship between sexual behaviour and the probability of STD clinic attendance, abortion and HIV testing.
- No relationship is detected between the numbers of heterosexual partners and experience of infertility or miscarriage.
- The likelihood of termination of pregnancy increases markedly with the numbers of heterosexual partners.

PERCEIVED RISK

- Fewer than 10% of the British public is at risk of unplanned pregnancy.
- The use of oral contraception declines steeply with age; condom use is most prevalent in the young; sterilization increases with age.

- The message to use condoms to prevent the risks of STD has been more acceptable than the message to restrict numbers of partners.
- The perceived risk of HIV infection is higher among those reporting higher risk behaviours.
- Despite the uptake of messages about condom use, there is little sign of the widespread adoption of other safer sex practices among those reporting heterosexual behaviour.

SEXUAL DYSFUNCTION

The normal sexual response cycle consists of: desire; arousal, mediated by the parasympathetic nervous system; plateau; orgasm, mediated by the sympathetic and central nervous system; resolution (longer in males and increases with age).

With sexual dysfunctioning the individual is unable to participate in a sexual relationship as he or she would wish. Both psychological and somatic processes are usually involved in the causation of sexual dysfunction. Women present more commonly with complaints about the subjective quality of sexual experience; men present with a failure of specific sexual response.

ICD-10 classification

ICD-10 categorizes *Sexual dysfunction not caused by organic disorder or disease* under 'Behavioural syndromes associated with physiological disturbances and physical factors', as follows:

- *Lack or loss of sexual desire.* This is not secondary to other sexual difficulties. It does not preclude sexual enjoyment or arousal, but makes initiation of sexual activity less likely.
- *Sexual aversion.* Sexual interaction is associated with strong negative feelings of sufficient intensity that sexual activity is avoided.
- *Lack of sexual enjoyment.* Sexual responses and orgasm occur normally but there is a lack of pleasure. This is much more common in women.
- *Failure of genital response.* In men this is primarily erectile dysfunction. In women it is primarily due to vaginal dryness.
- *Orgasmic dysfunction.* Orgasm does not occur or is delayed. It is more common in women than men.
- *Premature ejaculation.* This is the inability to control ejaculation sufficiently for both partners to enjoy the sex act.
- *Non-organic vaginismus.* This is occlusion of the vaginal opening caused by spasm of the surrounding muscles. Penile entry is either impossible or painful.
- *Non-organic dyspareunia.* Pain during intercourse may occur in both sexes. The term is used only if an organic cause is not present, and if there is no other primary sexual dysfunction.
- *Excessive sexual drive.* This usually occurs in men or women during late teenage or early adult years. If it is secondary to mental illness (e.g. mania) the underlying disorder is coded.

Sensate-focus therapy

Masters and Johnson (1970) described behavioural psychotherapy involving a couple in graded assignments which may be modified according to the particular problem presenting. The process is used extensively in the treatment of sexual disorders affecting both men and women. It consists of a combination of specified homework tasks together with setting specific limits to the extent of sexual contact allowed.

- Stage 1: Touching partner without genital contact for subject's own pleasure.
- Stage 2: Touching partner without genital contact for subject's and partner's pleasure.
- Stage 3: Touching partner with genital contact, but intercourse not permitted.
- Stage 4: Simultaneous touching of partner and being touched by partner with genital contact, but intercourse not permitted.
- Stage 5: If both feel ready, the female invites the male to put his penis into her vagina. Female in the top position heightens female control and allows the male to relax. No thrusting is allowed. Initial containment is brief, being lengthened with each session.
- Stage 6: Vaginal containment with movement is allowed. Different positions are encouraged. This does not inevitably lead to climax. The couple should practise stopping before climax. Provided physical contact is pleasurable orgasm is not necessary.

ERECTILE DYSFUNCTION

NORMAL PHYSIOLOGY

Erection is a neurovascular phenomenon requiring an intact arterial supply and intact venous valves, allowing cavernosal pressures to rise to those approaching systolic blood pressures. Vascular changes are brought about by the parasympathetic autonomic nervous system (S2, 3, 4) influenced by tactile stimuli and central limbic and cognitive mechanisms. Psychic erections are mediated by thoracic sympathetic outflow, whereas reflex erections result from sacral parasympathetic outflow. Androgens also influence erection, particularly those occurring in sleep, via the limbic system.

Epidemiology of erectile dysfunction

Studies with community samples indicate the prevalence of male erectile disorder of 4–9%. It comprises about 50% of male cases presenting to a psychosexual disorders service. The incidence rises with age, from about 1.3% at 35 years, to 55% at 75 years.

Aetiology of erectile dysfunction

The aetiology can be organic (in about 50%), psychological, or a combination.

ORGANIC CAUSES

Local organic causes

- *Peyronie's disease.* There is progressive fibrosis in the tunica albuginea and sometimes also in the cavernosa, resulting in curvature of the penis on erection. The cause is unknown.
- *Congenital deformities.* Examples are hypospadias and epispadias, or the absence of suspensory ligaments.
- *Priapism.* Although rare, priapism may result in impotence if not treated adequately within 24 hours.

Endocrine causes

- Diabetes causes a combination of arteriopathy and neuropathy. Two-thirds of diabetic males have erectile impotence. Of these it is complete in two-thirds and partial in the remaining third. A few also complain of other difficulties such as premature ejaculation. Onset is insidious, the course progressive with marked decline in sexual activity and desire.
- Nocturnal erections are androgen-dependent. Studies are conflicting on the role of androgens in erectile disorders. Effects are probably mediated through lowered sexual interest.
- Hyperprolactinaemia may be secondary to hypothalamic/pituitary disease. It occurs in those on phenothiazines, and sometimes in alcoholics.
- Naltrexone (endorphin) therapy significantly improves impotence in males with an apparent non-organic cause. Alteration in central opioid tone may be responsible.

Neurological causes

- There may be peripheral or autonomic neuropathy (e.g. in diabetes, alcoholism).
- Radical pelvic surgery may cause autonomic neurological disruption.
- There may be a spinal cord lesion (e.g. transection, multiple sclerosis).

Vascular causes

- Arterial disease can interfere with the blood supply to pelvic organs.
- Venous valves may be incompetent.

PHARMACOLOGICAL FACTORS

Alcohol has complex effects, including neuropathy and indirect effects on sex steroids and gonadotrophins. Oestrogen levels are raised causing gynacomastia and testicular atrophy in advanced liver disease. Raised blood alcohol levels inhibit sexual responses through central inhibitory effects. Psychosocial factors are also prominent in these patients.

Ganglion blockers (*antihypertensives*) interfere with both sympathetic and parasympathetic postganglionic transmission and cause both impotence and ejaculatory failure. Propranolol crosses the blood–brain barrier and may exert its effect centrally. Alpha-adrenergic blockers are not associated with erectile failure, but cause ejaculatory failure.

PSYCHOLOGICAL FACTORS

The classical history of the disorder that is suggestive of a psychological cause comprises lack of sexual interest but continued morning erections.

Psychoanalytic concepts

Sexual physiological changes result from the interplay between conscious and unconscious thoughts and feelings, and interpersonal relationships. Anxiety and fear, whether conscious or unconscious, can interfere with vascular changes required for erection. Arousal-phase disorders of erectile dysfunction in men are common. Interference with abandonment to erotic feelings can impair arousal in men and lead to difficulties with erection.

Psychoanalytic formulations of erectile disorders recognize anxiety about the persecutory object and unresolved Oedipal conflicts. Deep ambivalence about intimate involvement leading to fear of sexual failure is common.

In younger men with primary impotence, Oedipal conflicts are said to predominate, whereas in secondary impotence, neurotic partnership conflicts at a pre-Oedipal level, and narcissistic crises in middle age are said to predominate.

Cognitive concepts

Erectile disorder is considered to be a sign of negative self-image within a depressive view of the relationship, and is linked to abandonment fear.

Subjects with psychogenic erectile impotence have a situational sexual disorder in which sexual anxiety plays an important role. Compared to those with organic impotence or to controls, they view themselves as more insecure and tend to over-idealize their partners and their mothers.

Consideration should also be given to the following:

- fear of hurting the female
- fear of pregnancy
- distaste for female genitalia
- placing the partner on a pedestal
- non-sexual stress
- unsympathetic or angry partner
- trying too hard.

Assessment of erectile dysfunction

The assessment of erectile dysfunction includes the following:

- A full history is needed, including the nature of the problem, detailed sexual history, medical and psychiatric histories, medication and substance use.
- Assessment of the couple's relationship is essential. Difficulties such as hostility, lack of communication, unresponsive or unerotic partner may be important.
- Physical examination includes the external genitalia; laboratory investigations including blood glucose, tests of renal and hepatic function.
- A penile–brachial artery pressure index of less than 0.6 is indicative of arterial disease to the penis. Angiography may be necessary, especially in younger patients.
- Nocturnal penile tumescence monitoring can be used to measure circumference change in sleep erections. This can help distinguish organic from psychogenic; if the cause is organic, erections at night are abolished.
- Dynamic cavernometry, in which normal saline is infused into the corpus cavernosum, may detect venous incompetence.
- Intracorporeal injection of papaverine or phentolamine can be diagnostic to establish the capacity for erection and hence reduce the likelihood of a primarily arterial cause.

Management of erectile dysfunction

PHYSICAL TREATMENTS

Physical treatments are increasingly available which are efficacious for both physical and psychogenically induced erectile dysfunction. As a result the distinction is not always sought. Emotionally intensive sex therapy is often not considered, especially if it is managed by surgeons. Recently it has become possible to treat erectile disorders with oral drugs which increase the penile blood flow. Such drugs should be used with caution if the penis is deformed (for example, in angulation, cavernosal fibrosis, and Peyronie's disease).

Phosphodiesterase type 5 inhibitors

Orally administered phosphodiesterase type 5 inhibitors that are licensed for treatment of erectile dysfunction include sildenafil, tadalafil and vardenafil. These drugs should not be administered with other pharmacological treatments for erectile dysfunction. They should be used with caution in cardiovascular disease, anatomical deformation of the penis (e.g. angulation, cavernosal fibrosis, Peyronie's disease), and in those with a predisposition to prolonged erection (e.g. in sickle-cell anaemia, multiple myeloma, or leukaemia).

The drugs are contraindicated in patients:

- receiving nitrates
- in whom vasodilation is inadvisable
- in whom sexual activity is inadvisable
- with hypotension
- with a history of recent stroke
- with unstable angina
- with myocardial infarction.

The side-effects of these drugs include dyspepsia, vomiting, headache, flushing, dizziness, visual disturbances, raised intra-ocular pressure, and nasal congestion. Hypersensitivity reactions (including rash), priapism, and painful red eyes have also been reported.

Apomorphine

Sublingually administered apomorphine is licensed for the treatment of erectile dysfunction. Vasovagal symptoms (including sweating and syncope) can occur infrequently.

Intracavernosal injection of vasoactive drugs

Papaverine is commonly used to treat impotence. Self-injected, it gives an erection lasting about an hour, and may be used up to twice a week. Half those presenting to a sexual dysfunction clinic benefit from intracorporeal papaverine. Many decline the treatment because of the perception that injection is cumbersome and interrupts sexual foreplay, or because of objection to the use of needles. Intracorporeal pharmacotherapy provides a useful treatment option in the management of impotence but it is limited by the method of administration.

Complications include priapism which should be treated promptly by the withdrawal of 20–60 mL of blood and injection of an α-adrenergic agent such as phenylephrine 1–5 mg, or metaraminol 2 mg. Fibrosis is associated with prolonged use and rises in proportion to the total numbers of injections given. Haematomas and bruising are relatively common but of little significance.

Alprostadil (prostaglandin E_1) is administered by intracavernosal injection or intraurethral application for the management of erectile dysfunction (after exclusion of treatable medical causes); it is also used as a diagnostic test.

Alpha-adrenergic blocking agents

Phenoxybenzamine or phentolamine may also be used to give more prolonged erection.

Suction devices

Vacuum tumescence constriction therapy is efficacious and useful in those with organic as well as psychogenic impotence. These devices provide a safe method of obtaining an erection adequate for penetration in up to 90% of patients. Many couples derive substantial benefit from their use, but the disadvantages of a not fully rigid erection, lack of spontaneity, decreased sensation and delayed or absent ejaculation in some limit their acceptability.

Vascular surgery
Correction of venous leak may be successful if a specific leak is detected. Arterial surgery is less successful. Large vessel reconstruction for proximal arterial obstruction generally gives poor results, as most patients also have distal arterial disease.

Penile prosthetic implants
Surgically implanted penile prostheses are inserted into the corpus cavernosa. Three types are available: malleable, constructed of silastic with a malleable metal core giving permanent rigidity; self-contained inflatable; and multipart inflatable prostheses.

The psychological outcome of penile prosthesis implantation appears to be mediated by the nature of the marital relationship. Follow-up of recipients of penile implants 2.5 years following surgery found that those with organogenic impotence had no adverse sequelae, but some of those with psychogenic impotence had an exacerbation of pre-existing relationship difficulties. Ideally couple therapy should be offered as well as mechanical treatments, especially in those with a psychogenic cause.

PSYCHOLOGICAL TREATMENTS

Counselling
Practical advice about sexual technique is essential for all forms of treatment, even if the main treatment is physical.

Psychotherapy
Cognitive–behavioural methods report success rates of 70% for erectile impotence. Couple therapy appears to be superior to surrogate or individual therapies. Factors associated with successful outcome include the state of the marriage, better pre-treatment communication, better general sexual adjustment, female partner's interest and enjoyment of sex, absence of psychiatric history in the female partner, and early engagement in homework assignments.

Sensate focus therapy may need to be combined with other methods, such as improvement in communication skills. Once erections are starting to occur a form of 'paradoxical intent' may be used, in which the couple is instructed to get rid of the erection as soon as it occurs, and then to resume touching. The purpose is to demonstrate that erections do not need to be used as soon as they arise.

Psychodynamic therapists challenge disturbing fantasies, and prevent their re-enactment. The patient is offered a psychotherapeutic 'holding' to counteract the unsafe internal world. Gradually he becomes freed from his sexually disempowering psychic reality to respond to the external reality of erotic stimulation. Behavioural interventions may also be incorporated into the treatment.

PREMATURE EJACULATION

NORMAL PHYSIOLOGY

Orgasm, seminal emission and ejaculation are physiologically distinct processes, and are potentially separable.

Ejaculation is the forceful expulsion of semen from the urethra. If semen is released from the urethra without force it is emission. Before orgasm the male becomes aware that ejaculation is imminent and it follows within 1–3 seconds – 'ejaculatory inevitability'. Ejaculation and emission are mediated by the α-adrenergic sympathetic nervous system. Androgens have a role, since the first sexual consequence of castration is the inability to ejaculate, which is rapidly restored with androgen replacement.

In severe premature ejaculation, emission alone may occur with no ejaculatory component, minimal or absent orgasm and a long refractory period.

In youth, males have a tendency to ejaculate quickly. This usually diminishes with increasing age because of increasing control with experience, an ability to recognize the approach of ejaculatory inevitability, the dampening in responsiveness with age, and the lessening of novelty which arises in a stable relationship.

Epidemiology of premature ejaculation

Studies with community samples indicate the prevalence of 36–38% for premature ejaculation. Thirteen per cent of attendees at a sexual disorders clinic present primarily with this problem.

Aetiology of premature ejaculation

NON-PHYSICAL FACTORS

- Anxiety promotes emission but inhibits orgasm, and thus plays a crucial role in premature ejaculation.
- Primary premature ejaculation is always present. Secondary premature ejaculation develops after a period of satisfactory sexual functioning.
- Those with primary premature ejaculation are more impaired in sexual functioning, and are more anxious. Those with secondary premature ejaculation are more likely to have coexisting erectile disorder, a reduction in sex drive and a reduction in arousal.
- In psychological terms, whereas erectile disorder seems to belong to a depressive organization, premature ejaculation belongs to a phobic one.
- A variety of psychological factors may interfere with the learning process, impairing the ability to identify the point of impending ejaculation.

PHYSICAL FACTORS

There are few physical causes. Drugs do not cause premature ejaculation. It is possible that the autonomic control of ejaculation is very sensitive and therefore more difficult to control in some individuals.

Those with premature ejaculation do not have penile hypersensitivity compared to controls.

No differences in the pituitary gonadal system are found between those with erectile impotence, premature ejaculation and normal controls.

Management of premature ejaculation

Education in ejaculatory control using the 'pause' technique is the treatment of choice. During sensate-focus exercises, the male, when he predicts that he will ejaculate shortly, asks his partner to stop, allow his arousal level to subside slightly and then return to being caressed, repeating the process again when arousal increases.

If difficulty is experienced using this method, then the 'squeeze technique' is used. Just before ejaculation becomes inevitable, stimulation is stopped and the tip of the penis is grasped firmly for about 10 seconds, reducing the reflex ejaculatory response.

At therapeutic doses some antidepressants (e.g. fluoxetine) have a beneficial effect in men with premature ejaculation.

ANORGASMIA

NORMAL PHYSIOLOGY

The final stage of sexual excitement may be orgasm. In both sexes if no orgasm occurs, there is a slow resolution of physical and psychological changes associated with sexual excitement. Apart from ejaculation for which there is no female counterpart, the correlates of orgasm are similar in the sexes. Heart rate and blood pressure increase, there is a sudden increase in skeletal muscle activity involving almost all parts of the body. Rhythmic muscle contractions in the male genital tract expel semen; in females there is transient rhythmical contraction of the uterus and vagina. Psychologically there is an instant sense of relief; at its most extreme there can be a virtual loss of consciousness, and relaxation ensues.

The exact mechanism of orgasm is not known. In addition to local spinal mechanisms, the central nervous activity is also involved. EEG recordings during intense orgasm show changes which have been likened to those occurring during epileptic fits.

Epidemiology of anorgasmia

The prevalence in community samples is around 5–10% for inhibited female orgasm, and 4–10% for inhibited male orgasm. Among attendees at a sexual disorders clinic, 5% of males and 7% of females present primarily with orgasmic dysfunction. In females the prevalence of anorgasmia reduces with increasing age.

Aetiology of anorgasmia

Little is known.

PHYSICAL FACTORS

- In primary complete anorgasmia in both sexes, the bulbocavernosus reflex has been reported to be absent in a proportion; this is strongly correlated with the failure of treatment.
- Sometimes local pain, possibly secondary to muscle spasm, or in local viscera (uterus, rectum) can create fear of orgasm.
- Opiates appear to have a direct inhibitory effect, and antiserotonergic drugs inhibit orgasm.
- Female anorgasmia has been reported in association with tricyclic, MAOI, and SSRI antidepressants, and neuroleptic drugs.

PSYCHOLOGICAL FACTORS

The aetiology of anorgasmia is usually psychological. Anxiety inhibits orgasm in women but can hasten emission in men. Sex may be viewed as bad, disgusting or threatening the need to remain in control at all times. There may be a fear of pregnancy or venereal disease.

Management of anorgasmia

Sociocultural expectations and deficits in skills and sexual techniques are the two most important factors present in most cases. Direct masturbation training is the treatment of choice.

Treatment may take place in individual, couple or group settings. Tasks include relaxation, fantasizing and masturbation. Treatment is often successful, but the generalization of orgasm induced by masturbation to that induced by intercourse does not always occur.

VAGINISMUS

NORMAL PHYSIOLOGY

When sexually aroused, the upper two-thirds of the vagina are lax and capacious, whereas the lower third is closely invested by the surrounding musculature of the pelvic floor. The strongest of these muscles is the levator ani which forms a U-shaped sling around the posterior and lateral vaginal wall. Intense spasm in a nulliparous woman can virtually occlude the vagina. If these muscles are too tense, vaginal entry is impaired and painful – a condition known as vaginismus. A vicious circle ensues; pain or anticipation of pain causes further muscle contraction thereby increasing the likelihood of experiencing pain.

Epidemiology of vaginismus

Ten per cent of women presenting to a sexual disorders clinic have a primary presentation of vaginismus.

Aetiology of vaginismus

The majority of cases are primary. The problem was evident at first attempt at intercourse, and usually the woman has been reluctant to introduce anything to her vagina previously.

Occasionally onset can be related to a traumatic episode such as a painful vaginal examination or rape.

Sometimes vaginismus results from ambivalence about the relationship, or it may be secondary to reluctance to assume the mature adult's role. Irrational fears may also underlie the condition.

Management of vaginismus

Emphasis is upon helping the woman to gain comfort in exploring her own genitalia and inserting her finger. Finger insertion may be all that is required, combined with sensate-focus techniques.

Additional dilatation may be required using graded dilators. Initially carried out on her own, the partner is included when her confidence has increased.

DISORDERS OF GENDER IDENTITY

Classification

The ICD-10 classification codes *Gender identity disorders* under 'Disorders of adult personality and behaviour'.

TRANSSEXUALISM

There is the desire to live as a member of the opposite sex; discomfort with anatomic sex; a wish to change body into that of the preferred sex.

It must have been persistently present for two years; it must not be a symptom of another mental disorder such as schizophrenia, or be associated with an intersex, genetic or sex-chromosomal abnormality.

DUAL-ROLE TRANSVESTISM

This includes the wearing of clothes of the opposite sex for part of the time to enjoy the temporary experience of membership of the opposite sex, without the desire for a more permanent sex change. No sexual excitement accompanies this cross-dressing, distinguishing it from fetishistic transvestism.

GENDER IDENTITY DISORDER OF CHILDHOOD

This is persistent, intense distress about assigned sex, together with desire to be of the other sex, usually manifest during early childhood, and always before puberty. It is relatively uncommon. There is a profound disturbance of the sense of maleness or femaleness.

Between one- and two-thirds of boys with gender identity disorder of childhood show homosexual orientation during and after adolescence. However, very few exhibit transsexualism in later life, although most adults with transsexualism report having had a gender identity problem in childhood. Some girls retain male gender identification in adolescence and some go on to homosexual orientation. Most, however, do not.

It is more common in boys than girls in clinic samples.

Treatment of disorders of gender identity

Sex-reassignment treatment for transsexuals is a process of active rehabilitation into the new gender role, the provision and monitoring of opposite-sex hormones, and after a reasonable period of successful cross-gender living, sex-reassignment surgery is performed. The majority of transsexuals do experience a successful outcome in terms of subjective wellbeing and personal happiness.

SEXUAL DEVIATION

Classification

The ICD-10 classification codes sexual deviation as *Disorders of sexual preference* under 'Disorders of adult personality and behaviour'.

FETISHISM

Fetishism is the reliance on some non-living object as a stimulus for sexual arousal and gratification. It is often an extension of the human body such as clothing or footwear. It is often characterized by texture such as plastic, rubber or leather.

Fetishism is diagnosed only if the fetish is the most important source of sexual stimulation. Fantasies are common but do not amount to disorder unless they are so compelling that they interfere with sexual intercourse and lead to distress.

FETISHISTIC TRANSVESTISM

Fetishistic transvestism is the wearing of clothes of the opposite sex to obtain sexual excitement. More than a single item is worn, often an entire outfit. It is clearly associated with sexual arousal; there is no wish to continue cross-dressing once orgasm occurs, distinguishing this from transsexual transvestism.

EXHIBITIONISM

Exhibitionism is the recurrent or persistent tendency to expose the genitalia to strangers or people (usually of the opposite sex) in public places. There is usually sexual excitement at the time, often followed by masturbation. The tendency may only manifest at times of emotional stress or crisis, without such behaviour between.

It is almost entirely limited to heterosexual males, exhibiting to adult or adolescent females, usually from a safe distance in a public place. For some it is their only sexual outlet; for others they may also continue a normal sex life.

A reaction in the victim heightens the excitement in the perpetrator.

VOYEURISM

Voyeurism is the persistent tendency to look at people engaging in sexual behaviour or undressing. It usually leads to sexual excitement and masturbation. The victim is usually unaware.

PAEDOPHILIA

Paedophilia is the sexual preference for children, usually prepubertal or pubertal. Some are attracted to either one or both sexes.

It is rare in women. Included in this diagnosis are those men who retain a preference for adult sex partners, but when frustrated in their efforts turn to children as substitutes.

SADOMASOCHISM

Sadomasochism is the preference for sexual activity that involves the infliction of pain or humiliation. It is diagnosed only if this is the most important source of sexual stimulation.

MULTIPLE DISORDERS OF SEXUAL PREFERENCE

This is when more than one disorder of sexual preference occurs in one person and none is predominant.

OTHER DISORDERS OF SEXUAL PREFERENCE

This includes obscene telephone calls (telephone scatologia), frotteurism, sexual activity with animals (bestiality), the use of anoxia to heighten sexual pleasure (anoxophilia), and necrophilia.

SEXUAL ORIENTATION

Sexual disorientation alone is no longer classed as a disorder. ICD-10 allows for variations of sexual development or orientation that are problematic for the individual:

- heterosexual
- homosexual
- bisexual
- other, including prepubertal.

Evidence suggestive of a genetic basis to sexual orientation is provided in twin studies with 52% MZ to 22% DZ concordance in homosexual males, and 48% MZ to 16% DZ concordance in female homosexuals. Hamer *et al.* (1993) carried out a family pedigree study in which the distribution of homosexuality in the male relatives suggested a sex-linked inheritance. They found convincing evidence in this family of a correlation between homosexual orientation and the inheritance of polymorphous markers at the Xq28 region of the X chromosome.

ANTISOCIAL SEXUAL BEHAVIOUR

The acceptability of sexual behaviour is determined by society and is incorporated into the law. What constitutes unacceptable behaviour varies largely between cultures and within the same culture over time.

Antisocial sexual behaviours can be divided into two groups:

- 'normal' activities carried out inappropriately, without consent or with the wrong age group
- sexual activity which is morally perverse.

Specific antisocial sexual behaviours

RAPE

Rape is unlawful sexual intercourse with a person by force or against the person's will. Rapists are not a homogeneous group.

Classification of rapists (Trick & Tennant, 1981)

- *Situational stress rapist.* Otherwise sexually normal, these individuals commit rape when under extreme situational stress. There is much guilt and remorse afterwards.

- *Sociopathic rapist.* These have poor social adjustment with criminality, a poor work record, involve substance abuse, and have unstable relationships. Rape is often impulsive, with immediate gratification and little regard to the consequences. Threats of violence are common.
- *Sexually inadequate rapist.* These are shy, timid and insecure, lacking social skills. They often plan a rape against an attractive or sexually threatening woman.
- *Sadistic rapist.* These have a deep-rooted hatred of women arising from early relationships. The object of the rape is the infliction of humiliation and suffering; intercourse may be trivial in comparison to humiliating acts and the serious injuries inflicted. The rape is often carefully planned; precautions are taken to avoid detection.
- *Psychotic rapist.* These constitute a very small proportion of rapists. The rape is often bizarre, violent and terrifying for the victim.

PAEDOPHILIA

Paedophilia is the sexual attraction and preference for partners who are physically immature. Offenders are mostly men. Some prefer child victims of the opposite sex, some of the same sex. About 10% are bisexual in their preference.

Adolescent offenders have a better prognosis than older offenders.

The mentally immature offender with poor social skills may prefer child sexual partners because they are the only people with whom the person can relate at a general level.

The persistent middle-aged offender often has evidence of personality problems with poor relationships and unstable work patterns. These offenders usually have low rather than high sex drives. There is often an emotional bond between them and their child victims.

Some paedophiles are more dangerous than those described above. This offender has evidence of a serious personality disturbance affecting more aspects of his or her life than choice of sexual outlet.

Killing a child as part of a sexual offence is rare. It usually results from a state of panic, or from a desire to dispose of the evidence.

INCEST

Incest is generally forbidden across cultures. In law it is an offence for a man to have sexual intercourse with a woman he knows to be his daughter, grand-daughter, mother, sister or half-sister, and for a woman over 16 to allow a man whom she knows to be her son, father, grandfather, brother or half-brother to have sexual intercourse with her.

Sibling incest relationships are the most common, but father–daughter relationships are most commonly seen in court. They often reflect some breakdown in the marital relationship.

Incestuous families are characterized by alienation, disorganization and disintegration. They are rarely reported to the police.

Sibling incest is often the result of experimentation. It is more likely if there is a lack of parental control. Youngest sisters are the most vulnerable.

INDECENT EXPOSURE

Indecent exposure is an offence under the 1824 Vagrancy Act: 'openly, lewdly and obscenely exposing his person with intent to insult any female'. It is one of the most common sexual offences.

Exhibitionism, the exposing of genitals to the opposite sex, is categorized into the following two main groups:

- *Type I* – inhibited young men of relatively normal personality and good character who struggle against the impulse but find it irresistible. They expose with a flaccid penis and do not masturbate. They expose to individuals, not seeking a particular response. The frequency of exposure is often related to other sexual stresses and anxieties, such as marital conflict or pregnancy in the spouse.

- *Type II* – less inhibited, more sociopathic men. Individuals expose with erect penis in a state of excitement, and may masturbate. Pleasure is obtained and little guilt is shown. The person is more likely to expose to a group of women or girls, and may return repeatedly to the same place. The person seeks a response from the victim, either shock or disgust. There are fewer attempts to resist the urge to expose. The behaviour is associated with other psychosexual disorders and other types of offences. This may lead on to more serious sexual offences.

Eighty per cent do not reoffend if they are charged with a first offence. The chances of reconviction rise dramatically with the second offence. There is a small group of recidivists who persist, but these tend to reduce in their forties. It is generally a harmless non-violent offence, except in a minority who may progress to more violent offences.

There is a good prognosis associated with being married, good social relationships and work record.

Others

- *Fetishism* may come to the attention of the police if articles used are stolen (e.g. women's underwear).
- *Sadomasochism* may result in conviction for assault if extreme injury results, even if both parties consent.
- *Transvestites* may be charged with behaviour likely to cause a breach of the peace if they cross-dress in public.
- *Frotteurism* is the practice of rubbing the penis against another person in a clandestine way in a public place. It is liable to charges of either indecent assault or offence against public order.

Treatment of antisocial sexual behaviour

In a critical review of the literature, Marshall *et al.* (1991) concluded that some treatment programmes have been effective with paedophiles and exhibitionists but not with rapists.

In examining the value of the various treatment approaches they concluded that comprehensive cognitive–behavioural programmes were most likely to be effective with paedophiles and exhibitionists. There was also a clear value in the use of antiandrogens in those offenders who engage in excessively high rates of sexual activity.

BIBLIOGRAPHY

Bancroft, J. 1983: *Human Sexuality and its Problems.* Edinburgh: Churchill Livingstone.

Bancroft, J. 1994: Homosexual orientation: the search for a biological basis. *British Journal of Psychiatry* 164:437–440.

Bancroft, J. 1995: Sexual disorders. In Kendell, R.E. & Zealley, A.K. (eds) *Companion to Psychiatric Studies*, 5th edn. Edinburgh: Churchill Livingstone.

Brindley, G.S. & Gillian, P. 1982: Men and women who do not have orgasms. *British Journal of Psychiatry* 140:351–356.

Cooper, A.J., Cernovsky, Z.Z. & Colussi, K. 1993: Some clinical and psychometric characteristics of primary and secondary premature ejaculators. *Journal of Sex and Marital Therapy* 19:276–288.

Derogatis, L.R., Schmidt, C.W., Fagan, P.J. *et al.* 1989: Subtypes of anorgasmia via mathematical taxonomy. *Psychosomatics* 30:166–173.

Fabbri, A., Jannini, E.A., Gnessi, L. *et al.* 1989: Endorphins in male impotence: evidence for naltrexone stimulation of erectile activity in patient therapy. *Psychoneuroendocrinology* 14:103–111.

Gilbert, H.W. & Gingell, J.C. 1991: The results of an intracorporeal papaverine clinic. *Sex and Marital Therapy* 6:49–56.

Gregoire, A. 1992: New treatments for erectile impotence. *British Journal of Psychiatry* 160:315–326.

Hamer, D.H., Hu, S., Magnuson, V.L. *et al.* 1993: A linkage between DNA markers on the X chromosome and male sexual orientation. *Science* 261:321–327.

Hawton, K., Catalan, J. & Fagg, J. 1992: Sex therapy for erectile dysfunction: characteristics of couples, treatment outcome and prognostic factors. *Archives of Sexual Behaviour* 21:161–175.

Hiller, J. 1993: Psychoanalytic concepts and psychosexual therapy: a suggested integration. *Sex and Marital Therapy* 8:9–26.

Janssen, P.L. 1985: Psychodynamic study of male potency disorders: an overview. *Psychotherapy and Psychosomatics* 44:6–17.

Johnson, A.M., Wadsworth, J., Wellings, K. *et al.* 1994: *Sexual Attitudes and Lifestyles.* Oxford: Blackwell Scientific.

Kinsey, A.C., Pomeroy, W.B. & Martin, C.E. 1948: *Sexual Behaviour in the Human Male.* Philadelphia: W.B. Saunders.

Kinsey, A.C., Pomeroy, W.B., Martin, C.E. *et al.* 1953: *Sexual Behaviour in the Human Female.* Philadelphia: W.B. Saunders.

Kockett, G. 1980: Symptomatology and psychological aspects of male sexual inadequacy: results of an experimental study. *Archives of Sexual Behaviour* 9:457–475.

Marshall, W.L., Jones, R., Ward, T. *et al.* 1991: Treatment outcome with sex offenders. *Clinical Psychology Review* 11:465–485.

Masters, W.H. & Johnson, V.E. 1970: *Human Sexual Inadequacy.* London: Churchill Livingstone.

Mishra, D.N. & Shulka, G.D. 1988: Sexual disturbances in male diabetics: phenomenological and clinical aspects. *Indian Journal of Psychiatry* 30:135–143.

Pena, L.E. 1987: An analysis of female primary orgasmic dysfunction. *Revista de Analisis del Comportamiento* 3:151–163.

Pirke, K.M. *et al.* 1979: Pituitary gonadal system function in patients with erectile impotence and premature ejaculation. *Archives of Sexual Behaviour* 8:41–48.

Rowland, D.L., Haensel, S.M., Blom, J.H. *et al.* 1993: Penile sensitivity in men with premature ejaculation and erectile dysfunction. *Journal of Sex and Marital Therapy* 19:189–197.

Segraves, R.T., Taylor, R., Schoenberg, H.W. *et al.* 1982: Psychosexual adjustment after penile prosthesis surgery. *Sexuality and Disability* 5:222–229.

Snaith, P., Tarsh, M.J. & Reid, R. 1993: Sex reassignment surgery. *British Journal of Psychiatry* 162:681–685.

Spector, I.P. & Carey, M.P. 1990: Incidence and prevalence of the sexual dysfunctions: a critical review of the empirical literature. *Archives of Sexual Behaviour* 19:389–408.

Tondo, L., Cantone, M., Carta, M. *et al.* 1991: An MMPI evaluation of male sexual dysfunction. *Journal of Clinical Psychology* 47:391–396.

Trick, R.L. & Tennant, T.G. 1981: *Forensic Psychiatry: An Introductory Text.* London: Pitman Medical.

32

Sleep disorders

CLASSIFICATION

The ICD-10 classification of non-organic sleep disorders is:

F51.0   Nonorganic insomnia
F51.1   Nonorganic hypersomnia
F51.2   Nonorganic disorder of the sleep–wake schedule
F51.3   Sleepwalking
F51.4   Sleep terrors
F51.5   Nightmares

INSOMNIA

Insomnia is a disorder characterized by an insufficient quantity or quality of sleep. The estimated prevalence in adults ranges from 15% to over 40%. Prevalence is particularly high in the elderly.

CLINICAL FEATURES

The main result of true insomnia is daytime tiredness.

DIFFERENTIAL DIAGNOSIS

Important disorders that may cause insomnia, and that should therefore be excluded, include:

- depressive disorders
- mania
- anxiety disorders
- organic disorders (see Table 32.1).

Table 32.1   *Causes of insomnia*

Environmental	Poor sleep hygiene
	Change in time zone
	Change in sleeping habits
	Shiftwork
Physiological	Natural short sleeper
	Pregnancy
	Middle age
Life stress	Bereavement
	Exams
	House move etc.
Psychiatric	Acute anxiety
	Depression
	Mania
	Organic brain syndrome
Physical	Pain
	Cardiorespiratory distress
	Arthritis
	Nocturia
	GI disorders
	Thyrotoxicosis
Pharmacological	Caffeine
	Alcohol
	Stimulants
	Chronic hypnotic use
Parasomnias	Sleep apnoea
	Sleep myoclonus
Primary sleep disorders	

Reproduced with permission from Puri, B.K., Laking, P.J. & Treasaden, I.H. 2002: *Textbook of Psychiatry*, 2nd edn. Edinburgh: Churchill Livingstone.

AETIOLOGY

Table 32.1 gives the main causes of insomnia.

MANAGEMENT

The management of insomnia covers 'sleep hygiene', including:

- reduced lighting
- a comfortable bed
- a familiar and acceptable level of noise
- regular daytime exercise
- progressive muscle relaxation techniques for any associated anxiety
- a moderate intake of easily digested warm food
- sleep conditioning
- hypnotics (note the CSM guidelines on the prescription of benzodiazepines)
- behavioural approaches, particularly with children.

COURSE AND PROGNOSIS

Chronic insomnia may last through to old age.

HYPERSOMNIA

Daytime drowsiness occurs in 0.3–4% of the population.

CLINICAL FEATURES

Excessive daytime sleepiness and sleep attacks occur regularly or recurrently for short periods, causing a disturbance of social or occupational functioning.

DIFFERENTIAL DIAGNOSIS

Important differential diagnoses include:

- narcolepsy
- sleep apnoea
- organic disorders
- fatigue states
- Kleine–Levin syndrome.

AETIOLOGY

The common causes of hypersomnia are:

- as an early symptom of depressive disorder
- unknown cause: idiopathic.

MANAGEMENT

Treat any identified underlying cause. In idiopathic hypersomnia, amphetamines and other stimulants are occasionally used.

COURSE AND PROGNOSIS

The course is that of the underlying disorder. Idiopathic hypersomnia may improve with age.

DISORDERS OF THE SLEEP–WAKE CYCLE

Disorders of the sleep–wake cycle are characterized by sleep occurring out of phase with environmental and social cues (*Zeitgebers*).

DEFINITIONS

- *Entrainment failure* (rare). This refers to the independent running of the sleep–wake cycle.
- *Delayed sleep-phase syndrome* (rare). The sleep length is normal, there are no other psychiatric symptoms, but sleep takes place later than usual.
- *Advanced sleep-phase syndrome.* The sleep length is normal, there are no other psychiatric symptoms, but sleep takes place earlier than usual.

MANAGEMENT

Treat any primary disorder. If entrainment failure is secondary to a lack of sleep–wake cues in a modality such as vision (because of poor vision, say) then cues from other modalities and a careful routine may be employed. Advancing sleep in small increments may help in cases of delayed sleep-phase syndrome.

PARASOMNIAS

The parasomnias are phenomena occurring as part of or alongside sleep; they are shown in Table 32.2.

Table 32.2 *The parasomnias*

Sleepwalking (somnambulism)
Night terrors (pavor nocturnus)
Nightmares or dream anxiety
Bruxism (teeth grinding)
Nocturnal enuresis
Headbanging (jacatio capitis nocturnus)
Sleep paralysis
Nocturnal painful erections
Cluster headache
Physical symptomatology occurring at night, e.g. paroxysmal nocturnal dyspnoea, sleep epilepsy
Sleep myoclonus

Reproduced with permission from Puri, B.K., Laking, P.J. & Treasaden, I.H. 2002: *Textbook of Psychiatry*, 2nd edn. Edinburgh: Churchill Livingstone.

SOMNAMBULISM (SLEEP WALKING)

In this disorder there occurs a state of altered consciousness in which, while asleep, the individual arises and walks.

Sleep walking occurs at least once in 15% of children aged 5–12 years, and in 0.5% of adults. Females are more affected than men (sex ratio (F:M) = 4:3).

CLINICAL FEATURES

The sufferer is difficult to awaken during an episode, and may suffer injury if sleeping in an unfamiliar setting. Although complex behaviours, including attempted homicide, have been described as occurring during somnambulism, in general this is not common.

DIFFERENTIAL DIAGNOSIS

Important differential diagnoses include:

- psychomotor epilepsy during sleep
- fugue states
- sleep drunkenness.

AETIOLOGY

Somnambulism is familial in up to 20% of cases. There are no characteristic EEG changes. Sleep laboratory studies do *not* lend credence to the view that somnambulism represents the acting out of dreams.

MANAGEMENT

The person's night-time surroundings should be made safe in order to reduce the risk of injury during episodes. Reassurance and, sometimes, family work, anxiety-reduction techniques and small doses of hypnotics, may help.

NIGHT TERRORS

Night (sleep) terrors occur during sleep stages 3–4, and therefore usually one to two hours after sleep starts. In children, night terrors are common and occur on a frequent basis in 1–4%. They are far less common in adulthood.

CLINICAL FEATURES

The affected person, usually a child, awakes terrified and screaming, but little is recalled the following morning. Enuresis may occur during an episode.

DIFFERENTIAL DIAGNOSIS

The main differential diagnosis is nightmares.

AETIOLOGY

Aetiological factors that have been suggested include:

- stress
- previous loss of sleep
- familial
- induction by benzodiazepine antagonists (hence the theories about benzodiazepine receptor changes or endogenous substances acting on benzodiazepine receptors)
- upper airway obstruction in children.

MANAGEMENT

Methods that may be tried include:

- reassurance – of the child *and* the parents
- changing the settling routine
- keeping a diary and then waking the child just before each episode is expected.

Course and prognosis

These problems often resolve spontaneously.

NIGHTMARES

Nightmares are 'bad' (i.e. frightening) dreams. They occur universally.

CLINICAL FEATURES

Nightmares tend to occur during middle and late sleep; they usually occur during REM sleep, but occasionally during stages 1–2. They cause awakening, when the dream is remembered.

DIFFERENTIAL DIAGNOSIS

The main differential diagnosis is night (sleep) terrors.

AETIOLOGY

Aetiological factors that have been suggested include:

- negative dreams associated with:
  - daytime depression
  - daytime anxiety
  - daytime stress
- hypnotic withdrawal
- alcohol withdrawal
- medications:
  - β-adrenoceptor antagonists
  - reserpine.

MANAGEMENT

Any underlying disorder may require treatment. The nightmares themselves do not need to be treated.

BIBLIOGRAPHY

Laking, P.J. 2002: Sleep disorders. In Puri, B.K. Laking P.J. & Treasaden, I.H. (eds) *Textbook of Psychiatry*, 2nd edn. Edinburgh: Churchill Livingstone.

Parkes, J.D. 1985: *Sleep and its Disorders*. London: W.B. Saunders.

33

Personality disorders

HISTORY

- Hippocrates described four temperaments: melancholic, sanguine, phlegmatic, and choleric.
- In 1801, Pinel described *manie sans délire*.
- In 1835, Prichard described *moral insanity*.
- In 1906, Kraepelin described *psychopathic personality*: excitable, unstable, eccentric, liars, swindlers, antisocial and quarrelsome subtypes.
- Schneider subsequently extended the concept of psychopathic personality to include suffering to the self as well as to society.
- In 1939, Henderson's *psychopathic states* included three subtypes: aggressive, inadequate and creative psychopaths.
- In 1955, Cleckley described *sociopathy*: unreliable, untruthful, lacking remorse, poor motivation and antisocial behaviour.
- In 1978, Eysenck called for a dimensional rather than a categorical approach to the description of personality.

PERSONALITY DEVELOPMENT

- *Normothetic theories* are concerned with personality structure based on studies of populations.
- *Ideographic theories* relate to individual uniqueness, based on the study of the individual.

KELLY'S PERSONAL CONSTRUCT THEORY

Kelly considered every man to be a scientist, interpreting the world on the basis of past experience. Constructs are created and predictions are made accordingly. A system of constructs results, unique in each individual, existing at various levels of consciousness, those formed at earlier developmental stages being unconscious. Each construct has a range of convenience. Some are specific (e.g. chewy versus tender); others have a wider range of convenience.

Constructs are arranged into hierarchies. Superordinate constructs are central to the individual's sense of identity; subordinate constructs are less so.

According to this theory, anxiety results when the individual is presented with events outside the range of personal constructs. Hostility comprises the imposition of constructs upon another.

Bannister's repertory grid can be used to assess an individual's attitudes with respect to a series of bipolar constructs. (It can also be used to measure formal thought disorder.)

ROGER'S SELF-THEORY

Each individual has a drive to fulfil himself or herself and develop an *ideal self* within a *phenomenal field* of subjective experience. The most important aspect of personality is the congruence between the individual's view of the self and reality and his or her view of the self compared to the ideal self. If an individual acts at variance to his or her own self-image, anxiety, incongruence and denial result. The congruent individual is able to grow (self-actualization) and achieve personal potential both internally and socially.

PSYCHOANALYTIC THEORY

Behaviour and feelings are explained by unconscious drives and conflicts.

- The *id* is derived from the libido. Irrational, impulsive instincts are unable to postpone gratification, and are present at birth.
- The *ego* develops as the child grows. A conscious mind balances the demands of the id with the realities of the outside world. Anxiety results if the ego is unable to control the energies of the id.
- The *superego* comprises the internalization of the views of parents and society, like a conscience.

The id, the ego and the superego are in balance with each other.

Freud's stages of psychosexual development

Oral stage
- Age 0–1 years
- Gratification through sucking, biting
- Failure to negotiate leads to oral personality traits: moodiness, generosity, depression and elation, talkativeness, greed, optimism, pessimism, wishful thinking, narcissism

Anal stage
- Age 1–3 years
- Anus and defaecation are sources of sensual pleasure
- Failure to negotiate leads to anal personality traits: obsessive–compulsive personality, tidiness, parsimony, rigidity and thoroughness

Phallic stage
- Age 3–5 years
- Genital interest, relates to own sexuality: Oedipus/Electra complex
- Failure to negotiate leads to hysterical personality traits: competitiveness and ambitiousness

Latency stage
- Age 5–12 years

Genital stage
- Age 12–20 years
- Gratification from normal relations with people
- Able to relate to a partner.

Erikson's stages of development

Age	Sense of
0–1	Trust/security
1–4	Autonomy
4–5	Initiative
5–11	Duty/accomplishment
11–15	Identity
15–adult	Intimacy
Adulthood	Generativity
Maturity	Integrity.

Epigenesis is the process of development of the ego through these stages.

SITUATIONIST APPROACH

The external situation is considered the most powerful determinant of behaviour. Situationists maintain that traits result from differences in learning experiences. Behaviour changes according to the situation in which an individual finds himself or herself. Proponents dismiss the trait theory. Mischel (1983) argues against the existence of any stable personality dimension because of the poor correlation between behaviour or attitudes in one situation compared with another.

INTERACTIONIST MODEL

Behaviour depends upon the situation as well as personality traits.

CLASSIFICATION AND MEASUREMENT

The dimensional approach

Personality disorder differs from normal variation only in terms of degree. It assumes that universal traits are present in all people in differing degrees. Personality traits of some individuals are sufficiently maladaptive and abnormal as to constitute personality disorder.

Cattell's trait theory

Cattell identified 20 000 words describing personality. Using factor analysis he derived 16 first-order personality factors (PFs). Cattell's 16-PF test was devised on the basis of this work. Second-order factor analysis resulted in three broad dimensions similar to Eysenck's dimensions:

- sociability (extra/intra)
- anxiety
- intelligence.

Eysenck's theory

Factor analysis of rating scale data yields orthogonal dimensions, assumed to be normally distributed:

- neuroticism/stability
- extroversion/introversion

- psychoticism/stability
- intelligence.

Personality inventories have been used to measure these traits. The MPI (Maudsley Personality Inventory) was superseded by the EPI (Eysenck Personality Inventory), which in turn was superseded by the EPQ (Eysenck Personality Questionnaire) – measuring psychoticism and containing a lie scale.

Minnesota Multiphasic Personality Inventory (MMPI)
In this lengthy inventory, the subject answers 'true', 'false' or 'cannot say'. It is empirically constructed and measures traits. It is widely used.

Rorschach ink blot test
This is a projective test analysing fantasy material.

Rotter's internal–external locus of control
Individuals vary along a continuum in their perception of the locus of control of events. Those attributing events to an internal source are more confident about changing their life and environment.

The categorical approach

This approach groups people into discrete categories. It is simple and widely used but most individuals do not conform to categories.

- Kretschmer linked body-build with personality:
  - pyknic – sociable and relaxed
  - asthenic – self-conscious and solitary
  - athletic – robust and outgoing.
- Sheldon also linked build with personality:
  - endomorphic – viscerotonic personality
  - ectomorphic – cerebrotonic personality
  - mesomorphic – somatotonic personality.

ICD-10 AND DSM-IV-TR CLASSIFICATIONS

These are primarily categorical classifications, but they incorporate a dimensional approach, allowing the recording of personality traits subthreshold for a diagnosis of personality disorder.

ICD-10 classifications

Severe disturbance in characterological constitution and behavioural tendencies, involving several areas of the personality, is associated with personal and social disruption. This diagnosis is usually inappropriate before the age of 16–17 years.

GENERAL DIAGNOSTIC GUIDELINES

The condition is not attributable to brain damage, disease or other psychiatric disorder.

(a)   disharmonious attitudes and behaviours involving several areas of functioning
(b)   enduring, long-standing, not limited to episodes of mental illness
(c)   pervasive and maladaptive
(d)   appears during childhood or adolescence, continues into adulthood
(e)   personal distress
(f)   problems in occupational and social performance usual.

PARANOID PERSONALITY DISORDER

(a)   excessive sensitiveness to setbacks and rebuffs
(b)   bears grudges persistently
(c)   suspicious, misconstrues actions as hostile
(d)   combative, tenacious sense of personal rights
(e)   suspicions regarding fidelity of partner
(f)   excessive self-importance
(g)   conspiratorial explanations of events.

SCHIZOID PERSONALITY DISORDER

(a)   finds few activities pleasurable
(b)   emotional coldness, detachment or flattened affect
(c)   limited capacity to express feelings
(d)   apparent indifference to praise or criticism
(e)   little interest in sexual experiences with another person
(f)   preference for solitary activities
(g)   preoccupation with fantasy and introspection
(h)   lack of desire for close friends or confiding relationships
(i)   insensitivity to social norms and conventions.

DISSOCIAL PERSONALITY DISORDER

(a)   callous unconcern for feelings of others
(b)   gross and persistent irresponsibility and disregard for social norms, rules and obligations
(c)   incapacity to maintain enduring relationships
(d)   low tolerance to frustration; low threshold for aggression and violence
(e)   incapacity to experience guilt or to profit from experience, especially punishment
(f)   blames others.

Persistent irritability may be present. Conduct disorder during childhood and adolescence supports this diagnosis.

EMOTIONALLY UNSTABLE PERSONALITY DISORDER

Here the individual may act impulsively without consideration of consequences. There is affective instability. There is a minimal ability to plan ahead; outbursts of intense anger leading to violence are easily precipitated.

There are two variants:

- *Impulsive type.* There is emotional instability and lack of control. Outbursts of violence or threatening behaviour are common, especially in response to criticism.
- *Borderline type.* There is emotional instability. Self-image, aims and internal preferences are often unclear or disturbed. There are chronic feelings of emptiness. Intense unstable relationships cause repeated emotional crises; there are associated excessive efforts to avoid abandonment, suicidal threats or deliberate self-harm.

HISTRIONIC PERSONALITY DISORDER

(a) self-dramatization, theatricality, exaggerated expression of emotions
(b) suggestibility
(c) shallow and labile affect
(d) seeks excitement; centre of attention
(e) inappropriate seductiveness
(f) over-concern with physical attractiveness.

The individual is egocentric, self-indulgent, longing for appreciation, feelings easily hurt, manipulative.

ANANKASTIC PERSONALITY DISORDER

(a) feelings of excessive doubt and caution
(b) preoccupation with details, rules, lists, order, organization and schedule
(c) perfectionism interferes with task completion
(d) conscientiousness, scrupulousness, undue preoccupation with productivity to exclusion of pleasure and relationships
(e) pedantic
(f) rigid and stubborn
(g) insists others submit to their way of doing things, reluctant to allow others to do things
(h) intrusion of unwelcome, insistent thoughts or impulses.

ANXIOUS (AVOIDANT) PERSONALITY DISORDER

(a) persistent, pervasive tension and apprehension
(b) believe they are socially inept, unappealing or inferior to others
(c) preoccupation with being criticized or rejected in social situations
(d) unwillingness to become involved unless certain of being liked
(e) restrictions in lifestyle because of need for security
(f) avoidance of activities involving interpersonal contact because of fear of criticism, disapproval or rejection.

DEPENDENT PERSONALITY DISORDER

(a) allows others to make important life decisions
(b) subordination of own needs to those of others on whom they are dependent
(c) unwillingness to make demands on people on whom they are dependent
(d) uncomfortable or helpless when alone, fear inability to care for themselves
(e) fear of being abandoned
(f) unable to make decisions without excessive advice from others.

DSM–IV–TR classification

GENERAL DIAGNOSTIC CRITERIA

A   Enduring pattern of inner experience and behaviour, deviates markedly from expectations of individual's culture. Manifested in:
- 1 – cognition
- 2 – affectivity
- 3 – interpersonal functioning
- 4 – impulse control.

B   Inflexible and pervasive across a range of situations.
C   Leads to significant distress or impairment in social, occupational, or other areas.
D   Stable, of long duration, onset can be traced back to adolescence or early adulthood.
E   Not a manifestation or consequence of another mental disorder.
F   Not caused by the effects of a substance or a general medical condition.

Clusters

Personality disorders are grouped into three clusters:

- *Cluster A:* paranoid, schizoid, and schizotypal personality disorders – odd or eccentric
- *Cluster B:* antisocial, borderline, histrionic, and narcissistic personality disorders – dramatic, emotional, or erratic
- *Cluster C:* avoidant, dependent, and obsessive–compulsive personality disorders – anxious or fearful.

Axis

Personality disorders under DSM–IV are coded on Axis II, and listed in their order of importance. Specific maladaptive personality traits and the use of defence mechanisms may also be listed on Axis II.

PARANOID PERSONALITY DISORDER

A. Pervasive distrust and suspiciousness; beginning by early adulthood.
Four (or more) of the following:

1   suspects others are exploiting, harming, or deceiving him/her
2   doubts about loyalty or trustworthiness of friends
3   reluctant to confide in others, fears that information will be used maliciously
4   reads hidden meanings into benign remarks or events
5   persistently bears grudges
6   perceives attacks on character not apparent to others; quick to react angrily
7   recurrent suspicions regarding fidelity of partner.

B. Does not occur exclusively during the course of schizophrenia, mood disorder or other psychotic disorder; not caused by the direct effects of a general medical condition.

SCHIZOID PERSONALITY DISORDER

A. Pervasive detachment from social relationships; restricted expression of emotions; beginning by early adulthood.
Four (or more) of the following:

1   neither desires nor enjoys close relationships, including being part of a family
2   chooses solitary activities
3   has little interest in sexual experience with another person
4   takes pleasure in few activities
5   lacks close friends or confidants
6   is indifferent to praise or criticism of others
7   shows emotional coldness, detachment, or flattened affect.

B. Does not occur exclusively during the course of schizophrenia, mood disorder, other psychotic disorder, or pervasive developmental disorder; not caused by the effects of a general medical condition.

SCHIZOTYPAL PERSONALITY DISORDER

A. Pervasive social and interpersonal deficits; reduced capacity for close relationships; cognitive or perceptual distortions and eccentricities of behaviour; beginning by early adulthood.
   Five (or more) of the following:

1   ideas of reference
2   odd beliefs or magical thinking inconsistent with subcultural norms
3   unusual perceptual experiences
4   odd thinking and speech
5   suspiciousness or paranoid ideation
6   inappropriate or constricted affect
7   behaviour or appearance odd, eccentric, or peculiar
8   lack of close friends or confidants
9   excessive social anxiety; does not diminish with familiarity.

B. Does not occur exclusively during the course of schizophrenia, mood disorder, other psychotic disorder, or pervasive developmental disorder; not caused by the effects of a general medical condition.

ANTISOCIAL PERSONALITY DISORDER

A. Pervasive disregard for and violation of rights of others occurring since the age of 15 years.
   Three (or more) of the following:

1   failure to conform to social norms with respect to lawful behaviours
2   deceitfulness; repeated lying, use of aliases, conning others
3   impulsivity, failure to plan ahead
4   irritability and aggressiveness
5   reckless disregard for safety of self or others
6   consistent irresponsibility; repeated failure to sustain work or honour financial obligations
7   lack of remorse.

B. At least age 18 years.
C. Evidence of conduct disorder before the age of 15 years.
D. Not exclusively during the course of schizophrenia or mania.

BORDERLINE PERSONALITY DISORDER

Pervasive instability of interpersonal relationships, self-image and affects; marked impulsivity beginning by early adulthood.

Five (or more) of the following:

1   frantic efforts to avoid real or imagined abandonment
2   unstable, intense relationships alternating between extremes of idealization and devaluation
3   identity disturbance: markedly and persistently unstable self-image
4   impulsivity in at least two areas that are potentially self-damaging
5   recurrent suicidal behaviour, gestures, or threats, or self-mutilating behaviour
6   affective instability caused by a marked reactivity of mood
7   chronic feelings of emptiness
8   inappropriate, intense anger
9   transient, stress-related paranoid ideation or severe dissociative symptoms.

HISTRIONIC PERSONALITY DISORDER

Pervasive excessive emotionality and attention-seeking, beginning by early adulthood.
     Five (or more) of the following:

1   uncomfortable if not centre of attention
2   inappropriate sexually seductive or provocative behaviour
3   rapidly shifting, shallow emotions
4   uses physical appearance to draw attention to self
5   style of speech is excessively impressionistic
6   self-dramatization, theatricality, exaggerated expression of emotion
7   suggestible
8   considers relationships more intimate than they are.

NARCISSISTIC PERSONALITY DISORDER

Pervasive grandiosity, need for admiration, lack of empathy; beginning by early adulthood.
     Five (or more) of the following:

1   grandiose sense of self-importance
2   fantasies of unlimited success, power, brilliance, beauty, or ideal love
3   believe they are 'special' and should associate with other special or high-status people
4   requires excessive admiration
5   sense of entitlement
6   interpersonally exploitative
7   lacks empathy
8   often envious of others
9   arrogant, haughty behaviours or attitudes.

AVOIDANT PERSONALITY DISORDER

Pervasive social inhibition, feelings of inadequacy, hypersensitivity to negative evaluation;
beginning by early adulthood.
     Four (or more) of the following:

1   avoids activities that involve interpersonal contact; fears of criticism, disapproval, or rejection
2   unwilling to get involved with people unless certain of being liked
3   shows restraint within intimate relationships because of the fear of being shamed or ridiculed
4   preoccupied with being criticized or rejected in social situations

5   inhibited in new interpersonal situations because of feelings of inadequacy
6   views self as socially inept, personally unappealing, or inferior to others
7   reluctant to take risks or engage in new activities because they may prove embarrassing.

DEPENDENT PERSONALITY DISORDER

Pervasive, excessive need to be taken care of; submissive, clinging behaviour and fears of separation; beginning by early adulthood.

Five (or more) of the following:

1   difficulty making everyday decisions
2   needs others to assume responsibility for most major areas of life
3   difficulty expressing disagreement; fear of loss of support
4   difficulty initiating projects or doing things on their own
5   goes to excessive lengths to obtain nurturance and support
6   feels uncomfortable or helpless when alone; fears of being unable to cope
7   urgently seeks another relationship as a source of care and support when a close relationship ends
8   preoccupied with fears of being left to take care of themselves.

OBSESSIVE–COMPULSIVE PERSONALITY DISORDER

Pervasive preoccupation with orderliness, perfectionism, and control, at the expense of flexibility, openness, and efficiency; beginning by early adulthood.

Four (or more) of the following:

1   preoccupied with details, rules, lists, order, organization or schedules to the extent that the point of the activity is lost
2   perfectionism interferes with task completion
3   excessively devoted to work and productivity to the exclusion of leisure activities and friendships
4   over-conscientious, scrupulous, inflexible
5   unable to discard worn-out or worthless objects
6   reluctant to delegate tasks
7   miserly
8   rigid and stubborn.

PERSONALITY DISORDER NOT OTHERWISE SPECIFIED

This does not meet criteria for any specific personality disorder, but that it causes distress or impairment in one or more important areas of functioning (e.g. social or occupational).

EPIDEMIOLOGY OF PERSONALITY DISORDERS

METHODOLOGICAL PROBLEMS

Various methodological problems are encountered with prevalence studies:

- The diagnosis of a personality disorder may be during a psychiatric illness.
- There is often the lack of informants' accounts when making the diagnosis.
- An 'either/or' approach may be taken to diagnosis.
- The diagnosis may be made by variously reliable methods.
- There may be inconsistent recording of the presence of more than one personality disorder.

STATISTICS

A gradient exists in the prevalence of personality disorders from community to inpatient setting (see Table 33.1). The following are the approximate prevalences of personality disorder:

- community 10%
- general practice 20%
- psychiatric outpatients 30%
- psychiatric inpatients 40%.

Table 33.1 *Prevalence of personality disorders in different settings*

Personality disorder	Prevalence		
	Community	Outpatients	Inpatients
Paranoid	0.5–2.5%	2–10%	10–30%
Schizoid		Uncommon	
Schizotypal	3%		
Antisocial	3% in males	3–30%	
	1% in females		
Borderline	2%	10%	20%
Histrionic	2–3%		10–15%
Narcissistic	Less than 1%		2–16%
Avoidant	0.5–1.0%	10%	
Dependent	The most frequently reported		
Obsessive–compulsive	1%	3–10%	

It is generally more common in males than in females.

Certain personality disorders (e.g. antisocial personality disorder) are diagnosed more frequently in men, others (e.g. borderline, histrionic and dependent personality disorders) in women.

The American Epidemiologic Catchment Area (ECA) study found, using a diagnostic interview schedule, a prevalence of personality disorder in the community of 6%.

Antisocial personality disorder

- There is a lifetime prevalence of 2.3–3.6%.
- The male to female sex ratio is 7:1.
- It is twice as prevalent in inner cities compared to rural areas.
- Antisocial behaviours usually start at age 8–10 years. They do not develop after age 18.
- The highest lifetime prevalence is in the 25- to 44-year-old group, followed by the 18 to 24-year-old group.
- Spontaneous remission may occur in middle age. There is a correlation between increasing age and remission rate.
- There is excess mortality.

- Subjects are less likely to be married, less well educated.
- There is a highly significant correlation between antisocial personality disorder and drug and alcohol dependence.
- A high proportion (90%) have at least one lifetime psychiatric diagnosis.

AETIOLOGY OF PERSONALITY DISORDERS

ENVIRONMENTAL FACTORS

Psychodynamics

The failure to negotiate stages of psychosexual development and the characteristic use of defence mechanisms are said to result in disorders of personality. For example:

- Paranoid personality is the result of the projection of homosexual impulses. Later it was thought that excessive parental rage causing feelings of inadequacy resulted in projection on to others of hostility and rage.
- Borderline personality results from early traumatic experiences occurring within a context of sustained neglect resulting in enduring rage and self-hatred.
- Histrionic personality results from difficulties in the Oedipal phase of psychosexual development.
- Dependent personality results from fixation at the oral stage of psychosexual development.
- Obsessive–compulsive personality results from difficulties in the anal stage of psychosexual development.

Object relations

Personality is taken to be shaped by the child's early parental relationships. Dependent personality traits are thought to result from parental deprivation, obsessive–compulsive traits from the struggle with parents for control, and hysterical traits from parental seduction and competition.

For example, borderline personality is the result of a lack of stable involved attachment during development. This leads to an inability to maintain a stable sense of self or others without ongoing contact.

NEUROLOGICAL FACTORS

Eighty per cent of children with minimal brain dysfunction syndrome suffer from various personality disorders in adult life.

EEG studies in antisocial personality disorders demonstrate abnormalities which have led to speculation that psychopathic behaviour reflects cortical immaturity. Abnormalities found in this group more often than in normals include:

- generalized widespread slow (θ) wave activity
- 'positive spike' abnormality over temporal lobes
- localized temporal slow wave activity.

These abnormalities are more likely to occur in highly impulsive and aggressive psychopaths.

Psychopaths have lower cortical arousal, measured by slower cortical evoked potentials. Autonomic arousal is also lower, leading to speculation that sensation-seeking behaviour may be an attempt to increase cortical arousal.

Goyer *et al.* (1994) in a PET scanning study of personality disordered subjects found a significant inverse correlation between a history of aggressive impulse difficulties and regional cerebral metabolic rates in the frontal cortex. Those subjects with borderline personality disorders had significantly reduced frontal cortex metabolism.

GENETIC FACTORS

Normal personality appears to be at least moderately heritable:

- Breeding over generations of animals (e.g. dogs) produces strains with more or less aggressive temperaments.
- Psychophysiological characteristics are partly genetically inherited. For example, EEGs of monozygotic (MZ) twins are easily distinguished from those of dizygotic (DZ) twins, even when they are reared apart; the habituation of galvanic skin response is largely genetically determined.
- Large representative twin studies using model-fitting approaches consistently find a heritability of 35–50% for traits measured by questionnaire. Although 50% of the variance in personality traits is environmental, a shared family environment has consistently shown a negligible contribution to the variance.
- Monozygotic twins reared apart are more alike on personality measures than those raised together. It is suggested that twins reared together react against one another in an attempt to establish individual identities.

Antisocial personality disorder

Most twin and adoption studies suggest that antisocial personality disorder has a partial genetic aetiology. See Table 33.2. The heritable form of criminality is associated with petty recidivism and property offences rather than violent crime.

Mednick *et al.* (1984) studied 14 427 adoptees and their biological and adoptive parents. The effect was stronger when the biological mother was convicted than if the biological father was convicted. Association was for property offences only, playing a significant role in repeat offences; it did not apply to violent offences.

Robins (1966) found that the father's criminal behaviour was the single best predictor of antisocial behaviour in a child.

MZ to DZ concordance rates for adult criminality are 52%:22%. This suggests a definite genetic contribution. However, concordance rates of 87%:72% for juvenile delinquency are suggestive of a familial but not a genetic component to aetiology.

Within a family that has a member with antisocial personality disorder, males more often have antisocial personality disorder and substance-related disorders, whereas females more often have somatization disorder. However, in such families, there is an increase in the prevalence of all of these disorders in both males and females compared with the general population.

Table 33.2 *Percentages of convictions in male adoptees and the biological and adoptive parents*

	Conviction rate
Neither biological nor adoptive parent convicted	13.5%
Adoptive parents convicted. Biological parents not convicted	14.7%
Adoptive parents not convicted. Biological parents convicted	20.0%
Adoptive and biological parents convicted	24.5%

It is suggested that family background plays a part in subsequent criminality, but only when there is already a genetic predisposition. The risk of criminality is increased in those with prolonged institutional care, multiple temporary placements and those where the socioeconomic status of their adoptive home is low.

Schizotypal personality disorders

Kety *et al.* (1971) in an adoption study demonstrated that abnormalities were more common in the biological relatives of schizophrenics than in adoptive relatives or controls ('schizophrenia spectrum disorders'). From this derived the operational criteria for schizotypal personality disorder. Almost all studies of the families of schizophrenic probands have found an excess of both schizophrenia and schizotypal personality disorder among relatives (22% in the biological relatives of schizophrenics versus 2% of adoptive relatives and controls).

The heritability found in anxious personalities is probably related to trait anxiety, in obsessional personalities to a more general neurotic tendency as measured by the Eysenck Personality Inventory, and in hysterical personalities to extroversion.

Coccaro *et al.* (1993) examined the heritability of personality traits (impulsiveness, irritability and inhibition of assertive behaviour) in 500 healthy MZ and DZ twin pairs raised together and apart. The results showed substantial genetic influences, and were consistent with a genetic, but not a shared environmental influence.

ASSESSMENT OF PERSONALITY DISORDERS

Assessment can be difficult. Personality traits are egosyntonic, such that patients are often not aware of them and will not complain of them. In the diagnosis of personality disorder, multiple sources of information should be used, including an informant who has known the patient for a considerable time.

Personality traits should:

- be enduring, not transient
- be pervasive across situations
- be early in onset
- cause distress or impairment.

Account should be taken of social and cultural norms when considering behaviour or symptoms.

Axis I symptom disorder and medical illness should be identified since they may complicate the diagnosis.

Many difficulties of adolescence resolve as the person matures. Personality disorder should be diagnosed with care in adolescence.

MANAGEMENT OF PERSONALITY DISORDERS

Most research focuses upon the management of 'borderline' patients, partly because these are the patients commonly presenting in clinical practice. It is usually the case that both psychotherapy and drug therapy will be used in a patient with personality disorder.

Psychotherapy

PSYCHOANALYSIS

Psychoanalysis or intensive *psychoanalytic psychotherapy* is considered by many psychotherapists to be the treatment of choice for borderline individuals. The duration of therapy is 2–7 years. Treatment consists of interpretation of the transference and primitive defence mechanisms, the neutrality of the therapist and a consistent limit setting. Attention is particularly focused on the present rather than interpreting childhood experience.

An alternative is *supportive psychotherapy* which aims to strengthen a patient's adaptive functioning through education, suggestion and a facilitating interpersonal relationship. The interpretation of transference, defence mechanisms and regression and dependency are avoided, since they are considered likely to lead to suicide or other forms of acting out.

GROUP PSYCHOTHERAPY

Group psychotherapy has been traditionally avoided because borderline patients are considered too demanding and disruptive. However, gentle confrontation delivered by a group is considered by some to be effective, rendering egosyntonic traits more egodystonic.

Most groups can contain no more than one or two borderline patients. Apart from the cost, there is no evidence to recommend group therapy over individual therapy.

FAMILY THERAPY

This is frequently offered to borderline adolescent patients, and is regarded by many as the treatment of choice for these patients.

INPATIENT TREATMENT AND THERAPEUTIC COMMUNITIES

This is controversial. Currently there is a trend away from long-term admissions for borderline patients, probably driven by cost-containment. There is evidence to support the value of therapeutic communities such as the Henderson or the Cassel Hospitals. The therapeutic community approach is a multi-component treatment programme, incorporating individual therapy, ward groups, and patient participation in the maintenance of the community.

The risks of hospitalization to the patient include:

- stigma
- disruption of social and occupational roles
- loss of freedom
- hospital-induced behavioural regression.

Some consider the drawing up of a contract between the patient and doctor essential to the success of inpatient care. Miller (1989) considers a good treatment contract to incorporate the following:

- mutual agreement by all involved parties
- specific, focused, achievable goals with strategies to achieve them
- specific responsibilities of patient and staff
- provision of the minimum degree of structure necessary
- patient foregoing his or her usual means of managing intolerable feelings; alternative strategies are provided

- positive reinforcement of desirable behaviour
- not being drawn up when staff have unresolved punitive wishes towards the patient
- strictly enforced, but room for negotiated modification.

The alternative approach of brief admissions at the time of crisis is increasingly popular.

COGNITIVE–BEHAVIOURAL THERAPY (CBT)

Linehan *et al.* (1991) randomly allocated cognitive–behavioural therapy or 'treatment as usual' over a period of one year, to chronically parasuicidal borderline patients. During the year the CBT group showed fewer and less severe incidents of parasuicide, and had fewer inpatient days.

Physical treatments

Placebo-controlled drug trials among those with personality disorder show small specific drug effects as well as large placebo effects.

Neuroleptic drugs

Low-dose neuroleptic treatment has been shown to be beneficial particularly in the management of borderline subjects in a majority of trials. Low-dose flupenthixol significantly reduced the number of suicide attempts by 6 months when compared to placebo and mianserin in a mixed group of parasuicidal personality-disordered subjects.

Low-dose neuroleptics improve a broad spectrum of neurotic symptoms as well as reducing behavioural dyscontrol and numbers of suicide attempts, compared to placebo.

Antidepressants

Some patients with borderline or schizotypal personality disorder improve with tricyclic antidepressants on ratings of depressed mood, impulsive and manipulative behaviour, but there is significant potential for paradoxical effects and rage reactions. As a result they are not particularly recommended in the management of personality disorders unless major depression co-occurs. Depression complicated by personality disorder is only half as likely to respond to tricyclic drug treatment compared to pure major depression, however.

Selected borderline subjects respond to monoamine oxidase inhibitors (MAOIs), particularly where there is a history of childhood hyperactivity.

Serotonergic dysfunction has been implicated in key symptoms, particularly depression, impulsivity and obsessive–compulsive phenomena. Selective serotonin re-uptake inhibitors (e.g. fluoxetine) at doses of 20–80 mg per day result in the improvement in depressed mood and impulsivity as well as reducing self-mutilation. Sertraline used in impulsive aggressive patients results in marked improvements in overt aggression and irritability, evident from the fourth week of treatment.

Electroconvulsive therapy

The immediate response is good in depressed borderline subjects, but the relapse rate is high.

Lithium

In male convicts with a pattern of recurring easily triggered violence, a marked reduction in infractions resulted from treatment with lithium. The reduction in aggressive episodes requires lithium levels above 0.6 mmol/L. Major infractions such as assault or threatening behaviour are responsive to lithium in about 60%; minor infractions are unresponsive.

Lithium is helpful in a small numbers of patients with diverse personality disorders. Affective features, a family history of affective disorder or alcoholism may help selected subjects. A 2-month trial of lithium may be necessary to establish responders.

Carbamazepine
Impulsive aggression is the most serious symptom of personality disorder. In patients with behavioural dyscontrol, aggressive acts are reduced by about two-thirds and the severity of the outburst is improved. It is helpful even in the absence of epileptic, affective or organic features.

Benzodiazepines
These are contraindicated in personality disorder because of their propensity to disinhibit, induce rage reactions and states of dependence.

Psychostimulants
Psychostimulants such as dexamphetamine and pemoline may occasionally, sometimes dramatically, help personalities with aggression and hostility, particularly where there is an earlier history of drug-responsive attention-deficit disorder. However, because of their psychotogenic effects and addictive properties, extreme caution is used in prescribing.

OUTCOME

The personality disorders have a high morbidity and mortality. The standardized mortality ratio for the 20- to 39-year-old age group is raised six-fold, similar to that rise reported for the major functional psychoses.

Patients with personality disorder have high rates of comorbidity with both axis I and axis II conditions. Response to treatment of an axis I disorder is almost always worse in the presence of personality disorder. Patients are at a high risk of suicide.

In those borderline cases treated with psychotherapy, the aim of supportive psychotherapy may be to diminish suicidal behaviour and impulsive acts while awaiting a remission since the long-term prognosis of this disorder is good. A 15-year follow-up of 100 borderline personality-disordered patients found that 75% were no longer diagnosed as borderline. All scales showed a reduction of symptomatic behaviour, with a clear functional improvement. However, there is a high risk of suicide, with 8.5% completing suicide in the 15-year follow-up period. Those patients with chronic depression, good motivation, a psychological attitude, low impulsiveness and a stable environment are most responsive to treatment.

In those with antisocial personality disorders there is a significant association between the ability to form a relationship with the therapist and treatment outcome. In confined settings such as prison or in the military, confrontation by peers may bring changes in social behaviour. Prevalence seems to decrease with increasing age.

Schizotypal personality disorder has a relatively stable course, with only a small proportion of individuals going on to develop schizophrenia.

Some types of personality disorder (antisocial and borderline) tend to become less evident or to remit with age, whereas this appears to be less true for some other types (obsessive–compulsive and schizotypal).

BIBLIOGRAPHY

American Psychiatric Association 1994: *Diagnostic and Statistical Manual of Mental Disorders*, 4th edn. Washington, DC: APA.

Brennan, P.A. & Mednick, S.A. 1993: Genetic perspectives on crime. *Acta Psychiatrica Scandinavica* (Suppl.) 370:19–26.

Coccaro, E.F., Bergeman, C.S. & McClearn, G.E. 1993: Heritability of irritable impulsiveness: a study of twins reared together and apart. *Psychiatry Research* 48, 229–242.

DeBattista, C. & Glick, I.D. 1995: Pharmacotherapy of the personality disorders. *Current Opinion in Psychiatry* 8:102–105.

Freeman, C.P.L. 1995: Personality disorders. In Kendell, R.E. & Zealley, A.K. (eds) *Companion to Psychiatric Studies*, 5th edn. Edinburgh: Churchill Livingstone.

Gelder, M., Gath, D. & Mayou, R. 1985: *Oxford Textbook of Psychiatry*. Oxford: Oxford University Press.

Goyer, P.F., Andreason, P.J., Semple, W.E. *et al.* 1994: Positron emission tomography and personality disorders. *Neuropsychopharmacology* 10:21–28.

Higgitt, A. & Fonagy, P. 1992: Psychotherapy in borderline and narcissistic personality disorder. *British Journal of Psychiatry* 161:23–43.

Kety, S.S., Rosenthal, D., Wender, P.H. *et al.* 1971: Mental illness in the biological and adoptive families of adopted schizophrenics. *American Journal of Psychiatry* 128:302–306.

Linehan, M.M., Armstrong, H.E., Svarez, A. *et al.* 1991: Cognitive–behavioural treatment of chronically parasuicidal borderline patients. *Archives of General Psychiatry* 48:1060–1064.

McGuffin, P. & Thapar, A. 1992: The genetics of personality disorder. *British Journal of Psychiatry* 160:12–23.

Mednick, S.A., Gabrielli, W.F. & Hutchings, B. 1984: Genetic influences on criminal convictions: evidence from an adoption cohort. *Science* 224:891–894.

Miller, L.J. 1989: Inpatient management of borderline personality disorder: a review and update. *Journal of Personality Disorders* 3:122–134.

Mischel, W. 1983: Alterations on the pursuit of predictability and consistency of persons: stable data that yield unstable interpretations. *Journal of Personality* 51:578–604.

Paris, J., Brown, R. & Nowis, D. 1987: Long-term follow-up of borderline patients in a general hospital. *Comprehensive Psychiatry* 28:530–535.

Robins, L.N. 1966: *Deviant Children Grown Up*. Baltimore: Williams & Wilkins.

Stein, G. 1992: Drug treatment of the personality disorders. *British Journal of Psychiatry* 161:167–184.

Swanson, M.C.J., Bland, R.C. & Newman, S.C. 1994: Antisocial personality disorders. *Acta Psychiatrica Scandinavica* (Suppl.) 376:63–70.

Tyrer, P. & Ferguson, B. 1987: Problems in the classification of personality disorder. *Psychological Medicine* 17:15–20.

World Health Organization 1992: *Tenth Revision of the International Classification of Diseases*. Geneva: WHO.

34

Child and adolescent psychiatry

CHILD AND ADOLESCENT PSYCHIATRIC DISORDER

CLASSIFICATION

The ICD-10 classification of behavioural and emotional disorders with onset usually occurring in childhood and adolescence is shown in Table 34.1.

EPIDEMIOLOGY

Preschool

The main epidemiological study is the Waltham Forest Study (by Richman and colleagues) in the early 1970s of 3-year-olds, carried out in the London borough of that name. The Vineyard study (Martha) essentially confirmed its findings. The main findings included:

- 7% prevalence of moderate to severe behavioural and emotional problems, slightly greater in boys than girls
- 15% prevalence of mild behavioural and emotional problems
- strong associations found with:
  - maternal depression
  - poor parental marriage
  - delayed development of language
- strong continuities of behaviour and language disorders over the early school years.

Middle childhood

The main epidemiological studies are the Isle of Wight and Inner London Borough studies (by Rutter and colleagues) in the 1960s, of 10- and 11-year-olds. Recent studies in Norway and Puerto Rico essentially confirmed the findings. The main findings included:

- 6.8% overall point prevalence of child psychiatric disorder in the Isle of Wight
- 4% prevalence of conduct disorder
- 2.5% prevalence of emotional disorder
- male to female sex ratio of 1.9:1

Table 34.1 *F90–F98: Behavioural and emotional disorders with onset usually occurring in childhood and adolescence (ICD-10)*

F90 Hyperkinetic disorders	F90.0 Disturbance of activity and attention F90.1 Hyperkinetic conduct disorder F90.8 Other hyperkinetic disorders F90.9 Hyperkinetic disorder, unspecified
F91 Conduct disorders	F91.0 Conduct disorder confined to the family context F91.1 Unsocialized conduct disorder F91.2 Socialized conduct disorder F91.3 Oppositional defiant disorder F91.8 Other conduct disorders F91.9 Conduct disorder, unspecified
F92 Mixed disorders of conduct and emotions	F92.0 Depressive conduct disorder F92.8 Other mixed disorders of conduct and emotions F92.9 Mixed disorder of conduct and emotions, unspecified
F93 Emotional disorders with onset specific to childhood	F93.0 Separation anxiety disorder of childhood F93.1 Phobic anxiety disorder of childhood F93.2 Social anxiety disorder of childhood F93.3 Sibling rivalry disorder F93.8 Other childhood emotional disorders F93.9 Childhood emotional disorder, unspecified
F94 Disorders of social functioning with onset specific to childhood and adolescence	F94.0 Elective mutism F94.1 Reactive attachment disorder of childhood F94.2 Disinhibited attachment disorder of childhood F94.8 Other childhood disorders of social functioning F94.9 Childhood disorders of social functioning, unspecified
F95 Tic disorders	F95.0 Transient tic disorder F95.1 Chronic motor or vocal tic disorder F95.2 Combined vocal and multiple motor tic disorder (Gilles de la Tourette's syndrome) F95.8 Other tic disorders F95.9 Tic disorder, unspecified
F98 Other behavioural and emotional disorders with onset usually occurring in childhood and adolescence	F98.0 Nonorganic enuresis F98.1 Nonorganic encopresis F98.2 Feeding disorder of infancy and childhood F98.3 Pica of infancy and childhood F98.4 Stereotyped movement disorders F98.5 Stuttering (stammering) F98.6 Cluttering F98.8 Other specified behavioural and emotional disorders with onset usually occurring in childhood and adolescence F98.9 Unspecified behavioural and emotional disorders with onset usually occurring in childhood and adolescence

- an overall point prevalence of child psychiatric disorder in inner London twice that in the Isle of Wight.

Adolescence

- 10–20% prevalence of psychiatric disorder
- a male to female sex ratio of approximately 1:1.5.

AETIOLOGY

In general the aetiology of psychiatric disorders in children and adolescents is multifactorial.

ASSESSMENT

The information to be obtained in a child psychiatric interview is shown in Table 34.2.

DEPRESSION IN YOUNG PEOPLE

Depressive disorder occurs in 0.5–8% of 14- to 15-year-olds. Compared with adults, depressive disorder in childhood and early adolescence is more likely to present with:

- running away from home
- lowered academic performance
- separation anxiety/school refusal
- somatic pain, particularly of head, abdomen or chest
- antisocial behaviour (mostly in males).

Note: no antidepressant is licensed for use in under 18s in the UK. There is little or no evidence of tricyclic efficacy.

- 2003: SSRIs (not fluoxetine) + venlafaxine contraindicated for MDD in youth.

SCHOOL REFUSAL

School refusal is refusal to attend or stay at school because of anxiety and in spite of parental or other pressure.

EPIDEMIOLOGY

Boys and girls are equally represented. There are three main incidence peak ages:

- separation anxiety at age 5 years
- at age 11 years, which may be precipitated by the change from junior to secondary schooling
- at age 14–16 years, which may be a symptom of a psychiatric disorder:
  - depressive disorder
  - a phobia (e.g. social phobia).

The most common presentation is the one at 11 years.

Table 34.2 *Information to be amassed in a child psychiatric interview*

Source and nature of referral
Who made referral?
Who initiated referral?
Family attitudes to referral

Description of presenting complaints
Onset, frequency, intensity, duration, location (home, school etc.)
Antecedents and consequences
Ameliorating and exacerbating factors
Specific examples
Parental and family beliefs about causation
Past attempts to solve problem

Description of child's current general functioning
School:
   behaviour and emotions
   academic performance
   peer and staff relationships
Peer relationships generally
Family relationships

Personal/developmental history
Pregnancy, labour, delivery
Early developmental milestones
Separations/disruptions
Physical illnesses and their meaning for parents
Reactions to school
Puberty
Temperamental style

Family history
Personal and social histories of both parents, especially:
   history of mental illness
   their experience of being parented
History of family development:
   how parents came together
   history of pregnancies
   separations and effects on children
Who lives at home currently
Strengths/weaknesses of all at home
Current social stresses and supports

Information from observation of family interaction
Structure, organization, communication, sensitivity

Information from observation of child at interview
Motor, sensory, speech, language, social relating skills

Mental state, concerns, and spontaneous account if age appropriate

Results of physical examination

Plan for future investigation and management

Reproduced with permission from Puri, B.K., Laking, P.J. & Treasaden, I.H. 2002: *Textbook of Psychiatry*, 2nd edn. Edinburgh: Churchill Livingstone.

DIFFERENCES FROM TRUANCY

Truancy is an important differential diagnosis. Truancy differs from school refusal in that it is:

- ego-syntonic and intended
- often accompanied by other antisocial symptoms
- more likely to be associated with a family history of antisocial behaviour
- more likely to be associated with poor academic school performance
- more likely to be associated with larger family size.

MANAGEMENT

The mechanisms underlying the school refusal should be identified. If the condition is acute, a return to school should be arranged as soon as possible (the Kennedy approach), whereas, if the condition is chronic, a graded return to school should be arranged. Any specific problems (e.g. social phobia) should be addressed. If the individual does not return to school, then inpatient treatment may be necessary.

COURSE AND PROGNOSIS

Younger children have a better prognosis. Most children and adolescents do return to school, but approximately one-third of older patients seen in clinics develop neurotic difficulties or social impairment or social withdrawal in adulthood.

HYPERKINETIC DISORDERS

EPIDEMIOLOGY

- There is a point prevalence of 1.7%.
- They occur more often in males.
- The incidence decreases with increasing age group.
- The incidence increases with social adversity.

CLINICAL FEATURES

The cardinal features are:

- impaired attention
- over-activity
- impulsivity.

These should:

- occur in more than one environmental situation
- begin before the age of 6 years
- be of long duration.

The diagnosis is made far more commonly in the USA than it is in Britain.
Other associated features that may occur include:

- social disinhibition
- recklessness

- learning difficulties
- clumsiness.

DIFFERENTIAL DIAGNOSIS

The main differential diagnoses are:

- pervasive development disorders
- conduct disorder
- anxiety disorder.

AETIOLOGY

Possible causes that have been proposed include:

- brain abnormality
- genetic contribution
- dietary factors
- food allergy.

MANAGEMENT

A full assessment, including psychometric testing, should be carried out. Behavioural management approaches and pharmacotherapy with stimulants (methylphenidate or dexamfetamine) may be used (but beware side-effects). Atomoxetine was approved by the FDA in January 2003 for ADHD, and is awaiting a UK license. Selective noradrenaline reuptake inhibitor, non-stimulant, non-controlled. Second-line drugs that are occasionally used include tricyclic antidepressants and haloperidol.

COURSE AND PROGNOSIS

With development, there is usually an improvement of restlessness and impaired attention. However, poor self-esteem may result from the disorder, leading in turn to the possibility of affecting the development of personality. The presence of other disorders, such as conduct disorder, leads to a worse prognosis.

CONDUCT DISORDERS

EPIDEMIOLOGY

- The point prevalence was 4% in 10- and 11-year-olds in the Isle of Wight study (higher in inner London); with aggressive components in 1.1%.
- They occur more often in males.
- Aggressive (rather than antisocial) symptoms are more common in younger children.

DIAGNOSIS

According to ICD-10, conduct disorders are characterized by a repetitive and persistent pattern of dissocial, aggressive or defiant conduct, which when at its most extreme amounts to major violations of age-appropriate social expectations, and is therefore more severe than ordinary childish mischief or adolescent rebelliousness.

DIFFERENTIAL DIAGNOSIS

Conduct disorder overlaps with hyperkinetic disorders and emotional disorders. In the former case, the diagnosis should be hyperkinetic disorder if the criteria for this are met, whereas in the latter case in ICD-10 a diagnosis should be made of mixed disorder of conduct and emotions.

CLINICAL FEATURES

The antisocial behaviour may manifest in different ways, such as:

- temper tantrums in early and middle childhood
- oppositional defiant behaviour in older children.

AETIOLOGY

Possible causes that have been proposed include:

- life events:
  - bereavement
  - parental divorce
  - separation from parents
- social:
  - poor school
  - aberrant peer group
  - socially disadvantaged
- parental:
  - rejection
  - inconsistency
  - punitiveness
  - negativism
  - modelling of aggression
  - failure to set rules
  - failure to monitor
  - maternal depression
- individual:
  - anxiety
  - depression
  - difficult temperament
  - low IQ
  - educational retardation
  - neurological impairment.

MANAGEMENT

A full assessment should be carried out. Management strategies that may be employed include:

- behavioural management techniques
- cognitive therapy
- group therapy.

COURSE AND PROGNOSIS

Aggressive behaviour in middle childhood (but not that occurring in the preschool years) is associated with later sociopathy, particularly if there is also poor academic achievement. Fifty per cent of highly antisocial children become antisocial adults. Of adult sociopaths:

- 60% manifest highly antisocial behaviour as children
- another 30% manifest moderately antisocial behaviour as children.

ELECTIVE MUTISM

EPIDEMIOLOGY

Elective mutism usually manifests in early childhood, and boys and girls are equally represented. The prevalence is below 0.8 per 1000 children.

DIAGNOSIS

According to ICD-10, elective mutism is characterized by a marked, emotionally determined selectivity in speaking, such that the child demonstrates language competence in some situations but fails to speak in other (definable) ones.

CLINICAL FEATURES

In addition to the features given above, elective mutism tends to be associated with personality features such as:

- social anxiety
- withdrawal
- sensitivity
- resistance.

MANAGEMENT

Management approaches include:

- excluding any speech abnormalities
- behavioural approaches
- use of tape recordings or the telephone
- play therapy
- art therapy
- family therapy.

COURSE AND PROGNOSIS

In general, in the long term the prognosis is good unless other disorders are also present.

TIC DISORDERS

EPIDEMIOLOGY

Between 10% and 24% of children manifest tics during development. *Tourette's syndrome* (combined vocal and multiple motor tic disorder) accounts for a lifetime prevalence of 1.01–1.6%, with a male to female ratio of about 2:1. The average age of onset is 7 years (range 2–15 years).

CLINICAL FEATURES

Common simple motor tics include (ICD-10):

eye-blinking	shoulder-shrugging
neck-jerking	facial grimacing.

Common simple vocal tics include (ICD-10):

throat-clearing	sniffing
barking	hissing.

Common complex motor tics include (ICD-10):

hitting oneself	hopping
jumping.	

Common compex vocal tics include (ICD-10):

coprolalia	repeating certain words
palilalia.	

AETIOLOGY

The causes of tics are shown in Table 34.3.

Table 34.3   *Aetiology of tics*

Family	Individual
Family clusters reported, especially Tourette's	No gross neurological abnormalities
Prevalence of multiple tics in 14–24% of first-degree relatives of patients with Tourette's	Increased incidence of 'soft' neurological signs and 'non-specific' EEG changes
Increased family psychopathology in families of ticqueurs, although may be cause or effect	Some verbal–performance discrepancies in functioning
	Some neuroleptic medications effective in controlling tics
	Tics exacerbated by dopamine agonists
	Wide range of psychological mechanisms proposed for tic disorders, from the psychoanalytic to the classically behavioural
	Tic movement have been shown to mimic involuntary startle responses to sudden stimulus

Reproduced with permission from Puri, B.K., Laking, P.J. & Treasaden, I.H. 2002: *Textbook of Psychiatry*, 2nd edn. Edinburgh: Churchill Livingstone.

MANAGEMENT

Points in the management of tic disorders include:

- a full assessment, including a physical and detailed neurological examination
- reassurance of the patient and family
- advice to the family or other carers not to be annoyed or anxious at the occurrence of potentially embarrassing tics such as coprolalia
- liaison with the school
- psychological treatments
  - behavioural techniques such as massed practice
  - relaxation therapy
  - hypnotherapy
- pharmacotherapy (but beware side-effects)
  - haloperidol
  - pimozide
  - sulpiride
  - SSRIs.

COURSE AND PROGNOSIS

In most cases the tics disappear spontaneously within a few months. In a minority, however, there may be a progression from simple tics to Tourette's syndrome. One-third of cases of the latter present initially with vocal tics.

NON-ORGANIC ENURESIS

DEFINITION

According to ICD-10, non-organic enuresis is characterized by the involuntary voiding of urine, by day and/or by night, which is abnormal in relation to the individual's mental age and which is not a consequence of a lack of bladder control resulting from any neurological disorder, epilepsy, or a structural urinary tract abnormality. It is generally not diagnosed before the age of 5 years, and may be subdivided into:

- *primary:* urinary continence never achieved
- *secondary:* urinary continence has been achieved in the past.

EPIDEMIOLOGY

- *Prevalence.* The prevalence at different ages has been found to be:
  - 7 years – 6.7% in boys and 3.3% in girls
  - 9–10 years – 2.9% in boys and 2.2% in girls
  - 14 years – 1.1% in boys and 0.5% in girls.
- *Sex ratio:*
  - Male to female = 1:1 at the age of 5 years; approximately 2:1 in adolescence.
  - Secondary enuresis is more common in boys.

CLINICAL FEATURES

Non-organic enuresis may be associated with emotional problems, although it should be noted that the latter may be secondary to the enuresis itself.

AETIOLOGY

Possible causes that have been proposed include:

- genetic – 70% have a first-degree relative with late attainment of continence
- stressful life events – a doubling of frequency
- delayed toilet training
- developmental delay – twice as common in enuretic children as in controls
- bladder structure – enuretic children are more likely than non-enuretics to have a different shape of bladder baseplate and to have a reduced functional bladder volume.

MANAGEMENT

Points in the management include:

- a full assessment including a physical assessment to exclude a physical cause; look for evidence of:
  - urinary frequency
  - haematuria
  - dysuria
  - urgency
- urinary microscopy and microbiological analysis
- observation period
- star chart – relapse rate of approximately 40%
- pad and buzzer or, in older children, a pants alarm – relapse rate of approximately 40%
- low-dose tricyclic antidepressants – but there are side-effects and there is a high rate of relapse on discontinuation; can be useful for short time periods (e.g. school trips)
- nasal desmopressin – should not be continued for more than 3 months without stopping for a week for full reassessment
- exercises to increase the functional capacity of the bladder
- habit training.

COURSE AND PROGNOSIS

In general the prognosis is very good.

NON–ORGANIC ENCOPRESIS

DEFINITION

According to ICD-10, non-organic encopresis is the repeated voluntary or involuntary passage of faeces, usually of normal or near-normal consistency, in places not appropriate for that purpose in the individual's own sociocultural setting. It may be subdivided into:

- *continuous encopresis:* bowel control has never been achieved
- *discontinuous encopresis:* there has been a period of normal bowel control in the past.

EPIDEMIOLOGY

- *Prevalence.* At the age of 5 years, the prevalence is 1.5%. In 12-year-olds, the Isle of Wight study found a prevalence of 1.3% in boys and 0.3% in girls.
- The male to female sex ratio is between 3:1 and 4:1.

CLINICAL FEATURES

The presentation of this disorder is summarized in Table 34.4.

Table 34.4   *Presentation of faecal soiling (encopresis)*

Consistency of faeces	Normal, loose or constipated
Place deposited	In pants, hidden or in 'significant' places (e.g. in a particular person's cupboard)
Development	Never continent (continuous), after period of continence (discontinuous) or regression (in various contexts – see below)
Activity	Smearing, anal fingering, or masturbation
Context	Power battle, upsetting life events (e.g. sexual abuse, divorce) and/or other psychiatric disorder
Physical	With soreness, anal fissures etc., or with normal anus

Reproduced with permission from Puri, B.K., Laking, P.J. & Treasaden, I.H. 2002: *Textbook of Psychiatry*, 2nd edn. Edinburgh: Churchill Livingstone.

AETIOLOGY

Causes of non-organic encopresis are shown in Table 34.5.

Table 34.5   *Causes of encopresis*

Congenital	Constitutional variability can include bowel control
Individual	Developmental delay
	Physical trigger – anal fissure – constipation (low-roughage diet) – other bowel disorders
Parent–child	Coercive toilet training
	Emotional abuse or neglect
	'Battleground' for relationship problems
Wider environment	Sexual abuse
	Family disharmony

Reproduced with permission from Puri, B.K., Laking, P.J. & Treasaden, I.H. 2002: *Textbook of Psychiatry*, 2nd edn. Edinburgh: Churchill Livingstone.

MANAGEMENT

Points in the management include:

- a full assessment, but take care in carrying out an anal and rectal examination as informed consent is required from the child who may have been sexually abused (if there is evidence of sexual abuse, the appropriate procedures should be brought into play)

- assessment of family relationships and the home circumstances
- education of the carers with respect to the mechanics of defaecation
- improving the child's self-esteem
- individual therapy
- family therapy
- pharmacotherapy to soften the stools or to promote gastrointestinal motility.

If the above procedures fail, an intense behavioural programme in hospital may be required.

COURSE AND PROGNOSIS

In general the prognosis is very good.

BIBLIOGRAPHY

Black, D. & Cottrell, D. (eds) 1993: *Seminars in Child and Adolescent Psychiatry*. London: Gaskell.

Graham, P. 1986: *Child Psychiatry: A Development Approach*. Oxford: Oxford University Press.

Hoare, P. 1993: *Essential Child Psychiatry*. Edinburgh: Churchill Livingstone.

Laking, P.J. 2002: Child and adolescent psychiatry. In Puri, B.K., Laking, P.J. & Treasaden, I.H. (eds) *Textbook of Psychiatry*, 2nd edn. Edinburgh: Churchill Livingstone.

35

Learning disability

CLASSIFICATION

MENTAL RETARDATION

ICD-10 defines mental retardation as being a condition of arrested or incomplete development of the mind, which is especially characterized by impairment of skills manifested during the developmental period, which contribute to the overall level of intelligence; i.e. cognitive, language, motor and social abilities.

The following is a summary of the ICD-10 classification of mental retardation:

F70   *Mild mental retardation*
         IQ range 50–69
         Delayed understanding and use of language
         Possible difficulties in gaining independence
         Work possible in practical occupations
         Any behavioural, social and emotional difficulties are similar to the 'normal'

F71   *Moderate mental retardation*
         IQ range 35–49
         Varying profiles of abilities
         Language use and development variable (may be absent)
         Often associated with epilepsy, neurological and other disability
         Delay in achievement of self-care
         Simple practical work possible
         Independent living rarely achieved

F72   *Severe mental retardation*
         IQ range 20–34
         More marked motor impairment than F71 often found
         Achievements at lower end of F71

F73   *Profound mental retardation*
         IQ difficult to measure but <20

Severe limitation in ability to understand or comply with requests or instructions
Little or no self-care
Mostly severe mobility restriction
Basic or simple tasks may be acquired (e.g. sorting and matching)

DISORDERS OF PSYCHOLOGICAL DEVELOPMENT

These disorders, which have an onset in infancy/childhood and a steady course, may cause disability in adulthood. The ICD-10 diagnoses of disorders of psychological development are:

F80   *Specific developmental disorders of speech and language*
F80.0 Specific speech articulation disorder
F80.1 Expressive language disorder
F80.2 Receptive language disorder
F80.3 Acquired aphasia with epilepsy (Landau–Kleffner syndrome)
F80.8 Other developmental disorders of speech and language
F80.9 Developmental disorder of speech and language, unspecified

F81   *Specific developmental disorders of scholastic skills*
F81.0 Specific reading disorder
F81.1 Specific spelling disorder
F81.2 Specific disorder of arithmetical skills
F81.3 Mixed disorder of scholastic skills
F81.8 Other developmental disorders of scholastic skills
F81.9 Developmental disorder of scholastic skills, unspecified

F82   *Specific developmental disorder of motor function*

F83   *Mixed specific developmental disorders*

F84   *Pervasive developmental disorders*
F84.0 Childhood autism
F84.1 Atypical autism
F84.2 Rett's syndrome
F84.3 Other childhood disintegrative disorder
F84.4 Overactive disorder associated with mental retardation and stereotyped movements
F84.5 Asperger's syndrome
F84.8 Other pervasive developmental disorders
F84.9 Pervasive developmental disorder, unspecified

F88   *Other disorder of psychological development*

F89   *Unspecified disorder of psychological development*

EPIDEMIOLOGY OF LEARNING DISABILITY

EPIDEMIOLOGY OF IMPAIRMENT

The prevalence of learning disability – defined as having an intelligence quotient (IQ) of less than 70 – is 3.7%, which is considerably higher than would be expected from the normal distribution of IQ. The levels of coexistence of different impairments are shown in Table 35.1.

Table 35.1 *Levels of coexistence of different impairments*

	Severe mental retardation	Mild mental retardation
Cerebral palsy	approx. 20%	approx. 8%
Epilepsy	30–37%	12–18%
Hydrocephalus	5–6%	2%
Severe visual impairment	6–10%	1–9%
Severe hearing impairment	3–15%	2–7%
One or more major impairments	40–52%	24–30

EPIDEMIOLOGY OF SPECIFIC SYNDROMES

The frequencies (per 1000 births) of common specific syndromes are:

- cerebral palsy: 2.2
- fetal alcohol syndrome: 1.6
- Down's syndrome: 1.43
- fragile X syndrome: 0.92
- spina bifida: 0.6–3.0
- early infantile autism: 0.45
- phenylketonuria: 0.1
- Prader–Willi syndrome: 0.1
- Huntington's disease: 0.1.

PSYCHIATRIC DISORDER

The Isle of Wight study (see Chapter 34) found:

- The presence of a physical disorder not affecting the brain was associated with a two-fold increase in the prevalence of psychiatric disorder.
- Brain damage was associated with a five-fold increase in the prevalence of psychiatric disorder.
- Brain damage + epilepsy was associated with a ten-fold increase in the prevalence of psychiatric disorder.

CLINICAL FEATURES OF LEARNING DISABILITY

BEHAVIOURAL PHENOTYPES

The associations of behaviour with specific syndromes are summarized in Table 35.2.

CHALLENGING BEHAVIOURS

Common challenging behaviours that occur are shown in Table 35.3.

SELF-ESTEEM

Low self-esteem is common in people with learning disabilities.

Table 35.2 *Behavioural phenotypes: summary of associations of behaviour to specific syndromes*

Angelman syndrome	Happy disposition; laughing at minimal provocation; handflapping; inquisitiveness
Down's syndrome	Common obsessionality and stubbornness; 25% have attention deficit disorder in childhood
Fragile X syndrome	Idiosyncratic linguistic and interpersonal styles; disagreement about whether close association with autism
Klinefelter's syndrome	Passive and compliant in childhood; aggressive and antisocial past puberty
Lesch–Nyhan syndrome	Compulsive severely mutilating self-injurious behaviour
Sanfilippo syndrome (a mucopolysaccharidosis)	Prominent sleep disorder
Noonan's syndrome	Common problems in peer-relations; stubbornness and perseverative behaviour
Prader–Willi syndrome	Insatiable appetite (diagnostic); sleep abnormalities; frequent temper tantrums; self-injury through skin picking
Rett syndrome	Reduced interest in play in early infancy followed by autistic-like symptoms; stereotypic hand movements; self-injury; anxiety and depression common
Tuberous sclerosis	75% autism, hyperactivity or both.

Table 35.3 *Common challenging behaviours*

Violence to self or others	Biting, hitting, spitting, headbanging, scratching, pinching, tantrums, property damage
Behaviours out of usual context	Shouting, undressing, running away, masturbation, urination, defecation, sexual behaviours towards others, vomiting, passivity, oppositional behaviour
Generally inappropriate behaviours	Rocking, flapping, stealing, kleptomania

FAMILY CHANGES

Figure 35.1 shows the psychological processes that may occur in families having an impaired or disabled member.

CHILDHOOD AUTISM (KANNER'S SYNDROME)

This is characterized by the following triad:

- poor or absent social interaction
- language and communication disorder
- restricted and repetitive behaviour.

The abnormality is apparent before the age of 3 years, and there is a male to female ratio of between 3:1 and 4:1. Clinical features include:

- echolalia
- palilalia
- lack of social usage of language

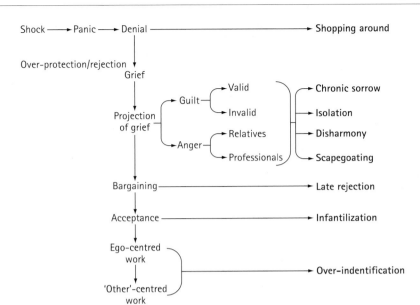

Figure 35.1 *Psychological processes in families with an impaired or disabled member.* (Reproduced, with permission, from Bicknell, J. 1983: The psychopathology of handicap. *Br J Med Psychol* 56:167–178.)

- relative lack of creativity and fantasy in thoughts
- poor eye contact
- lack of socioemotional reciprocity
- self-injury
- stereotyped behaviour
- epilepsy in adolescence
- resistance to change in routine
- attachments to unusual objects.

DOWN'S SYNDROME

The clinical features of Down's syndrome include:

- bradycephaly
- widely spaced eyes with epicanthic folds and oblique palpebral fissures
- Brushfield spots
- small nose and mouth
- horizontally furrowed tongue
- high arched palate
- malformed ears
- broadening and shortening of the neck and hands
- single transverse palmar crease
- curvature of the fifth finger
- an increased range of joint movements
- hypotonia
- increased incidence of cataract

- increased incidence of congenital cardiac disease
- increased incidence of umbilical herniae
- increased incidence of respiratory infections
- increased incidence of acute leukaemia
- IQ < 50 in approximately 85% of cases.

FRAGILE X SYNDROME

The clinical features of fragile X syndrome include:

- elongated facies
  - oedema
  - tissue thickening
  - prognathism
- large everted ears
- single transverse palmar crease
- soft velvety skin
- large forehead
- blue eye colour
- high arched palate
- increased incidence of connective tissue disorders
- hyperextensible joints
- flat feet
- delay in language acquisition with cluttering speech
- learning disability
- mitral valve prolapse in 80%
- macro-orchidism in 70% after puberty.

AETIOLOGY OF LEARNING DISABILITY

The causes of learning disability are summarized in Table 35.4.

Table 35.4 *Aetiology of disability*

Prenatal	Perinatal	Postnatal
Inborn errors of metabolism	Asphyxia/hypoxia at birth	Meningitis/encephalitis
Chromosomal abnormalities	Mechanical birth trauma	Head injury (accidental or inflicted)
Congenital infections (rubella, cytomegalavirus syphilis, HIV, toxoplasmosis)	Small babies	Lead poisoning (and other heavy metals)
	Hyperbilirubinaemia (kernicterus)	
	Hyperoxia (iatrogenic)	Malnutrition
Irradiation	Hypoglycaemia	Other infections (e.g. whooping cough)
Drugs (e.g. thalidomide)	Prematurity (intraventricular haemorrhage etc.)	
Maternal alcohol intake		Environmental chemicals
Malnutrition, including vitamin deficiencies		

MANAGEMENT OF LEARNING DISABILITY

Management must be tailored to the individual case and may include:

- behavioural treatments
- family therapy
- modified individual psychotherapy
- modified group psychotherapy
- pharmacotherapy:
  - for a diagnosed psychiatric disorder
  - for a challenging behaviour.

BIBLIOGRAPHY

Clarke, A.M., Clarke, A.D.B & Berg, J.B. (eds) 1985: *Mental Handicap: The Changing Outlook.* London: Methuen.

Laking, P.J. 2002: Psychiatry of disability. In Puri, B.K., Laking, P.J. & Treasaden, I.H. *Textbook of Psychiatry,* 2nd edn. Edinburgh: Churchill Livingstone.

Russell, O. 1985: *Mental Handicap.* Edinburgh: Churchill Livingstone.

<h1>36</h1>

Eating disorders

ANOREXIA NERVOSA

Classification

ICD–10

This condition is characterized by deliberate weight loss resulting in under-nutrition with secondary endocrine and metabolic disturbance. It requires the presence of all the following:

(a) Bodyweight maintained at 15% below expected; Quetelet's body mass index <17.5 kg/m². (Quetelet's body mass index = mass/height²; age 16 or over.)
(b) Weight loss self-induced by the avoidance of fattening foods and one or more of the following: self-induced vomiting; self-induced purging; excessive exercise; the use of appetite suppressants and/or diuretics.
(c) Body-image distortion: a specific psychopathology comprising a dread of fatness which persists as an intrusive, over-valued idea; a low weight threshold is imposed on self.
(d) Amenorrhoea in women; loss of sexual interest and potency in men; endocrine disorder of hypothalamus–pituitary–gonadal axis (HPA); elevated growth hormone and cortisol levels; abnormal peripheral metabolism of thyroid hormone; abnormalities of insulin secretion.
(e) If onset is prepubertal, the sequence of pubertal events delayed or arrested; puberty is often completed with recovery, but menarche late.

DSM–IV–TR

Diagnostic features

A Individual refuses to maintain minimally normal bodyweight (< 85% normal weight)
B Intense fear of gaining weight (loss of appetite rare)
C Disturbance in perception of shape or size of body
D Amenorrhoea (absence of at least three consecutive menstrual cycles).

Subtypes

These are used to specify the presence or absence of regular binge eating or purging during the current episode.

- *Restricting type.* Weight loss is accomplished through dieting, fasting or excessive exercise.
- *Binge eating/purging type.* There is regular binge eating or purging (or both) during the current episode. Most engage at least weekly. This group are more likely to have other impulse-control problems, to abuse alcohol or drugs, to exhibit mood lability, and be sexually active.

Differential diagnosis of anorexia nervosa

Other causes of weight loss should be considered, especially when presenting features are atypical (e.g. an onset of illness after the age of 40 years).

In medical conditions such as gastrointestinal disease, brain tumours, occult malignancies, and acquired immunodeficiency syndrome (AIDS), serious weight loss may occur. In these cases the individuals do not have a distorted body image or a desire for futher weight loss.

Superior mesenteric artery syndrome (postprandial vomiting is secondary to intermittent gastric outlet obstruction) should be distinguished from anorexia nervosa, although it may develop in anorexia nervosa because of emaciation.

Depressives do not generally have a desire for excessive weight loss or a morbid fear of gaining weight.

Schizophrenics may exhibit odd eating behaviours and occasionally weight loss. However, they rarely fear weight gain or have body-image disturbance.

Clinical features of anorexia nervosa

PSYCHOLOGICAL SYMPTOMS AND SIGNS

The person may exhibit:

- morbid fear of fatness/excessive pursuit of thinness
- denial of the problem
- distorted body image
- fear of losing control of eating
- problems with separation and independence
- depressive feelings – insomnia, lack of concentration, irritability
- suicidal ideas
- obsessional thoughts and rituals which may improve with weight gain
- preoccupation with thoughts of food (enjoys cooking for others; does not like eating in public)
- withdrawn.

PHYSICAL SIGNS AND COMPLICATIONS

The person may exhibit:

- emaciation
- slowed metabolic rate (low blood pressure, slow pulse)
- lanugo hair
- cardiac arrhythmias and failure
- peripheral oedema

- amenorrhoea/loss of libido
- reproductive system atrophy (shrunken uterus and ovaries with cystic multifollicular ovarian changes)
- osteoporosis from low calcium intake and absorption, reduced oestrogen and increased cortisol secretion:
  - bone pain and deformity
  - bone density reduction with increasing years of amenorrhoea
  - pathological fractures after about 10 years
- hypoglycemia
- dehydration
- hypothermia, cold intolerance
- seizures
- delayed gastric emptying
- acute gastric dilatation
- pancreatitis
- tetany
- degeneration of myenteric plexus of bowel:
  - cathartic colon
  - constipation
- reduced growth, delayed puberty
- cardiac and skeletal muscle-wasting
- purpura secondary to reduced collagen in skin and bone marrow suppression
- mitral valve prolapse
- proximal myopathy
- impaired liver function
- impaired renal function caused by chronic dehydration and hypokalemia
- diffuse EEG abnormalities, reflecting metabolic encephalopathy (may result from fluid and electrolyte disturbances)
- increase in the ventricular:brain ratio secondary to starvation.

Effects secondary to repeated self-induced vomiting

There may be:

- erosion of tooth enamel
- dental caries
- parotid gland enlargement.

Common blood abnormalities

Look for:

- hypokalaemia (cardiac arrhythmias, cardiac arrest, renal damage)
- hypoglycaemia
- metabolic alkalosis
- hypomagnesaemia
- hypozincaemia
- hypophosphataemia
- raised serum amylase
- hypercholesterolaemia
- hypercarotaemia
- leucopenia with relative lymphocytosis

- normochromic normocytic anaemia
- low T_3
- raised cortisol and growth hormone
- low plasma gonadotrophins and gonadal steroids; in females, low serum oestrogen, in males low serum testosterone.

The 24-hour pattern of secretion of luteinizing hormone resembles that normally seen in the prepubertal individual.

Epidemiology of anorexia nervosa

Incidence and prevalence estimates vary depending on the diagnostic criteria used, and the population studied. However, the following can be stated:

- It is rare (prevalence about 1–2 per thousand women). The Epidemiological Catchment Areas (ECA) study found only 11 cases in 20 000 persons studied.
- The peak age of onset is 15–19 years.
- The incidence is 10 times higher in females compared to males.
- There is a higher prevalence in higher socioeconomic classes and Western Caucasians, and a significant association with greater parental education. Rates in private schools are 1% – much higher than in state schools (0.15%). Rates are much higher again in ballet or modelling schools (7%).
- The suggestion of increasing prevalence over time is probably not supported, although greater numbers are coming to the attention of services.

Aetiology of anorexia nervosa

GENETIC FACTORS

Family studies show an increased incidence of eating disorders among first- and second-degree relatives of those suffering from anorexia nervosa.

Twin studies have shown higher concordance rates for monozygotic (MZ) than for dizygotic (DZ) twins. Holland *et al.* (1988) found a MZ to DZ concordance ratio of 56:5. Five per cent of first-degree relatives are affected. This suggests that genetic factors are significant in the aetiology. This study suggested 80% of variance in liability to anorexia nervosa was genetic.

Walters and Kendler (1995), in a population-based twin study, found higher concordance rates among DZ twins than among MZ twins.

Data suggest a familial component to anorexia nervosa, but the very low prevalence in the general population has prevented determination of whether this is genetic or environmental.

There is an increased risk of mood disorders among first-degree biological relatives, particularly of those with binge eating/purging type. The morbid risk of affective disorder in families of the eating-disordered is similar to that of families of bipolar probands, and is significantly greater than that in families of schizophrenics or those with borderline personality disorder. This supports growing evidence that anorexia nervosa and bulimia nervosa (see below) are closely related to affective disorder.

ENVIRONMENTAL FACTORS

Non-genetic factors are thought to play a crucial role in the aetiology of anorexia nervosa.

The family

Minuchin *et al.* (1978) found that relationships in families of anorexics are characterized by over-protection and enmeshment. Kendler found that a typical anorexic came from an inward, often over-protected and highly controlled family.

Higher rates of childhood sexual abuse are reported by eating-disordered patients than by controls. Childhood sexual abuse appears to be a vulnerability factor for psychiatric disorder in general, not for eating disorders in particular.

Sociocultural factors

There is a cult of thinness. Anorexic and bulimic women viewing fashion images of women show a 25% increase in their body size estimation afterwards. The media presentation of idealized women is likely to have some effect upon eating-disordered subjects.

Among 15-year-old schoolgirls, the relative risk of developing anorexia nervosa was eight times greater in those who dieted compared to those who did not in a prospective study.

Immigrants from low-prevalence to high-prevalence cultures may develop anorexia nervosa as thin-body ideals are assimilated. Cultural factors influence the manifestation of the disorder: in some cultures, for example, body-image disturbance may not be prominent and the expressed motivation for food restriction may have a different content, such as epigastric discomfort or distaste for food.

Physical illness

An excess of physical illnesses in childhood has been found in those with anorexia nervosa. Physical illness may be a risk factor for the later development of anorexia nervosa, possibly by inducing pathology in the family dynamics.

Cases of anorexia nervosa have been reported with onset immediately related to a glandular fever-like illness. The disruption of the central CRH regulation has been suggested as the mediator of this.

Psychological factors

Psychodynamic theories include: fantasies of oral impregnation; dependent relationships with a passive father; guilt over aggression toward ambivalently regarded mother.

Operant conditioning theories include: phobic avoidance of food resulting from sexual and social tensions generated by physical changes associated with puberty.

Personality

Anorexics have a high prevalence of defined personality disorders and an excess of obsessive, inhibited and impulsive traits. It is suggested that in an environment that emphasizes thinness as a criterion for self-worth, vulnerable individuals cope with the challenges of adolescence by repetitive reward-seeking behaviour.

Braun *et al.* (1994) found that 69% of eating-disordered patients had at least one personality disorder; these were also more likely to have an affective disorder or substance dependence than those without personality disorder.

Anorexics are more likely to suffer from anxious–avoidant personality disorders (cluster C), whereas dramatic–erratic personality disorders (cluster B) are more common in bulimics.

NEUROTRANSMITTERS

Brain serotonin systems are implicated in the modulation of appetite, mood, personality variables and neuroendocrine function. An increase in intrasynaptic serotonin reduces food consumption; a reduction in serotonin activity increases food consumption and promotes weight gain.

Kaye *et al.* (1991) found increased cerebrospinal fluid concentrations of major serotonin metabolite 5-HIAA in long-term weight-restored anorectics, which may indicate an increased serotonin activity contributing to pathological feeding behaviour.

It has been suggested that amenorrhoea is caused by primary hypothalamic dysfunction. This is supported by the fact that a return to normal menstruation lags behind the return of bodyweight, and amenorrhoea sometimes precedes weight loss. This, however, is not proven.

Amenorrhea is caused by abnormally low levels of oestrogen, because of the diminished pituitary secretion of follicle-stimulating hormone and luteinizing hormone (LH). This is usually a consequence of weight loss but, in a minority of individuals, it may actually precede it. In prepubertal females, menarche may be delayed.

Management of anorexia nervosa

Weight restoration and psychotherapy are the main treatments. If a person is very emaciated, inpatient care may be necessary because of physical danger. A full physical assessment is required, including electrolytes. Nursing support, too, is important.

FEEDING

While the person is emaciated the initial aim of therapy is weight gain. Aim for 1 kg, and not more than 2 kg, weight gain per week. The premorbid weight, or the weight at which periods stopped plus 5 kg, are guides to a healthy weight. Psychotherapy at this stage is difficult, so wait until the weight has ceased to be dangerously low.

There is slowed gastric emptying, so meals must be introduced slowly to reduce the risks of gastric dilatation or rupture. If the patient is very emaciated, liquid feeds may be better initially. Gradually build up from 1000 to 3500 kcal per day.

There may be reduced circulating oestrogens, a shrunken uterus, and small amorphous ovaries. As weight is gained, the uterus increases in size and the ovaries become multifollicular. At normal weight the ovaries become follicular; this is detected by pelvic ultrasound and can be used to indicate correct weight.

PSYCHOTHERAPY

Family therapy is the treatment of choice, particularly in young restricting anorexics (age under 22 years) with a duration of illness less than 4 years. Therapy is directive, and parents are encouraged to take control of eating. Work also covers issues of individuation and separation. Parental counselling also may be effective.

For older anorexics, cognitive–behavioural therapy is the treatment of choice.

PHARMACOTHERAPY

Chlorpromazine is sometimes used to promote weight gain. Beware of postural hypotension, arrhythmias and hypothermia.

Prognosis in anorexia nervosa

The course and outcome are variable. Some patients recover fully after a single episode. Some exhibit fluctuating patterns of weight gain followed by a relapse. Others experience a chronically deteriorating course of the illness over many years.

Anorexia nervosa is a serious disorder with substantial mortality. Hsu *et al.* (1979), in a 4- to 8-year follow-up of 100 cases of severe anorexia nervosa treated at a specialist centre, found 48 had good outcome, 30 intermediate, 20 poor; two had died of inanition.

Poor outcome is associated with a longer duration of illness, an older age of onset and presentation, lower weight at onset and at presentation, the presence of bulimia, anxiety when eating with others, vomiting, poor childhood social adjustment and poor parental relationships. The more intractable the illness, the poorer the outcome.

Sullivan (1995) found that the aggregate mortality rate for anorexia nervosa is 5.6% per decade. This is 12 times the annual death rate due to all causes for females aged 15–24. The aggregate mortality rate for anorexia nervosa is substantially greater than that reported for psychiatric inpatients and the general population.

The causes of death were complications of eating disorder in 54% and suicide in 27%. Suicide rates are 200 times greater than in the general population.

BULIMIA NERVOSA

Classification

ICD-10

Bulimia nervosa is characterized by repeated bouts of over-eating, excessive preoccupation with the control of bodyweight, leading to extreme measures to mitigate against the fattening effects of food. It shares the same specific psychopathology of fear of fatness as anorexia nervosa.

A diagnosis under ICD-10 requires all of the following:

(a) Persistent preoccupation with eating and an irresistable craving for food; episodes of over-eating in which large amounts of food are consumed in short periods of time.
(b) Attempts to counteract the fattening effects of food by one or more of the following: self-induced vomiting; purgative abuse; alternating periods of starvation; use of drugs (appetite suppressants, thyroid preparations, diuretics). Diabetic bulimics may neglect insulin treatment.
(c) Morbid dread of fatness. Patient sets weight threshold well below healthy weight. Often there is a history previously of anorexia nervosa.

DSM-IV-TR

Diagnostic features

A Recurrent episodes of binge eating, characterized by the following:
- 1 – eating, in a discrete period of time (e.g. within any 2-hour period), an amount of food that is definitely larger than most people would eat during a similar period of time and under similar circumstances
- 2 – a sense of lack of control over eating during the episode.

B Recurrent inappropriate behaviour to prevent weight gain (e.g. self-induced vomiting; misuse of laxatives, diuretics, enemas, or other medications; fasting; or excessive exercise).

C Binge eating and inappropriate compensatory behaviours both occurring, on average, at least twice a week for 3 months.

D Self-evaluation unduly influenced by body shape and weight.

E Disturbance not occurring exclusively during episodes of anorexia nervosa.

Subtypes

- *Purging type.* There is regularly self-induced vomiting or misuse of laxatives, diuretics, or enemas during the current episode.
- *Nonpurging type.* The individual has used inappropriate compensatory behaviours, such as fasting or excessive exercise, but has not regularly engaged in self-induced vomiting or the misuse of laxatives, diuretics or enemas during the current episode.

BINGE–EATING DISORDER

In this variation, there are recurrent episodes of binge eating in the abscence of the regular use of inappropriate compensatory behaviours characteristic of bulimia nervosa.

Differential diagnosis of bulimia nervosa

In certain medical conditions, such as the Kleine–Levin syndrome, there is disturbed eating behaviour, but characteristic psychological features of bulimia nervosa such as over-concern with body shape and weight are not present.

Over-eating is common in atypical depression, but suffers do not engage in inappropriate compensatory behaviour or exhibit over-concern with body shape and weight.

Binge eating is included in the impulsive behaviour criterion that is part of the DSM-IV definition of borderline personality disorder. If full criteria for both discorders are met, both diagnoses are given.

Clinical features of bulimia nervosa

PSYCHOLOGICAL SYMPTOMS AND SIGNS

The person may exhibit:

- morbid fear of fatness
- distorted body image – over-concern with shape and weight
- an overwhelming urge to over-eat, with subsequent guilt and disgust
- self-induced vomiting (90%), using fingers and, later, reflex vomiting, which results in relief from physical discomfort and reduction of fear of gaining weight
- laxative abuse (30%), excessive exercise and food restriction
- depression, irritability, poor concentration, suicidal ideas
- older than the anorectic, more socially competent and sexually experienced
- possibly normal weight, or just slightly under-weight or over-weight
- menstrual abnormalities (<50%)
- more insight than in anorexia nervosa, often eager for help
- depressive symptoms (in the majority), anxiety, impulsive and compulsive behaviours and problems with interpersonal relationships
- stealing and dependence upon substances.

There is also a high prevalence of depression, self-mutilation, attempted suicide, substance abuse and low self-esteem.

PHYSICAL SIGNS AND COMPLICATIONS

- *Related to vomiting:*
  - dental erosion and toothache

- parotid gland enlargement
- callouses on backs of hands: Russell's sign
- oedema
- conjunctival haemorrhages caused by raised intrathoracic pressure
- oesophageal tears
- ipecacuanha intoxication causing cardiomyapathy and cardiac failure, usually fatal.
- *Related to purgative abuse:*
  - rectal prolapse
  - constipation
  - diarrhoea
  - cathartic colon, damaged myenteric plexus.
- *Related to binges:*
  - acute dilatation of stomach (medical emergency).

Common biochemical abnormalities
These include:

- hypokalaemic alkalosis
- raised serum bicarbonate
- hypokalaemia – direct potassium loss from vomiting, indirect renal loss in response to raised aldosterone secondary to volume depletion
- hypochloraemia
- hypomagnesaemia
- metabolic acidosis with reduced serum bicarbonate in those abusing laxatives
- raised serum amylase (salivary isoenzyme) – monitoring serum amylase can be used to monitor vomiting behaviour.

Electrolyte disturbances can cause weakness, lethargy, arrhythmias and cardiac arrest.

Epidemiology of bulimia nervosa

- The prevalence among adolescent and young adult females is approximately 1–3%.
- The lifetime prevalence for strictly defined bulimia nervosa is 1.1% in females and 0.1% in males.
- Kendler *et al.* (1991) estimate a heritability of liability to bulimia nervosa of 50%.
- The social class distribution is more even than for anorexia nervosa (see above).
- The average age of onset is 18 years, slightly older than in anorectics.
- The female to male ratio is 10:1.
- It is reported more frequently in Caucasians in Western Europe, North America and Australasia.
- There are reports of increasing prevalence with time.

Aetiology of bulimia nervosa

GENETIC FACTORS

In twins, the MZ to DZ concordance rate for narrowly defined bulimia nervosa is 23:9.

ENVIRONMENTAL FACTORS

Prior to illness onset, bulimics are more likely to be over-weight than their peers.

Rigid dieting is the most common precipitant of binge eating. Gross bingeing is the most common precipitant for self-induced vomiting. Dieting may affect appetite and satiety mechanisms. Second World War veterans who had been prisoners of war and suffered weight loss report more binge eating afterwards than veterans who had not been prisoners. Data is supportive of an aetiological role for eating restraint in promotion of bingeing.

Many normal-weight bulimics are the eldest or only daughters. Lacey *et al.* (1991) postulates that at times of parental marital discord the mother can use her daughter as an easily available therapist, burdening the child at an age when she cannot deal with the expressed emotions.

Bulimics report more sexual abuse in childhood than controls.

NEUROTRANSMITTERS

Many abnormalities in eating disorders are secondary to dieting, weight loss, and binge/purge behaviour.

Serotonin is involved in the mediation of satiety responses to feeding as well as the regulation of mood, anxiety and impulsive behaviour. There is evidence in normal-weight bulimics of altered post-synaptic $5HT_{1c}$ receptor sensitivity, and depression associated with dysregulation of pre-synaptic 5HT function.

There is further support for the 5HT dysregulation hypothesis from findings that cerebrospinal fluid (CSF) concentrations of the serotonin metabolite 5HIAA and dopamine metabolite HVA are inversely correlated with a frequency of binge eating in the month prior to admission.

Beta-endorphin concentration in CSF of bulimics is significantly reduced, possibly related to chronic activation of the HPA axis secondary to dieting.

Cholecystokinin-8 (CCK-8) is involved in regulating satiety and anxiety. It is dependent upon an intact 5HT function. Bulimics have lower CSF CCK-8 concentrations than controls. A central, but not peripheral CCK dysfunction is implicated in bulimia nervosa.

Arginine–vasopressin (AVP) CSF concentrations are high in bulimics. An increased central AVP may be related to obsessive preoccupation with the aversive consequences of eating and weight gain. It also interacts with 5HT.

There is a general reduction of sympathetic responsivity and activation of HPA activity in bulimia nervosa, probably as a result of long-term neuroendocrine adaptation to caloric restriction.

PERSONALITY

- Personality disturbance is more common in patients with eating disorders than in the general population. On the Eysenck Personality Inventory, bulimics score higher for psychoticism and neuroticism than do anorexics and controls. On the MMPI, bulimics have elevated scores for psychopathic deviance.
- Low self-esteem, low paternal care, external locus of control and high neuroticism scores are risk factors for bulimia.
- Bulimics are more likely than anorexics to abuse substances (20%). Lifetime rates of alcohol dependence are high.
- The prevalence of social phobia in eating-disordered subjects, especially in bulimics, far exceeds that in the general population.
- Bulimics have high rates (40%) of major depression. There is significant comorbidity between anorexia and bulimia.

Management of bulimia nervosa

PSYCHOTHERAPY

Freeman *et al.* (1988) conducted a controlled trial of psychotherapy. The controls were left significantly worse than all treatment groups at the end of the trial. Behavioural, cognitive–behavioural and group therapy were all effective; 77% stopped bingeing. Improvements were maintained at 1 year. Behavioural therapy was the most effective, with the lowest drop-out rate and earlier onset of improvement. There seemed to be no advantage in adding a cognitive element.

Psychotherapy produces a wider range of changes with more stable maintenance than does drug therapy (see below).

BEHAVIOURAL THERAPY

This aims to stop bingeing and purging by restricting exposure cues that trigger binge/purge behaviour, developing alternative behaviours and delaying vomiting.

COGNITIVE–BEHAVIOURAL THERAPY

This includes psychoeducation, self-monitoring and cognitive restructuring. Eating regular meals is very important.

PHARMACOTHERAPY

Imipramine, phenelzine, amitriptyline, nortriptyline, desipramine and fluoxetine are all superior to placebo in double-blind controlled trials. The dose required is similar to the antidepressant dose. There is a 50–70% reduction in bingeing. The magnitude of the change is smaller than with psychotherapy.

Lithium, anticonvulsants, serotonin promoters and opiate antagonists have all been used successfully.

Cognitive and/or behavioural therapies are the treatment of choice. Antidepressants alone are not adequate.

Prognosis in bulimia nervosa

The outcome for bulimia nervosa improves with time. The majority of patients make a full recovery or suffer only moderate abnormalities in eating attitudes after 10 years.

There is comorbidity with depression, and prominent anoretic features increase the likelihood of a poor response.

In a 10-year follow-up of treated bulimics, 52% recovered fully, 39% continued to suffer some symptoms, and 9% continued to suffer the full syndrome.

In terms of prognostic factors, there is evidence from a number of studies that the following factors may be associated with poor outcome (Keel & Michell, 1997; Quadflieg & Fichter, 2003):

- depression
- personality disturbance
- greater severity of symptoms
- longer duration of symptoms

- low self-esteem
- substance abuse.

Bulimics with multi-impulsive personality disorder do less well than those with bulimia alone.

BIBLIOGRAPHY

Braun, D.L., Sunday, S.R. & Halmi, K.A. 1994: Psychiatric comorbidity in patients with eating disorders. *Psychological Medicine* 24:859–867.

Brewerton, T.D. & Ballenger, J.C. 1994: Biological correlates of eating disorders. *Current Opinion in Psychiatry* 7:150–153.

Collings, S. & King, M. 1994: Ten-year follow-up of 50 patients with bulimia nervosa. *British Journal of Psychiatry* 164:80–87.

Fahy, T.A., Eisler, I. & Russell, G.F.M. 1993: Personality disorder and treatment response in bulimia nervosa. *British Journal of Psychiatry* 162:765–770.

Fairburn, C.G. 1993: Eating disorders. In Kendell, R.E. & Zealley, A.K. (eds), *Companion to Psychiatric Studies*. Edinburgh: Churchill Livingstone.

Fombonne, E. 1995: Anorexia nervosa: no evidence of an increase. *British Journal of Psychiatry* 166:462–471.

Freeman, C.P.L., Barry, F., Dunkeld-Turnbull, J. & Henderson, A. 1988: Controlled trial of psychotherapy for bulimia nervosa. *British Medical Journal* 296:521–525.

Garfinkel, P.E., Lin, E., Goering, P. *et al.* 1995: Bulimia nervosa in a Canadian community sample: prevalence and comparison of subgroups. *American Journal of Psychiatry* 152:1052–1058.

Hamilton, K. & Waller, G. 1993: Media influences on body size estimation in anorexia and bulimia: an experimental study. *British Journal of Psychiatry* 162:837–8340.

Holland, A.J., Sicotte, N. & Treasure, J.L. 1988: Anorexia nervosa: evidence for a genetic basis. *Journal of Psychosomatic Research* 32:561–571.

Hsu, L.K.G., Crisp, A.H. & Harding, B. 1979: Outcome of anorexia nervosa. *Lancet* i:61–65.

Hudson, J., Pope, H.G., Jenas, J.M. *et al.* 1983: Family history of anorexia nervosa and bulimia nervosa. *British Journal of Psychiatry* 142:133–138.

Kaye, W.H., Gwirtsman, H.E., George, D.T. *et al.* 1991: Altered serotonin activity in anorexia nervosa after long-term weight restoration. *Archives of General Psychiatry* 48:556–562.

Keel, P.K. & Mitchell, J.E. 1997: Outcome in bulimia nervosa. *American Journal of Psychiatry* 154:313–321.

Kendler, K.S., Maclean, C., Neale, M. *et al.* 1991: The genetic epidemiology of bulimia nervosa. *American Journal of Psychiatry* 148:1627–1637.

Lacey, H.J., Gowers, S.G. & Bhat, A.V. 1991: Bulimia nervosa: family size, sibling sex and birth order. A catchment area study. *British Journal of Psychiatry* 158:491–494.

Minuchin, S., Rosman, B.C. & Baker, L. 1978: *Psychosomatic Families: Anorexia Nervosa in Context*. Cambridge, MA: Harvard University Press.

Palmer, R.L. & Robertson, D.N. 1995: Outcome in anorexia nervosa and bulimia nervosa. *Current Opinion in Psychiatry* 8:90–92.

Park, R.J., Lawrie, S.M. & Freeman, C.P. 1995: Post-viral onset of anorexia nervosa. *British Journal of Psychiatry* 166:386–389.

Patton, G.C., Johnson-Sabine, E., Wood, K. *et al.* 1990: Abnormal eating attitudes in London schoolgirls (a prospective epidemiological study): outcome at twelve months follow-up. *Psychological Medicine* 20:383–394.

Patton, G.C., Wood, K. & Johnson-Sabine, E. 1986: Physical illness and anorexia nervosa. *British Journal of Psychiatry* 149:756–759.

Quadflieg, N. & Fichter, M.M. 2003: The course and outcome of bulimia nervosa. *European Journal of Child and Adolescent Psychiatry* 12 (Suppl. 1):99–109.

Robins, L.N. & Regier, D.A. (eds) 1991: *Psychiatric Disorders in America: The Epidemiologic Catchment Area Study.* New York: Free Press.

Sohlberg, S. & Strober, M. 1994: Personality in anorexia nervosa: an update and a theoretical integration. *Acta Psychiatrica Scandinavica* 89 (Suppl. 378):1–15.

Sullivan, P.F. 1995: Mortality in anorexia nervosa. *American Journal of Psychiatry* 152:1073–1074.

Vize, C.M. & Cooper, P.J. 1995: Sexual abuse in patients with eating disorders, patients with depression and normal controls: a comparative study. *British Journal of Psychiatry* 167:80–85.

Walters, E.E. & Kendler, K.S. 1995: Anorexia nervosa and anorexia-like syndromes in a population-based female twin sample. *American Journal of Psychiatry* 152:64– 71.

37

Cross-cultural psychiatry

For the purposes of this chapter, culture is defined as the learned way of life of a group of people bound together by a common social heritage. People of the same cultural group behave, think and give meaning to life in a similar way, and share a set of values and beliefs.

INTERNATIONAL COMPARISONS

Schizophrenia

Kraepelin delineated dementia praecox and manic depression. In 1904 he visited the asylum of Buitenzorg in Java to examine the similarities and differences between European patients and those from another culture. He was satisfied that he could recognize cases of dementia praecox in Java, giving credence to his diagnostic distinction. This represents one of the first investigations in transcultural psychiatry.

INTERNATIONAL PILOT STUDY OF SCHIZOPHRENIA (IPSS)

This study (WHO, 1973) was devised to determine whether schizophrenia could be recognized as the same condition in a wide variety of cultural settings. Nine centres (Columbia, Czechoslovakia, Denmark, India, Nigeria, Russia, Taiwan, the UK and the USA) participated. The Present State Examination was translated into seven languages, and psychiatrists trained in its use interviewed 1200 patients. Diagnoses were then generated using the computer program CATEGO. The main findings were:

- When narrow criteria of Schneider's first-rank symptoms were applied, an incidence of schizophrenia was found which did not differ significantly across cultural settings. Therefore schizophrenia is recognizable as the same condition across a wide variety of cultures.
- Broadly defined, schizophrenia has an incidence which differs significantly from one country to another.
- The outcome of schizophrenia was found to vary inversely with the social development of the

society. Those from developing countries had a better prognosis than those from the developed world.

DETERMINANTS OF OUTCOME STUDY

This study (Sartorius et al., 1986) extended its case-finding techniques to include rural primary healthcare centres, traditional healers, police stations, and prisons as well as the more conventional psychiatric settings. More than 1300 cases were interviewed in 12 centres across 10 countries. The main findings were:

- The incidence of narrowly defined schizophrenia was stable across a wide range of cultures, climates and ethnic groups, confirming findings of the IPSS. The *form of presentation* of schizophrenia varied across cultures.
- Catatonic schizophrenia was a common form of presentation in the under-developed world, but has become much rarer in the West. Catatonia presented in 10% of cases in developing countries but in only a handful of those in developed countries.
- Hebephrenic schizophrenia was diagnosed in 13% of cases from developed countries, but in only 4% of cases from developing countries.
- In developing countries, acute schizophrenia was diagnosed more often than in developed countries.

To identify the cause of the good prognosis for schizophrenia in the less-developed world, Leff et al. (1990) determined the levels of expressed emotion (EE) in a subsample of the Chandigarh cohort of first-contact schizophrenic patients from the WHO determinants of the outcome study. At 1-year follow-up, a dramatic reduction had occurred in each of the EE components. No rural relative was rated as high EE at follow-up. It was concluded that the better outcome of this cohort of schizophrenic patients is partly attributable to tolerance and acceptance by family members.

Neurosis

Using standardized interviewing and case-finding techniques, the prevalence rates for neurosis in developing countries are comparable with or higher than those found in the West, contrary to what was previously believed.

In many Third World countries, hysteria represents a high proportion of psychiatric practice. In the West there has been a substantial decrease in the numbers of patients with hysteria, and a compensatory rise in the incidence of anxiety and depression. It is suggested that this can be seen as a shift from a somatic to a psychological mode of communication of emotional distress. The tendency to express distress in a psychological form is associated with higher social class and education. Catatonia could similarly be viewed as a non-verbal manifestation of schizophrenia.

Orley and Wing (1979) investigated the rates of psychiatric illness in two villages in East and West Africa. The rates of depression and anxiety showed large differences (22% and 10% respectively). Compared to rates in Western countries (10–12%) these rates are high. Communities in the developed and undeveloped world are heterogeneous, a point emphasized by the 'new cross-cultural psychiatry' (see below).

In comparing the psychopathology of Jewish and gentile East London depressives, hypochondriasis and tension are much more common in the Jewish group, whereas guilt is more common in the gentiles. Guilt is culturally determined and more common in Christians.

Somatic symptoms of depression appear to be universal, but the concept of depression of mood is not recognized in all cultures; many cultures do not have the language to express the feeling of depression as described in the West. Instead such terms as 'sinking heart' or 'soul loss' are found. In China, 87% of people suffering from neurasthenia fulfil the criteria for major depression and respond to treatment with antidepressants.

THE 'NEW CROSS-CULTURAL PSYCHIATRY'

Kleinman (1977) described the 'new cross-cultural psychiatry'. He criticized as a category fallacy the assumption that Western diagnostic categories were themselves culture-free entities.

Anthropologists have criticized the older transcultural epidemiological research for imposing Western concepts of psychopathology on non-Western people. These studies have also been criticized on the grounds of translation difficulties, the poor quality of questionnaire-generated diagnosis, a disregard for various understandings of the self, and for ignoring the cultural variation for broadly defined illness.

Beliefs about the mechanisms of illness among people in the under-developed world have been divided into three main ideas:

- *Object intrusion.* This is illness caused by a physical object being intruded into the person's body.
- *Spirit intrusion.* A spirit is believed to take possession of the person's body.
- *Soul loss.* The soul of the person is believed to have been stolen by spirits.

TRANSLATION AND VALIDITY OF RATING SCALES

In the translation of rating scales, five types of problem in validity arise:

- *Content validity.* The content of instruments must be relevant in the culture into which the instrument is translated. For example, coca paste abuse is common in Peru, so the substance-abuse schedule should reflect this.
- *Semantic validity.* Words used in the original and new instruments must have the same meanings.
- *Technical validity.* Where languages are not written or illiteracy rates are high, answering a questionnaire may elicit answers that represent a misunderstanding of the intention.
- *Criterion validity.* Do responses to similar items measure the same concept in two cultures? For example, in American Indians hallucinations normally occur during the course of bereavement, but this is not the case in North Americans generally; this must thus be accommodated.
- *Conceptual validity.* This requires that responses relate to a theoretical construct within the culture.

CLASSIFICATORY SYSTEMS

Europe and North America have greatly influenced the models of mental illness and the classification of mental illness over the last century. ICD-10 has been criticized in cross-cultural terms. The international group of psychiatrists involved in drawing up the first draft consisted of 47, only two of whom were from Africa. Thus conditions encountered in many other cultures which do not resemble Western categories have been assigned the title 'culture bound' conditions, or 'masked' representations of 'real' illness.

CULTURE-BOUND SYNDROMES

Debate exists about what constitutes a culture-bound syndrome. The term is used to describe disorders which are considered unique to a given culture (cultural determinist view). However, the question of whether the classically described 'culture-bound syndromes' are actually unique to the given culture, or are in fact universal phenomena merely influenced by culture (universalist view), has not been settled. The following syndromes are frequently cited.

Amok

Occurring in Malays, amok consists of a period of withdrawal, followed by a sudden outburst of homicidal aggression in which the sufferer will attack anyone within reach. The attack typically lasts for several hours until the sufferer is overwhelmed or killed. If alive, the person typically passes into a deep sleep or stupor for several days, followed by amnesia for the event. It almost always occurs in men.

It was first described in Malays in the mid-sixteenth century. It is believed to have originated in the cultural training for warfare among Malay warriors. Later it became a personal act by an isolated individual, apparently motiveless, but the motive could be understood as the restoration of self-esteem or 'face'.

It was very common in Malaya at the beginning of the nineteenth century, but the incidence was reduced when the British took over the administration of Malaya. Today it has virtually disappeared.

It is most common in Malays, but reports of amok from other countries exist, questioning its position as a culture-bound syndrome; it is clear, however, that there is a strong cultural element.

Among Malay cases in mental hospitals, the most common diagnosis is schizophrenia. Depression, acute brain syndrome and hysterical dissociation have also been found in some cases. The majority do not have a mental illness. Attacks are often preceded by interpersonal discord, insults or personal loss, and social drinking.

Koro

This is common in south-east Asia and China; it may occur in epidemic form. It involves the belief of genital retraction with disappearance into the abdomen, accompanied by intense anxiety and the fear of impending death.

Cases of a similar condition have been described in non-Chinese subjects. In these cases the syndrome is often only partial, such as the belief of genital shrinkage, not necessarily with retraction into the abdomen; it usually occurs within the context of another psychiatric disorder and resolves once the underlying illness has been treated.

Debate about the cultural specificity of this disorder continues. Some argue that the culturally determined syndrome is clearly different from the symptom of genital retraction occurring in some non-Chinese psychotic subjects.

The development of koro has been associated with psychosexual conflicts, personality factors and cultural beliefs in the context of psychological stress.

Dhat

This is commonly recognized in Indian culture, and is also widespread in Nepal, Sri Lanka, Bangladesh and Pakistan. It includes vague somatic symptoms (fatigue, weakness, anxiety, loss of appetite, guilt, etc.) and sometimes sexual dysfunction (impotence or premature ejaculation) which the subject attributes to the passing of semen in urine as a consequence of excessive indulgence in masturbation or intercourse.

Patients are typically from a rural area, from a family with conservative attitudes towards sex and of average or low socioeconomic status. Literacy and religion are unimportant.

Bhatia and Malik (1991) studied male patients attending a sexual problems clinic in New Delhi. They found that 65% arrived with a primary complaint of dhat syndrome. Twenty-three per cent of these also complained of impotence or premature ejaculation. The age of presentation is early twenties, with about 50% unmarried. Most are literate. Although some suffered from depression and anxiety, those with dhat syndrome differed from the others only in the relative absence of depression and anxiety. Treatment with anxiolytics or antidepressant drugs resulted in significant improvement, however.

Dhat syndrome is considered by many to be a true culture-bound condition. The belief in the precious properties of semen is ingrained in Indian culture.

Windigo
This is described in North American Indians, and ascribed to depression, schizophrenia, hysteria or anxiety. It is a disorder in which the subject believes he or she has undergone a transformation and become a monster who practises cannibalism. However, it has been suggested that windigo is in fact a local myth rather than an actual pattern of behaviour.

Latah
This usually begins after a sudden frightening experience in Malay women. It is characterized by a response to minimal stimuli with exaggerated startles, coprolalia, echolalia, echopraxia and automatic obedience. It has been suggested that this is merely one form of what is known to psychologists as the 'hyperstartle reaction' and is universally found.

Piblokto
This dissociative state is seen among Eskimo women. The patient tears off her clothing, screams and cries and runs about wildly, endangering her life by exposure to the cold. It may result in suicidal or homicidal behaviour.

Brain fag syndrome
This is a widespread low-grade stress syndrome described in many parts of Africa and also in New Guinea. It is commonly encountered among students, probably because of the high priority accorded to education in African society, and is particularly prevalent at examination times.

Five symptom types have been described as comprising brain fag syndrome:

- head symptoms – aching, burning, crawling sensations
- eye symptoms – blurring, watering, aching
- difficulty in grasping the meaning of spoken or written words
- poor retentivity
- sleepiness on studying.

Guinness (1992) found the rates to be highest in rural areas serving peasant populations (34% of students), compared to periurban schools (22%) and schools for the professional élite (6%).

Sufferers of brain fag syndrome are resistant to psychological interpretation of their condition. It is suggested that brain fag syndrome is a form of depression in which depressive features are not articulated in Western psychological terms.

PSYCHIATRY AND BLACK AND ETHNIC MINORITIES IN BRITAIN

Britain is a multiracial society. In some large cities, ethnic minorities represent 20% or more of the total population. Ethnic minority groups are of two types:

- immigrants
- second- or third-generation residents.

The stresses incurred by these two groups are different. Ethnic minority groups are heterogeneous in terms of religion and cultural background.

Immigrants

People migrate for various reasons, and so adjustment will depend on many factors including those operating before migration, the reasons for migration and factors operating in the host society.

Types of migrant

- *Settlers* are likely to be prepared for a new way of life.
- *Exiles* have been forced to migrate. This may result in grief reaction for their old way of life. They may have suffered torture or other atrocities before migration.
- *Migrant workers* are less likely to put down roots in the host country. They may be supporting their family financially at home.
- *Other:* students, business people etc.

Stresses involved in migration

There are various social stresses:

- culture shock and readjustment to the host society
- downward social mobility, poor housing, unemployment or job dissatisfaction, unfulfilled aspirations, and lack of opportunities
- racial prejudice and discrimination in the host society
- loss of extended family support
- intergenerational difficulties as children integrate, bringing cultural conflict into the home.

In a 3-year follow-up study of Vietnamese boat people given asylum in Norway, Hauff and Vaglum (1995) found there was no decline in psychological distress over time. One in four suffered psychiatric disorder and the prevalence of depression at 3 years was 18%. Female gender, extreme traumatic stress in Vietnam, negative life events in Norway, and chronic family separation were the predictors of psychopathology. Thus the effects of war and persecution were long-lasting, and compounded by adversity in exile.

Some studies have found that the mental health of refugees improves over time, and it is possible that adverse factors in the host environment have significant effects on the readjustment and mental health of refugees.

Mental illness among ethnic minorities

SCHIZOPHRENIA

The higher than expected rates of schizophrenia among Afro-Caribbean people born in Britain have been noted since the 1960s. Studies of hospital admissions have demonstrated high rates of schizophrenia in this group compared to British whites and Asians.

The highest rates of schizophrenia in the Afro-Caribbean group occur in UK-born second-generation subjects (up to nine times that among Europeans). Differences persist even when age and socioeconomic status are taken into account.

These results have caused controversy, with criticisms of misdiagnosis due to unfamiliar culturally determined patterns of behaviour, acute psychotic reactions being mistaken for schizophrenia, or racism accounting for the observed differences. However, well-designed studies dealing with methodological problems fail to substantiate these criticisms. Harvey *et al.* (1990) studied consecutive Afro-Caribbean and white British psychotic inpatients prospectively and found no differences in the course of illness or the pattern of symptoms. This caused them to reject the hypothesis that misdiagnosis accounts for the higher rates of schizophrenia in this group.

Schizophrenia as defined by operational research criteria is more common in people of Afro-Caribbean origin living in the UK.

Sugarman and Craufurd (1994) found a lifetime morbid risk of schizophrenia in the parents of Afro-Caribbean subjects to be the same as the risks to parents of British white schizophrenic subjects (8.9% and 8.4% respectively). However, for the siblings of Afro-Caribbean probands the risk was 15% compared to 1.8% for white siblings. Among the siblings of UK-born Afro-Caribbean probands, the risk was even higher at 27.3%. These observations suggest that schizophrenia in Afro-Caribbean patients is no less familial than the rest of the population (as evidenced by the similar risks to parents), but that the increased risk is caused by environmental factors capable of precipitating schizophrenia in those who are genetically predisposed to it.

The environmental factor postulated has not been identified to date. There is no evidence of increased rates of schizophrenia in the West Indies and therefore no evidence that Afro-Caribbeans carry a greater genetic loading for schizophrenia.

Admission rates for Asians are similar to Europeans, except for the 16- to 29-year age group, who tend to have lower psychiatric admission rates than Europeans. This gives rise to concerns that services are not reaching this particular group.

SUICIDE

Raleigh and Balarajan (1992) reported suicide rates among British ethnic minority groups compared to the indigenous British white population.

- Suicide rates were high among young Indian women (age-specific SMRs of 273 and 160 at ages 15–24 and 25–34 respectively), but low among Indian men (SMR 73).
- Suicide rates were low in Caribbeans (SMRs 81 and 62 in men and women respectively).
- Suicide rates were high in East Africans (SMRs 128 and 148 in men and women respectively), and were largely confined to the younger age groups.
- Immigrant groups had a higher rate of suicide by burning, with a nine-fold excess among Indian women.

High suicide rates among young Indian women are reported within India and in countries where Indian immigrants have settled. High expectations of academic and economic success, the stigma of failure, the authority of their elders and the expected unquestioning compliance of younger family members is thought to predispose to suicide in this culture. Among Indian women these pressures are accentuated by expected submission and deference to males and elders. Rates of suicide and attempted suicide in this group are not greatly different from those in the country of origin, suggesting that the increased rates are not particularly related to issues of migration. In India, dowry-related self-burning is well known. The common causes of suicide by burns in young women include marital problems and interpersonal difficulties with other family members.

In contrast, suicide rates among older Indian women are low, which is thought to accord with the greater respect given to them by virtue of their age.

CHILD AND ADOLESCENT PSYCHIATRIC PRESENTATIONS

Second-generation Afro-Caribbean children presenting to child and adolescent psychiatric services differ in their patterns of presentation when compared to British white children of comparable age and socioeconomic status.

Psychotic and autistic disorders are over-represented in Afro-Caribbean children compared to whites, with psychotic disorders present in 3.4% and 0.8% respectively, and autistic disorders present in 3.4% and 0.6% respectively. Studies also find that the autistic children of immigrant parents are more likely than their white counterparts to be severely or profoundly mentally handicapped. Mental handicap is also over-represented in Afro-Caribbean children (19% vs 11%).

Afro-Caribbean children present with a significantly higher rate of conduct disorder (35% vs 25%) and a significantly lower rate of emotional disorder (18% vs 27%) when compared to white counterparts.

Use of psychiatric services by ethnic minorities

Young, male, black, schizophrenic Afro-Caribbeans have high psychiatric admission rates compared to white British, and a higher rate of compulsory admissions. In inner-city London, the ratio of black Afro-Caribbeans to whites among admissions is higher than the equivalent proportion in the population (three times higher in Hammersmith and Fulham).

Part of the explanation for this is the higher rates of schizophrenia in black Afro-Caribbeans. Bebbington *et al.* (1994) concluded that ethnicity was not of major importance in decisions to use the Mental Health Act in two regions in London. The use of compulsion was strongly linked with challenging behaviour and diagnosis of schizophrenia, but not with ethnicity *per se*.

Dunn and Fahy (1990), studying police admissions under Section 136 of the Mental Health Act 1983 to a South London psychiatric hospital, found an excess of admissions of blacks. However, clinicians judged that more than 90% of detained black and white subjects were suffering from a psychiatric disorder, and were therefore appropriately detained. The judgement of the police in this study was not biased towards apprehending black people as a result of unconscious racist attitudes, as previously suggested by some.

Cole *et al.* (1995) found that for first-episode patients the route to psychiatric care in Haringey (North London) was different from those for chronic patients. While compulsory admission was more likely for black patients, the excess was less striking than in other studies. Black patients were no more likely to have police involvement than other patients. The most important factors in avoiding adverse pathways to care were having a supportive family or friend, and the presence of a general practitioner. Having a GP or close person avoided the need for compulsory detention, an effect seen in both black and white subjects.

Suggestions to account for the over-representation of compulsory admissions among Afro-Caribbeans include the possibility that the stigma of mental illness is greater in this community, thus resulting in delays before cases come to the attention of the services. Afro-Caribbean patients with previous psychotic episodes are more likely than their white counterparts to deny they had a problem at all; these patients are more likely to be non-compliant with anti-psychotic medication and to require compulsory readmission.

APPROACHES TO MANAGEMENT

Communication

In areas with large numbers of ethnic minorities, the service should provide for interpreters to be available for translation. It is preferable that these people have training in psychiatric and sociological terms and concepts, as well as competence in both languages. *Cultural competence* is required as well as a knowledge of the language. Relatives may need to be used, but caution must be taken to ensure that the patient's best interests are being represented.

Family
Involve the family and mobilize the community for support. They may assist in the process of assessment in helping to understand the context of experience and circumstances.

Psychotherapy
Religious leaders and healers can provide important alternative sources of support. Psychotherapy with ethnic minority groups needs to recognize a different philosophical framework and personal development. Thus the Western concern with personal autonomy and independence may not be relevant in those cultures which emphasize the interdependence of the family and the community. Culturally consonant therapy should be offered.

BIBLIOGRAPHY

Ball, R.A. & Clare, A.W. 1990: Symptoms and social adjustment in Jewish depressives. *British Journal of Psychiatry* 156:379–383.

Bebbington, P.E., Feeney, S.T., Flannigan, C.B. *et al.* 1994: Inner London collaborative audit of admissions in two health districts: II. Ethnicity and the use of the Mental Health Act. *British Journal of Psychiatry* 165:743–749.

Bhatia, M.S. & Malik, S.C. 1991: Dhat syndrome: a useful diagnostic entity in Indian culture. *British Journal of Psychiatry* 159:691–695.

Cole, E., Leavey, G., King, M. *et al.* 1995: Pathways to care for patients with a first episode of psychosis: a comparison of ethnic groups. *British Journal of Psychiatry* 167:770–776.

Dunn, J. & Fahy, T.A. 1990: Police admissions to a psychiatric hospital: demographic and clinical differences between ethnic groups. *British Journal of Psychiatry* 156:373–378.

Goodman, R. & Richards, H. 1995: Child and adolescent psychiatric presentations of second-generation Afro-Caribbeans in Britain. *British Journal of Psychiatry* 167:362–369.

Guinness, E.A. 1992: Profile and prevalence of the brain fag syndrome: psychiatric morbidity in school populations in Africa. *British Journal of Psychiatry* 160 (Suppl. 16):42–52.

Harvey, I., Williams, M., McGuffin, P. *et al.* 1990: The functional psychoses in Afro-Caribbeans. *British Journal of Psychiatry* 157:515–522.

Hauff, E. & Vaglum, P. 1995: Organised violence and the stress of exile: predictors of mental health in a community cohort of Vietnamese refugees three years after resettlement. *British Journal of Psychiatry* 166:360–367.

Hotopf, M. & Mullen, R. 1992: Koro and Capgras syndrome in a non-Chinese subject. *British Journal of Psychiatry* 161:577.

Kleinman, A. 1977: Depression, somatisation and the new 'cross-cultural psychiatry'. *Social Science and Medicine* 11:3–10.

Kleinman, A. 1987: Anthropology and psychiatry: the role of culture in cross-cultural research on illness. *British Journal of Psychiatry* 151:447–454.

Kon, Y. 1994: Amok. *British Journal of Psychiatry* 165:685–689.

Leff, J., Wig, N.N., Bedi, H. *et al.* 1990: Relatives' expressed emotion and the course of schizophrenia in Chandigarh: a two-year follow-up of a first-contact sample. *British Journal of Psychiatry* 156:351–356.

Littlewood, R. 1990: From categories to contexts: a decade of the 'new cross-cultural psychiatry'. *British Journal of Psychiatry* 156:308–327.

Murphy, J.M. 1994: Anthropology and psychiatric epidemiology. *Acta Psychiatrica Scandinavica* (Suppl.) 385:48–57.

Orley, J. & Wing, J.K. 1979: Psychiatric disorders in two African villages. *Archives of General Psychiatry* 36:513–521.

Patel, V. & Winston, M. 1994: 'Universality of mental illness' revisited: assumptions, artefacts and new directions. *British Journal of Psychiatry* 165:437–440.

Raleigh, V.S. & Balarajan, R. 1992: Suicide and self-burning among Indians and West Indians in England and Wales. *British Journal of Psychiatry* 161:365–368.

Sartorius, N., Jablensky, A., Korten, A. *et al.* 1986: Early manifestations and first contact incidence of schizophrenia in different cultures. *Psychological Medicine* 16:909–928.

Shepherd, M. 1995: Two faces of Emil Kraepelin. *British Journal of Psychiatry* 167:174–183.

Smyth, M.G. & Dean, C. 1992: Capgras and koro. *British Journal of Psychiatry* 161:121–123.

Sugarman, P.P.A. & Craufurd, D. 1994: Schizophrenia in the Afro-Caribbean community. *British Journal of Psychiatry* 164:474–480.

Thomas, C.S., Stone, K., Osborn, M. *et al.* 1993: Psychiatric morbidity and compulsory admission among UK-born Europeans, Afro-Caribbeans and Asians in central Manchester. *British Journal of Psychiatry* 163:91–99.

World Health Organization 1973: Report of the International Pilot Study of Schizophrenia. Geneva: WHO.

38

Old-age psychiatry

EPIDEMIOLOGY

Fifteen per cent of the population of England and Wales is aged over 65. The age dependency ratio (defined as the population aged over 65 as a percentage of the working population) is projected to rise, so as the aged population rises there will be fewer people of working age to support them.

Within the elderly population, disability rises steeply with age, from 16 per 1000 who are in their sixties to 133 per 1000 who are aged over 80.

The prevalence of psychiatric morbidity in those aged over 65 is:

- dementia 5%
- depression 13.5%
- phobic disorders 10%
- generalized anxiety 4%
- personality disorder 1%
- paranoid states 0.5%
- panic disorder – rare.

The prevalence of dementia rises exponentially with age, doubling every 5.1 years. Thus the prevalence in the over-65s is 5%, and in the over-80s it is 20%.

PHYSICAL PROCESSES OF AGEING

The cause of ageing is not known.

GENETIC FACTORS

Programmed ageing is supported by the observation of the *Hayflick limit*: human diploid cells cultured *in vitro* have a finite lifespan. Upon repeated subculture of normal cells, mitosis ceases independently of culture conditions. This evidence supports theories of genetically programmed ageing. Cells derived from tumour tissue do not display this limit.

It is speculated that this effect is caused by the progressive loss of DNA sequences in the telomere involved in the maintenance of DNA stability and replication.

Changes in ageing probably do not involve defects in DNA, but may involve errors in the control of DNA expression: *epigenetic defects*.

NON-GENETIC THEORIES

Wear-and-tear theories
Age-related decline in organ function is thought to be responsible for ageing. It is no longer thought tenable as a central cause of ageing; it is probably secondary to ageing.

Mitochondrial decline
Across species, mitochondria show a reduction in numbers, an increase in size and structural changes in old organisms. Damage to mitochondrial membranes caused by free radicals is thought to contribute to these changes.

Free radical theories
Free radicals commonly result from oxidative reactions in normal cellular processes, particularly in the inner membranes of mitochondria and during phagocytosis. The resulting damage includes lipid peroxidation which can result in cell death. In animal experiments, antioxidants (free-radical scavengers) have been shown to increase life expectancy but not to increase maximum lifespan, raising doubt about the role of free radicals in the primary ageing process.

The only method proven to increase the maximum lifespan in experimental animals is calorie restriction. This mechanism is unknown but it may involve the delayed maturation of the immune system or reduced free-radical damage secondary to reduced metabolic rate.

NEUROBIOLOGY OF AGEING

In normal ageing there is a slow reduction in weight and volume of the human brain, with a proportionate increase in the size of the ventricles and subarachnoid space after the age of 50 years.

The brain is over-provided with nerve cells, so a loss of cells does not necessarily result in a loss of function. Some parts of the brain show no loss in nerve-cell numbers with normal ageing (e.g. dentate nucleus of cerebellum). Nerve-cell loss is known to occur in parts of the cerebral cortex, the pyramidal and granule cells of the hippocampus, substantia nigra and Purkinje cells of cerebellum. In normal ageing, especially after the age of 85, a shrinkage of nerve cells is known to occur in the cerebral cortex and putamen.

Nerve-cell connections are reduced in some cells with compensatory increases seen in others in normal ageing.

Lipofuscin accumulates in the cytoplasm of nerve cells from childhood.

Tau protein, involved in linking neurofilaments and microtubules, accumulates in a small proportion of ageing nerve cells particularly in the hippocampus and entorhinal cortex, resulting in neurofibrillary tangles. Senile plaques are made up of a core of extracellular amyloid surrounded by abnormal collections of neuritic processes. In the normal ageing brain these are found in the neocortex, amygdala, hippocampus and entorhinal cortex.

Rod-shaped Hirano bodies are found near the hippocampal pyramidal cells. These comprise the microfilament actin. Accompanying their presence is a granulovacuolar degeneration in the pyramidal nerve cells.

Abnormal intracellular inclusions called Lewy bodies are found in the substantia nigra and locus ceruleus in some normal old people. They comprise a spherical body in the cytoplasm of a nerve cell. They have a laminated appearance with a dense granular core and fibrillary material radiating to the periphery.

In normal old brains amyloid can be found deposited in the walls of blood vessels. Deposits are usually small, widespread, in superficial cortical and leptomeningeal vessels overlying the cerebral lobes. Amyloid is also deposited in irregular patches in the normal ageing cerebral cortex. It is called β amyloid (A4 amyloid) and is the same as that located at the centre of neuritic or senile plaques.

All the above neuropathological changes occur in Alzheimer's disease but to a much greater extent.

THE PSYCHOLOGY OF AGEING

COGNITION

Intellectual functioning
Intelligence peaks at the age of 25 years. It levels off until the age of 60–70 and declines thereafter. Many studies have demonstrated an accelerated decline in cognitive functioning in those who are closest to their death. This has been referred to as the *terminal drop*, and poor health may be the cause.

Using the WAIS-R, a classic pattern of intellectual decline is seen, with performance IQ declining more rapidly than verbal IQ. Factors thought to account for this pattern include the following:

- *Speed of processing.* This makes some contribution to the age-related decline but is not the whole explanation.
- *Familiarity/novelty.* Tasks that have been learnt over a lifetime, relying on over-learned abilities, are most resistant to age-related changes (*crystallized intelligence*). Tasks requiring the less-practised processing of new information are most sensitive to age-related decline (*fluid intelligence*).

Although intelligence declines with age, there are considerable individual differences.

- *Problem-solving.* The ability to abstract a concept and apply it to a new situation declines with age, most prominently after the age of 70. The elderly have more problems if tasks are presented in an abstract manner.
- *Creativity.* Scientific creativity peaks in the 30s, whereas artistic creativity peaks in the 50s. Humans seem to be most creative when they are producing the greatest volume of work: *intellectual vigour.*

PSYCHOMOTOR SPEED

Reaction time increases with age, with most slowing occurring in the central processing of information. Older people are less able to maintain a state of readiness, and less likely to choose flexible active information-processing than younger people.

MEMORY

- *Short-term memory.* Short-term memory as tested by the digit span does not change with age.
- *Working memory.* Memory tasks requiring monitoring or complex decision-making are performed more poorly in the elderly than in the young. Decline is increased with the complexity of the task or increased memory load.

- *Long-term memory.* The retrieval of information in the elderly is impaired; thus uncued recall shows an age-related decrement, but cued recall reduces the extent of the decrement. Memory is more durable if it is encoded at a semantic level, rather than at a phonological or orthographic level. Older subjects are less likely to code at the semantic level. Memory performance in the elderly is best if the meaning is easily extracted.

Memory of source is impaired in the elderly, which is thought to be related to deficits in frontal lobe functioning.

Memory of distant events becomes poorer the more remote the patient is from the event.

Retention of knowledge is retained with age. Knowledge-based skills are relatively preserved into old age.

IMPORTANCE OF LOSS

People experience unique problems after the age of 65. Activities are limited by declining physical strength and some suffer debilitating illness. Loss of employment with retirement may result in feelings of reduced self-worth and low self-esteem. The ageing individual increasingly suffers the loss of family and friends through death.

Erikson describes the psychosocial changes that individuals negotiate as they develop. The last of these – *integrity versus despair* – is concerned with the way the individual approaches death. A well-lived life is more likely to result in a sense of integrity and wholeness at this time of reflection upon life achievements. Those with regrets and thoughts of opportunities missed are more likely to approach death with a sense of despair.

PERSONALITY CHANGES

Most studies of personality in older age support the concept of the stability of personality with age.

Adjustment to ageing can be explained by different models which may apply in different individuals. The activity theory entails the successfully adjusted individual as being fully engaged with life, with interests and social contact. The disengagement theory suggests that the individual focuses increasingly on his or her inner world as adjustment is made to diminished family and social roles.

High anxiety levels in the elderly are correlated with physical ill-health, but most chronic neurotic conditions improve in old age. Anxiety-prone personalities arise from a more biological origin, whereas insecure personalities arise more from early environmental events. Dysthymic personalities seem to persist into old age.

SOCIAL AND ECONOMIC FACTORS IN OLD AGE

ATTITUDES

Popular Western culture devalues old age, with women perceived more negatively than men. Children are least likely, and young/middle-aged adults are most likely, to devalue the elderly.

Most elderly people are able to lead independent lives, are financially secure and are not lonely. However, the common perception of the elderly is as dependent, confused, lonely, rigid, depressed and passive people.

The majority of old people cope well with ageing, reporting high life satisfaction, good cognitive skills, openness to new experience and a positive view of themselves. These are considered to display an integrated personality. Those that cope less well display either passive–dependent or disintegrated personalities.

Factors that influence a person's self-view include personality, gender, health and socioeconomic status.

Deviance from social norms generally decreases with age, while the prevalence of stigmatizing conditions increases.

STATUS

As people age the number of social roles they occupy decreases. This may reduce their social worth. Much of the decline in the status of the elderly is associated with their reduced socioeconomic circumstances.

The status of elderly people is high in preliterate societies and low in modern societies. The factors thought to contribute to this effect include the reduction in the usefulness of the elderly as repositories of knowledge, the break-up of the extended family, and the reduced importance of land inheritance.

In modern society, industrial capitalism is thought to have contributed to the declining social status of the elderly mainly through the imposition of a retirement age and stigmatizing age-related financial provision. The proportion of over-65s with a wage has steadily declined through state-imposed retirement for all, irrespective of their ability to work. This has led to poverty and the stigmatization of the old, with a loss of work role and work-related life satisfaction.

RETIREMENT AND INCOME

State pensions were introduced in the early twentieth century following work by Booth revealing impoverishment among the elderly.

Retirement in itself is not a cause of increased morbidity. The main problem experienced in retirement is substantial income reduction: the relative value of pensions today has fallen compared with 50 years ago. In addition to the loss of earnings there is the loss of status, companionship and job satisfaction.

ACCOMMODATION

The likelihood that elderly people will live alone, away from their families, depends on a number of factors, and is relatively common in Britain. The ageing population is living longer and is thus more likely to live alone at some stage in their later years. Increasing home ownership increases the chances that the elderly will live alone for longer.

For health reasons, large proportions of the very old live in institutional care or with relatives or friends. Old people living alone make more use of statutory services than those living with others.

Disengagement theories which hold that older people gradually withdraw from society in preparation for death have now lost favour. Instead, activity theories encourage the maintenance of social interaction and role. Elderly people do maintain a high level of social contact with others. Unhappiness is associated with a lack of friends in a social network.

SOCIOCULTURAL DIFFERENCES

Gender

Ageing women are more stigmatized than ageing men. They are more likely to live alone and are more likely to be poor.

Social class

Almost half of pensioners from social classes I and II have money in addition to the state pension, from private pension schemes and savings, compared to only 5% of those in social classes IV and V.

Ethnicity

There are competing theories about the effect of ethnicity and ageing:

- The *age as leveller hypothesis* argues that, because all old people are socially disadvantaged, the relative disadvantage experienced by ethnic minorities reduces in old age.
- The *double jeopardy hypothesis* argues that disadvantages are exacerbated with age.

Problems experienced by the ageing ethnic minority subject are no different from those facing all ethnic minority groups. Language difficulties are common, and lack of income is most common in Asian people who have travelled from abroad to join their families and lack pension entitlement.

PSYCHOPHARMACOLOGY OF OLD AGE

PHARMACOKINETICS AND PHARMACODYNAMICS

Age-related changes in drug handling

Changes with ageing that may affect pharmacokinetics include:

- ↓ total body mass
- ↓ proportion of body mass that is composed of water
- ↓ proportion of body mass that is composed of muscle
- ↑ proportion of body mass that is composed of adipose tissue
- ↑ gastric pH
- ↓ rate of gastric emptying
- ↓ blood flow in splanchnic circulation
- ↓ gastrointestinal absorptive surface
- changes in plasma protein concentration: this may be the result of illness
- ↓ metabolically active tissue
- ↓ hepatic biotransformation
- ↓ glomerular filtration rate
- ↓ renal tubular function.

Clearance

This is the major determinant of steady-state plasma drug concentration. Reduced renal clearance is particularly important with respect to lithium. The reduction of renal clearance is predictable with age but the reduction with age of hepatic clearance is not as straightforward. All other psychotropic drugs are cleared by hepatic biotransformation, which is variably reduced with age.

Distribution

This is determined by the drug's relative solubility in lipid as opposed to water, proclivity for various body tissues, and plasma protein binding. Most psychotropic drugs, being lipophilic, have a relatively small plasma concentration compared to the total amount of drug in the body.

Absorption

Although structural and functional changes in the gastrointestinal tract are known to occur in ageing, there is no evidence that the rate or extent of absorption of orally administered psychotropic medications is changed in the elderly.

DRUG INTERACTIONS

The incidence of side-effects and adverse drug reactions increases with age. The causes that may contribute to this include:

- ↑ incidence of coexisting physical illness
- ↑ number of prescriptions with age
- ↓ compliance
- changed pharmacokinetics and pharmacodynamics exposing the body to higher drug levels
- ↑ risk for acute organic brain syndrome with age.

PRACTICAL CONSIDERATIONS

Antipsychotics

The elderly are more sensitive to antimuscarinic (anticholinergic) side-effects. Parkinsonian side-effects are more likely in the elderly, in women, and in those with organic brain disease. The prevalence of tardive dyskinesia increases with age and is more common in women. The length of treatment is more strongly related than the absolute dose. Acute dystonias, although common in the young, are rare in the elderly.

An alert has been issued on the use of risperidone and olanzapine in dementia related psychosis and dementia related behavioural disturbance. They are no longer approved for these indications because of:

1. A twofold increase in mortality compared to placebo
2. A threefold increase in cerebrovascular adverse events compared to placebo.

Prescribers should consider carefully the risk of cerebrovascular events before treating any patient with a previous history of stroke or TIA. Consideration should also be given to risk factors for cerebrovascular disease including hypertension, diabetes, current smoking and atrial fibrillation.

Tricyclic antidepressants

With ageing there occurs:

- ↑ plasma half-life
- ↑ steady-state levels
- ↑ volume of distribution
- ↑ postural hypotension.

Heart disease is a relative contraindication. Again, the elderly are particularly prone to antimuscarinic (anticholinergic) side-effects, which may result in acute brain syndromes, urinary retention, and glaucoma.

MAOIs

Extreme caution is needed if considering prescribing these to patients with hypertension and cardiovascular disease.

Lithium

Because of lowered renal clearance, lithium doses in the elderly are approximately 50% lower than in the young. Diuretics may reduce renal clearance even further, increasing the risk of lithium toxicity.

Benzodiazepines

Accumulation in the elderly is not more likely to occur than in the young. The elderly are at an increased risk of delirium and falls.

DISTRICT SERVICE PROVISION

THE NEED FOR SPECIALIZATION

In Britain the specialization of psychogeriatric services started in the 1960s. Mentors included Post and Roth who distinguished between types of dementia and increased the academic standing of the discipline. Specialization has allowed the development of a professional identity with academic departments, journals and a section of the Royal College of Psychiatrists concerned exclusively with the problems facing the elderly.

The elderly display a number of concomitant problems. Those with mental illness often have physical illness and social problems as well. The provision of adequate care for the elderly requires liaison with primary care, geriatric medicine and social services, as well as with informal carers and voluntary agencies. Finally, without specialization, old age psychiatry would be in direct competition for resources with adult psychiatry.

PRINCIPLES OF SERVICE PROVISION

The planning of services for the elderly must take into account the age distribution of the population, including the numbers of the very elderly who are most likely to need the most costly institutional care.

The elderly require:

- accurate assessment – medical, psychological, social and functional
- specialist knowledge
- least disruptive solutions
- prompt interventions.

Informal carers should be considered and supported, and liaison between all aspects of service is paramount.

NEEDS OF CARERS

Community care of the mentally ill, especially dementia sufferers, results in significant strain on the informal carers. Families provide the most practical and emotional help to the elderly population. This is usually provided by a very close relative, such as a spouse or a daughter, and usually falls largely on one relative. Female carers outnumber males 2:1. Most carers are willing and wish to keep the patient at home, but the strain on them is great. The carers of demented elderly people have more problems than others, which increase with the degree of dementia. The sources of stress include:

- practical – e.g. elderly person requiring help with personal and household tasks and care
- behavioural – e.g. nocturnal disturbance, incontinence, wandering and aggression
- interpersonal
- social – e.g. restrictions on the carer's personal life.

The British government's *Health of the Nation* document recognizes the important role of carers and directs services specifically to their support.

ASSESSMENT OF A REFERRAL

Psychiatric assessment

Prior to assessment, establish what the referrer wishes to know, and what the patient and the carers have been told to expect. It is useful to interview an informant, and that is essential in those with organic brain syndromes.

The most informative setting for the initial assessment is within the person's home. Coordination is required to ensure that informants are available. The psychiatrist should be vigilant for unrecognized physical illness presenting with psychiatric symptoms, and if this is suspected should ensure that the patient receives the appropriate medical interventions. Examination at home allows an assessment of the patient's coping in the immediate environment, including visuospatial orientation and the ability to manage independently. It also allows assessment of local resources such as neighbours' and relatives' availability, and any evidence of the unwise use of alcohol.

If the first assessment occurs on a medical ward as a liaison visit, the medical notes should be read and the medical and nursing staff should be interviewed before the patient is seen. Carers should be contacted to supplement the information gathered on the ward. The patient interview should take place in the most private conditions available.

PSYCHIATRIC HISTORY

Following the introduction of the psychiatrist, the patient should be asked whether he or she has any problems to discuss. An assessment of how the patient deals with questioning is made throughout. The interview should be unhurried, allowing the patient to relate a full family and personal history.

Details of past medical and past psychiatric history are very important, as are any medications the patient is currently taking. It is also helpful to have some understanding of the patient's premorbid personality, which is best accessed through informants.

Establish whether the patient has a history of heavy drinking either currently or at some time in the past. A history of smoking is also needed.

Mental state examination

Appearance and behaviour

If the patient has difficulties with verbal exchange (caused for example by severe dementia, delirium, aphasia, severe hearing and/or visual impairments), then careful observation can provide much information. Poor hygiene, incontinence or inadequate nutrition gives an indication of the patient's ability to live independently. Distinguish whether the problem is recent or chronic. Any evidence of physical illness such as cerebrovascular disease may also be observed.

The patient's behaviour may be suggestive of pathology. Observe for signs of psychomotor retardation or agitation, perplexity or behavioural disturbance. An inability to focus or sustain attention appropriately may be a sign of clouded consciousness.

Patients with acute or chronic brain syndromes often display a number of behaviours which can jeopardize their placement in the community. Examples of such behaviours include day/night reversal, wandering, aggression, sliding or throwing themselves to the floor, stripping off their clothes and the smearing of faeces.

Speech

Cognitive impairment may result in circumlocution, paraphrasia and polite evasions hiding a lack of depth and detail in speech. Severe hearing impairment may be overcome by communication through gesture and/or writing.

The elderly with mixed affective states may demonstrate a 'slow flight of ideas'.

Thought

Early dementia may be noticeable only after a lengthy interview with a repetition of themes, a lack of internal logic, and a limitation of discussion inconsistent with the level of intelligence.

Mood

Depression is common and is often missed in the elderly. Mania, too, is easily missed in the elderly and should always be considered.

Hallucinations and delusions

These do not differ substantially in old age compared to the young.

Cognitive examination

If a patient is unable to give a reasonable account of himself or herself, it is often helpful to conduct the cognitive assessment earlier in the interview. If the person has given a history, aspects of cognitive functioning will already have been indirectly assessed.

THE EXAMINATION

The following aspects are assessed:

- *orientation* – to time, place and person
- *attention and concentration* – assessed using 'serial sevens' or naming months of the year backwards if numerical abilities are not good
- *immediate memory* – assessed using digit span (normal 7 6 2)
- *short-term verbal memory* – assessed using name and address with six parts, repeated immediately to assess registration, then again after 5 minutes with intervening distraction to prevent rehearsal, also using Babcock sentence
- *short-term non-verbal memory* – assessed by immediate recall (registration) of a geometric shape, then recall after 5 minutes with intervening distraction to prevent rehearsal
- *long-term memory* – assessed during history-taking (ask date and place of birth)
- *general knowledge* – assessed by asking historical and recent commonly known facts (e.g. the current prime minister, monarch and family, the president of the USA, the colours of the Union Jack, the names of capital cities)

- *verbal fluency* – number of words beginning with T in one minute, or the number of four-legged animals in one minute
- *calculation* – assessed by asking a simple calculation such as a subtraction
- *writing*
- *spatial* – including bodily awareness
- *recognition* – of objects and faces
- *appropriate use of everyday objects*
- *naming things* – to detect nominal dysphasia
- *receptive and expressive use of written and spoken language*
- *perseveration* – suggestive of frontal lobe dysfunction
- *tests of praxis* – such as drawing a square or a clock face (constructional apraxia), asking the patient to make a fist, oppose thumb and little finger, fold a piece of paper and place it in an envelope
- *tests of gnosis* – such as picture recognition, tactile recognition.

Physical examination

All elderly people presenting to psychiatry should have a full physical examination. Check the person's temperature (using a low-reading thermometer) and state of hydration if clouding of consciousness is suspected.

Primitive reflexes are found mostly in dementing patients, although they may occur transiently in acute confusional states. Examples include the palmomental reflex, grasp reflex, pout reflex, sucking reflex and glabellar tap.

Tremors and involuntary movements are more common in old age, but be alert to the possibility of a cerebrovascular event, the onset of Huntington's or Wilson's disease or, more commonly, treatment with dopaminergic preparations such as L-dopa for Parkinson's disease.

Increasing sensory impairments in old age, particularly of hearing and vision, predispose to paranoid states. Closed angle glaucoma is a contraindication to the use of drugs with anticholinergic side-effects, such as phenothiazines and tricyclic antidepressants.

Investigations

A chest X-ray is required in all sick elderly people, even if the chest is apparently clear on physical examination. Pneumonia, tuberculosis and carcinoma can all present with acute confusional states, or depression. An ECG is also required.

The prevalence of thyroid disease increases in old age. Physical signs are often unreliable in the elderly, so TSH screening should be performed in all. Hyperthyroidism can be mistaken for anxiety states, hypomania or delirium. Hypothyroidism can present as depression with psychomotor retardation, dementia or delirium.

Routine investigations in the hospitalized elderly should include FBC with differential WCC, ESR, U&E, creatinine, LFTs with calcium and proteins, glucose, TSH, ECG, chest X-ray, and a mid-stream urine examination.

STRUCTURAL IMAGING

In normal ageing there is progressive cortical atrophy and increasing ventricular size. Imaging can identify potentially treatable intracranial lesions.

Structural imaging is helpful in discovering the aetiology of dementia, although it does not establish the diagnosis, which is determined clinically. The distribution of cerebral atrophy helps to distinguish different types of dementia.

Alzheimer's disease
Normal CT scans of brain do not reliably differentiate normals from those with Alzheimer's disease, with approximately 20% overlap between these groups. This limits the usefulness of scanning in the individual patient. Generally cortical atrophy and ventricular enlargement are greater than in controls, with increasing cognitive dysfunction correlating with increasing cerebral atrophy, but more so with increasing ventricular size. An increase in ventricular size over a span of one year is suggestive of Alzheimer's disease.

The clinical usefulness of neuroimaging can be improved by using a temporal lobe orientation in CT scanning which allows an accurate measurement of the medial temporal lobe. Using conventional angle CT scans it is almost impossible to measure this. In Alzheimer's disease a dramatic thinning of the width of the medial temporal lobe in the region of the brainstem is seen. SPET scans also reveal significantly reduced parietotemporal perfusion in these subjects. Combining SPET scans with temporal-lobe-oriented CT scans improves the diagnostic accuracy of Alzheimer's disease by an order of magnitude over that derived using clinical criteria (likelihood ratio 30 vs 2.6).

Pick's disease
Gross atrophy is seen in the frontotemporal regions (knife-blade atrophy), but the diagnosis cannot be made on this evidence alone.

Huntington's disease
Gross shrinkage of the caudate nucleus ('loss of shouldering') supports a clinical diagnosis of this disease.

Multi-infarct dementia
Focal pathology suggestive of cerebrovascular infarcts and/or white matter changes suggestive of small vessel vascular disease supports this diagnosis.

Normal-pressure hydrocephalus
Enlarged ventricles without cortical atrophy in the presence of normal CSF pressure on lumbar puncture supports this diagnosis.

ELECTROENCEPHALOGRAPHY (EEG)

In normal ageing (after the age of 60) the following changes occur in the EEG:

- slowing of α rhythm
- increased θ activity particularly in the left temporal region
- increased δ activity particularly in the anterior regions
- diminished β activity (only in those aged over 80).

Dementias
In *Alzheimer's disease* the EEG may be normal (6%) or show minor non-specific changes. The following changes may occur:

- diffuse slowing in early stages
- reduced α and β activity, plus increased θ and δ activity as the disease progresses
- paroxysmal bifrontal δ waves (more common than in normal ageing).

In *Pick's disease* the EEG is more likely than in Alzheimer's disease to be normal, and shows less slowing of the α waves.

In *vascular dementia* the tracing shows asymmetry and localized slow waves, with a sparing of background activity.

In *Creutzfeld–Jacob disease* a slow background rhythm with paroxysmal sharp waves is characteristic.

In *Huntington's disease* a low-voltage pattern may be seen.

Delirium

Most conditions causing delirium cause slowing of the EEG tracing:

- Metabolic causes:
  - *hepatic encephalopathy* – slowing of rhythm with posterior preservation; triphasic waves are highly indicative
  - *acute renal failure* – low-voltage activity with posterior slowing
  - *bursts of θ activity*
  - *hypocalcaemia* – slowing with bursts of spikes
  - *hypercalcaemia* – runs of 1- to 2-second waves
  - *hyperthyroidism* – acceleration of α rhythm
  - *hypothyroidism* – low-voltage EEG.
- Drugs:
  - *phenothiazines* – increase voltage, slow α activity, reduce β activity; in overdose, paroxysmal slow waves are characteristic
  - *antidepressants* – increase EEG activity but reduce α rhythm; in overdose, widespread α activity and spikes
  - *benzodiazepines* – increase β waves, especially frontal; in overdose, prominent fast activity unresponsive to stimuli
  - *lithium* – slow α rhythm with occasional, sometimes focal, spikes; in overdose, diffuse slowing, triphasic waves and paroxysmal abnormalities.

Of those with delirium, 90% of patients have abnormal traces. Delta activity, asymmetry in δ waves and localized spike and sharp wave complexes occur more frequently in those with intracranial pathology. Alpha activity correlates with cognitive functioning, and δ activity correlates with the length of illness.

Psychological assessment

Changes in psychological functions such as mood, personality, behaviour and cognition are often the first signs of psychiatric illness in the elderly. Various scales have been devised to provide for the accurate and objective assessment of all aspects of psychological functioning in the elderly. The simpler tests can be used by non-psychologist disciplines in their assessment and monitoring of the elderly mentally ill. Psychologists can help other disciplines in their roles, and take on the psychometric assessments of those patients with confusing or particularly demanding clinical pictures.

PSYCHOMETRIC TESTING

This quantifies the level and range of ability. Serial measures can be used to monitor the effect of interventions, or to measure progress of the patient's condition over time.

It is essential, when any particular test is used in the elderly, that it has been validated in the elderly population, and that its predictions have also been validated.

EXPERIENTIAL ASSESSMENT

This tries to clarify the nature of impairment. By understanding the nature of the impairment it is possible to develop interventions which ameliorate the impairment.

Psychometric measures of function

These are used to clarify the diagnosis, to predict outcome, to predict need, and to monitor change.

- *Clarifying the diagnosis.* Batteries of tests have been devised to distinguish between different diagnostic groups: The *Kendrick Battery* was developed to distinguish normal, functionally impaired and demented elderly groups. The *Geriatric Depression Scale* is a 30-item self-administered rating scale, with cut-off score determining whether depressed (extensively validated and highly discriminant).
- *Predicting outcome.* Various scales, such as the *Clifton Assessment Procedures for the Elderly* (CAPE), can predict survival, placement and decline in elderly subjects. The *Kew Cognitive Map* assesses parietal lobe function and language functions in the dementing patient. This successfully predicts 6-month survival (McDonald, 1969).
- *Predicting need.* The CAPE assesses the level of disability and thus allows for prediction of need for support services. Identification of impairments allows for interventions which may overcome the problems posed by the impairment. Assessments can be used to provide objective evidence for allocation of resources.
- *Monitoring change.* The *National Adult Reading Test* (NART) is used to determine premorbid IQ, thus aiding in the initial assessment of apparent cognitive impairment. Premorbid function is compared to current functioning using the *Wechsler Adult Intelligence Scale* (WAIS).

Repeating tests over time can give an estimate of deterioration, but this can be unreliable since even the elderly with dementia can show practice effects with repeated testing.

Experiential analysis of function

These are used to explain dysfunction and to develop strategies for intervention.

- *Explaining dysfunction.* A finding in a psychometric test may conclude that a patient is unable to carry out a task, but does not try to establish why. The decomposition of impaired performance is used to establish which ability is impaired. A hypothesis of what the disability comprises is tested before a conclusion is reached.
- *Developing strategies for interventions.* A behavioural approach may be used with an ABC (antecedents, behaviour and consequences) analysis before attempting an intervention.

Social assessment

This involves a detailed assessment of:

- living conditions
- personal care
- dynamics of family/carer
- support network
- financial situation

- family structure
- level of independence
- physical functioning in the person's environment.

Assessment is usually conducted by a social worker, but it may also be undertaken by other disciplines in the multidisciplinary team with appropriate training and supervision.

Occupational therapy assessment

Occupational therapists assess personal independence, social, recreational and leisure activities, and interpersonal functioning with a view to maximizing functioning level and independence in all aspects of daily life.

With the elderly, assessment of *activities of daily living* (ADLs) forms the main emphasis. This provides a baseline of functioning in areas of personal hygiene and grooming, cooking, cleaning and shopping, based on interview, observation and checking performance. An important part of the assessment is to identify strengths which can be built on to overcome deficits.

The best place to conduct ADL assessments is within the person's own home, as early in the illness as possible in order to establish baselines. ADL assessment is invaluable in helping to establish the most appropriate placement on discharge, and to determine those packages of care which are most likely to enable ongoing independent living.

PSYCHOLOGICAL REACTIONS TO PHYSICAL DISEASE

Theories of 'successful ageing' maintain that elderly people select a range of activities they want or need to do, then optimize their performance of these activities, and compensate for losses of physical or mental abilities.

Because of the increased prevalence of multiple pathology, adverse social circumstances and loss in old age, the understanding of the psychological consequences of physical disease must take into account physical, mental and social factors.

ADJUSTING TO PHYSICAL ILLNESS

Several factors contribute to the experience of a physical illness:

- the meaning of the illness, both generally and specifically to that patient
- the response of those close to the patient
- physical symptoms
- social consequences of the illness
- coincidental life events and difficulties.

RESPONSES TO PHYSICAL ILLNESS

There are three components to coping style:

- the exercise of autonomy and independence
- the sense of personal responsibility, or locus of control
- activity versus passivity.

Factors affecting psychological response to a physical illness include:

- characteristics of the individual
- characteristics of the physical illness.

Psychiatric disorder may arise as a consequence of the stresses imposed by the physical condition, but it may also arise as a direct physical consequence of the pathological process. For example:

- Hyperthyroidism may give rise to an anxiety state.
- Hypercalcaemia, infection, hypoxia or organ failure may give rise to delirium.
- Steroids may give rise to depression, elation or emotionalism.
- Frontal lobe lesions are likely to result in apathy.

PSYCHIATRIC CONSEQUENCES OF SPECIFIC PHYSICAL DISORDERS

Cerebrovascular disease

Mood disorders may follow a stroke. These are mixed and affect different patients differently. General dysphoria and worry are common. Post-stroke depression and anxiety are recognized. Mania following stroke is described but is rarely seen in practice. Apathy and social withdrawal are seen in the absence of depression.

Syndromes more characteristic of stroke include emotional lability and the denial of handicap (anosognosia).

Sensory impairment

Most commonly seen are impairment of hearing and/or vision. These have a dramatic impact upon the individual's ability to communicate with others which may cause social withdrawal, reduced activity and apparent cognitive decline. They may increase the risks of depression and paraphrenia in the elderly although this is not proven.

DEMENTIA IN OLD AGE

Dementia is defined as a global deterioration in brain functions in clear consciousness, which is usually progressive and irreversible. It results in the deterioration of all higher brain functions including memory, thinking, orientation, comprehension, calculation, the capacity to learn, language and judgement, and is accompanied by deterioration in emotional control, behaviour and motivation.

The dementias become more prevalent with increasing age. The most common dementia in the elderly is Alzheimer's disease, followed by multi-infarct dementia.

Alzheimer's disease

CLINICAL FEATURES

Alzheimer's disease (AD) is a diagnosis that can be made with accuracy only at post-mortem. However, it is possible to make a reasonably accurate diagnosis on the basis of clinical findings.

AD may present at any stage of the illness. Clinical features are most easily considered in stages:

- *Early stage* – until about 2 years:
  - impaired concentration

- memory impairment
- fatigue and anxiety
- fleeting depression of mood
- exaggeration of pre-existing personality traits
- unusual incidents cause increasing concern
- occasional difficulty with word-finding
- altered handwriting
- perseveration of words and phrases.
- *Intermediate stage:*
  - further deterioration in above
  - neurological abnormalities start to appear
  - 5–10% develop epilepsy
  - apraxias and agnosias develop
  - disorientation in time and space
  - get lost in familiar surroundings
  - speech problems with nominal dysphasia, receptive dysphasia, expressive dysphasia, dysarthria, reduced vocabulary
  - groping for words, mispronunciation, reiteration of parts of words (logoclonia), echolalia
  - reduced ability to read and write
  - concurrent progressive memory loss involving recent and past events
  - misidentification (e.g. mirror sign)
  - emotional lability
  - catastrophic reaction (extreme anxiety and tearfulness when unable to complete a task)
  - motor restlessness or inertia.
- *Late stage:*
  - all intellectual functions grossly impaired
  - considerable neurological disability
  - increased muscle tone
  - wide-based unsteady gait
  - personality changes, often with fatuous gross euphoria
  - no communication
  - failure to recognize self or family
  - speech replaced by jargon dysphasia.
- *Final stage:*
  - no personality
  - no communication
  - emaciated
  - incontinent
  - limb contractures
  - death often from pneumonia and inanition.

AETIOLOGY

As mentioned in Chapter 11, the neuropathological findings in Alzheimer's disease include:

- intracytoplasmic neurofibrillary tangles
- extracellular senile (argyrophilic) plaques which comprise a central core of amyloid, silica and aluminium
- granulovacuolar degeneration
- amyloid deposited in walls of blood vessels.

These are found in normal ageing but are more extensive in Alzheimer's disease. Similar neuropathology is observed in the brains of those with Down's syndrome (trisomy 21) who survive into middle age.

There is significant loss of neurones in the brains of Alzheimer's disease patients compared to controls. Most neuronal loss is found in the superior, middle and inferior frontal gyri, superior and middle temporal gyri and the cingulate gyrus.

The cause of Alzheimer's disease is not known but there are several theories.

Ageing

There is no clear neuropathological division between Alzheimer's disease and normal ageing, leading to speculation as to whether Alzheimer's disease is a discrete disease entity or the extreme end of a normal spectrum of age-related decline. However, the distribution of neurohistological findings suggests the former. Plaques and tangles are commonly found in the ageing hippocampus, but much more rarely in the neocortex as is seen in Alzheimer's disease.

Neurotransmitter abnormalities

Neurotransmitter abnormalities include a wide range of changes in catecholamines and neuropeptides. Of most interest is the low cortical cholinergic activity and reduced choline acetyltransferase especially in the temporal cortex. This is thought to be secondary to the degeneration of neurones in the nucleus basalis of Meynert which provides the cortex with its cholinergic projection.

Genetic factors

Genetic factors must account for the disease in some patients. It is familial in some families, especially those in which the onset is early (under 65, presenile dementia). It is also hypothesized that late-onset Alzheimer's disease is an autosomal dominant trait with age-dependent expression and low penetrance, resulting in apparent sporadic cases. The finding of Alzheimer's disease in many patients with Down's syndrome who reach middle age has focused interest on chromosome 21 on which is located the amyloid precursor protein gene. Research has demonstrated that a defect in this gene is not the cause of Alzheimer's disease, but there is increasing agreement that in both familial and sporadic Alzheimer's disease the post-translational processing of amyloid precursor protein is abnormal. Work is now ongoing to investigate other genetic modifications on chromosome 21 which may contribute to the abnormal deposition of amyloid.

Environmental factors

Aluminium. The brains of those with Alzheimer's disease contain more total aluminium than those of controls. Aluminium is found in the areas of the brain most affected in Alzheimer's disease, particularly in the neurones containing tangles, and in the core of senile plaques. Some studies have reported higher concentrations of aluminium in drinking water associated with a higher prevalence of Alzheimer's disease, but these are not consistent. Those receiving haemodialysis accumulate aluminium from the dialysate. Before this was recognized patients developed severe dementia. Steps are now taken to reduce the burden of aluminium accumulation in those receiving haemodialysis. Aluminium probably accumulates in the brains of those with Alzheimer's disease secondary to the disease process rather than being directly causative. It remains possible that aluminium is a contributory factor in some cases of Alzheimer's disease.

Head injury. In sporadic Alzheimer's disease there is an increased risk in those who have experienced head injury within the preceding 10 years.

Infection. It is hypothesized that an infectious agent entering via the transolfactory route may be responsible for some cases of Alzheimer's disease. Herpes simplex type 1 is known to have a predilection for those brain areas particularly affected in Alzheimer's disease and is suspected by some as a possible cause. However, this remains speculative.

MANAGEMENT

A multidisciplinary team is essential, as are close links with physicians, general practitioners, social services and the voluntary sector. The Alzheimer's Disease Society can provide carers with valuable information about local facilities, and often run local counselling and sitting services.

Driving should cease as soon as there is any evidence that it may be unsafe. The patient should be asked to inform the DVLC, but if they fail to do so, the doctor has a duty to inform them.

Small doses of neuroleptic medication may be needed in those patients who are agitated, distressed, aggressive or who have sleep reversal. The elderly, and particularly those with organic brain syndromes, can be exquisitely sensitive to the adverse effects of psychotropic drugs, so caution should be taken with starting doses. Caution with atypical antipsychotics which have been withdrawn for this indication.

Those with Alzheimer's disease are predisposed to developing depression which may require treatment with antidepressant medication, preferably using preparations with few antiadrenergic and anticholinergic (antimuscarinic) side-effects (e.g. SSRIs).

Psychological approaches include the behavioural management of problem behaviours, reality orientation, reminiscence therapy and music therapy.

Those with Alzheimer's disease are more sensitive to cerebral insults and are more prone to developing superimposed acute organic brain syndromes (delirium) than healthy people. A sudden deterioration in functioning should prompt a search for superimposed potentially treatable pathology.

See Appendix 2 for a summary of the NICE technology appraisal guidance for Alzheimer's disease.

PROGNOSIS

Disease progression varies considerably from subject to subject. The younger the age of onset the more rapid the decline. In those aged under 50 the mean survival time is about 7 years, whereas in those aged between 55 and 74 the mean survival is increased to about 9 years.

Poor prognostic factors include:

- significant language impairment
- poor cognitive functioning
- clinical evidence of parietal lobe involvement
- CT scan showing reduced density of left parietal region.

Vascular dementia

CLINICAL FEATURES

Vascular dementia is characterized by a stepwise deteriorating course with a patchy distribution of neurological and neuropsychological deficits. There is evidence of vascular diseases on physical examination (hypertension, hypertensive changes on fundoscopy, carotid bruits, enlarged heart, focal neurological signs suggestive of cerebrovascular accident).

Three presentations occur:

- dementia follows a stroke
- dementia gradually develops following multiple asymptomatic cerebral infarcts
- neuropsychiatric symptoms gradually become evident.

Distinguishing between vascular dementia and Alzheimer's disease can be difficult; indeed, in a certain proportion of cases both coexist. A more insidious onset with a continuous rather than stepwise course, less insight, fewer affective symptoms and lack of hypertension or neurological signs is more suggestive of Alzheimer's disease. Vascular dementia is more likely than Alzheimer's disease to produce coexistent depression, persecutory delusions, anxiety and emotional disturbance.

Based on clinical presentation, history and CT scan findings the vascular dementias have been subdivided into Binswanger's disease, leuko-araiosis, and multiple lacunar states.

Binswanger's disease

This is a progressive subcortical vascular encephalopathy with CT scan revealing markedly enlarged ventricles secondary to infarction in hemispheric white matter. Infarcts are observed to affect periventricular and central white matter. The age of onset is 50–65, with a gradual accumulation of neurological signs, dementia and disturbances in motor function including pseudobulbar palsy. There is often a history of severe hypertension, systemic vascular disease and stroke.

Leuko-araiosis

This was used by Hachinski to describe CT scan appearances of reduced density of white matter. It differs from infarcts in that it affects only white matter, is patchy and diffuse and does not result in the enlargement of cerebral sulci or ventricles. It is found in non-demented subjects as well as those with degenerative and vascular dementia.

Multiple lacunar states

These are CT scan appearances of small well localized subcortical infarcts. It is associated with dementia characterized by dysarthria, incontinence and explosive laughing, secondary to frontal lobe disturbance.

AETIOLOGY

There is an excess of vascular dementia in males, which is probably caused by an increased prevalence of *cardiovascular disease* in men. Hypertension is the most frequent risk factor among those with vascular dementia. Risk factors known to increase the risk of stroke also increase the risk of vascular dementia; e.g. cigarette smoking, heart disease, hyperlipidaemia, and moderate alcohol consumption.

MANAGEMENT

As well as the general management of the dementing patient and carers as outlined earlier in the chapter, with vascular dementia it is worth attempting to treat the underlying cardiovascular condition in order to slow or halt the progression of the condition. The treatment of hypertension is important. Depression may respond to an antidepressant.

PROGNOSIS

The rate of progression to death is similar in this group to those suffering from Alzheimer's disease (see above). Poor prognostic factors include:

- severity of dementia
- bedridden
- urinary incontinence.

Frontal lobe dementias

Dementia of frontal lobe type and Pick's disease both mainly affect the frontal and anterior temporal areas of the brain. Alzheimer's disease and vascular dementia may also have extensive frontal involvement but they are distinguishable on clinical, radiological and histopathological grounds.

In a large-scale neuropathological study over 20 years, 10% of dementia cases had dementia of the frontal lobe type, and a further 2.5% had Pick's disease (the Lund study, 1987).

CLINICAL FEATURES

Frontal lobe dementias have a younger age of onset than Alzheimer's disease, with a larger proportion presenting in the under-65 group. There is a slow insidious onset with marked frontal lobe features including disinhibition with reduced social awareness and lack of judgement. Shallowness, lability of affect, inappropriate jocularity (*Witzelsucht*) and apathy are typical. Persistent pain, hyperalgesia, and Kluver–Bucy syndrome may also occur. Obsessionality in daily routine and language difficulties characterized by reduced spontaneity, reduced output, stereotyped phrases, perseveration, echolalia and finally mutism are seen. Memory loss is variable, and not as marked as in Alzheimer's disease, and agnosias and dyspraxias are less common.

CT scan reveals frontotemporal atrophy.

AETIOLOGY

Genes are clearly implicated, with one-half of cases showing a family history. Little else is known about the aetiology of these conditions.

MANAGEMENT AND PROGNOSIS

The management is similar to that of Alzheimer's disease (see above). There is a slow deterioration of functions. The mean duration of dementia of frontal lobe type is 8 years, and of Pick's disease 11 years.

Parkinson's disease dementia

It is difficult to distinguish dementia specifically associated with Parkinson's disease from other causes of dementia which are likely to occur coincidentally in elderly people suffering from Parkinson's disease. It is estimated that dementia occurs in 15–20% of those with Parkinson's disease, compared to 5–10% of the normal population, corrected for age.

CLINICAL FEATURES

Cognitive deficits seem to occur in most subjects with Parkinson's disease; it is possible that those considered to be suffering from dementia are simply those at the extreme end of cognitive decline in this condition.

Cognitive deficits in Parkinson's disease include:

- slowness in comprehension and response (bradyphrenia)
- impaired abstract reasoning
- memory impairment, including poor retrieval and poor short-term memory, especially frontal lobe working memory
- impaired remote memory (only in the late stages).

Patients with typical extrapyramidal signs of Parkinson's disease who later develop cognitive impairment, especially of a subcortical type, are given a diagnosis of dementia of Parkinson's disease.

AETIOLOGY

This is not known. It is known that in Parkinson's disease there is damage to the ascending monoaminergic system affecting central dopamine, serotonin and noradrenaline systems. There is also damage to substantia innominata, causing cortical cholinergic disruption.

All patients with Parkinson's disease have Lewy bodies in their cerebral cortex, with a subset having more Lewy bodies than most. Not all of these have dementia, although it appears that all have some evidence of cognitive decline.

MANAGEMENT

Exclude treatable pathology, such as depression or acute brain syndrome.

Treatment with anti-parkinsonian drugs does not improve the cognitive manifestations of the disease. Avoid anticholinergic drugs if possible.

Transplants of fetal nerve cells is experimental and may improve the outlook for those with Parkinson's disease. It is not known how helpful this will be in the treatment of dementia of Parkinson's disease.

Cortical Lewy body disease

It is not clear whether this type of dementia should be separated from the dementia of Parkinson's disease. Some patients who suffer from a condition almost indistinguishable clinically from Alzheimer's disease have diffuse Lewy bodies in the cerebral cortex on postmortem examination. In some patients the neurohistology is mixed with features of this and Alzheimer's disease.

CLINICAL FEATURES

Memory impairment progresses into dementia and a motor disorder often suggestive of Parkinson's disease. The dementia is often like that of Alzheimer's disease but is more likely to have features suggestive of an acute brain syndrome such as a fluctuating mental state, altered conscious level and hallucinations.

Cortical Lewy body disease is diagnosed in those presenting with dementia suggestive of Alzheimer's disease, but in whom parkinsonian features develop.

PROGNOSIS

There is terminal decline.

Normal-pressure hydrocephalus

CLINICAL FEATURES

There is insidious onset of dementia with psychomotor retardation, unsteady gait and urinary incontinence. Onset is usually in the 60s or 70s. Behavioural disturbance, hallucinations and paranoia are uncommon.

The diagnosis is made on the basis of clinical presentation, with a CT scan of the brain revealing dilated ventricles (especially the third ventricle) without cortical atrophy, with normal CSF pressures.

AETIOLOGY

There is obstruction to outflow of cerebrospinal fluid from the subarachnoid space, but the ventricular system remains in communication with the subarachnoid space thus allowing CSF to flow out of the ventricular system. This scenario is associated with:

- subarachnoid haemorrhage
- cerebrovascular disease
- meningoencephalitis
- post-intracranial surgery.

MANAGEMENT

Insertion of a shunt will allow the drainage of CSF from the ventricles to the heart.

PROGNOSIS

The best results are seen in those with a full clinical syndrome, a short history and an obvious cause for their condition. Mental and physical improvement is likely after surgery.

One-third of those undergoing surgery will develop complications such as:

- shunt infection and malfunction
- epilepsy
- subdural haematoma.

Creutzfeldt–Jakob disease (CJD)

This is a very rare cause of a rapidly progressive dementia.

CLINICAL FEATURES

There may be a brief prodromal period of anxiety, depression or hallucinations. Sudden onset and rapid progression of dementia, pyramidal and extrapyramidal deficits present usually in the 50- to 60-year age group.

Physical features include limb spasticity, muscular wasting and fasciculation, tremor, rigidity, choreiathetoid movements, myoclonus, dysarthria and dysphagia. Convulsions may occur.

In addition to the above classic form, three variant forms are described:

- *Heidenhain form*. Prominent visual defects may result in cortical blindness. Extrapyramidal symptoms and myoclonus occur.
- *Ataxic form*. There is rapidly progressive cerebellar ataxia, with involuntary movements and myoclonic jerks. Finally muteness and generalized rigidity occur.
- *Cortical form*. This includes parietal lobe symptoms.

The EEG is always abnormal in CJD, showing an increase in slow-wave activity, a reduction in α rhythm; as the disease progresses, bilateral slow spike wave discharges may accompany myoclonic jerks.

AETIOLOGY

Microscopy of brain material reveals vacuolar changes in grey matter particularly in cerebral and cerebellar cortex, creating characteristic spongiform appearances. There is a loss of nerve cells and reactive astrocytosis. About 10% of cases appear to be familial.

The disease is transmissible to laboratory animals by intracerebral inoculation, with symptoms developing years later. The efect is similar to spongiform encephalopathies observed in animals (scrapie in sheep, bovine spongiform encephalopathy (BSE) in cows). Prion protein is responsible for transmission. This is an unusual infective agent since it does not appear to contain nucleic acid, being made up entirely of protein. It differs from normal cell-membrane-derived proteins in that it is highly resistant to degradation by cellular proteases, heat or conventional chemical disinfectants.

CJD has been transmitted in man through dural grafts; through human pituitary-derived growth hormone used to treat children with growth hormone deficiency; and through cross-contamination from instruments used in brain biopsy. Pathologists and those handling human brain tissue are also at increased risk of developing this condition.

A form of CJD known as the *BSE variant* has been identified in humans. It has a slightly different clinical presentation. There can be onset in younger people. It is rapidly progressive and is thought to be associated with eating or being otherwise exposed to cattle infected with BSE.

Other human diseases related to CJD in humans include kuru and Gerstmann–Sträussler syndrome. Kuru results from eating human brain and causes a cerebellar degeneration. Gerstmann–Sträussler syndrome is inherited with cerebellar ataxia forming a prominent clinical feature. Both are extremely rare.

PROGNOSIS

There is terminal decline.

Human immunodeficiency virus (HIV) dementia

This is one of the most prominent features of HIV encephalopathy.

CLINICAL FEATURES

There is initial lethargy, apathy, cognitive disturbance, reduced libido and general withdrawal. As the condition progresses evidence of dementia becomes apparent with cognitive disturbance, incontinence, ataxia, hyperreflexia and increased muscle tone.

AETIOLOGY

Although HIV infection results in complications such as opportunistic cerebral involvement of cytomegalovirus, and cerebral lymphoma, the encephalopathy of HIV is thought to be directly caused by HIV which is a neurotropic virus.

Pathology is found in the white matter of cerebral and cerebellar hemispheres and in deep grey matter. Multinucleated giant cells deriving from macrophages are found in the affected brain tissue.

MANAGEMENT AND PROGNOSIS

Therapeutic trials of antiviral treatment suggest that improvement in HIV dementia may occur, but the prognosis is poor.

Huntington's disease (chorea)

This is a genetic disorder resulting in a condition characterized by continuous involuntary movements and a slowly progressive dementia. There are 5 cases per 100 000 in the UK.

CLINICAL FEATURES

The onset is usually between the ages of 35 and 45, but childhood onset accounts for 10–20% of cases. The onset is insidious, with fidgety movements or non-specific psychiatric symptoms in the early stages.

Movement disorder consists of choreiform movements in the head, face and arms, ill-sustained and jerky voluntary and involuntary movements affecting all muscles, and a distinctive wide-based gait with sudden lurching.

Psychiatric disturbance is variable but common. Initial insight may result in depression. Prodromal personality changes, antisocial behaviour with substance misuse, affective and schizophreniform disorders are sometimes seen. Insight gives way to mild euphoria with explosive outbursts, irritability and rage. There is a slowly progressive intellectual impairment, with some patients profoundly demented in the final stages, whereas others remain reasonably aware.

AETIOLOGY

Transmission is mostly by a fully penetrant single autosomal-dominant gene (located on chromosome 4), affecting 50% of offspring (see Chapter 19 for more details). Occasionally sporadic cases occur.

Pathological appearances include a marked atrophy of head of caudate nucleus and putamen, severe generalized neuronal loss resulting in cortical atrophy which is most marked over the frontal lobes, with ventricular dilatation.

MANAGEMENT

Tetrabenazine helps to reduce the movement disorder. Antidepressants, ECT and minor tranquillizers may be helpful in the early stages, with phenothiazines in low dose in later stages to control behavioural disturbance.

Genetic counselling for family members should be offered.

PROGNOSIS

The duration to death is 12–16 years.

General paralysis of the insane (GPI)

This is a rare condition and can be missed.

CLINICAL FEATURES

The condition develops 5–25 years after primary infection with *Treponema pallidum*. The onset is usually gradual with depression a dominant symptom. There is then slowly progressive memory and intellectual impairment. Frontal lobes are particularly involved, resulting in characteristic personality change with disinhibition, uncontrolled excitement, and over-activity which may be mistaken for hypomania. Grandiose delusions are present in only 10%.

Physically there is slurred speech, a tremor of lips and tongue and Argyll Robertson pupil in 50%. As the condition progresses there is increasing leg weakness leading to spastic paralysis.

The Wasserman Reaction on CSF examination is always positive, with lymphocytosis, raised protein and raised globulin.

AETIOLOGY

The disease is a terminal consequence of syphilis. There is marked cerebral atrophy with meningeal thickening, resulting from neuronal loss and astrocyte proliferation. The presence of iron pigment in microglia and perivascular spaces is specific for the disease. Spirochaetes are found in the cortex in 50% of cases.

MANAGEMENT AND PROGNOSIS

Treatment is with high-dose penicillin under steroid cover to prevent Herzheimer reaction. Following treatment, mental symptoms may diminish.

DELIRIUM IN OLD AGE

This is a state of fluctuating global disturbance of the cerebral function, abrupt in onset and of short duration, arising as a consequence of physical illness or toxic effects.

It is most common at the extremes of life both in the very young and the elderly. This may be caused by reduced cerebral reserve, a concurrence of multiple physical problems and a higher prevalence of polypharmacy in the elderly.

It affects 10–25% of the over-65s admitted to medical wards. Those with dementia are particularly vulnerable to developing superimposed delirium.

CLINICAL FEATURES

- There is rapid onset with a fluctuating course. Lucid intervals occur.
- The delirium tends to be more marked at night particularly in conditions of poor illumination.
- Awareness is always impaired. Alertness tends to fluctuate and can be both increased or decreased.

- Orientation is always impaired, particularly for time.
- Recent and immediate memory is impaired with poor new learning and lack of recall for events occurring during the delirious period. However, the knowledge base remains intact.
- Thinking may be slowed or accelerated.
- Misperceptions, particularly visual, are common.
- Hallucinations and delusions may occur.
- Heightened anxiety and fear are often prominent.
- The sleep–wake cycle is always disturbed, with daytime drowsiness and nocturnal insomnia.
- Physical illness or drug intoxication is usually present.

AETIOLOGY

Although delirium presents with global disturbance of cognitive function, certain neurological pathways seem to be specifically involved. Autonomic disturbance implicates the brainstem. Cholinergic and adrenergic pathways are also thought to mediate delirium.

Any physical insult can result in delirium particularly in a predisposed individual. In the elderly the following causes are the most common:

- hypoxia
- infection
- metabolic disturbance
- iatrogenic
- CNS disease
- epilepsy.

MANAGEMENT

Delirious patients should be fully investigated physically. The treatment of delirium is the treatment of the underlying condition.

Hydration and nutrition should be monitored. Vitamin supplements, particularly thiamine, should be administered if there is any possibility of previous alcohol abuse or malnutrition.

Confusion is minimized if the delirious patient is nursed as consistently as possible by the same staff, in a well-illuminated environment. The patient should be aided in his or her orientation by providing environmental cues such as signposting and repeating information slowly and regularly.

Drugs known to exacerbate delirium should be avoided if possible. Sleep reversal may respond to small doses of temazepam or thioridazine. Disturbed behaviour not amenable to other interventions, such as gentle reassurance, may respond to treatment with a neuroleptic. Haloperidol is the most frequently used in this situation because it is effective and safe.

PROGNOSIS

Between 30% and 40% of delirious patients on medical wards die of the underlying condition. However, those who recover have a good prognosis, and only 5% go on to develop dementia.

DEPRESSION IN OLD AGE

Depressive symptoms affect 11–16% of the over-65s. About 3% suffer major depression.

Female first admissions for affective illness peak at age 80, then fall off. Male first admissions continue to climb until the end of life, overtaking women at the age of 85.

The prevalence of depression declines with advancing age despite the above findings. This may be because of a survivor effect with fewer young depressed surviving to old age, or it may imply that depression in older age is more likely to require inpatient admission.

CLINICAL FEATURES

Elderly depressives present with much the same features of depression as younger people, but the following may be more common in the elderly:

- hypochondriacal preoccupations
- psychomotor retardation or agitation
- paranoid and delusional ideation
- neurovegetative symptoms
- depressive pseudodementia
- behavioural disturbance (e.g. food refusal, aggressive behaviour, shoplifting, alcohol abuse)
- minimization/denial of low mood
- complaints of loneliness
- complaints disproportionate to organic pathology and pain of unknown origin
- onset of neurotic symptoms.

DIAGNOSIS

Because the elderly commonly suffer from coexistent physical disorders affecting neurovegetative functioning, the diagnosis of depression can prove more difficult than in the young. A careful history usually suffices to address this difficulty. The *Geriatric Depression Scale* is helpful since it focuses almost entirely on cognitive rather than physical symptoms of depressive disorder and is easy to administer.

AETIOLOGY

Genetic factors

The genetic contribution to depressive illness reduces with age. The risk of depression in first-degree relatives is lowered with the increasing age of onset of depression in the proband. The risks to relatives are also lower if there has been only a single episode, whereas they are increased with recurrent depression in the proband.

Neurobiological factors

Felix Post (1968) suggested that subtle cerebral changes may make ageing persons increasingly liable to affective disorders.

A subgroup of elderly depressives have ventricular enlargement on a CT scan of the brain. They are characterized as being older, with a later age of onset, more neurovegetative symptoms, and a higher death rate at 2 years than elderly depressives without ventricular enlargement. CT scan appearances in late-onset depressives are more comparable to those with Alzheimer's disease than to those with early-onset depression or normal controls. Thus early- and late-onset depression may be different disorders, and the late-onset type may have a stronger association with neurological dementing disorders than the early-onset type.

Depressed patients with ischaemic brain lesions have more vascular risk factors and less family history of mood disorders than those without.

In a proportion of elderly depressives, subtle brain disease is a risk factor.

Physical illness

Depression can present secondary to a variety of physical conditions, and may sometimes be the first indication of ill-health. The following are the main causes of secondary depression which is more common in the elderly:

- occult carcinoma, particularly of lung and pancreas
- chronic obstructive airways disease (COAD)
- cerebrovascular accident (CVA)
- myocardial infarction (MI)
- hypercalcaemia
- Cushing's disease
- hypo- and hyperthyroidism
- alcoholism
- pernicious anaemia
- iatrogenic – steroids, β-blockers, methyl-dopa, reserpine, clonidine, nifedipine, digitalis, L-dopa, tetrabenazine
- infections – brucellosis, neurosyphilis, influenza.

Personality

It is suggested that personality dysfunction is associated with some late-life depression.

Environmental factors

Murphy (1982) found an association between the onset of depression and severe life events occurring significantly more commonly in the previous year compared to healthy controls. These included physical illness, separation, bereavement, financial loss and enforced change of residence.

MANAGEMENT

The depressed elderly person should be treated in much the same way as a depressed younger person, with antidepressants in an adequate dose for an adequate duration. The choice of antidepressant will depend on concurrent physical morbidity, and the dose is generally lower, particularly when commencing a new drug.

Although tricyclic antidepressants are not absolutely contraindicated in the elderly, they have cardiotoxic properties and cause sedation and confusion in some. Thus lofepramine is often preferred. Alternatively trazodone and SSRIs are sometimes better tolerated.

Deluded depressed patients require the addition of a neuroleptic.

ECT remains the most effective treatment for depression and is the treatment of choice in those with life-threatening depression. It is generally well tolerated, although memory problems may follow, so unilateral electrode placement is sometimes considered preferable. It is contraindicated in those with raised intracranial pressure, and is inadvisable within 3–6 months of a cerebrovascular accident, pulmonary embolus or myocardial infarction. However, the anaesthetist's views should be sought in any patient over whom there is particular concern. The liable consequences of inadequately treated or resistant depression should be weighed against the potential adverse effects of a general anaesthetic and ECT. Monoamine oxidase inhibitors should be discontinued at least 10 days prior to giving ECT.

About two-thirds of cases resistant to first-line therapy show an improvement with lithium augmentation. Generally this is well tolerated, although the levels need careful monitoring in those with impaired renal function or those on diuretics.

Psychotherapy can be considered, although this should usually be in addition to drug therapy.

Socially isolated elderly depressed patients are at a high risk of committing suicide, so it is important that they be treated energetically.

PROGNOSIS

Depression in old age is a heterogeneous condition and therefore has a heterogeneous outcome. Seventy per cent of elderly depressives recover within a year, but 20% relapse. The death rate is higher for late-life depressives than for non-depressed patients.

Chronicity in late-life depression is more common in those with:

- active medical illness
- high severity of depression
- melancholic features
- delusions
- cognitive impairment
- morphologic brain abnormalities.

The development of a transient dementia syndrome during a depressive episode, the onset of the first depressive episode in very old age, and abnormalities in brain morphology may be predictors of dementia in an elderly person with major depression.

MANIA IN OLD AGE

In most elderly people suffering from mania, the age of onset was usually in their young adult life. However, in the elderly population, the onset of the first manic episode is bimodally distributed with peaks at ages 37 and 73. Mania in the elderly is relatively uncommon, comprising about 5% of elderly psychiatric admissions.

AETIOLOGY

Genetic factors
Late-onset cases appear to have less genetic loading than younger-onset cases, with fewer of the former giving a family history of affective disorder.

Organic factors
Secondary mania is that arising in a patient with no previous history of affective disorder, soon after a physical illness such as cerebral tumour or infection. However, evidence suggests that this is more likely to arise in those genetically predisposed to a bipolar affective disorder by virtue of a family history of such.

People with late-onset mania have a greater number of large subcortical hyperintensities on brain magnetic resonance imaging (MRI) compared to controls. It is thought that some cases of late-onset mania are a subtype of secondary mania attributable to changes in the brain's deep white matter.

CLINICAL FEATURES

These are similar to the features in younger adults, but it is thought that the following are more common in elderly manic patients:

- garrulousness
- slow flight of ideas
- cognitive impairment
- irritable surliness
- mixed affective states
- depression following soon after mania recovers.

MANAGEMENT

Most patients require treatment in hospital. Treatment is with neuroleptics and/or lithium, with the addition of carbamazepine if this is not fully effective. If the person is unresponsive or intolerant to this combination, ECT can be effective for manic or mixed affective states. Lithium prophylaxis is advisable in the longer term.

PROGNOSIS

The outlook is the same as in bipolar disorder. Recurrence is usual and therefore mood stabilizers are advisable in the longer term.

PARAPHRENIA IN OLD AGE

EXPLANATORY NOTE

Paraphrenia is a term introduced originally by Kraepelin in 1909 to describe a psychotic condition characterized by the relatively late age of first onset, chronic delusions and hallucinations, the preservation of volition and a lack of personality deterioration. The term quickly lost favour until Roth reintroduced it in 1955 to describe *late paraphrenia*, a condition with age of first onset after 60 years, well-organized delusions with or without hallucinations, and a well-preserved personality and affective response.

ICD-9 allowed the diagnosis of paraphrenia, but this has been dropped from ICD-10. In ICD-10, late-onset disorders are not differentiated from early-onset disorders, so most paraphrenias are coded in ICD-10 under schizophrenia or delusional disorders.

Despite this development in the ICD-10 classification of late-life psychoses, evidence suggests that some late-onset delusional disorders are distinct from schizophrenia, and the use of the term *late paraphrenia* therefore persists.

EPIDEMIOLOGY

Good epidemiological studies in this area have not been completed. It is estimated that in Camberwell (London) there is an annual incidence of late paraphrenia of 17–26 per 100 000. There is a well-established preponderance of females over males in late paraphrenia. Late paraphrenics are more likely to be unmarried, and have a lower fecundity than controls.

CLINICAL FEATURES

Osvaldo *et al.* (1995) studied the psychopathology of late paraphrenics and found the following:

- All had at least one type of delusion. These most frequently involved persecution and self-reference; delusions of thought broadcast, sin, guilt and grandiosity were also present.
- Forty-six per cent had at least one Schneiderian first-rank symptom.
- Eighty-three per cent had some hallucinatory experience, most commonly auditory, but also visual, somatic, and olfactory.
- Thought disorder and catatonic symptoms were almost never seen.
- Inappropriate affect was not seen.
- Negative symptoms were seen frequently but were mild.
- Other psychiatric symptoms such as worry, irritability, poor concentration, self-neglect and obsessive features were all seen more commonly in late paraphrenics than in controls.

AETIOLOGY

Genetic factors

There is an increased risk of schizophrenia in the first-degree relatives of paraphrenics, but it is less than the risk to the relatives of younger-onset schizophrenics.

Paraphrenia is partly genetically determined, but the part played by inheritance requires further study.

Personality

In a subset of paraphrenic patients there is a history of those who have long-standing paranoid personalities which are thought to predispose to the development of paraphrenia in old age.

Sensory impairment

Hearing impairment is associated with the development of paranoid symptoms. The characteristics most strongly associated with late paraphrenia are the early age of onset of hearing impairment, long duration and profound hearing loss. Auditory hallucinations are most consistently associated with hearing loss. It is thought that deafness may exert its action through increased social isolation, withdrawal and suspiciousness. Late paraphrenia has also been associated with visual impairment.

Brain disease

Compared to normal controls, late paraphrenics have significantly larger cerebral ventricles and are more cognitively impaired.

Miller *et al.* (1991), in an MRI study of non-demented late paraphrenics, found that organic brain pathology was common. In a group selected to exclude obvious organic pathology, the following abnormalities were found:

- Forty-two per cent had structural brain abnormalities, with white matter lesions particularly evident in temporal, occipital and frontal areas.
- Fifty-eight per cent had neuromedical illness, such as tumours and metabolic disorders.
- Twenty-five per cent had evidence of silent cerebral vascular disease, most commonly associated with hypertension.
- Neuropsychological testing revealed deficits in intellectual, frontal lobe and verbal memory functions.

MANAGEMENT

Assessment and management are usually best undertaken in the patient's home where the psychopathology is most likely to be evident. Time must be spent developing a rapport and trying to engage with the patient. Day-centre attendance may be helpful in increasing socialization.

If sensory impairment is present there is evidence that the condition can improve upon treatment of the deficit (e.g. a hearing aid for the deaf person).

The treatment of metabolic disorders or other physical conditions may bring about an improvement in the mental state. The treatment of hypertension may prevent a deterioration if this is caused by silent cerebrovascular disease.

Neuroleptic medication may bring about an improvement. A substantial minority show no significant response, and about one-quarter show a full response to treatment. Treatment response is associated with improved compliance, the use of depot medication, an involvement of a CPN, and lower medication doses.

PROGNOSIS

Some patients make little or no response to treatment, while others make a full response. Long-term contact with psychiatric services is required.

ANXIETY IN OLD AGE

Anxiety disorders are often chronic, but about one-third of cases in the elderly have an onset after the age of 65 years.

Phobias

Phobias are quite evenly distributed across the age groups, with lower rates in the over-75s compared to the 65- to 75-year group. Phobias are the most common psychiatric disorder in elderly women in a community sample. Specific phobias are more common than agoraphobia or social phobia. The 1-month prevalence for phobic disorders is approximately 10%.

Generalized anxiety disorder (GAD)

Prevalence increases with age and is more common in women. The 1-month prevalence for GAD is approximately 4%.

Panic disorder

This is rarely encountered in the elderly. The 1-month prevalence for panic disorder in <1%.

CLINICAL FEATURES

Features are generally similar to those seen in younger adults, but the following are more common in the elderly:

- anxious preoccupation with physical illness, finance, crime and family
- subjectively impaired sleep which may be a normal part of ageing
- somatic symptoms of anxiety may be misattributed to physical causes
- abuse and over-prescription of sedative drugs.

AETIOLOGY

Environmental factors

Early parental loss is associated with phobic disorders in younger and older adults.

Physical illness

Anxiety disorders and neuroses are associated with increased mortality and increased cardiovascular, respiratory and gastrointestinal morbidity.

The onset of agoraphobia after the age of 65 is often associated with a physical insult such as a myocardial infarction, surgery or a fracture.

Anxiety symptoms can be caused by a number of physical disorders, and a full physical examination should form a part of the assessment of the elderly anxious patient. Causes include:

- cardiovascular (e.g. myocardial infarction, cardiac arrhythmia, postural hypotension)
- respiratory (e.g. pulmonary embolism, asthma, hypoxia, COAD)
- endocrine (e.g. hyper/hypothyroidism, hypoglycaemia, phaeochromocytoma)
- neurological (e.g. epilepsy, cerebral tumour, vestibular disease)
- drug-induced (e.g. caffeine, sympathomimetics, sedative withdrawal).

Comorbidity

There are high levels of comorbidity with other psychiatric conditions, particularly depression. Late-onset cases of anxiety are almost always associated with depression, which may be either a primary or secondary association.

MANAGEMENT

Although there is less formal evaluation of therapies for anxiety disorders in the elderly, there is evidence that they do respond to psychological interventions including behavioural, cognitive and anxiety-management training.

Benzodiazepines and other sedatives are not generally indicated in the treatment of persistent anxiety disorders, particularly not in the elderly because of the problems of tolerance, dependence, confusion and falls.

Some anxiety disorders will respond to treatment with an antidepressant, particularly the SSRIs which are specifically helpful in depression associated with anxiety, and panic disorder.

Neuroleptics are sometimes helpful for their anxiolytic properties, but caution is required when prescribing any sedative in the elderly.

FURTHER CONSIDERATIONS IN OLD-AGE PSYCHIATRY

Personality change

Introversion increases with ageing. At an extreme level this can result in the 'senile squalor' or *Diogenes syndrome* in which the elderly recluse lives a limited life in advanced squalor with extreme hoarding of rubbish. Alcohol or frontal lobe dysfunction may play a part in this condition, although characteristically the syndrome is unaccompanied by any psychiatric disorder sufficient to account for the state in which the patient lives. Thus it is usually inappropriate to invoke the Mental Health Act; instead, Section 47 of the Public Health Act is usually used to deal with these situations if required.

The prognosis is poor with almost inevitable relapse. Day-care may help, and institutional care is often required.

Suicide and attempted suicide

Suicide is over-represented in the elderly. The elderly comprise 15% of the UK population, yet they account for 25% of all completed suicides, and only 5% of attempted suicides. Ninety per cent of those completing suicide in old age were depressed, and two-thirds of those attempting suicide in old age had a psychiatric disorder. Suicide rates increase with age until very old age, when they seem to tail off, more so for women.

The suicide rate is greater in men than in women; men are more likely to use a violent method and to use alcohol.

The depressed elderly who complete suicide tend to suffer from a moderate, often first-episode depression with the clinical picture often comprising agitation, hopelessness, guilt, insomnia and hypochondriasis. The times of highest risk include:

- bereavement and their anniversaries
- the first few weeks after antidepressant treatment when the person develops the ability to enact his or her thoughts prior to full recovery
- in the first few weeks after discharge from hospital.

Eighty per cent of those completing suicide had seen their general practitioner before their death. The incidence of physical illnesses in completed elderly suicides is higher than expected. Chronic pain is often a contributory factor, particularly post-herpetic neuralgia. Living alone, a widowed or separated status, and alcohol abuse are also risk factors.

Cultural factors probably play a role since suicide rates among some elderly populations, such as elderly Indian people, are extremely low.

Thus suicidal elderly patients should always be taken seriously. Depression should be adequately treated, isolation ameliorated if possible and pain should be properly managed.

Alcohol and drug abuse

ALCOHOL

Alcohol abuse reduces with ageing, especially in men. However, about 3% of the over-75s in a general practice survey drank above the safe limits.

The reasons for this apparent decline in alcohol abuse with age include the selective death of early-onset alcoholics, reduced tolerance to the effects of alcohol secondary to reduced liver enzymes, and increased sensitivity of the ageing brain to sedatives, increased poverty in old age, and reduced opportunities to drink in elderly social circles.

New cases of alcoholism in old age tend to be more neurotic with less evidence of personality disorder than in younger-onset cases. Physical ill-health and psychiatric illness may be a trigger to excessive alcohol use in old age.

DRUGS

Illicit drug abuse is not a great problem in the elderly, but addiction to prescribed benzodiazepines, opiates and other analgesics, barbiturates and laxatives is problematic. In the USA where the very elderly comprise 12% of the population, they are responsible for the consumption of 50% of prescribed hypnotics.

Doctors need to take care in their prescribing, to prevent the initiation of prescribed drug addiction. It is often worth attempting to wean even elderly persons from their drug of addiction, since abstinence can greatly improve the quality of life. However, there is a group, particularly the very elderly, who are better left on the drug if they strongly object to withdrawal.

Sexual activity

NORMAL SEXUAL BEHAVIOUR IN OLD AGE

Sixty per cent of married couples aged 60–75 and 25% of those over 75 are sexually active. One-fifth of men aged over 80 have sexual intercourse at least once a month. Thus sexual activity and sexual interest continue into old age.

The determinants of sexual activity in old age include:

- age
- gender – men are more sexually active than age-matched women
- married status
- own physical health
- physical health of partner
- enjoyment of sex.

Loss of, or illness in, a partner is a common reason for the cessation of sexual activity in the elderly.

PHYSIOLOGICAL CHANGES WITH AGEING

The female genitalia atrophy with age particularly after the menopause. Blood flow is also reduced during arousal, resulting in reduced vaginal lubrication. However, regular sexual intercourse or masturbation protects the female genitalia from these changes. Clitoral sensitivity and orgasm do not change with ageing.

In the male, erections are slower to develop and require more tactile stimulation than in youth. The erection is less firm and persistent than in youth. The plateau phase can be prolonged longer and, although ejaculation is less forceful, orgasm remains unaltered. The refractory period is much longer than in youth.

SEXUAL PROBLEMS IN OLD AGE

Physical illness may impair sexual activity because of:

- fear of the risk involved in sexual intercourse (e.g. myocardial infarction)
- difficult or painful intercourse (e.g. arthritis)
- impaired responsiveness of genitalia (e.g. neuropathy)
- reduced feelings of sexual attractiveness (e.g. after mastectomy or colostomy)
- reduced sexual desire (e.g. dementia)
- drug effects (e.g. antidepressants, antipsychotics, antihypertensives, thiazide diuretics, benzodiazepines).

Elderly people in residential homes or hospitals should be provided with the privacy required to continue sexual expression with a consenting partner or by masturbation if they wish. The attitudes of staff and family may need to change through a process of education and discussion.

Sleep disorders

Forty per cent of older adults complain of chronic sleep problems, and use a disproportionate amount of night-time sedation, often on a long-term basis.

The cause of sleep disturbance in the elderly is multifactorial. Assessment therefore requires a careful history, with selective investigation.

PRIMARY SLEEP DISORDERS

These include sleep apnoea and nocturnal myoclonus, both of which are age-related.

Sleep apnoea

Sleep apnoea is an extremely common disorder affecting a quarter of independently living old people, and higher proportions of those in institutional care. However, the presence of sleep-related breathing disturbance in the absence of daytime sleepiness or impaired daytime functioning is probably not clinically significant.

Sleep apnoea is associated with increased morbidity and mortality. It is associated with daytime fatigue, memory problems, hypertension and cardiac arrhythmias. It is further associated with the increased risk of a stroke, even after controlling for other risk factors such as hypertension, cardiac arrhythmia and obesity.

Circadian rhythms

Some sleep disturbance in old age is associated with changes in the systems that regulate circadian rhythm.

In older age the body's circadian rhythms lose strength, with a breakdown in timing and amplitude. Proposed interventions include:

- fitness training
- evening bright-light exposure
- melatonin supplementation in those deficient.

All these methods have brought about an improvement but are of only limited usefulness. Fitness training and bright-light exposure require a lot of time and effort, and are continued after trials in only a minority of subjects. Melatonin is not commercially available in reliable formulations, and in some can cause depression.

SECONDARY SLEEP DISORDERS

The significant numbers of complaints of disturbed sleep are secondary to other conditions such as medical or psychiatric illness, drug and alcohol use, behavioural and environmental factors. It is essential that the primary problem be identified and treated, rather than treating the secondary sleep disturbance. The use of hypnotics should be avoided whenever possible. Sleep disturbance is typically associated with poor physical health and depression.

In some elderly people the apparent sleep disturbance is simply the unrealistic expectation that they should sleep for as long and as soundly as when they were younger. This often responds well to reassurance. In other patients, attention to issues of sleep hygiene is required. This involves addressing behaviour such as the excessive use of caffeine-containing drugs, and environmental conditions improving the conduciveness to sleep, such as ensuring the bedroom is peaceful and dark, without stimulation, and keeping regular sleep hours without daytime napping.

Bereavement

Mood disorders associated with bereavement are prevalent in later life and are associated with morbidity and chronicity similar to other late-life depression. In a study of late-life widows, 24% were depressed at 2 months after the loss, 23% at 7 months, and 16% at 13 months. Risk factors for depression at 13 months included a past history of mood disorder, intense grief or depression early after the loss, and few social supports.

PSYCHOTHERAPY WITH OLDER ADULTS

INDIVIDUAL PSYCHODYNAMIC THERAPY

Traditionally psychoanalysts have been sceptical about the treatment of people over the age of 50 years. Sigmund Freud argued that older adults were too far removed in time from the formative childhood experiences, that there was too little time left to work with problems, and that older adults were too rigid to allow therapeutic change. A minority of psychotherapists work with older adults, demonstrating that these views are still pervasive. However, a view also exists that these notions do not derive from evidence, rather from conflicts within therapists regarding ageing and dealing with older subjects.

Older adults can be treated with psychodynamic therapy. Conditions suitable for treatment include neurotic and personality disorders rooted in unconscious, unresolved childhood conflict.

ADAPTATIONS IN THERAPY

Patients treated include those suffering from depression, phobias, anxiety neurosis and hysteria. Psychosomatic disorders in patients over the age of 60 are not considered treatable with psychotherapy.

It is suggested that the treatment of choice for neurotic disorders in the 55- to 75-year age group is one to two 50-minute sessions per week for between several months to two years. In those with reactive crises, short-term low-frequency dynamic therapy of 5–20 sessions is indicated until the age of about 80.

Older adults have completed their psychosexual and psychosocial development, but still have to cope with psychosocial tasks such as retirement, loss of partner, ill-health and impending death. They also have to struggle with unresolved unconscious psychological conflict and intergenerational difficulties.

With age the ego adapts by deploying increasingly mature defence mechanisms. The superego similarly adapts. However, the unconscious id is largely unchanged with time. Inner psychological conflict can persist from childhood.

TRANSFERENCE AND COUNTERTRANSFERENCE

Early in therapy with elderly patients the transference and countertransference are likely to be reversed compared to therapy with younger patients. With the younger patient the therapist unconsciously assumes the position of a powerful parent. With the elderly patient the transference is likely to be reversed whereby the therapist experiences the unconscious transference of their own parental relationships. It is essential that supervision be provided such that the therapist is aware of these issues as they arise in therapy. Similarly, early in therapy the patient is likely to transfer past experiences with younger people, such as his or her own children; but as the therapy progresses the patient will develop the more classical transference relationships.

COMMON THEMES

In older age an increasing number of threatening and loss events occur. The therapist must work with the patient to mourn the losses, thus freeing the patient to continue to take up new opportunities and relationships. Decreasing independence and increasing dependence are often central themes in therapy. Coming to terms with the past and changed relationships and power structures are also relevant.

For the isolated elderly person, group work may be more appropriate than individual therapy.

MEDICOLEGAL ISSUES IN OLD AGE PSYCHIATRY

ELDER ABUSE

The abuse of elderly people by their carers has received increasing attention since the 1970s. Its prevalence is difficult to estimate and depends on the definition of abuse – which can range from irritability and verbal abuse, to sexual and physical abuse.

Among patients referred for respite care to geriatric wards in London, there was a high morbidity for dementia. Almost half of the carers admitted to some form of abuse, verbal more commonly than physical. Verbal abuse was associated with poor pre-morbid relations between patient and carer, and depression and anxiety in the carer. Physical abuse was associated with poor communication by the patient and high alcohol consumption in the carer. Few patients admitted to any abuse by their carers.

MANAGEMENT OF FINANCIAL AFFAIRS

Mental disorder from whatever cause can restrict a person's ability to deal with money, pay bills or buy or sell property. This can affect people in any age group but is more common in the elderly, particularly among those suffering from dementing conditions. Various options exist to help deal with the financial affairs of people unable to do so themselves because of mental disorder. See Chapter 21 in which advocacy, appointeeship, the powers of attorney, the Court of Protection and testamentary capacity are considered. The effect of psychiatric disorders on driving capability is also considered in that chapter.

BIBLIOGRAPHY

Brun, A. 1987: Frontal lobe degeneration of the non-Alzheimer type: I. neuropathology. *Archives of Gerontology and Geriatrics* 6:193–208.

Department of Health 1991: *Epidemiological Overview of the Health of Elderly People*. London: Central Health Monitoring Unit.

Jacoby, R. & Oppenheimer, C. (eds) 1991: *Psychiatry in the Elderly*. London: Oxford University Press.

Kay, D.W.K., Beamish, P. & Roth, M. 1964: Old age mental disorders in Newcastle upon Tyne: I. A study of prevalence. *British Journal of Psychiatry* 110:146–158.

McDonald, C. 1969: Clinical heterogeneity in senile dementia. *British Journal of Psychiatry* 115:267–271.

Miller, B.L., Lesser, I.M., Boone, K.B. *et al.* 1991: Brain lesions and cognitive function in late-life psychosis. *British Journal of Psychiatry* 158:76–82.

Murphy, E. 1982: Social origins of depression in old age. *British Journal of Psychiatry* 141:135–142.

Lindesay, J., Briggs, K. & Murphy, E. 1989: The Guy's/Age Concern survey: prevalence rates of cognitive impairment, depression and anxiety in an urban elderly community. *British Journal of Psychiatry* 155:317–329.

Osvaldo, P., Almeida, R., Howard, R.J. *et al.* 1995: Psychotic states arising in late life (late paraphrenia): psychopathology and nosology. *British Journal of Psychiatry* 166:205–214.

Osvaldo, P., Almeida, R., Howard, R.J. *et al.* 1995: Psychotic states arising in late life (late paraphrenia): the role of risk factors. *British Journal of Psychiatry* 166:215–228.

Post, F. 1968: The factor of ageing in affective illness. In Coppen, A. & Walk, A. (eds) *Recent Developments in Affective Disorders*. Ashford: Headley Brothers, 105–116.

Schneider, L.S. 1993: Treatment of depression, psychosis, and other conditions in geriatric patients. *Current Opinion in Psychiatry* 6:562–567.

Zisook, S. & Peterkin, J.J. 1993: Mood disorders and bereavement in late life. *Current Opinion in Psychiatry* 6:568–573.

39

Forensic psychiatry

EPIDEMIOLOGY OF OFFENDING

Relationship with age
In the UK the peak age of offending is 14 years in girls and 17–18 years in boys. Half of all indictable crimes are committed by people aged under 21 years. By the age of 30 years, 30% of males in the UK have been convicted of an indictable offence.

Sex ratio
The sex ratio of convicted males to females in the UK is approximately 5:1.

JUVENILE DELINQUENCY

Juvenile delinquency is defined as law-breaking behaviour by 10- to 21-year-olds.

AETIOLOGY

The aetiology is multifactorial and is not associated with an established psychiatric disorder. Factors associated with the development of delinquency include:

- unsatisfactory child-rearing
- low IQ
- conduct disorder in childhood
- parental criminality
- large family size.

MANAGEMENT AND PROGNOSIS

Factors that may improve the prognosis with respect to adult criminality include:

- counselling
- establishing a good relationship with a parent or counsellor
- improvement in the home environment
- a good experience in school
- a good peer group
- successful employment
- a good relationship or marriage.

Approximately 50% have stopped their delinquent behaviour by the age of 19 years.

CRIMINAL RESPONSIBILITY IN THE UK

In England and Wales, criminal responsibility starts at the age of 10 years. In Scotland it starts at the age of 8 years.

Definitions

- *Dolci incapax.* Criminal responsibility is partial between the ages of 10 and 14 years. After the age of 14 years an individual is legally responsible for his or her actions unless caused by:
  - a mistake
  - an accident
  - duress
  - necessity
  - mental disorder.
- *Actus rea.* This is an unlawful act.
- *Mens rea.* This is guilty intent, and is required in addition to an unlawful act for certain offences, such as murder and rape.

MENTALLY ABNORMAL OFFENDERS

EPIDEMIOLOGY

The prevalence of mental abnormality in all offenders is estimated to be 1%. The prevalence of mental abnormality in those in prison in the UK is estimated to be up to 33%.

FORENSIC PSYCHIATRIC ASSESSMENT AND COURT REPORTS

These should include:

- a full history and mental state examination
- obtaining an objective account of the offence
- obtaining an objective account of previous offences
- additional information from relatives, friends, social workers, probation officers, etc.
- a review of previous psychiatric and other relevant records.

Table 39.1 details a model psychiatric court report.

Table 39.1 *Model psychiatric court report*

Para 1	**Introduction:** Inform the court of when and where the patient was seen, at whose request, what information was available, e.g. statements related to the case, who were the informants, and sometimes what information was not available. State the current offences(s) with date for which charged.
Para 2	Inform the court of his/her past medical history and of the result of medical examination, e.g. 'Physical examination revealed no abnormality'.
Para 3	Report the important, relevant points of the family history, including family psychiatric disorder and criminality.
Para 4	**Personal history:** Report the important points of his/her personal history, i.e. physical development, e.g. birth, milestones, bedwetting (enuresis), schooling (e.g. bully/bullied, truancy), occupational history (which will include difficulties sustaining employment or with colleagues at work).
Para 5	Report his/her sexual and marital history: be reasonably discreet as the report may be read in open court.
Para 6	Report details of his/her personality in terms of social interaction, emotions, habits, e.g. drinking, gambling, drugs.
Para 7	Report past forensic history, e.g. past convictions. This is, however, inadmissible.
Para 8	Report past psychiatric history (dates, diagnoses, relevant details and relationship of mental disorder and treatment to offending).
Para 9	Report circumstances leading to current offence(s) and the defendant's state of mind at the time of the offence. Restrict discussion to the phenomena observed, e.g. 'For the time of the offence he gives a history of tearfulness, loss of hope, poor sleeping', etc., 'These are symptoms of the mental illness of depressive disorder', etc.
Para 10	Report the result of the interview: 'He showed/did not show evidence of mental illness or mental impairment'. Then give a brief outline of the evidence, e.g. 'He muttered to himself, looked around the room as though hallucinating' etc., or list symptoms detected and say 'These are symptoms of the severe mental illness of schizophrenia' etc. Information in paragraphs 1–10 should be factual, verifiable and ideally agreed by all, even if others' opinions of these facts differ from your own.
Para 11	The final paragraph should express your opinion. The court will be interested particularly in your opinion regarding: (a) Is the defendant fit to plead and stand his/her trial? (b) Is he/she suffering from a mental disorder, i.e. mental illness, a form of mental impairment or psychopathic disorder? (c) Where appropriate, comment on issues of responsibility, e.g. not guilty by reason of insanity; diminished responsibility in cases of homicide. (d) If suffering from mental disorder, can arrangements be made for his/her treatment in the National Health Service (arrange this if you think they can). Make suggestions to the court about which Mental Health Act order would be appropriate, e.g. Sections 37/41 in England and Wales, or suggest treatment as a condition of a Probation Order, e.g. 'In my opinion this man suffers from the severe mental illness schizophrenia, characterized by delusions (false beliefs) and hallucinations (voices, or visions). I consider he would benefit from treatment in a psychiatric hospital. I have made arrangements for a bed to be reserved for him at X hospital under Section 37 of the Mental Health Act 1983 if the court considers that this would be appropriate. I additionally recommend, if the court so agrees, that he be made subject to restrictions under Section 41 of the Mental Health Act 1983 to protect the public from serious harm and to facilitate his long-term psychiatric management, including specifying the conditions of his discharge from hospital, e.g. of residence and compliance with out-patient psychiatric treatment'. As an alternative: 'In my opinion this man does not suffer from mental illness, mental impairment nor psychopathic disorder and is not detainable in hospital under the Mental Health Act 1983. He has an anxious and dependent personality disorder, requires considerable support and

would benefit from group psychotherapy as an out-patient. The court may consider that it would be an appropriate disposal to help this man if he were to attend an out-patient group under my direction at X Health Centre as a condition of probation.'

Comment should be made on any mitigating circumstances, e.g. marital/work stress, and on the prognosis. Express any doubts you may have as to the likelihood of benefit from treatment.

If you have no psychiatric recommendation, say so, e.g. 'I have no psychiatric recommendation to make in this case'.

Finally, if essential information is lacking or if time is not sufficient to make the necessary arrangements for a hospital bed, then do not hesitate to state your findings up to date, state what you would like to do, and ask for a further period of remand.

Reproduced with permission from Puri, B.K., Laking, P.J. & Treasaden, I.H. 2002: *Textbook of Psychiatry*, 2nd edn. Edinburgh: Churchill Livingstone.

OUTCOME OF SENTENCING

The outcome of sentencing of mentally abnormal offenders in England and Wales is shown in Table 39.2.

Table 39.2 *Outcome of sentencing of mentally abnormal offenders*

(a)	The law takes its course, e.g. a fine, prison
(b)	Conditional or absolute discharge, possibly with voluntary psychiatric treatment
(c)	Probation order, with or without condition of psychiatric treatment (e.g. under Section 3 of the Powers of the Criminal Courts Act 1973 in England & Wales)
(d)	Detention under the Mental Health Act, e.g. under Section 37 with or without a Section 41 Restriction order under the Mental Health Act 1983 of England & Wales

Reproduced with permission from Puri, B.K., Laking, P.J. & Treasaden, I.H. 2002: *Textbook of Psychiatry*, 2nd edn. Edinburgh: Churchill Livingstone.

MENTAL DISORDER

Mental disorders that may be associated with offending include:

- *Schizophrenia*. This is mostly associated with minor offending secondary to deterioration in personality and social functioning.
- *Depressive disorder*. This is under-represented in offenders. It is associated with homicide and shoplifting.
- *Epilepsy*. This is over-represented in prisoners but offending in epileptics is rarely ictal.
- *Morbid delusional jealousy* (Othello syndrome). This is associated with repetitive and serious injury to the spouse/partner.

Alcohol and drugs that have been taken voluntarily do not, in general, lessen the individual's full legal responsibility. While amnesia is not a legal offence, its underlying cause may well be.

FITNESS TO PLEAD

A mentally disordered offender is unfit to plead if, at the time of the trial (but not necessarily at the time of the offence), he or she is unable to carry out one or more of the following:

- instruct counsel
- appreciate the significance of pleading

- challenge a juror
- examine a witness
- understand and follow the evidence of court procedure.

McNAUGHTEN RULES

To be found not guilty by reason of insanity, it has to be proved to a court that, at the time of the offence, the offender laboured under such defect of reason that he or she met these Rules, namely:

- that by reason of such defect from disease of the mind, the individual did not know the nature or quality of his or her act
- the individual did not know that what he or she was doing was wrong.

Diminished responsibility

In the case of a charge of murder, a defence of diminished responsibility (Homicide Act 1957) may be brought in; whereupon it has to be shown that, at the time of the offence, the offender suffered from:

> such abnormality of mind, whether caused from a condition of arrested or retarded development of mind or any inherent causes or induced by disease or injury, as substantially impaired [the individual's] mental responsibility for [his or her] act.

INFANTICIDE

In England and Wales, infanticide is a type of unlawful homicide in which:

> a woman by any wilful act caused the death of her child under the age of 12 months, but at the time of the act or omission the balance of her mind was disturbed by reason of her not being fully recovered from the effect of giving birth to the child, or the effect of lactation consequent upon the birth of the child.

AUTOMATISM

In this rare plea, usually in cases of homicide, the defendant pleads that, at the time of the offence, his or her behaviour was automatic.

DANGEROUSNESS

Dangerous individuals are people who have caused or who might cause serious harm to others. Its features include:

- repetition
- incorrigibility
- unpredictability
- untreatability
- infectiousness.

The best predictor of future dangerous behaviour is the individual's past behaviour. Shorter-term prediction is better than longer-term prediction. Dangerousness is associated with the availability of weapons, morbid jealousy, and the sadistic murder syndrome.

CIVIL ASPECTS

TESTAMENTARY CAPACITY

This is considered in Chapter 21.

TORT

A mentally disordered person is considered incapable of committing a tort (a civil wrong to an individual or to the reputation or estate of an individual) unless the disorder did not preclude an understanding of the nature or probable consequences of the act.

CONTRACTS

A contract requires free full consent and is void if an individual was of unsound mind at the time of making the contract.

MARRIAGE

Being a contract, marriage is void if an individual had a mental disorder at the time of marriage such that the nature of the contract was not appreciated at that time. A marriage may be annulled for any of the following reasons:

- The partner has a mental disorder at the time of marriage so as not to appreciate the nature of the contract.
- One partner did not disclose that he or she suffered from epilepsy or a communicable venereal disease.
- Either party was under 16 years at the time of marriage.
- Pregnancy by another male at the time of marriage was not disclosed.
- There was non-consummation.
- One of the partners was forced to agree to the marriage by duress.

BIBLIOGRAPHY

Faulk, M. 1988: *Basic Forensic Psychiatry.* Oxford: Blackwell.

Puri, B.K., Brown, R., McKee, H. & Treasaden, I.H. 2004: *Mental Health Law Handbook.* London: Arnold.

Treasaden, I.H. 2002: Forensic psychiatry. In Puri, B.K., Laking, P.J. and Treasaden, I.H. *Textbook of Psychiatry,* 2nd edn. Edinburgh: Churchill Livingstone.

Appendix 1

NICE GUIDANCE

Core interventions in the treatment and management of schizophrenia in primary and secondary care.

The treatment and management of schizophrenia is divided into 3 phases:

1. initiation of treatment at first episode
2. acute phase
3. promoting recovery.

- Patients should be assessed and receive help at the earliest opportunity.
- Clear information should be given to patients and their families.
- Obtain informed consent before treatment is initiated.
- Encourage advance directives.

INITIATION OF TREATMENT (FIRST EPISODE)

- If there is a suspicion of schizophrenia, individuals should be assessed urgently by a consultant psychiatrist.
- Atypical antipsychotic drugs should be introduced at the earliest convenience by the GP.
- Atypical drugs at the lower end of the dose range should be used in the first episode of schizophrenia.

TREATMENT OF THE ACUTE EPISODE

- Community mental health teams are an acceptable way of organising community care.
- Crisis resolution and home treatment teams should be used to manage crises of patients and should augment services provided by early intervention and assertive outreach teams.
- Alternatives to acute in-patient care should be developed.
- Antipsychotic therapy should be initiated as part of a comprehensive package of care.
- The minimum effective dose should be used.
- Massive loading doses (rapid neuroleptization) should be avoided.
- Where a potential to cause weight gain or diabetes has been identified for the atypical antipsychotic prescribed, there should be routine monitoring for these potential risks.

EARLY POST-ACUTE PERIOD

- Patients should be helped to understand their illness and should be encouraged to write an account of their illness in their notes.
- The assessment of needs for health and social care for people with schizophrenia should be comprehensive and address medical, social, psychological, occupational, economic, physical and cultural issues.

PSYCHOLOGICAL TREATMENTS

- Cognitive behavioural therapy should be available to patients with schizophrenia.
- Family interventions should be available.
- Counselling and supportive psychotherapy are not recommended in routine care.

MEDICATION ADVICE

- Continuation of antipsychotic drugs for 1 or 2 years after a relapse is recommended.
- Withdrawal of antipsychotic medication should be gradual and monitored.
- Following the withdrawal of drugs, patients should continue to be monitored for signs of relapse for at least 2 years after the last acute episode.

PROMOTING RECOVERY

Primary care

- General practices should develop case registers for people with schizophrenia.
- GPs should regularly monitor the physical health of patients with schizophrenia. Particular attention should be paid to endocrine disorders, e.g. diabetes, hyperprolactinaemia, blood pressure, lipds, side effects of medication and lifestyle risk factors, e.g. smoking.
- GPs should re-refer patients to secondary care particularly if:
  - treatment adherence is problematic;
  - there is poor response to treatment;
  - co-morbid substance misuse is suspected;
  - level of risk to self or others is raised;
  - when patient first joins the practice.

Secondary Care

- A full assessment of health and social care needs should be made regularly.
- Carers should have their needs assessed.

SERVICE INTERVENTIONS

- Assertive outreach teams should be developed for patients who engage poorly with services, are high users of in-patient care, or are homeless.
- Crisis resolution and home treatment teams should be available for those in acute crisis.
- The CPA ensures services are managed and integrated.

PSYCHOLOGICAL INTERVENTIONS

Cognitive behavioural and family interventions should be available.

PHARMACOLOGICAL INTERVENTIONS

Antipsychotics are indispensable to prevent relapse.

- Continuous dosage regimens are preferred.
- Depots should be considered an option.

TREATMENT RESISTANT SCHIZOPHRENIA (TRS)

- In TRS clozapine should be introduced at the earliest convenience.
- The addition of a second antipsychotic may be considered if clozapine alone is ineffective.

EMPLOYMENT

Employment schemes should be developed to help those with schizophrenia to work.

RAPID TRANQUILLISATION

Staff should be trained in de-escalation and rapid tranquillisation. Offer oral medication first. If intramuscular administration is necessary, lorazepam, haloperidol and olanzapine are preferred. Vital signs should be monitored regularly.

This appendix is a summary of the following NICE guideline:

National Institute for Clinical Excellence (2002) Core interventions in the treatment and management of schizophrenia in primary and secondary care. NICE Clinical Guideline No. 1. London: National Institute for Clinical Excellence. Available from: www.nice.org.uk.

Appendix 2

NICE TECHNOLOGY APPRAISAL GUIDANCE

Alzheimer's disease

NICE has recommended that, for the adjunctive treatment of mild and moderate Alzheimer's disease in patients with a mini-mental state examination (MMSE) score above 12 points, donepezil, galantamine and rivastigmine should be available under the following conditions:

- Alzheimer's disease must be diagnosed in a specialist clinic.
- Treatment is initiated by specialists but continued by GPs under a share-care protocol.
- Carers views are sought before and during drug treatment.
- The patient is reassessed 2-4 months after treatment is started; treatment should be continued only if MMSE has improved.
- Patient should be assessed every 6 months. Treatment continues only if MMSE score remains above 12 points.

Memantine is an NMDA receptor antagonist that affects glutamate transmission. It is licensed for treating moderate to severe Alzheimer's disease.
Donepezil is a reversible inhibitor of acetylcholinesterase that can be given once daily.
Rivastigmine is a reversible non-competitive inhibitor of acetylcholinesterases, given twice daily.
Galantamine is a reversible inhibitor of acetylcholinesterase and it also has nicotinic receptor agonist properties. It is given twice daily.
   Acetylcholinesterase inhibitors can cause unwanted dose-related cholinergic effects and should be started at a low dose and the dose increased according to response and tolerability.

This appendix is a summary of the following NICE technology appraisal guidance:

National Institute for Clinical Excellence (2001) Guidance on the use of donepezil, rivastigmine and galantamine for the treatment of alzheimer's disease. NICE Technology Appraisal Guidance No. 19. London: National Institute for Clinical Excellence. Available from: www.nice.org.uk.

Index